Encyclopedia of
Nutritional Supplements

The Essential Guide for Improving
Your Health Naturally

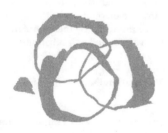

Michael T. Murray, N.D.

PRIMA PUBLISHING

PRIMA PUBLISHING and colophon are registered trademarks of Prima Communications, Inc.

Warning—Disclaimer
Prima Publishing has designed this book to provide information in regard to the subject matter covered. It is sold with the understanding that the publisher and the author are not liable for the misconception or misuse of information provided. Every effort has been made to make this book as complete and as accurate as possible. The purpose of this book is to educate. The author and Prima Publishing shall have neither liability nor responsibility to any person or entity with respect to any loss, damage, or injury caused or alleged to be caused directly or indirectly by the information contained in this book. The information presented herein is in no way intended as a substitute for medical counseling.

Library of Congress Cataloging-in-Publication Data

Murray, Michael T.
   Encyclopedia of nutritional supplements : the essential guide for improving your health naturally / Michael T. Murray.
      p.   cm.
   Includes index.
   ISBN 0-7615-0410-9
   1. Vitamins in human nutrition—Encyclopedias.   2. Minerals in human nutrition—Encyclopedias.
3. Dietary supplements—Encyclopedias.   I. Title
QP771.M87   1996
612.3'9—dc20   96-3804
                                                                                          CIP

96 97 98 99 DD 10 9 8 7 6 5
Printed in the United States of America

How to Order:
Single copies may be ordered from Prima Publishing, P.O. Box 1260BK, Rocklin, CA 95677; telephone (916) 632-4400. Quantity discounts are also available. On your letterhead, include information concerning the intended use of the books and the number of books you wish to purchase.

Visit us online at http://www.primapublishing.com

This book is dedicated to the legacy of the true pioneers of nutritional science—Linus Pauling, Roger Williams, Albert Szent-Gyorgi, and Adelle Davis—and to those who continue to carry the torch of truth—Jonathan Wright, Jeffrey Bland, Alan Gaby, Joseph Pizzorno, Gladys Block, Abram Hoffer, Melvyn Werbach, Patrick Quillin, Shari Lieberman, and all of the others.

Contents

Preface

This book was written to help you make sense of the often confusing and conflicting information regarding nutritional supplements. It is designed to empower you with respect to your health care decisions; it is *not* designed to replace appropriate medical care. With that in mind, here are some important recommendations:

- Do not self-diagnose. Proper medical care is critical to good health. If you have symptoms suggestive of an illness discussed in this book, please consult a physician, preferably a naturopath, holistic M.D. or D.O., chiropractor, or other natural health care specialist.
- If you are currently on a prescription medication, you absolutely must work with your doctor before discontinuing any drug. Furthermore, you must make your physician aware of all the nutritional supplements you are currently taking and why.
- If you wish to try a nutritional supplement as a therapeutic measure, discuss it with your physician. Since your physician is most likely unaware of the nutritional supplement that you may want to use, you may need to educate him/her. Bring this book along with you to the doctor's office. Most of the therapeutic recommendations given in this book are based on published studies in medical journals. Key references are provided, from which you or your physician may find additional information.
- Remember, although many nutritional supplements are effective on their own, they work even better if they are part of a comprehensive natural treatment plan that focuses on diet and lifestyle factors.

I hope you enjoy the *Encyclopedia of Nutritional Supplements* and find good health as a result!

Michael T. Murray, N.D.

Acknowledgments

Most of all I would like to acknowledge all the researchers, physicians, and scientists who over the years have sought to better understand the use of nutritional supplements and other natural medicines. Without their work, this book would not exist, and medical progress would halt. My role is simply to translate their efforts into a practical format.

I would also like to acknowledge the many special blessings in my life. Chief among them are my beautiful wife, Gina, and our first child, Alexa Michelle. I have also been blessed with loving and supportive parents, Cliff and Patty Murray, and some absolutely phenomenal friends. I am truly humbled by all my blessings in this life and give thanks to God.

PART ONE

Introduction to
Nutritional Supplements

*W*elcome to the world of nutritional supplements!

Terminology

To help you more fully understand the chapters that follow, here are a number of terms that you will come across repeatedly throughout this book—it's worth taking the time to become familiar with them.

A *study* is a very broad term that covers almost every type of objective analysis. A *case study* is a report on anecdotal evidence. Case studies can either be single case studies involving one patient or a series of case studies involving five or more case studies.

An *epidemiological study* is an analysis of large populations that looks at patterns of disease and the factors that influence those patterns. *Prevalence* refers to the number of people who have a particular condition at given time. How many new cases of a condition that occur over a given period of time is called its *incidence*.

A *retrospective study* looks to the past for clues. For example, in studying people with lung cancer, researchers found a high number of smokers in the group. A *prospective study* is one in which subjects are enrolled in a study and followed forward in time. For example, one of the more famous prospective studies is the Nurses' Health Study in which 100,000 nurses have been answering questionnaires annually since 1976. This study has already produced a number of interesting results, such as benefit in the prevention of heart disease with vitamin E supplementation and an increase in the risk of breast cancer with hormone replacement therapy. The association or correlation between a factor and disease incidence can either be positive or negative (inverse). An example of a *positive correlation* is the more cigarettes a person smokes, the greater his or her risk for developing lung cancer. An example of an *inverse correlation* is the more fruits and vegetables a person consumes, the lower his or her risk for developing lung cancer.

A *clinical trial* is a study in which human subjects receive treatment. Since you can treat only in the present, not in the past, clinical trials are always prospective. In a *controlled trial*, at least two groups are compared. The treated or experimental group receives treatment, while the control group receives no treatment. In a placebo-controlled trial, an inactive pill or procedure—the *placebo*—is given to the control group. Placebo is Latin for "I will please [you]." Placebos got their name because any treatment, even simple attention, tends to make people feel better. Overall, the placebo effect is an astonishing 33 percent, although it varies depending upon the condition. In other words, an average of one out of three subjects report significant improvement after receiving a placebo (usually a sugar pill).

A *randomized trial* is a trial in which the subjects are randomly assigned to either the treatment group or control group. A *crossover trial* is one in which each patient receives both the treatment and the placebo during the trial. For example, Group A starts out receiving the treatment while Group B receives the placebo. Midway through the trial (usually after a wash-out period where no treatment or placebo is given), the subjects are crossed over—i.e., Group A now receives the placebo and Group B receives the treatment.

A *blind study* means that either the researchers and/or subjects don't know which group each subject is in. In a typical *single-blind study*, the subjects don't know what they are receiving but the researchers do. In a *double-blind study*, neither the researchers nor the subjects know what they are receiving; all information is coded, and the code is not broken until the end of the trial. Double-blind testing is important because in a single-blind study, researchers can give unconscious signals to test subjects. The double-blind study is the gold standard; however, a good double-blind study must have a large enough sample size (the bigger the better) to produce *statistically significant* results, which means the results are unlikely to have occurred as a result of chance. Often a *probability value (p value)* is given. A p value less than 0.1 means that the probability that the results occurred by chance is less than 1 out of 100 (1 percent). A p value of less than 0.5 is generally regarded as being statistically significant. The lower the p value, the more significant the results.

A *meta-analysis* refers to analysis of the combined results from a number of selected trials in order to arrive at a general conclusion. A meta-analysis is particularly useful when a number of small trials have given conflicting or inconclusive results. By combining the results from the well-designed trials, there may be enough subjects to yield more statistically significant results.

Chapter Organization

Each chapter is organized using the following headings as logical divisions.

Deficiency Signs and Symptoms
Recommended Dietary Allowance
Beneficial Effects
Available Forms
Principal Uses
Dosage Ranges
Safety Issues
Interactions

The Emerging Role of Nutritional Supplementation in Medicine

An evolution is occurring in health care as more natural medicines gain acceptance. Interestingly, this acceptance is largely a result of increased scientific investigation and the public's awareness of this research. It appears that medical researchers now have in their possession the technology and understanding necessary to more fully appreciate the value of "natural" therapies. In essence, many natural therapies are being improved or refined through scientific investigation. Science is paving the way for the medicine of the future—a medicine that recognizes the healing power of nature.

What Exactly Is Science?

The term *science* refers to "possession of knowledge as distinguished from ignorance or misunderstanding." Scientific knowledge is based upon the scientific method, meaning that the understanding is based on the collection of data through observation and experiment. We must keep in mind that while science is evolutionary, the underlying natural laws it tries to explain are constant. In other words, gravity existed long before Sir Isaac Newton was around to explain it.

We use science to explain the nature of the human body and the environment. Breakthrough developments in many areas of science are occurring at an incredible pace, particularly in areas of medicine. What was once considered scientific medicine is often discarded when a deeper understanding is achieved. For example, in the 1800s scientific medicine involved bloodletting and the administration of very toxic substances. Likewise, many current medical treatments involving the use of drugs and surgery in all probability will be discarded in the future.

There is a trend toward using substances found in nature, including compounds that are found in the human body—such as interferon, interleukin, insulin, and human growth hormone—as well as foods, food components, herbs, and herbal compounds. More and more researchers are discovering the tremendous healing properties of these natural compounds and their advantages over synthetic medicines and surgery in the treatment of many health conditions. Through these scientific investigations, a trend toward natural medicine is emerging.

Science and Natural Medicine

Most natural healing therapies are based upon scientific investigation. In most cases, the initial investigation was of an empirical or observational nature. However, in the past 20 plus years there have been tremendous advances in the understanding of how many natural therapies work to promote health or treat disease. This increased understanding is a result of more strict scientific investigation.

Scientific studies and observations have not only held up the validity of diet, nutritional supplements, herbal medicines, chiropractic adjustments, and massage, but also some of the more esoteric natural healing treatments such as acupuncture, biofeedback, meditation, and homeopathy. In many instances, the scientific investigation has not only validated the natural approach but has also led to significant improvements.

The Emerging Philosophy of Medicine

While science is important in the expansion of our knowledge of natural medicine, five time-tested principles remain crucial These principles serve as the foundation upon which the emerging philosophy of both naturopathic or allopathic medicine should be based:

- **Principle 1: Remember the Healing Power of Nature.** The body has considerable power to heal itself. It is the role of the physician or healer to facilitate and enhance this process, preferably with the aid of natural, nontoxic therapies. Above all, the physician or healer must do no harm.

- **Principle 2: View the Whole Person.** An individual must be viewed as a whole composed of a complex interaction of mind, body, and spirit.

- **Principle 3: Identify and Treat the Cause.** It is important to seek the underlying cause of a disease rather than simply suppress the symptoms. Symptoms are expressions of the body's attempt to heal, but causes can spring from physical, mental or emotional, and spiritual levels.

- **Principle 4: The Physician Is a Teacher.** A physician should be foremost a teacher, educating, empowering, and motivating the patient to assume more personal responsibility for his or her health by adopting a healthy attitude, lifestyle, and diet.

- **Principle 5: Prevention Is the Best Cure.** Prevention of disease is best accomplished through dietary and life habits that support health and prevent disease.

We are seeing evidence of an increased acceptance of these principles and the practice of natural medicine, an acceptance that is a direct result of increased scientific investigation. Scientists are validating the time-tested principles of naturopathic medicine and other natural therapies. This validation of natural medicine is not entirely surprising. After all, if these principles and techniques are based upon truth, they should stand up to strict scientific scrutiny.

Scientific investigation in the area of natural medicine will likely lead to further improvements, particularly in the area of prevention. Most conditions being treated by medicines are entirely preventable. It is estimated that over 70 percent of the $838 billion spent on health care in 1992 was spent on chronic degenerative diseases that have been clearly linked to diet and lifestyle, diseases which are the major killers of Americans—heart disease, cancer, strokes, and diabetes.

Science is redirecting medicine back to those ancient truths. Perhaps the famous words of Thomas Edison will turn out to be truly prophetic: "The doctor of the future will give no medicine, but will interest his patient in the care of the human frame, in diet and in the cause and prevention of disease."

Functions of Vitamins and Minerals

Although Edison doesn't specifically mention nutritional supplementation, in today's world we recognize it as an integral part of our diet. The term *nutritional supplementation* includes the use of vitamins, minerals, and other food factors to support good health and prevent or treat illness.

The key function of nutrients like vitamins and minerals in the human body is to serve as essential components in enzymes and coenzymes. Enzymes are molecules involved in speeding up chemical reactions necessary for human bodily function. Coenzymes are molecules that help the enzymes in their chemical reactions.

Enzymes and coenzymes work to either join molecules together or split them apart by making or breaking the chemical bonds that join molecules together. A key concept in nutritional medicine is learning how to supply the necessary support or nutrients that allow enzymes of a particular tissue to work at their optimum levels.

Most enzymes are composed of a protein along with an essential mineral and possibly a vitamin. If an enzyme is lacking the essential mineral or vitamin, it cannot function properly. By providing the necessary mineral through diet or a nutritional formula, the enzyme is then able to perform its vital function. For example, zinc is necessary for the enzyme that activates vitamin A in the visual process. Without zinc in the enzyme, the vitamin A cannot be converted to the active form. This deficiency can result in what is known as night blindness. By supplying the enzyme with zinc, we are performing "enzymatic therapy" and allowing the enzyme to perform its vital function.

Many enzymes require additional support in order to perform their functions. The support is in the form of a coenzyme, a molecule that functions along with the enzyme. Most coenzymes are composed of vitamins and/or minerals. Without the coenzyme, the enzyme is powerless. For example, vitamin C functions as a coenzyme to the enzyme proline hydroxylase, which is involved in collagen synthesis. Without vitamin C, there is impaired collagen synthesis, resulting in failure of wounds to heal, bleeding gums, and easy bruising. There may be plenty of proline hydroxylase (the enzyme), but in order for it to function it needs vitamin C.

Growing Popularity of Nutritional Supplementation

In the last few years more Americans than ever are taking nutritional supplements. Estimates state that over 100 million Americans take dietary supplements on a regular basis. Despite the fact that there is tremendous scientific evidence to support the use of nutritional supplementation, many medical experts and researchers have not endorsed nutritional supplementation—even though 98 percent of them take supplements themselves.

Why are so many Americans taking supplements? They know they are not getting what they need from their diets, and they realize that supplements make them feel healthier.[1] Numerous studies have demonstrated that most Americans consume a diet inadequate in nutritional value. Comprehensive studies sponsored by the U.S. government (HANES I and II, Ten-State Nutrition Survey, USDA nationwide food consumption studies, etc.) have revealed marginal nutrient deficiencies exist in a substantial portion of the U.S. population (approximately 50 percent and that for some selected nutrients in certain age groups, more than 80 percent of the group consumed less than the RDA (Recommended Dietary Allowance).[2]

These studies indicate the chances of consuming a diet meeting the RDA for all nutrients is extremely unlikely for most Americans. In other words, while it is theoretically possible that a healthy individual can get all the nutrition he or she needs from foods, most Americans do not even come close to meeting all their nutritional needs through diet alone. In an effort to increase their intake of essential nutrients, many Americans look to vitamin and mineral supplements.

While most Americans are deficient in many vitamins and minerals, the level of deficiency is usually not to a point where obvious nutrient deficiencies are apparent. A severe-deficiency disease like scurvy (lack of vitamin C) is extremely rare, but marginal vitamin C deficiency is thought to be relatively common. The term *subclinical deficiency* is often used to describe marginal nutrient deficiencies. A subclinical or marginal deficiency indicates a deficiency of a particular vitamin or mineral that is not severe enough to produce a classic deficiency sign or symptom. In many instances the only clue of a subclinical nutrient deficiency may be fatigue, lethargy, difficulty in concentration, a lack of well-being, or some other vague symptom. Diagnosis of subclinical deficiencies is an extremely difficult process that involves detailed dietary or laboratory analysis. Such tests are usually far more expensive than taking a year's supply of the vitamin being tested for and are therefore not cost effective.

RDA Is Not Enough

The Food and Nutrition Board of the National Research Council has been setting guidelines for Recommended Dietary Allowances for vitamins and minerals since 1941, originally with the intent of reducing the rates of severe nutritional deficiency diseases such as scurvy (deficiency of vitamin C), pellagra (deficiency of niacin), and beriberi (deficiency of vitamin B_1). Another critical point is that the RDAs were designed to serve as the basis for evaluating the adequacy of diets of groups of people, not individuals. Individuals simply vary too widely in their nutritional requirements to assume that the RDAs are identical for all people. As stated by the Food and Nutrition Board, "Individuals with special nutritional needs are not covered by the RDAs."[3]

A tremendous amount of scientific research indicates that the "optimal" level for many nutrients, especially the so-called antioxidant nutrients like vitamins C and E, beta-carotene, and selenium, may be much higher than their current RDAs. The RDAs focus on the prevention of nutritional deficiencies in population groups only; they do not define "optimal" intake for an individual.

Other factors the RDAs do not adequately consider are environmental and lifestyle factors that can destroy vitamins and bind minerals. For example, even the Food and Nutrition Board acknowledges that smokers require at least twice as much vitamin C as do nonsmokers; but what about other nutrients and smoking? And what about the effects of alcohol consumption, food additives, heavy metals (lead, mercury, etcetera.), carbon monoxide, and other chemicals associated with our modern society that are known to interfere with nutrient function? Dealing with hazards of modern living may be another reason why many people take supplements.

While RDAs have done a good job of defining nutrient intake levels to prevent nutritional deficiencies, we still have much to learn about the optimum intake of nutrients.

Accessory Nutrients

In addition to discussing essential nutrients in this book, I also address a number of food components and natural physiological agents that have demonstrated impressive health-promoting effects (See Part Five—Accessory Nutrient Profiles). They include flavonoids, probiotics, carnitine, and coenzyme Q_{10}. These compounds exert significant therapeutic effects with little, if any, toxicity. More and more research indicates that these accessory nutrients, although not considered "essential" in the classical sense, play a major role in preventing illness.

An Important Caveat

The very term *nutritional supplements* denotes that the beneficial compounds described in this book are supplementary measures to good health. A person cannot make up for poor dietary habits, a negative attitude, and a lack of exercise by taking pills—whether the pills are drugs or nutritional supplements. Although many nutritional supplements are effective in improving health, for the long term it is absolutely essential that individuals devote attention to developing a positive mental attitude, a regular exercise program, and a healthful diet.

2

Some Practical Recommendations

Since this book is filled with such exciting information about specific nutrients, I must make some practical recommendations. Otherwise, I can imagine a reader going into a health food store and coming out with single bottles of every nutrient described in this book. To simplify matters, I tend to recommend the following supplements to establish a strong nutritional foundation upon which to build:

• Take a high-quality multiple vitamin and mineral supplement.

• Take extra antioxidants.

• Take one tablespoon of flaxseed oil daily.

Recommendation 1—Take a High-Quality Multiple Vitamin and Mineral Supplement

Taking a high-quality multiple vitamin and mineral supplement that provides all of the known vitamins and minerals serves as the foundation of a nutritional supplementation program. Dr. Roger Williams, one of the premier biochemists of our time, states that healthy people should use multiple vitamin and mineral supplements as an "insurance formula" against possible deficiency. This does not mean that a deficiency will occur in the absence of the vitamin and mineral supplement any more than not having fire insurance means that your house is not going to burn down. But given the enormous potential for individual differences and the varied mechanisms of vitamin and mineral actions, supplementation with a multiple formula seems to make sense. The recommendations in the table on the next page provide an optimum intake range for selecting a high-quality multiple supplement.

Recommendation 2—Take Extra Antioxidants

Most health-minded individuals are familiar with the terms *antioxidants* and *free radicals*. Loosely defined, a free radical is a highly reactive molecule that can bind to and destroy body components. Free radical or "oxidative" damage is what makes us age.

Recommended Vitamin Intake in International Units (I.U.), Milligrams (mg.), or Micrograms (mcg.)

Vitamin	Range for Adults	Comments
Vitamin A (retinol)	5,000 I.U.	Women of child-bearing age should not take more than 2,500 I.U. of retinol daily due to the possible risk of birth defects if they become pregnant.
Vitamin A (from beta-carotene)	5,000–25,000 I.U.	
Vitamin D	100–400 I.U.	Elderly people in nursing homes living in northern latitudes should supplement at the high range.
Vitamin E (d-alpha tocopherol)	100–800 I.U.	It may be more cost effective to take vitamin E separately.
Vitamin K (phytonadione)	60–300 mcg.	
Vitamin C (ascorbic acid)	100–1,000 mg.	It may be easier to take vitamin C separately rather than in a multiple formula.
Vitamin B_1 (thiamin)	10–100 mg.	
Vitamin B_{12} (riboflavin)	10–50 mg.	
Niacin	10–100 mg.	
Niacinamide	10–30 mg.	
Vitamin B_6 (pyridoxine)	25–100 mg.	
Biotin	100–300 mcg.	
Pantothenic acid	25–100 mg.	
Folic acid	400 mcg.	
Vitamin B_{12}	400 mcg.	
Choline	10–100 mg.	
Inositol	10–100 mg.	

Free radicals have also been shown to be responsible for the initiation of many diseases, including the two biggest killers of Americans—heart disease and cancer.

Antioxidants, in contrast, are compounds that help protect against free-radical damage. Antioxidant nutrients like beta-carotene, selenium, vitamin E , and vitamin C are very important in protecting against the development of heart disease, cancer, and other chronic degenerative diseases. In addition, antioxidants are also thought to slow down the aging process.

Based on extensive data, it appears that a combination of antioxidants will provide greater antioxidant protection than any single nutritional antioxidant. Therefore, in addition to recommending that individuals consume a diet rich in plant foods, especially fruits and vegetables, I suggest using a combination of antioxidant nutrients rather than high dosages of any single antioxidant. Mixtures of antioxidant nutrients

Recommended Mineral Intake in International Units (I.U.), Milligrams (mg.), or Micrograms (mcg.)

Minerals	Range for Adults	Comments
Boron	1–6 mg.	
Calcium	250–1,250 mg.	Women at risk or suffering from osteoporosis may need to take a separate calcium supplement when trying to achieve higher dosage levels.
Chromium	200–400 mcg.	For diabetes and weight loss, patients can use dosages of 600 mcg.
Copper	1–2 mg.	
Iodine	50–150 mcg.	
Iron	15–30 mg.	Men and postmenopausal women rarely need supplemental iron.
Magnesium	250–500 mg.	When magnesium therapy is indicated, take a separate magnesium supplement.
Manganese	10–15 mg.	
Molybdenum	10–25 mcg.	
Potassium	200–500 mg.	
Selenium	100–200 mcg.	
Silica	1–25 mg.	
Vanadium	50–100 mcg.	
Zinc	15–45 mg.	

appear to work together harmoniously to produce the phenomena of synergy. In other words, 1 + 1 = 3.

The two primary antioxidants in the human body are vitamin C and vitamin E. Vitamin C is an *aqueous phase* antioxidant. This means that it is found in body compartments composed of water. In contrast, vitamin E is a *lipid phase* antioxidant because it is found in lipid- (fat-) soluble body compartments such as cell membranes and fatty molecules. If you are taking a high-potency multiple vitamin and mineral formula, many of the supportive antioxidant nutrients such as selenium, zinc, and beta-carotene are provided for. Therefore, your primary concern may be simply to ensure beneficial levels of vitamin C and vitamin E. Here are my daily supplementation guidelines for these key nutritional antioxidants for supporting general health. Be sure to recognize how much your multiple vitamin and mineral formula is providing:

Recommended Antioxidant Supplementation in International Units (I.U.) or Milligrams (mg.)

Vitamin	Range for Adults
Vitamin E (d-alpha tocopherol)	400–800 I.U.
Vitamin C (ascorbic acid)	500–1,500 mg.

Recommendation 3—Take One Tablespoon of Flaxseed Oil Daily

In this day and age of concern over fat in our foods, my recommendation to supplement an individual's daily diet with one tablespoon of flaxseed oil may be puzzling. However, this recommendation makes perfectly good sense. While it is true Americans should not consume more than 30 percent of their daily calories as fats, a lack of the dietary essential fatty acids has been suggested to play a significant role in the development of many chronic degenerative diseases such as heart disease, cancer, and strokes.

Experts estimate that approximately 80 percent of our population consumes an insufficient quantity of essential fatty acids. This dietary insufficiency presents a serious health threat to Americans. In addition to providing the body with energy, the essential fatty acids—linoleic and linolenic acid—provided by plant foods function in our bodies as components of nerve cells, cellular membranes, and hormonelike substances known as prostaglandins. In addition to playing a critical role in normal physiology, essential fatty acids can actually be protective and therapeutic against heart disease, cancer, autoimmune diseases like multiple sclerosis and rheumatoid arthritis, many skin diseases, and others. Research indicates that over 60 health conditions benefit from essential fatty acid supplementation.

Many consider organic, unrefined flaxseed oil to be the answer to restoring the proper level of essential fatty acids. Flaxseed oil is unique because it contains both essential fatty acids—alpha linolenic (an omega–3 fatty acid) and linoleic acid (an omega–6 fatty acid)—in appreciable amounts. Flaxseed oil is the world's richest source of omega–3 fatty acids. At a whopping 58 percent by weight, it contains over two times the amount of omega–3 fatty acids as fish oils. Scientists have studied omega–3 fatty acids extensively with regard to their beneficial effects in cardiovascular disease, inflammation and allergies, and cancer.

PART TWO

Vitamins

There are 13 different known vitamins, each with its own special role to play. Vitamins are classified into two groups: fat-soluble (A, D, E, and K) and water-soluble (the B vitamins and vitamin C). I have added another category, "unofficial" B vitamins, for choline and inositol.

Vitamins are essential to good health; without them, key body processes would halt. Low levels of vitamins and minerals in our bodies may be preventing many of us from achieving optimal health. Vitamins function along with enzymes in chemical reactions necessary for human bodily function, including energy production. Vitamins and enzymes work together, acting as catalysts that speed up the making or breaking of chemical bonds that join molecules together.

Fat Soluble Vitamins

Vitamin A
Vitamin D
Vitamin E
Vitamin K

Water-Soluble Vitamins

Vitamin C
Thiamin (Vitamin B_1)
Riboflavin (Vitamin B_2)
Niacin (Vitamin B_3)
Pyridoxine (Vitamin B_6)

Biotin
Pantothenic Acid and Pantethine
Folic Acid
Vitamin B_{12}

"Unofficial" B Vitamins

Choline
Inositol

3

Vitamin A and Carotenes

Vitamin A was the first recognized fat-soluble vitamin. Although identified as a necessary growth factor in 1913, it was not chemically characterized until 1930. Two groups of researchers, McCollum and Davis at the University of Wisconsin, and Osborne and Mendel at Yale University, made the initial discovery of vitamin A almost simultaneously. They found that young animals fed a diet deficient in natural fats became very unhealthy, as evidenced by their inability to grow and their poor immune function. These researchers also noted that the animals' eyes became severely inflamed and infected on the restricted diet—conditions quickly relieved by the addition of butterfat or cod liver oil to the diet. Once known as the "anti-infective vitamin," vitamin A recently regained recognition as a major determinant of immune status. Carotenes, some of which can be converted into vitamin A, are also gaining a great deal of attention as immune system enhancers. Because of the vitamin A activity of some carotenes, this chapter explores both vitamin A and carotenes.[1]

Carotenes

Carotenes represent the most widespread group of naturally occurring pigments in nature. They are an intensely colored (red and yellow) group of fat-soluble compounds. All organisms that transform sunlight into chemical energy via the process of photosynthesis do so with the help of carotenes. These compounds not only play a role in the process of photosynthesis, but also play a crucial role in protecting the organism or plant against the tremendous amount of free radicals produced during photosynthesis.

Scientists have characterized over 600 carotenoids, of which only 30 to 50 seem to have vitamin A activity. Biological activity of a carotene has historically been considered synonymous with its corresponding vitamin A activity. However, recent research suggests that this function of carotenes has been overemphasized, and carotenoids have been found to exhibit many other activities. Researchers have described beta-carotene as the most active of the carotenoids because of its higher provitamin A activity, but several other carotenes exert greater antioxidant effects.

Retinol

When isolated in its pure form, vitamin A is a pure yellow crystal that is fat-soluble. Vitamin A is termed retinol, signifying that it is an alcohol involved in the function of the retina of the eye. We find retinol in nature primarily as long-chains. The aldehyde form of retinol is commonly designated retinaldehyde or retinal, while the acidic form is termed retinoic acid. Some scientists suggest that retinol serves only as a precursor to these two active forms of vitamin A—retinal being primarily involved with vision and reproduction, retinoic acid being important in other body functions, such as growth and differentiation.

Synthetic derivatives of retinoic acid have been developed to treat many skin conditions and, more recently, certain forms of cancer. Isotretinoin (13-cis retinoic acid; trade name, Accutane) is used in treating severe cystic acne and disorders of keratinization, such as Darier's disease and lamellar ichthyosis. Etretinate, an aromatic derivative of retinoic acid, has no appreciable activity against acne, but some consider it more potent than isotretinoin in the treatment of psoriasis. These compounds, however, are not without side effects such as liver damage, nausea and vomiting, and muscle pain.[1,2]

Food Sources

The most concentrated sources of preformed vitamin A are liver, kidney, butter, whole milk, and fortified lowfat and skim milk, while the leading sources of provitamin A carotenes are dark green leafy vegetables (collards and spinach) and yellow-orange vegetables (carrots, sweet potatoes, yams, and squash) (see Table 3.1).

The carotenes in green plants are found in the chloroplasts along with chlorophyll, usually in complexes with a protein or fat. Beta-carotene is the predominant form in most green leaves and, in general, the greater the intensity of the green color the greater the concentration of beta-carotene. Orange colored fruits and vegetables—carrots, apricots, mangoes, yams, squash, etcetera—typically have higher concentrations of provitamin A carotenoids, the amount of provitamin A again is directly related to the intensity of the color. Yellow vegetables have higher concentrations of xanthophylls, hence a lowered provitamin A activity. In the orange and yellow fruits and vegetables, beta-carotene concentrations are high, but other provitamin A carotenoids typically predominate. The red and purple vegetables and fruits—such as tomatoes, red cabbage, berries, and plums—contain a large portion of non–vitamin A-active pigments, including flavonoids. Legumes, grains, and seeds are also significant sources of carotenoids.

We also find carotenoids in various animal foods, such as salmon and other fish, egg yolks, shellfish, milk, and poultry. Carotenoids are frequently added to foods as colorants (see Tables 3.2 and 3.3).

Absorption

A variety of factors influence the absorption efficacy of vitamin A and carotenes. Unlike retinol, carotenes require bile acids to facilitate absorption. Other factors that affect vitamin A and carotene absorption include: the presence of fat, protein, and

TABLE 3.1   Vitamin A Content of Selected Foods, in International Units per 3½-oz. (100-g.) Serving

Liver, beef	43,900	Sweet potatoes	8,800
Liver, calf	22,500	Parsley	8,500
Chili peppers	21,600	Spinach	8,100
Dandelion root	14,000	Mustard greens	7,000
Chicken liver	12,100	Mangoes	4,800
Carrots	11,000	Hubbard squash	4,300
Apricots, dried	10,900	Cantaloupe	3,400
Collard greens	9,300	Apricots	2,700
Kale	8,900	Broccoli	2,500

TABLE 3.2   Provitamin A Carotenoids and Food Sources

Carotenoid	Activity (Percent)	Food Sources
Beta-carotene	100	Green plants, carrots, sweet potatoes, squash, spinach, apricots, green peppers
Alpha-carotene	50–54	Green plants, carrots, squash, corn, watermelons, green peppers, potatoes, apples, peaches
Gamma-carotene	42–50	Carrots, sweet potatoes, corn, tomatoes, watermelons, apricots
Beta-zeacarotene	20–40	Corn, tomatoes, yeast, cherries
Cryptoxanthin	50–60	Corn, green peppers, persimmons, papayas, lemons, oranges, apples, apricots, paprika, poultry
Beta-apo-8'-carotenal	72	Citrus fruit, green plants
Beta-apo-12'-carotenal	120	Alfalfa meal

TABLE 3.3   Nonprovitamin A Carotenoids and Food Sources

Carotenoid	Food Source
Lycopene	Tomatoes, carrots, green peppers, apricots, pink grapefruit
Zeaxanthin	Spinach, paprika, corn, fruits
Lutein	Green plants, corn, potatoes, spinach, carrots, tomatoes, fruits
Canthaxanthin	Mushrooms, trout, crustaceans
Crocetin	Saffron
Capsanthin	Red peppers, paprika

antioxidants in the food; the presence of bile and a normal complement of pancreatic enzymes in the intestinal lumen; and the integrity of the mucosal cells. The absorption efficiency of dietary vitamin A is usually quite high (80 to 90 percent) with only a slight reduction in efficiency at high doses. In contrast, beta-carotene's absorption efficiency is much lower (40 to 60 percent) and it decreases rapidly with increasing dosage.[1,2] Carotene supplements are better absorbed than the carotenes from foods.[3]

Transformation in the Intestinal Lining

The majority of absorbed retinol is complexed with palmitic acid or some other free fatty acid within the cells of the intestinal lining. The retinol–fatty acid complex is then incorporated, along with other fatty substances (e.g., triglycerides, phospholipids, and cholesterol) into a large sphere of fatty substances called a chylomicron. The chylomicron is transported through the lymphatic channels into the general circulation and eventually is removed from the circulation by the liver. Carotenes, unless they are converted to vitamin A, are absorbed unchanged and transported by chylomicrons.[4,5]

Conversion of Carotenes into Vitamin A

The conversion of provitamin A carotenes to vitamin A depends on several factors, including protein status, thyroid hormones, zinc, and vitamin C.[6] The conversion diminishes as carotene intake increases and when serum retinol levels are adequate.[7] Scientists originally believed beta-carotene and other provitamin A carotenes were cleaved by an enzyme (carotene dioxygenase) in a manner that would yield two molecules of retinal. However, they currently believe that the enzyme nonspecifically attacks any one of the double bonds of the beta-carotene. Therefore, it sometimes may result in the formation of two retinal molecules, but most often it does not. The retinal formed is then converted to retinol.

Transport, Storage, and Excretion

Upon reaching the liver, vitamin A is stored primarily in special cells known as Ito cells. Although we find small amounts of vitamin A in most tissues (see Table 3.4), the liver stores more than 90 percent of the total body vitamin A content. It is stored as a complex consisting of 96 percent retinyl esters (retinol plus a fatty acid) and 4 percent unesterified retinol. When the body needs more vitamin A, an enzyme that transfers the released retinol to the retinol-binding protein (RBP) breaks down the retinyl esters. The bound retinol is then processed and secreted into the blood, where it forms a 1:1 complex with a protein (prealbumin).[1,2]

Adequate dietary protein and zinc are necessary for proper retinal mobilization. The half-life of RBP and prealbumin is less than 12 hours, making them particularly likely to be deficient during protein-calorie malnutrition or other situations in which protein metabolism is abnormal. A zinc or vitamin E deficiency severely impairs vitamin A metabolism because these two nutrients function synergistically in many physiological processes of vitamin A metabolism (absorption, transport, and mobilization in particular).[2]

TABLE 3.4 **Distribution of Vitamin A and Carotenes (Micrograms) in Some Human Tissues (Kilograms)**

Tissue	Vitamin A	Carotenes	Beta-carotene
Adrenal	10.4	20.1	10.8
Liver	149	8.3	Not determined
Testis	1.14	5.0	4.7
Fat	1.46	3.9	1.3
Pancreas	0.52	2.3	1.1
Spleen	0.89	1.6	1.2
Lung	0.91	0.6	Not determined
Thyroid	0.43	0.6	Not determined

Retinol is transferred into the cell after RBP binds to a cell surface receptor. The retinol is then quickly bound by cellular retinol-binding protein (CRBP) within the cell.

The body metabolizes retinoic acid differently than it does retinol. Retinoic acid is absorbed and transported in the blood bound to a different protein (albumin). It does not accumulate within the liver or other tissue in any appreciable amounts. It is metabolized quite rapidly to more polar oxygenated compounds. Within cells, it is bound to the cellular retinoic acid binding protein (CRABP).[1]

Vitamin A metabolites are excreted mainly through the feces (via the bile) and the urine. During periods of deficiency, an adaptation in utilization takes place, as evidenced by a reduction in the rate of vitamin A catabolism.[1,2]

No specific carrier protein exists in the blood for carotenes. These compounds are typically transported in human plasma in association with the plasma lipoproteins, particularly by low-density lipoprotein (LDL). As a consequence, patients with high serum cholesterol or LDL levels tend to have high serum carotene levels. The concentrations found in the plasma usually reflect the dietary concentration, with beta-carotene typically comprising only 20 to 25 percent of the total serum carotene level.[8]

Carotenes may be stored in adipose tissue, the liver, other organs (the adrenals, testes, and ovaries have the highest concentrations), and the skin (see Table 3.4). Deposition in the skin results in a yellowing of the skin known as carotenodermia. This is a benign (and probably very beneficial) state. Carotenodermia not directly attributable to dietary intake or supplementation, however, may be indicative of a deficiency in a necessary conversion factor, i.e., zinc, thyroid hormone, vitamin C, or protein.[2,5]

Deficiency Signs and Symptoms

Vitamin A deficiency may be because of inadequate dietary intake (primary deficiency) or some secondary factor that interferes with the absorption, storage, or transportation of vitamin A. Some factors known to induce a vitamin A deficiency include: malabsorption because of bile acid or pancreatic insufficiency, protein-energy malnutrition, liver disease, zinc deficiency, and abetalipoproteinemia.[1]

Immune system abnormalities associated with a vitamin A deficiency include impaired ability to mount an effective antibody response, decreased levels of helper T-cells, and alterations in the mucosal linings of the respiratory and gastrointestinal tract. Vitamin A deficient individuals are more susceptible to infectious diseases and have higher mortality rates. In addition, during the course of an infection vitamin A stores are severely depleted. Thus, a vicious cycle ensues. Infectious conditions associated with vitamin A deficiency include the measles, chicken pox, respiratory syncytial virus (RSV), AIDS, and pneumonia.

Prolonged vitamin A deficiency results in the characteristic signs of follicular hyperkeratosis (buildup of cellular debris in the hair follicles, giving the skin a goose-bump appearance; occurs most often at the back of the upper arm), night blindness, and increased rate of infection. As the condition worsens, it also affects the mucous membranes of the respiratory tract, gastrointestinal tract, and genitourinary tract . Soon the classic eye disease known as xerophthalmia ensues because of vitamin A deficiency. Even a mild vitamin A deficiency is associated with a significant increase in mortality. This is extremely significant because vitamin A deficiency is particularly widespread in developing countries, particularly in Asian countries where as many as 10 million children per year develop xerophthalmia.[1,2]

Xerophthalmia

We use the term *xerophthalmia* to cover all the eye-related manifestations of vitamin A deficiency. Blindness is one of the most serious consequences of vitamin A deficiency. Although xerophthalmia rarely occurs in the United States, it is the major preventable cause of blindness in Asia.

In an effort to prevent vitamin A deficiency in underdeveloped countries, the World Health Organization (WHO) administers large prophylactic doses (200,000 I.U.) to children every six months.

Exposure to Toxic Chemicals Increases Vitamin A Degradation

Studies have demonstrated a link between exposure to toxic chemicals and vitamin A nutrition. Administration of compounds such as polybrominated biphenyls, dioxin, and other toxic chemicals to rats results in a decrease in the hepatic content of vitamin A. Administration of vitamin concurrently with the xenobiotics partially prevents the symptoms of toxicity. Exposure to these compounds results in an increased vitamin A requirement because of the enhanced degradation of vitamin A in the liver.[9,10]

Recommended Dietary Allowance

Vitamin A activity was originally measured in International Units (I.U.) One I.U. is defined as .3 micrograms of crystalline retinol or .6 micrograms of beta-carotene. In

1967, an FAO/WHO Expert Committee (Food and Agriculture Organization of the United Nations/World Health Organization) recommended that vitamin A activity be referred to in terms of retinol equivalents rather than in I.U., with 1 microgram of retinol being equivalent to 1 retinol equivalent (R.E.). The amount of beta-carotene required for 1 R.E. is 6 micrograms, while the amount required for other provitamin A carotenes is 12 micrograms. In 1980, The Food and Nutrition Board of the NRC/NAS (National Research Council/National Academy of Sciences) adopted this recommendation. Therefore, the 1980 RDA for vitamin A is stated in micrograms and retinol equivalents.

Recommended Dietary Allowance of Vitamin A

Group	Retinol Equivalents	International Units
INFANTS UNDER 1 YEAR	375	1,875
CHILDREN		
1–3 years	400	2,000
4–6 years	500	2,500
7–10 years	700	3,500
YOUNG ADULTS AND ADULTS		
Males 11+ years	1,000	5,000
Females 11+ years	800	4,000
Pregnant females	800	4,000
Lactating females	800	4,000

Beneficial Effects

Science best understands the role of vitamin A with regard to its effects on the visual system. The human retina has four kinds of vitamin A containing photopigments: rhodopsin, present in the rods (the retinal cells responsible for night vision); and three iodopsins, present in each of the different cones that are responsible for day vision (blue, yellow, and red). The vitamin A form found in these pigments is the 11-cis isomer of vitamin A aldehyde (retinal). When a photon of light strikes the rod, the 11-cis retinal splits from the rhodopsin molecule to yield opsin and all-trans retinol. This reaction leads to a change in membrane potential and subsequent transmission of the visual impulse.[1]

When there is bright flash of light (such as oncoming headlights), there is a temporary bleaching of rhodopsin. It may take a moment or two before the retinal is regenerated and sight is returned. It takes longer to adapt if vitamin A levels are low.[1,2] Poor adaptation to changes in light and poor vision at night are some of the initial findings in low vitamin A states.[1]

Growth and Development

We believe Vitamin A affects growth and development by its necessary role in the synthesis of many glycoproteins (e.g., mucus), some of which may control cellular differentiation and gene expression.[1,2]

The adhesion between cells is apparently related to the manufacture of molecules known as glycoproteins. The synthesis of these compounds is markedly depressed in vitamin A deficiency. Consequently, during deficiency there is a loss of normal stimuli for cellular growth and differentiation. In addition, cellular retinol-binding protein (CRBP) is transferred directly into the nucleus of the cell and may function in a fashion similar to some of the steroid hormones in stimulating cellular processes.

The effects of a vitamin A deficiency most readily appear in tissues that have a rapid turnover rate, i.e., the epithelial cells that line the oral cavity, respiratory tract, urinary tract, and ducts of secretory glands.[1,2]

The role of vitamin A and carotenes in the development and maintenance of epithelial tissue cannot be overstated. Vitamin A status determines whether mucin or keratin is synthesized in epidermal cells; the presence of adequate vitamin A results in mucin production, while a lack results in hyperkeratinization of the skin, cornea, upper respiratory tract, and genitourinary tract.[1,2]

Reproduction

Since 1922, scientists have been aware of the necessity of vitamin A in the reproductive functions in higher animals.[2] Beta-carotene also seems have a specific effect in fertility distinct from its role as a precursor to vitamin A.[11-13] In bovine nutritional studies, cows fed beta-carotene-deficient diets exhibited delayed ovulation and an increase in the number of follicular and luteal cysts.[11,12] The corpus luteum has the highest concentration of beta-carotene in any organ measured.[13] The carotene cleavage activity changes with the ovulation cycle, with the highest activity occurring during the midovulation stage. Some researchers speculate that a proper ratio of carotene to retinol must be maintained to ensure proper corpus luteum function.

Because the corpus luteum produces progesterone, inadequate corpus luteum function could have significant deleterious effects. Inadequate corpus luteum secretory function is one of the characteristic features of infertile and/or irregular menstrual cycles.[14] Furthermore, an increased estrogen to progesterone ratio has been implicated in a variety of clinical conditions, including ovarian cysts, premenstrual tension syndrome, fibrocystic breast disease, and breast cancer.[15] Since supplemental beta-carotene given to cows significantly reduced the incidence of ovarian cysts (42 percent in the control group versus 3 percent in the beta-carotene group), it may have a similar effect in humans.[12,13] Cystic mastitis is another bovine condition that benefited from increased dietary beta-carotene levels.[16] The annual monetary loss from bovine mastitis in the United States is estimated at $1.5 to 2 billion, and ovarian cysts represent the major cause of infertility in cattle. Perhaps farmers have a greater appreciation of beta-carotene than do many nutritionists.

Immune system

Vitamin A is essential to proper immune function. First, it affects the immune system because it plays an essential role in maintaining the epithelial and mucosal surfaces and their secretions. These systems constitute a primary nonspecific host defense mechanism. In addition, vitamin A stimulates and/or enhances numerous immune processes, including induction of antitumor activity, enhancement of white blood cell function, and increased antibody response.[17] These effects are not due simply to a reversal of vitamin A deficiency since many of these effects apparently are further enhanced by excessive amounts of vitamin A. Retinol has also demonstrated significant antiviral activity and has prevented the immunosuppression induced by glucocorticoids, severe burns, and surgery. Some of these effects are probably related to vitamin A's ability both to prevent stress-induced thymic involution and promote thymus growth. Because carotenes are better antioxidants, they may prove be better in protecting the thymus gland than vitamin A, particularly since the thymus gland is susceptible to free-radical and oxidative damage.

Beta-carotene appears to enhance thymus gland function and increase interferon's stimulatory action on the immune system.[18] Interferon is a powerful immune-enhancing compound that plays a central role in protection against viral infections.

Antioxidant Activity

In general, carotenes exert significant antioxidant activity compared to that of vitamin A.[19] The antioxidant activity of carotenes is probably the factor responsible for the anticancer effects noted in population studies. Since aging is also associated with free-radical damage, perhaps carotenes also protect against aging. Evidence seems to support this hypothesis. Carotenoid content of tissue is the most significant factor in determining maximal life span potential (MLSP) of mammalian species.[20] For example, human MLSP of approximately 90 years correlates with a serum carotene level of 50 to 300 micrograms per deciliter while other primates, such as the rhesus monkey, have a MLSP of approximately 34 years correlating with a serum carotene level of 6 to 12 micrograms per deciliter (see Figure 3.1).

While beta-carotene has received most of the attention, many carotenes that have low or no vitamin A activity exert much greater protection. For example, while beta-carotene generates vitamin A much more efficiently than alpha-carotene, alpha-carotene is approximately 38 percent stronger as an antioxidant and 10 times more effective in suppressing liver, skin, and lung cancer in animals.[21] Even more powerful is lycopene.[22] Lycopene exhibits the highest overall singlet oxygen-quenching carotenoid. Its activity is roughly double that of beta-carotene. Furthermore, lycopene may exert even more impressive anticancer effects.

To evaluate the role of lycopene as a protective factor in digestive-tract cancers, researchers in northern Italy conducted a case-control study Although tomato intake in northern Italy is high, it is also heterogeneous—some people eat a lot of tomatoes while others eat very few, if any. Tomatoes are a perfect food to study because they are quite high in lycopene but very low in carotene.

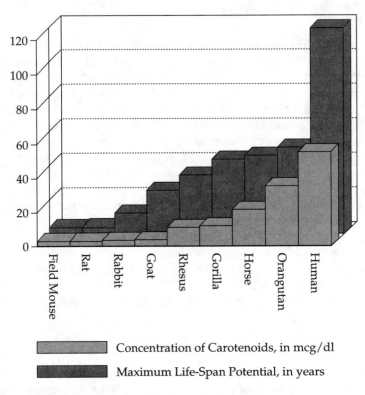

Concentration of Carotenoids, in mcg/dl

Maximum Life-Span Potential, in years

SOURCE: Cuder RG: Carotenoids and retinol: their possible importance in determining longevity of primate species. *Proc Natl Acad Sci* 81:7627–31, 1984.

FIGURE 3.1   Carotenes and maximum life-span potential.

The researchers obtained their data from a series of hospital-based studies of various cancers of the digestive tract that took place between 1985 and 1991.[23] They divided the frequency of consumption of raw tomatoes into four levels—less than two, three to four, five to six, and more than seven servings per week. Results showed a consistent pattern of protection as a result of high intake of raw tomatoes in all examined cancer sites of the digestive tract. The degree of protection was similar to, but somewhat more marked than, that afforded by green vegetable and fruit studies carried on in the same areas. The results support the findings of other researchers who found such things as a 40 percent reduction in the risk of esophageal cancer by simply consuming one serving of raw tomatoes per week and a 50 percent reduced rate for cancers of all sites among elderly Americans reporting a high tomato intake. The results of this study indicate that increasing dietary lycopene levels may be a significant protector against cancer.

According to a detailed analysis of the levels of carotenoids in 120 fruits and vegetables, very few contained lycopene.[24] The table below illustrates lycopene levels in some of those foods. These values indicate food processing does not destroy lycopene levels.

Milligrams of Lycopene per 100 Grams of Fruit or Vegetable

Name	Amount of Lycopene
Apricot, canned	0.06
Apricot, dried	0.8
Grapefruit (pink and raw)	3.4
Guava juice	3.3
Tomato, raw	3.1
Tomato juice, canned	8.6
Tomato paste, canned	6.5
Tomato sauce, canned	6.3
Watermelon, raw	4.1

Available Forms

Natural vitamin A is available either as retinol or retinyl-palmitate. Either micelliza-tion or emulsification improve absorption. Micellization is the process of making the fat-soluble vitamin A into very small droplets (micelles) so that the material is dis-persed in water. Emulsification is the process of emulsifying the vitamin A with another chemical (such as lecithin) so that it can mix with water. Despite manufactur-ers' claims, regular vitamin A is absorbed at a rate of 80 to 90 percent. I am particular-ly amused by one company's claim that its micellized vitamin A is absorbed up to 520 percent better than other forms of vitamin A. Since regular vitamin A is absorbed at a rate of 80 to 90 percent, such a claim is impossible.

There are three primary sources of carotenes on the market—synthetic all-trans beta-carotene, beta- and alpha-carotene from the algae *Dunaliella*, and mixed carotenes from palm oil. Of these three, palm oil carotenes are the best form. First, let's take a look at the antioxidant activities (see Table 3.5).

Palm oil carotenes appear to give the best antioxidant protection. The carotene complex of palm oil closely mirrors the pattern in high-carotene foods. In particular, unlike the synthetic version—which only provides the trans configuration of beta-carotene—natural carotene sources provide beta-carotene in both a trans and cis configuration:

60 percent beta-carotene (both trans and cis isomers)
34 percent alpha-carotene
3 percent gamma-carotene
3 percent lycopene

Palm oil carotenes are absorbed four to ten times better than synthetic all-trans beta-carotene.[25–27] Carotenes from *Dunaliella* are also absorbed well.[28]

The widespread health concerns concerning the use of "tropical oils" like palm and coconut do not apply to carotene products extracted from palm oil because the fat content is minimal. In addition, the real problem with palm oil occurs when it is processed, i.e., partially hydrogenated.

TABLE 3.5   Antioxidant Potential of Carotene Products

Source	Quenching Rate	Percent in Source	Mg/25,000 I.U.	Antioxidant Potential
PALM OIL ANALYSIS				
Alpha-carotene	1.9	33	7.36	2.60
Beta-carotene	1.4	63	14.04	3.66
Gamma-carotene	2.5	2.5	0.56	0.26
Lycopene	3.1	0.1	0.02	0.01
Total				6.54
ALGAL CAROTENE ANALYSIS				
Alpha-carotene	1.9	4.0	0.61	0.22
Beta-carotene	1.4	96.0	14.69	3.83
Total				4.05
SYNTHETIC BETA-CAROTENE ANALYSIS				
Beta-carotene	1.4	100	14.97	3.90
Total				3.90

Principal Uses

Vitamin A is used primarily as an immune enhancer in viral illnesses and in the treatment of numerous skin disorders. Carotenes are used as antioxidants in the prevention of cancer and cardiovascular disease, as immune-enhancing agents, and in the treatment of photosensitivity disorders.

Vitamin A in Viral Illnesses

Vitamin A is absolutely critical to a healthily functioning immune system. Vitamin A–deficient individuals are susceptible to infectious diseases, particularly viral infections. Then during the course of the ensuing infections, the already low vitamin A stores are severely depleted.

Vitamin A Supplementation in Measles

Vitamin A deficiency is a major problem in many developing countries as evidenced by the fact that five to ten million children in these countries exhibit severe vitamin A deficiency. Recently a number of well-designed studies have confirmed an effect first noted in 1932—Vitamin A supplementation can significantly reduce infant mortality among measles patients by at least 50 percent. Typically the dosage of vitamin A in double-blind studies has been 200,000 to 400,000 I.U. administered only once or twice to replenish body stores.[28,29]

Now, you may be thinking that the use of vitamin A supplementation in the treatment of measles is only indicated in Third-World countries. However, a study of "well-nourished" children in Long Beach, California, suffering from measles indicated that 50 percent were deficient in vitamin A.[30] This finding supports the use of vitamin A supplementation even in the U.S.

Vitamin A Therapy for Infants with RSV Infections

Wide-scale immunization programs have reduced the risk of measles in children. However, vitamin A therapy appears appropriate for other childhood viral illnesses. One of the most common viruses nowadays is respiratory syncytial virus (RSV), a common cause of severe respiratory disease in young children. Children with RSV have low serum vitamin A levels. Furthermore, the lower the vitamin A level, the greater the severity of the disease—similar to the relationship shown in measles. Because vitamin A supplementation diminishes the morbidity and death caused by measles, a group of researchers decided to determine vitamin A's safety and absorption pattern in RSV as a first step in determining its therapeutic effectiveness.[31]

Twenty-one children with a mean age of 2.3 months (range, 1 to 6 months) with mild RSV infection were treated with 12,500 to 25,000 I.U. of oral micellized vitamin A. Baseline vitamin A levels were low; but within 6 hours after receiving a minimum of 25,000 I.U. of vitamin A, normal levels were re-established. Despite their young ages, none of the children experienced any obvious signs or symptoms of vitamin A toxicity. Although the study was not designed as a therapeutic trial, the subjects receiving vitamin A had hospital stays shorter than those of children with a similar severity of illness who were not enrolled in the study.

Placebo-controlled trials are necessary to determine the true effectiveness of vitamin A in RSV infection. Vitamin A supplementation is an attractive treatment of RSV infections for many reasons, including its low cost, wide availability, and ease of administration.

Vitamin A Deficiency in AIDS Linked to Increased Mortality

Another viral illness that may benefit from vitamin A supplementation is AIDS. Vitamin A deficiency is quite common during HIV infection and is clearly associated with a decreased level of circulating helper T-cells, one of the hallmark features of AIDS.[32]

Analysis of vitamin A levels, helper T-cells, and other blood parameters in HIV individuals indicates that more than 15 percent of the subjects tested had deficient vitamin A levels in their blood. When vitamin A levels were low, helper T-cell levels were much lower than the levels in HIV-infected individuals who had normal levels of vitamin A. Vitamin A deficiency is also associated with a higher rate of mortality because of HIV.

Beta-carotene may be the preferred form of vitamin A for supplementation in HIV patients because retinoic acid, the active form of vitamin A, may actually increase HIV replication in humans. Low beta-carotene levels are common in AIDS, presumably as a result of fat malabsorption, and are associated with greater impairment of immune function.[33]

Vitamin A in the Treatment of Other Skin Disorders

In the late 1930s, dermatologists introduced the use of high-dose vitamin A therapy for a wide variety of dermatological conditions. It is still used by a few dermatologists; however, since the advent of the synthetic retinoids, this type of therapy is not as popular as it once was. Vitamin A therapy is quite effective in treating skin conditions associated with excessive formation of keratin (hyperkeratosis), a skin protein that can clog the pores of the skin to produce a "goose-bump" effect. Examples of some skin conditions associated with hyperkeratosis include acne, psoriasis, ichthyosis, lichen planus, Darier's disease, palmoplantar keratoderma, and pityriasis rubra pilaris. The dosages of vitamin A used to treat these conditions are typically quite high—300,00 to 500,000 I.U. per day for five to six months in the treatment of acne, and 1 to 3.5 million I.U. per day for one to two weeks for the other conditions.[34-38] The use of these high dosages usually results in the development of significant toxicity. Although there is some evidence that carotenes may be more useful and less toxic in some of these conditions, the pharmacological effect responsible for the effects of vitamin A in hyperkeratosis probably result when serum retinol levels exceed serum retinol–binding protein capacity, causing destabilization of membranes and destruction of the keratin-producing cells.[34]

In monitoring for vitamin A toxicity, laboratory tests appear unreliable until obvious toxicity symptoms are apparent. The first significant toxic symptom is usually headache followed by fatigue, emotional instability, and muscle and joint pain. Chapped lips (cheilitis) and dry skin (xerosis) generally occur in the majority of patients, particularly in dry weather. Because high doses of vitamin A during pregnancy can cause birth defects, women of child-bearing age should use effective birth control during vitamin A treatment and for at least one month after discontinuation of treatment.

High doses of vitamin A may not be necessary if other nutritional factors like zinc and vitamin E are included. These nutrients work with vitamin A in promoting healthy skin. A safe and effective recommendation for vitamin A in the treatment of acne is less than 25,000 I.U. per day.

Topical Vitamin A in the Treatment of Dry Eyes

Dry-eye disorders are complex diseases that can be characterized by a localized water deficiency in the tear ducts, a mucin deficiency, or a combination of both. Despite the diversity of underlying causes, the changes in the conjunctiva of the eye are similar in all cases, i.e., loss of goblet cells (mucin-producing cells), abnormal enlargement of nongoblet epithelial cells, and an increase of cellular layers and keratin deposition, stratification, and keratinization.

Other than topical vitamin A therapy, all other nonsurgical therapies of dry eye—frequent application of artificial tears, lubricants, or slow-releasing polymers, and the therapeutic use of soft contact lenses—are not directed toward reversing the underlying process but rather toward alleviating the symptoms.

The hypothesis that a localized vitamin A deficiency in the lining of the outer eye may be responsible for dry eye is obvious, considering vitamin A's vital role in epithelial tissue. Clinical studies featuring commercial vitamin A eyedrops (Viva-

Drops from Vision Pharmaceuticals, 1-800-325-6789) have yielded impressive clinical results in the treatment of dry eyes.[39,40] Unlike other dry-eye preparations, however, topical vitamin A reverses the underlying cellular changes causing the dry eye. Viva-Drops is available in many pharmacies and some health food stores. However, I would recommend calling the company to find a store near you that carries the product.

Carotenes in Cancer Prevention

Population-based epidemiological studies clearly demonstrate a strong inverse correlation between dietary carotene intake and a variety of cancers involving epithelial tissues (lung, skin, uterus, cervix, gastrointestinal tract, etcetera).[41,42] The epidemiological association is much stronger for carotene than for vitamin A. This may reflect carotene's superior antioxidant, immune-potentiating activity and anticarcinogenic activity.[43]

No one would argue that a diet high in carotenes is not protective against cancer (except, perhaps, Victor Herbert, M.D., a longtime crusader against nutritional supplementation). The big question is, can beta-carotene supplementation reduce the risk of cancer? The answer appears to be no, that on its own beta-carotene supplementation does not reduce the risk of cancer. Three highly publicized reports on cancer prevention trials featuring synthetic all-trans beta-carotene in high-risk groups have produced negative results. However, before we close this issue, let's take a closer look at each of these studies to help put things into perspective.

Alpha-tocopherol, Beta-carotene Cancer Prevention Study Group

Here researchers studied 29,000 men in Finland who smoked and drank alcohol.[44] The men took beta-carotene (20 milligrams daily) and/or vitamin E. The results of this study indicated an 18 percent increase in lung cancer in the beta-carotene group. This result was not unexpected. Studies in primates have demonstrated that when animals ingest alcohol and beta-carotene, they experience an increase in liver damage as a result of oxidative damage.[45] Other researchers have pointed out that beta-carotene is very susceptible to oxidative damage.[46] To protect against oxidative damage of beta-carotene, other antioxidant nutrients need to be present.[47] Absence of these protective nutrients could result in the formation of cancer-causing compounds, which further stresses the importance of relying on foods and broader-spectrum nutritional antioxidant support. For example, the group that received both beta-carotene and vitamin E did not show an increase in cancer. In addition, the group that did not receive beta-carotene supplements demonstrated a strong protective effect of high dietary beta-carotene and blood carotene levels against lung cancer. All together this data strongly suggests that the protection offered by beta-carotene is apparent only when other important antioxidant nutrients are present.

The CARET Study

The second trial reporting on the role of beta-carotene in a high-risk group is the Carotene and Retinol Efficacy Trial (CARET).[48] Over 18,000 U.S. male and female smokers and asbestos workers participated in the study, which halted 21 months prematurely on January 13, 1996. At that time, 4 years of intervention indicated that beta-carotene supplementation (30 milligrams daily) increased lung cancer by 28 percent and overall deaths by 17 percent. Let's put these numbers and percentages into their proper perspective. Among active smokers, the risk of lung cancer during the CARET study was 5 out of every 1,000. The 28 percent increase found with beta-carotene supplementation increased this number to roughly 6 out of 1,000.[45]

Once again, in the group not taking beta-carotene, researchers found the lowest rate of cancer in individuals with the highest blood beta-carotene levels. In former smokers, beta-carotene supplementation actually reduced cancer risk by 20 percent.

Physicians' Health Study

In the Physicians' Health Study, 22,071 U.S. male physicians took either 50 milligrams of beta-carotene or a placebo every other day for 12 years. Results demonstrated no significant effect, positive or negative, on cancer or cardiovascular disease—even in the group (11 percent) who smoked.[49]

General Comments on the "Negative" Studies

The results of these three studies indicate that synthetic beta-carotene supplementation may have adverse effects in high-risk groups for cancer and cardiovascular disease. These studies do not erase the hundreds of studies showing the effect of a diet rich in carotenes and nutritional antioxidants with regard to cancer and cardiovascular disease. These results indicate the need for a diet high in carotenes. If people desire to supplement their diets with carotene, they should not smoke and they should protect beta-carotene against the formation of toxic derivatives by taking extra vitamin C, vitamin E, and selenium

Other Prospective Studies

In addition to these three highly publicized studies, other prospective and double-blind studies show promising results. In particular, beta-carotene supplementation is especially effective in the treatment of early cancerous lesions of the oral cavity and esophagus.[50,51] Although beta-carotene exerts these benefits on its own (in dosages ranging from 15 to 180 milligrams per day), one of the most positive studies featured a broader supplement program. The Linxian Cancer Chemoprevention Study is a prospective study of 30,000 rural Chinese adults. In one of the substudies, subjects received one of four supplement programs—retinol and zinc; riboflavin and niacin; vitamin C and molybdenum; and beta-carotene, vitamin E, and selenium (dosages 1 to 3 times greater than the U.S. RDA). The latter group demonstrated 13 percent fewer cancer deaths and a reduction of 9 percent in overall deaths.[52,53] These results again support the notion that a combination of antioxidants is superior to high levels of any single antioxidant.

Carotenes in Prevention of Cardiovascular Disease

High carotene intake is also associated with lowering the risk of cardiovascular disease.[54] Like other antioxidants, beta-carotene may inhibit damage to cholesterol and the lining of the arteries.[55] However, it appears that beta-carotene is less effective in protecting against cardiovascular disease than vitamin E, probably because vitamin E protects against oxidative damage to cholesterol better than beta-carotene.[56]

Carotenes as Immune-Enhancing Agents

Carotenes have demonstrated a number of immune-enhancing effects in recent studies.[18] However, immune-enhancing effects were demonstrated as far back as 1931 when scientists discovered that a diet rich in carotenes (determined by blood carotene levels) were inversely related to the number of school days missed by children.[57] Originally researchers thought that the immune-enhancing properties of carotenes were because of their conversion to vitamin A. They now know that carotenes exert many immune-enhancing effects independent of any vitamin A activity.[18]

One of the most impressive studies was conducted on healthy human volunteers.[58] Results demonstrated that oral beta-carotene (180 milligrams/day, approximately 300,000 I.U.) significantly increased the frequency of OKT4+ (helper/inducer T cells) by approximately 30 percent after 7 days, and of OKT3+ (all T-cells) after 14 days.[51] T4+ lymphocytes play a critical role in determining host immune status. This study indicates that oral beta-carotene may be effective in increasing the immunological competence of the host where there is a selective diminution of the T4 subset of T-cells, such as in acquired immunodeficiency syndrome (AIDS) and cancer.

However, rather than supplementing the diet with synthetic beta-carotene, it may be more advantageous to use natural carotene sources or increase the intake of carotene-rich foods. In another study, 126 healthy college students were randomly assigned to one of the following groups: Group A, the control group; Group B, a group that used a 15-milligram (25,000 I.U.) beta-carotene supplement daily; and Group C, a group that consumed approximately 15 milligrams of beta-carotene per day from carrots. Group B achieved the best results—an increase in the white blood cell number and function.[59]

What is baffling about these results is that absorption studies show supplemental beta-carotene is better absorbed than the carotenes from carrots and other vegetables.[3]

Decreased Beta-carotene Levels in Epithelial Cells in Vaginal Candidiasis

When a woman's immune system is depressed, she is more susceptible to vaginal candidiasis than she is when her immune system is healthy. These immune system depressions may be because of low carotene levels. In a study that compared beta-carotene levels in exfoliated vaginal cells with vaginal candidiasis to exfoliated vaginal cells from a control group, the beta-carotene level per one million cells in the women with vaginal candidiasis was 1.46 ng (nanograms) compared to 8.99 ng in the control group. Hence, the beta-carotene level in women with vaginal candidiasis was one sixth that of normal.[60]

These results, coupled with beta-carotene's known effects on enhancing the immune system, suggest that low tissue levels of beta-carotene are associated with vaginal candidiasis. A high dietary or supplemental intake of beta-carotene may be protective against vaginal candidiasis.

Carotenes in the Treatment of Photosensitivity Disorders

Beta-carotene has become the treatment of choice for photosensitivity disorders (skin rashes induced by the sun). It is most effective in the treatment of a condition named erythropoietic protoporphyria (EPP), while its effectiveness in other photosensitivity disorders—polymorphous light eruption, solar urticaria, and discoid lupus erythematosis—has also been demonstrated but not to the same degree.[61-68] Beta-carotene also has a small but significant effect in increasing the exposure level at which manifestations of sunburn begin, thus allowing some subjects the opportunity to stay in the sun long enough to get a "tan" for the first time.[69]

Patients with EPP exhibit elevated levels of compounds known as porphyrins in blood, feces, and skin, and are sensitive to visible light. This sensitivity manifests itself after exposure to sunlight by a burning sensation followed by swelling and redness. Topical sunscreens are of no value. The photosensitivity is because of excitation of the porphyrin molecule by ultraviolet radiation, which results in production of free radicals that are very deleterious to the skin. Direct cell damage results in the release of chemical mediators, which in turn damage other cells, causing itching, burning, redness, and swelling.

In EPP, blood carotene levels of 600 to 800 micrograms per deciliter produce optimum effects, and the protective effect doesn't manifest after 4 to 6 weeks of therapy. The action of beta-carotene and other carotenes in human tissue is similar to their action in plant cells; i.e., they function as a cellular screen against sunlight-induced free-radical damage.

Dosage Ranges

Intent of use determines dosage ranges for vitamin A. For general health purposes, a dosage of 5,000 I.U. for men and 2,500 for women appears reasonable. During an acute viral infection, a single oral dosage of 50,000 I.U. for one or two days is safe even in infants.

> Women who might be pregnant must not use vitamin A supplements; instead, use beta-carotene.

Although high-dose therapy of vitamin A may be useful for the treatment of acne and hyperkeratotic skin disorders, a physician should closely monitor the therapy.

With carotenes, a daily dosage of 25,000 I.U. (15 milligrams of beta-carotene) appears to be reasonable for general health. For the treatment of precancerous lesions and immune enhancement, the dosage range is 25,000 to 300,000 I.U. In the treatment of EPP, the dosage should maintain blood carotene levels between 600 to 800 micrograms per deciliter.

Safety Issues

Women must avoid vitamin A supplementation during pregnancy. A recent study published in the prestigious *New England Journal of Medicine* demonstrated that dosages greater than 10,000 I.U. during pregnancy (specifically during the first 7 weeks after conception) have probably been responsible for 1 out of each 57 cases of birth defects in the United States. Women who are at risk for becoming pregnant should keep their supplemental vitamin A levels below 5,000 I.U. or, better yet, look to carotenes.[70]

Accidental ingestion of a single large dose of vitamin A (100,000 to 300,000 I.U) produces acute toxicity in children, resulting in raised intracranial pressure with vomiting, headache, joint pain, stupor, and occasionally papilledema. Symptoms rapidly subside upon withdrawal of the vitamin, and complete recovery always results.[1]

Vitamin A toxicity may occur in adults who take in excess of 50,000 I.U. per day for several years. Smaller daily doses may produce toxicity symptoms if there are defects in storage and transport of vitamin A, which occurs in cirrhosis of the liver, hepatitis, protein calorie malnutrition, and in children and adolescents.[71,72] Signs of vitamin A toxicity generally include dry, fissured skin; brittle nails; alopecia; gingivitis; cheilosis; anorexia; irritability; fatigue; and nausea. Serum levels of vitamin A of 250 to 6600 I.U. per deciliter are typical of toxicity. Prolonged, severe hypervitaminosis A results in bone fragility and thickening of the long bones.

Toxicity is typically encountered during high dose vitamin A therapy for various skin conditions. Although dosages below 300,000 I.U. per day for a few months rarely cause toxicity symptoms, early recognition is still very important. Cheilitis (chapped lips) and xerosis (dry skin) generally appear in the majority of patients, particularly in dry weather. The first significant toxicity symptom is usually headache, followed by fatigue, emotional lability, and muscle and joint pain. Laboratory tests are of little value in monitoring toxicity because serum vitamin A levels correlate poorly with toxicity, and SGOT and SGPT are elevated only in symptomatic patients.[34]

On the other hand, supplementing the diet with beta-carotene does not produce any significant toxicity despite its use in very high doses in the treatment of numerous photosensitive disorders. Occasionally, patients complain of "loose stools," but this usually clears up spontaneously and does not necessitate stopping treatment. Elevated carotene levels in the blood do not lead to vitamin A toxicity, nor do they lead to any other significant disturbance besides a yellowing of the skin (carotenodermia). The ingestion of large amounts of carrots or carrot juice (.45 to 1.0 kilograms of fresh carrots per day for several years) can, however, cause a neutropenia as well as menstrual disorders.[73,74] Although the blood carotene levels (221 to 1,007 micrograms per deciliter) of these patients did reach levels similar to those of patients taking high doses of beta-carotene (typically 800 micrograms per deciliter), the disturbances were because of some other factor in carrots. Neither these effects nor any others have been observed in subjects consuming very high doses of pure beta-carotene over long periods of time— e.g., 300,000 to 600,000 I.U. per day (180 to 360 milligrams beta-carotene, which is equivalent to 4 to 8 pounds of raw carrots).[75–79] Doses up to 1,000 milligrams per kilogram of body weight have been given to rats and rabbits for long periods of time with no signs of embryotoxicity, toxicity, tumori-genicity, or interference in reproductive functions.[80]

Interactions

Vitamin E and zinc are particularly important to the proper function of vitamin A. A deficiency of zinc, vitamin C, protein, or thyroid hormone impairs the conversion of pro-vitamin A carotenes to vitamin A.

4

Vitamin D

Since our bodies can produce vitamin D by the action of sunlight on the skin, many experts consider it more of a hormone than a vitamin. Nonetheless, by current definitions vitamin D is both a vitamin and a hormone.

Food Sources

There are two major food forms of vitamin D—vitamin D_2 (ergocalciferol) and vitamin D_3 (cholecalciferol). Vitamin D_2, the form most often added to milk and other foods is also the form most often used in nutritional supplements. Good natural sources of vitamin D are cod liver oil, cold-water fish (mackerel, salmon, herring, etcetera), butter, and egg yolks. Vegetables are low in vitamin D; the best sources are dark green leafy vegetables.

Deficiency Signs and Symptoms

Vitamin D deficiency results in rickets in children and osteomalacia in adults. Rickets, characterized by an inability to calcify the bone matrix, results in softening of the skull bones, bowing of legs, spinal curvature, and increased joint size. Once common, these diseases are now extremely rare.

Vitamin D deficiency is now most often seen in elderly people who do not get any sunlight, particularly those in nursing homes. The consequences are lack of bone strength and density, and joint pain.[1]

Recommended Dietary Allowance

Recommended Dietary Allowance for Vitamin D

Group	International Units
INFANTS UNDER 6 MONTHS	300
CHILDREN 6 MONTHS–10 YEARS	400
YOUNG ADULTS AND ADULTS	
Males 11–24 years	400
Males 25+	200
Females 11–24 years	400
Females 24+ years	200
Pregnant females	400
Lactating females	400

Beneficial Effects

Vitamin D is best known for its ability to stimulate the absorption of calcium. However, there are actually different forms of vitamin D, each form exerting a different level of activity on calcium metabolism.

In the skin, sunlight changes the precursor to vitamin D, 7-dehydrocholesterol, into vitamin D_3 (cholecalciferol). It is then transported to the liver and converted by an enzyme into 25-hydroxycholecalciferol, which is five times more potent than cholecalciferol. An enzyme in the kidneys then converts the 25-hydroxycholecalciferol to 1,25-dihydroxycholecalciferol $(1,25\text{-}(OH)_2D_3)$, which is ten times more potent than cholecalciferol and the most potent form of vitamin D_3 (see Figure 4.1).

Disorders of the liver or kidneys result in impaired conversion of cholecalciferol to more potent vitamin D compounds. Many patients with osteoporosis have high levels of 25-OHD_3, while the level of 1,25-$(OH)_2D_3$ is quite low.[2] This signifies an impairment of the conversion of 25-OHD_3 to 1,25-$(OH)_2D_3$ in osteoporosis. Researchers have proposed many theories to account for this decreased conversion, including relationships to estrogen and magnesium deficiency. Recently, scientists have theorized that the trace mineral boron plays a role in this conversion.

Vitamin D also exerts many anticancer properties, especially against breast and colon cancer.[3-6] The incidence of both colon and breast cancer is higher in areas where people are exposed to the least amount of light.

Available Forms

Vitamin D is available in all the forms described above. Vitamin D_2 is the most common nutritional supplement form. Calcitriol, the prescription drug form of

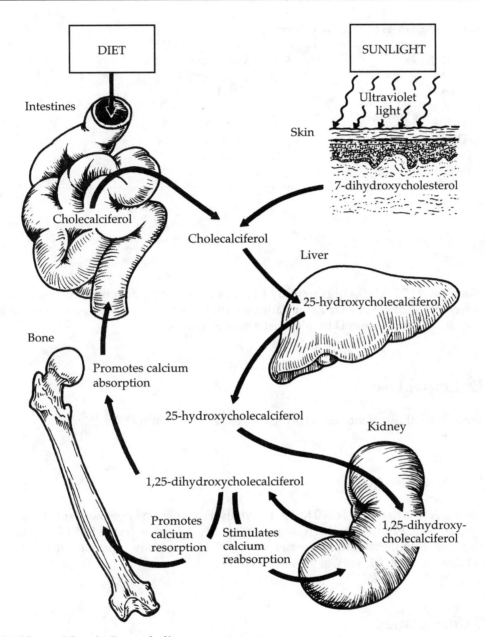

FIGURE 4.1   Vitamin D metabolism.

Relative Activities of Vitamin D Forms

Available Forms	Potency Multiplication Factor
Vitamin D_3	1
Vitamin D_2	1
25-OH-D_3	2 to 5
25-OH-D_2	2 to 5
1,25-$(OH)_2D_3$	10
1,25-$(OH)_2D_2$	10

vitamin D [1,25-$(OH)_2D_3$] is roughly 10 times as potent as vitamin D_2 or D_3. Doctors prescribe Calcitriol primarily for patients with kidney disease because these patients cannot convert vitamin D to this most active form.

Principal Uses

The principal use of vitamin D is the prevention of vitamin D deficiency.

Dosage Ranges

The RDA for vitamin D is 200 to 400 I.U. daily. For elderly people not exposed to sunlight or living in the northern latitudes, a daily intake of 400 to 800 I.U. is recommended. Supplementation greater than 400 I.U. per day in most adults, young children, and adolescents, is unwarranted.

Safety Issues

Vitamin D has the greatest potential among all the vitamins to cause toxicity. Dosages greater than 1,000 I.U. per day are certainly not recommended. Increased blood concentration of calcium (a potentially serious situation), deposition of calcium into internal organs, and kidney stones are some of the characteristics of vitamin D toxicity.

Many researchers suggest that long-term overconsumption of vitamin D in fortified foods contributes to atherosclerosis and heart disease, possibly as a result of decreasing magnesium absorption.[7]

Interactions

Vitamin D is intricately involved in calcium metabolism. The drugs cholestyramine, Dilantin, phenobarbital, and mineral oil all interfere with the absorption and/or metabolism of vitamin D.

5

Vitamin E

Most animal species, including humans, require vitamin E. In 1922 researchers discovered that when rats ate a purified diet without vitamin E, they became unable to reproduce. When wheat germ oil was added to their diet, fertility returned. Later, scientists isolated vitamin E and called it the "antisterility" vitamin. Alpha-tocopherol is the chemical name for the most active form of vitamin E. The term *tocopherol* comes from the Greek words *tokos*, which means "offspring," and *phero*, which means "to bear." Hence, *tocopherol* literally means "to bear children."

Food Sources

Although the RDA for vitamin E (alpha-tocopherol) is set at 10 milligrams (roughly 15 I.U. of vitamin E activity), the amount of vitamin E required is largely dependent upon the amount of polyunsaturated fats in the diet. The more polyunsaturated fats consumed, the greater the risk that they will be damaged. Since vitamin E prevents this damage, as the intake of polyunsaturated fatty acids increases, so does the need for vitamin E.

Fortunately, in nature, where there are high levels of polyunsaturated fatty acids, there are also higher levels of vitamin E. The best sources of vitamin E are polyunsaturated vegetable oils, seeds, nuts, and whole grains. Cooking and processing of foods, especially flour, reduce their vitamin C content. Good sources are asparagus, avocados, berries, green leafy vegetables, and tomatoes.

Deficiency Signs and Symptoms

Vitamin E functions primarily as an antioxidant in protecting against damage to the cell membranes. Without vitamin E, the cells of the body would be quite susceptible to damage, nerve cells in particular. Severe vitamin E deficiency is quite rare, but there are four major conditions where low levels of vitamin E are common:

- Fat malabsorption syndromes, such as celiac disease, cystic fibrosis, and post-gastrectomy syndrome
- Premature infants
- Hereditary disorders of red blood cells, such as sickle cell disease and thalassemia
- Hemodialysis patients

Symptoms of vitamin E deficiency in adults include nerve damage, muscle weakness, poor coordination, involuntary movement of the eyes, and breaking of red blood cells, leading to anemia (hemolytic anemia). In premature infants, vitamin E deficiency is characterized by hemolytic anemia and a severe eye disorder known as retrolental fibroplasia.

Recommended Dietary Allowance

Recommended Dietary Allowance of Vitamin E

Group	International Units
INFANTS UNDER 1 YEAR	4.5–6.0
CHILDREN 1–10 YEARS	9–10.5
YOUNG ADULTS AND ADULTS	
Males 11+ years	15
Females 11+ years	12
Pregnant females	15
Lactating females	18

Beneficial Effects

Vitamin E is the premier "lipid phase" antioxidant in the body. It is actually incorporated into the lipid (fatty) portion of cell membranes and carrier molecules, where it acts to stabilize and protect these structures from compounds such as lead, mercury, and other heavy metals; toxic compounds such as benzene, carbon tetrachloride, and cleaning solvents; drugs; radiation; and the body's free-radical metabolites. Because of Vitamin E's antioxidant effects, supplementation or a high vitamin E diet exerts a protective effect in many common health conditions.

Vitamin E is important to immune function. In addition to protecting the thymus gland and circulating white blood cells from damage, vitamin E is particularly important in protecting the immune system from damage during times of oxidative stress and chronic viral illnesses, such as AIDS and chronic viral hepatitis.

Available Forms

Vitamin E is available in many different forms, either natural or synthetic. Natural forms of vitamin E are designated *d-*, as in d-alpha-tocopherol, while synthetic forms are *dl-*, as in dl-alpha-tocopherol. The letters *d* and *l* reflect mirror images of the vitamin E molecule. An analogy is your hands—you have a right hand (d) and a left hand (l). They are mirror images of each other. In the human body, only the *d-* form is recognized. Although the *l-* form has antioxidant activity, it may actually inhibit the *d-* form from entering cell membranes.[1-3] Therefore, natural vitamin E (the *d-* form) has greater benefit than the synthetic (*dl*). I recommend avoiding synthetic vitamin E. Here are some of the names of each type of vitamin D:

Natural Forms	Synthetic Forms
d-alpha-tocopherol	dl-alpha-tocopherol
d-alpha-tocopheryl acetate	dl-alpha-tocopheryl acetate
d-alpha-tocopheryl succinate	dl-alpha-tocopheryl succinate

There are actually several natural tocopherols that demonstrate vitamin E activity. The most active tocopherol in terms of antioxidant activity is d-alpha-tocopherol, but d-beta-, d-gamma-, d-delta-tocopherol, and a group of related compounds known as tocotrienols also exert antioxidant activity. Natural sources of vitamin E, like soy, typically are composed of only about 10 percent alpha-tocopherol; the remainder of their vitamin E content is mainly because of other "less active" tocopherols. However, the benefits of these other tocopherols are only now being discovered. For example, while the vitamin E activity of alpha-tocotrienol is rated at 30 percent compared to alpha-tocopherol's 100 percent, alpha-tocotrienol actually demonstrated greater antitumor activity.[4] In a study of men with coronary artery disease, d-gamma-tocopherol was low, not d-alpha-tocopherol, suggesting that d-gamma may be just as important as d-alpha-tocopherol in preventing heart disease.[5]

Natural vitamin E supplements containing mixed tocopherols, including the tocotrienols, appear to offer the greatest benefit. The best forms of natural vitamin E in these products may be those where the d-alpha-tocopherol is bound to either acetate or succinate—two natural weak acids used in cellular metabolism. Binding results in the formation of d-alpha-tocopheryl acetate and d-alpha-tocopheryl succinate, respectively. These forms of vitamin E may be more advantageous because they are more stable than free d-alpha tocopherol. Once the body ingests these forms, it splits the acetate or succinate off the molecule to reform alpha-tocopherol.[3]

Fat-soluble versus Water-soluble Vitamin E

Another commercial form of vitamin E is a water-soluble form known under various tradenames (e.g., Trolox and Aquasol E). This form of vitamin E is much more expen-

TABLE 5.1   Vitamin E Activities of Various Tocopherols

Compound	Activity (International Units of Compound per Milligram)
d–Alpha-tocopherol	1.49
d–Alpha-tocopheryl acetatel	1.36
dl–Alpha-tocopherol	1.1
dl–Alpha-tocopheryl acetate	1.0
d–Beta-tocopherol	0.60
d–Gamma-tocopherol	0.15–0.45
d–Alpha-tocotrienol	0.3
d–Delta-tocopherol	0.015

sive than the fat-soluble form (10 times), but is it worth it? Clinical research in patients with cystic fibrosis indicates that it is not.[6] Patients suffering from cystic fibrosis, a genetic disorder characterized by severe pancreatic insufficiency and fat malabsorption, often suffer from deficiencies of fat-soluble vitamins, particularly vitamin E. Children and adults with cystic fibrosis need to supplement with vitamin E. Although many physicians recommend the expensive water-soluble form, the reality is that the fat-soluble form (regular vitamin E supplements) can provide results that are just as good at considerably less cost. A double-blind study comparing fat-soluble vitamin E produced results just as good as the water-soluble form. Since both forms are equally effective, the choice should be based on economics. At current prices, the use of the fat-soluble form would lead to a savings of about $500 per year. Since individuals with cystic fibrosis require long-term, indefinite vitamin E supplementation, over a 20-year period this would result in a $10,000 savings.

Principal Uses

The principal use of vitamin E is as an antioxidant in the protection against heart disease, cancer, and strokes—the three leading killers of Americans. In addition to this application, vitamin E supplementation is useful in a long list of other health conditions, particularly in cardiovascular diseases, diabetes, fibrocystic breast disease, menopausal symptoms, and tardive dyskinesia. I discuss several other applications for vitamin E in depth elsewhere, such as the treatment of Parkinson's disease, the prevention of premature rupture of membranes during pregnancy, and the treatment of arthritis; the following, however, is an extensive list of conditions where vitamin E supplementation is commonly used.

- Acne
- AIDS
- Alcohol-induced liver disease

- Allergy
- Anemia
- Angina
- Arrhythmias
- Atherosclerosis
- Autoimmune disorders
- Cancer
- Capillary fragility
- Cardiomyopathy
- Cataract
- Cervical dysplasia
- Diabetes
- Dysmenorrhea
- Eczema
- Epilepsy
- Gallstones
- Hepatitis
- *Herpes simplex*
- *Herpes zoster*
- Immunodepression
- Infections
- Inflammation
- Intermittent claudication
- Lupus
- Macular degeneration
- Menopause
- Multiple sclerosis
- Myopathy
- Neuralgia
- Neuromuscular degeneration
- Osteoarthritis
- Parkinson's disease
- Peptic ulcers
- Periodontal disease
- Peripheral vascular disease
- Pregnancy

- Premenstrual syndrome
- Raynaud's disease
- Rheumatoid arthritis
- Scleroderma
- Seborrheic dermatitis
- Skin ulcers
- Ulcerative colitis
- Wound healing

Antioxidant Protection against Heart Disease and Strokes

Vitamin E provides significant benefit in protecting against heart disease and strokes. Confirmed antiantherosclerotic effects of vitamin E include an ability to reduce LDL cholesterol peroxidation with an improvement in plasma LDL breakdown; inhibition of excessive platelet aggregation; increase in HDL cholesterol levels; and increase fibrinolytic activity. Diabetics who are not insulin-dependent have experienced improvements in insulin sensitivity and plasma lipids (see Diabetes in this chapter).

Several large populations have demonstrated that vitamin E levels may be more predictive of developing a heart attack or stroke than total cholesterol levels.[7-9] One study indicated that low vitamin E levels are far more predictive of heart disease than the factors most people associate with heart disease.[7] High blood cholesterol was predictive 29 percent of the time and high blood pressure 25 percent of the time, but low levels of vitamin E in the blood were predictive of a heart attack almost 70 percent of the time. While many suggest that the consumption of red wine is the reason behind the "French Paradox"—i.e., why the French have a lower rate of heart disease and strokes than Americans despite a higher cholesterol and fat intake—higher vitamin E levels provide an explanation.[7,10]

Vitamin E prevents the oxidation of cholesterol and its carrier proteins and prevents the initial damage to the artery, which can ultimately lead to the process of atherosclerosis. Fats and cholesterol are particularly susceptible to free-radical damage. When damaged, fats and cholesterol form toxic derivatives known as lipid peroxides and oxidized cholesterol, respectively. Vitamin E and other antioxidants block the formation of these damaging compounds. Of all the antioxidants, vitamin E may offer the greatest protection against the oxidation of LDL cholesterol because of its ability to be easily incorporated into the LDL molecule. Furthermore, there is a clear-cut dosage effect; i.e., the higher the dosage of vitamin E the greater the degree of protection against oxidative damage to LDL cholesterol (see Table 5.2). Although dosages as low as 25 milligrams are effective in offering some protection, doses greater than 400 I.U. are required to produce clinically significant effects.[11] Dosages as high as 200 I.U. simply do not provide the same degree of protection as 400 to 800 I.U., especially in smokers and people exposed to greater oxidative stress.[11-13]

Some studies have shown that relatively low dosages of vitamin E supplements can significantly reduce the risk of dying from a heart attack or a stroke. One study

TABLE 5.2   Effect of Increasing Doses of Vitamin E on Oxidation Parameters

Dose (mg/day)	Lag Time[a]	Propagation Rate[a]
0	94	7.8
25	99	8.0
50	100	7.9
100	106	7.7
200	111	7.5
400	116	6.8
800	120	6.5

[a]Lag time is the time before oxidation occurs after the addition of an oxidizing agent. The higher the number, the greater the beneficial effect.

[b]Propagation rate is the rate at which lipid peroxidation progresses. The lower the number, the greater the beneficial effect.

looked at 87,245 nurses. It concluded that nurses who took 100 I.U. of vitamin E daily for more than two years had a 41 percent lower risk of heart disease compared to nonusers of vitamin E supplements.[14] Another study involved 39,910 male healthcare professionals. The results were similar—a 37 percent lower risk of heart disease with the intake of more than 30 I.U. of supplemental vitamin E daily.[15]

A recent study demonstrates more clearly the benefits of "low dosage" vitamin E supplementation in preventing heart disease.[16] The study utilized the extensive dietary and nutritional supplement database collected in the Cholesterol Lowering Atherosclerosis Study. Researchers studied a total of 156 men aged 40 to 59 years with previous coronary artery bypass graft surgery. The study measured by antiography the change in the percentage of vessel diameter obstruction because of hardening of the arteries after 2 years of randomized therapy of either (a) a cholesterol-lowering diet or (b) a cholesterol-lowering drug (colestipol-niacin combination) or placebo in association with supplemental antioxidant vitamins.

Overall, the results of the study indicated that subjects in the group taking 100 I.U. or greater of vitamin E demonstrated significantly less coronary artery lesion progression than did subjects taking less than 100 I.U. The placebo group demonstrated no benefit from vitamin E supplementation. These results indicate that vitamin E supplementation, even at a relatively low dosage (100 I.U.), can reduce the progression of coronary artery disease when used in conjunction with cholesterol-lowering therapy (preferably natural).

These recent studies on vitamin E only confirm what people in the health-food industry and nutritionally minded physicians have known for more than 50 years. Vitamin E is good for the cardiovascular system. However, based on studies on the protective effects of different dosages of vitamin E, dosages of at least 400 I.U. would have produced even more spectacular results.

In addition to offering protection against cardiovascular disease, vitamin E supplementation also plays a major role in the treatment of heart disease, recovery from stroke, and peripheral vascular diseases like intermittent claudication. The "Mecca" for vitamin E research in cardiovascular disease is Shute Institute and Medical Clinic in London, Ontario, Canada. The Shute Institute has been active in the use of vitamin E therapy since the 1940s. The Shute brothers, Drs. Evan and Wilfred Shute, brought to light many of the now-substantiated cardiovascular benefits of vitamin E. It was the Shute brothers' contention that vitamin E is vital to cardiovascular health. They felt it is important to supplement the diet with high doses of vitamin E in many health conditions, especially those involving the cardiovascular system. Once scorned in mainstream medical circles, now the Shute brothers have been vindicated. For over a half century the Shute Institute has successfully treated over 60,000 patients with vitamin E and other natural therapies. Vitamin E holds center stage in their treatment programs.

Antioxidant Protection against Cancer

Like other antioxidants, such as vitamin A and beta-carotene, vitamin E offers significant protection against cancer when taken in high doses. Over a dozen studies have shown that low vitamin E levels (especially if combined with low selenium levels) increase the risk of certain types of cancer (particularly cancers of the gastrointestinal tract and lungs).[17,18] In one of these studies, researchers found that individuals with a low level of vitamin E in the blood had a 50 percent greater risk of developing cancer than those with a high level. Although not all studies show that vitamin E protects against all cancers, supplementation appears very much worthwhile given its excellent safety profile and possible benefits.

Diabetes

Diabetics appear to have an increased requirement for vitamin E for a number of reasons, probably because oxidative stress is a major factor in diabetes. Vitamin E improves insulin action and exerts a number of beneficial effects that may aid in preventing the long-term complications of diabetes, especially cardiovascular disease.

Several studies show E supplementation is beneficial. For example, in one study examining vitamin E's role on glucose metabolism and insulin action, 10 control (healthy) subjects and 15 non–insulin-dependent diabetics underwent an oral glucose-tolerance test before and after taking 1,350 I.U. of vitamin E per day for 4 months. In the healthy subjects, vitamin E supplementation improved glucose tolerance and insulin sensitivity. In the diabetics given vitamin E, improvements in glucose metabolism and insulin action were even more obvious. The authors of the study concluded "Our study demonstrates that in diabetic patients daily oral vitamin E supplements may reduce oxidative stress, thus improving membrane physical characteristics and related activities in glucose transport."[19]

In another double-blind study conducted at the University of Naples, moderately obese elderly persons (average age 74 years) with stable-effort angina and insulin insensitivity were given vitamin E supplementation (1,350 I.U. per day of d-alpha-tocopheryl acetate). Vitamin E supplementation lowered fasting and 2-hour plasma insulin concentrations from 88 to 68 pmol/L (picomole per liter) and 348 to 263 pmol/L, respectively; plasma triglycerides from 1.34 to 1.07 mmol/L (millimole per liter); and the ratio of plasma LDL to HDL cholesterol from 7.64 to 5.52 mmol/L. These results should provide additional evidence to the mainstream medical community of the benefits of high-dose vitamin E supplementation in patients with cardiovascular disease.[20] Given the possible benefit and lack of risk of toxicity at the proper dosage, vitamin E supplementation is a particularly wise choice in diabetics.

Fibrocystic Breast Disease

Fibrocystic breast disease (FBD) is a mildly uncomfortable to severely painful benign cystic swelling of the breasts. Typically cyclic, it usually precedes a woman's menses. It is the most frequent disease of the breast (affecting 20 to 40 percent of premenopausal women), usually a component of the premenstrual syndrome (PMS), and considered a risk factor for breast cancer.

Several double-blind clinical studies show vitamin E (alpha-tocopherol) relieves many PMS components, particularly fibrocystic breast disease.[21,22] Researchers have not yet discovered the vitamin's precise biochemical role in doing so, but studies indicate vitamin E (600 I.U. per day) normalizes hormone levels in PMS and FBD patients.

Menopausal Symptoms

In the late 1940s, controlled clinical studies demonstrated that vitamin E is effective in relieving hot flashes and menopausal vaginal complaints.[23-25] Unfortunately, there have been no further clinical investigations. However, many nutritionists recommend that menopausal patients take 800 I.U. of vitamin E daily. After the hot flashes subside, they can reduce the dosage to 400 I.U.

Tardive Dyskinesia

Tardive dyskinesia is a syndrome characterized by involuntary movements of the face and mouth, most often caused by a reaction to drugs used in the treatment of schizophrenia. These drugs may lead to free-radical damage to nerve cells involved in the control of the facial muscles. Vitamin E protects cells from free-radical damage, and several studies show it is very effective in the treatment of tardive dyskinesia.[26-28]

In the most recent double-blind study, vitamin E at a dose of 1,600 I.U. per day significantly improved the symptoms of tardive dyskinesia.[28] As with most other studies involving schizophrenia, vitamin E was most effective when administered to patients who had been taking the antipsychotic drugs for less than 5 years. When patients have been using the drugs for more than 5 years, their level of improvement is about half that in patients taking the drugs for less time.

Dosage Ranges

The typical dosage for vitamin E for general and therapeutic purposes is 400 to 800 I.U. per day. However, I doubt if dosages greater than 400 I.U. are really necessary in most people taking a high-potency multiple and extra vitamin C. Vitamin C regenerates oxidized vitamin E in the body and potentiates its antioxidant benefits.

Safety Issues

Although vitamin E is a fat-soluble vitamin, it has an excellent safety record. Recent clinical trials of vitamin E supplementation at doses as high as 3,200 I.U. daily in a wide variety of subjects for periods of up to 2 years have not shown any unfavorable side effects. Several studies have carried out detailed safety assessments. For example, one double-blind trial of 32 elderly (more than 60 years old) people assessed the effect of daily supplementation of 800 I.U. of d,l-alpha-tocopheryl acetate for 30 days by measuring general health, nutrient status, liver and kidney function, metabolism, blood cell status, blood nutrient and antioxidant status, thyroid hormones, and urinary function.[29] The only significant effect was a significant increase in serum vitamin E levels. Vitamin E at this dose was extremely well tolerated, and no one reported side effects The results of this study are not surprising and are consistent with a large body of knowledge demonstrating that vitamin E supplementation is extremely safe.

Interactions

Vitamin E interacts extensively with other antioxidant nutrients, especially vitamin C and selenium. Vitamin E also improves the use of vitamin A, may be necessary in the conversion of vitamin B_{12} to its most active form, and protects essential fatty acids from becoming damaged.

Vitamin E may potentiate the effects of anticoagulant drugs like Coumadin and Warfarin and augment the coagulative functions of vitamin K. Vitamin E may also increase the inhibition of platelet aggregation caused by aspirin.

6

Vitamin K

Vitamin K is an often-neglected vitamin because deficiency is quite rare. Vitamin K's most famous role is in the manufacture of clotting factors. However, recent studies show that vitamin K is also necessary for building healthy bones and may play a role in treating and preventing osteoporosis.

There are three major forms of vitamin K—vitamin K_1 (phylloquinone), the natural vitamin K from plants; vitamin K_2 (menaquinone), derived from bacteria in the gut; and vitamin K_3 (menadione), a synthetic derivative.

Food Sources

Dark green leafy vegetables, broccoli, lettuce, cabbage, spinach, and green tea are rich sources of vitamin K. Good sources are asparagus, oats, whole wheat, and fresh green peas (see Table 6.1). The RDA for vitamin K is 1 microgram per 2.2 pounds body weight. You can study Table 6.1 to see the specific vitamin K content of these foods.

Deficiency Signs and Symptoms

Signs and symptoms of vitamin K deficiency are rare because gut bacteria can produce vitamin K_2. When vitamin K deficiency does present itself (easy bruising, appearance of ruptured capillaries, etcetera), it is usually a result of taking anticoagulant

TABLE 6.1   Vitamin K Content of Selected Foods, in Micrograms per 3 $^1/_2$-oz. (100-g.) Serving

Kale	729	Lettuce	129	Green peas	19
Green tea	712	Cabbage	125	Whole wheat	17
Turnip greens	650	Watercress	57	Green beans	14
Spinach	415	Asparagus	57		
Broccoli	200	Oats	20		

drugs like Coumadin and Warfarin or long-term antibiotics. Since newborns do not yet have gut bacteria, they are particularly susceptible to vitamin K deficiency; therefore, vitamin K is often administered intramuscularly to newborns to prevent hemorrhagic disease. An alternate therapy is vitamin K_1 for the mother during the pregnancy and orally for the child after birth.

Recommended Dietary Allowance

Recommended Dietary Allowance of Vitamin K

Group	Micrograms
INFANTS	
Under 6 months	5
6–12 months	10
CHILDREN	
1–3 years	15
4–6 years	20
7–10 years	30
YOUNG ADULTS AND ADULTS	
Males 11–14 years	45
Males 15–18 years	65
Males 19–24 years	70
Males 25+ years	80
Females 11-14 years	45
Females 15–18 years	55
Females 19–24 years	60
Females 25+ years	65
Pregnant females	65
Lactating females	65

Beneficial Effects

Vitamin K's primary role is in the manufacture of clotting factors like prothrombin and clotting factors VII, IX, and X. The three vitamin Ks function similarly in helping with blood clotting, but in other important functions vitamin K_1 appears to be substantially superior. For example, vitamin K_1 plays an important role in bone health because it is responsible for converting a bone protein from its inactive form to its active form. Osteocalcin is the major noncollagen protein found in our bones. As Figure 6.1 illustrates, vitamin K is necessary for allowing the osteocalcin molecule to join with the calcium and holding the calcium into place within the bone.[1]

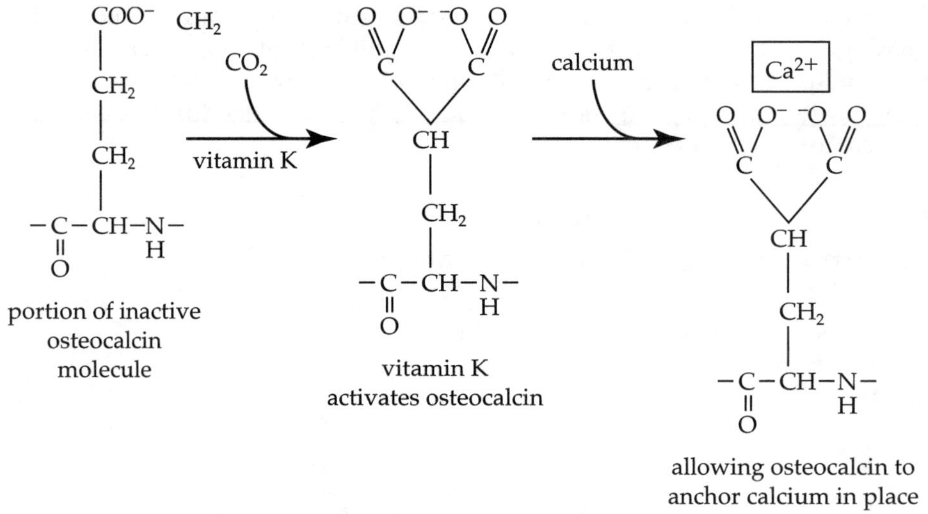

FIGURE 6.1   Activation of osteocalcin.

Available Forms

There are three major forms of vitamin K—vitamin K_1 (phylloquinone), the natural vitamin K from plants; vitamin K_2 (menaquinone), derived from bacteria in the gut; and vitamin K_3 (menadione), a synthetic derivative. Vitamin K_1 is the preferred form.

One of the best sources of vitamin K_1 is fat-soluble chlorophyll. Chlorophyll is the green pigment of plants found in the chloroplast compartment of plant cells. The conversion of electromagnetic energy (light) into chemical energy takes place in the chloroplast via photosynthesis. The chlorophyll molecule is essential for this reaction to occur.

The natural chlorophyll found in green plants is fat soluble. Most of the chlorophyll products found in health stores, however, contain water-soluble chlorophyll. Because water-soluble chlorophyll is not absorbed from the gastrointestinal tract, its use is limited to ulcerative conditions of the skin.[2,3] Its astringent qualities, coupled with an ability to stimulate wound healing, make it an excellent healer. These healing effects are also found with the topical administration of water-soluble chlorophyll in the treatment of skin wounds. Water-soluble chlorophyll is also used medically to help control body, fecal, and urinary odor.[4,5]

In order to produce a water-soluble chlorophyll, the natural chlorophyll molecule must be altered chemically. The fat-soluble form, the natural form of chlorophyll as found in fresh juice, offers several advantages over water-soluble chlorophyll. This is particularly true regarding chlorophyll's ability to stimulate hemoglobin and red blood cell production and to relieve excessive menstrual blood flow.[6,7] In fact, the chlorophyll molecule is very similar to the heme portion of the hemoglobin molecule of our red blood cells.

The rest of the body absorbs fat-soluble chlorophyll quite well. In addition, fat-soluble chlorophyll contains other components of the chloroplast complex (including beta-carotene and vitamin K_1), which possess significant health benefits. Like the other plant pigments, chlorophyll also possesses significant antioxidant and anti-cancer effects.[8] Water-soluble chlorophyll products do not provide all these additional benefits.

Principal Uses

Vitamin K_1 and fat-soluble chlorophyll supplements are used in the prevention and treatment of osteoporosis, excessive menstrual bleeding, and hemorrhagic disease of newborns.

Osteoporosis

A deficiency of vitamin K_1 leads to impaired mineralization of the bone because of inadequate osteocalcin levels. Patients with fractures because of osteoporosis exhibit very low blood levels of vitamin K_1.[9] The severity of the fracture strongly correlates with the level of circulating vitamin K. The lower the level of vitamin K, the greater the severity of the fracture. Vitamin K_1's presence in green leafy vegetables may be one of the protective factors of a vegetarian diet against osteoporosis.[10]

Excessive Menstrual Bleeding

Excessive menstrual bleeding (menorrhagia) is a common female complaint. Even when clotting time is typically normal (ruling out a vitamin K deficiency), some scientists recommend the use of vitamin K (historically in the form of crude preparations of chlorophyll).[11]

Hemorrhagic Disease of the Newborn

Since 1961 the Committee on Nutrition of the American Academy of Pediatrics has recommended that physicians inject newborns with vitamin K_1 to prevent hemorrhagic disease, a condition that occurs because of a lack of vitamin K. A baby is born with a sterile intestinal tract . Because a major source of vitamin K (in the form of K_2) is synthesized from gut bacteria and most women do not have high concentrations of vitamin K_1 in their breast milk, the baby must rely on the amount of vitamin K delivered through the placenta until his or her own body establishes gut microflora

The practice of injecting vitamin K_1 (1 milligram intramuscularly at birth) into newborns significantly prevents hemorrhagic disease. Vitamin K_1 is used because administration of vitamin K_2 to infants is associated with the breaking of red blood cells (hemolysis), leading to anemia and liver toxicity. While injection of vitamin K_1 is extremely effective, physicians can achieve similar results using orally administered vitamin K_1 for those who want to avoid the injection. In these cases, the German

Pediatric Society recommends giving oral vitamin K_1 at a dosage of 5 milligrams twice weekly for the first 3 months of life.[12]

Dosage Ranges

In general, the best plan includes increasing green leafy vegetable intake and supplementing with a 150 to 500 microgram dosage of vitamin K_1

Safety Issues

There are no known side effects or toxicity with the administration of vitamin K_1.

Interactions

Vitamin K administration may counteract the anticoagulant actions of drugs like Warfarin and Coumadin, which work to prevent clot formation by blocking vitamin K's activation of prothrombin. Aspirin, certain antibiotics, Dilantin, and possibly high dosages of vitamin E (e.g., greater than 600 I.U.) also antagonize vitamin K action.

7

Vitamin C

Although vitamin C (ascorbic acid) is the most popular vitamin supplement in the United States, in many respects it is the most controversial. Over the years many respected scientists have shared polarized views on the importance of vitamin C supplementation to human health. While researchers and experts may argue just how much vitamin C we need to consume, one thing about vitamin C is not controversial—its essential role in human nutrition.

Food Sources

While most people think of citrus fruits as the best source of vitamin C, vegetables also contain high levels, especially broccoli, peppers, potatoes, and brussels sprouts (see Table 7.1). Exposure to air destroys Vitamin C, so it is important to eat fresh foods as quickly as possible. Although a salad from a salad bar is a healthier lunch choice than a hamburger, the vitamin C content of the fruits and vegetables from a salad bar is only a fraction of what it would be in a fresh salad. For example, freshly sliced cucumbers, if left standing, lose 41 percent and 49 percent of their vitamin C content within the first 3 hours. A sliced cantaloupe left uncovered in the refrigerator loses 35 percent of its vitamin C content in less than 24 hours.

Deficiency Signs and Symptoms

While most other animals can manufacture their own vitamin C, the human body does not have this luxury. Throughout history humans have suffered from the vitamin C–deficiency disease known as scurvy. The classic symptoms of scurvy are bleeding gums, poor wound healing, and extensive bruising. In addition to these symptoms, susceptibility to infection, hysteria, and depression are also hallmark features.

Scurvy affected many people in ancient Egypt, Greece, and Rome. Scurvy undoubtedly molded world history because rations supplied during military campaigns and long ocean voyages seldom contained adequate amounts of vitamin C.

TABLE 7.1   Vitamin C Content of Selected Foods, in Milligrams per 3¹/₂-oz. (100-g.) Serving

Acerola	1300	Strawberries	59	Okra	31
Peppers, red chili	369	Papayas	56	Tangerines	31
Guavas	242	Spinach	51	New Zealand spinach	30
Peppers, red sweet	190	Oranges & juice	50	Oysters	30
Kale leaves	186	Cabbage	47	Lima beans, young	28
Parsley	172	Lemon juice	46	Black-eyed peas	29
Collard leaves	152	Grapefruit & juice	38	Soybeans	29
Turnip greens	139	Elderberries	36	Green peas	27
Peppers, green sweet	128	Liver, calf	36	Radishes	26
Broccoli	113	Turnips	36	Raspberries	25
Brussels sprouts	102	Mangoes	35	Chinese cabbage	25
Mustard greens	97	Asparagus	33	Yellow summer squash	25
Watercress	79	Cantaloupe	33	Loganberries	24
Cauliflower	78	Swiss chard	32	Honeydew melons	23
Persimmons	66	Green onions	32	Tomatoes	23
Cabbage, red	61	Liver, beef	31	Liver, pork	23

SOURCE: U.S.D.A., Nutritive Value of American Foods in Common Units, Agriculture Handbook No. 456.

During some parts of history, scurvy hit a population just like the plague. Between 1556 and 1857, for example, 114 epidemics of scurvy were reported during the winter months, when fresh fruits and vegetables are not available. Even more severe was the devastating scurvy associated with long sea voyages.

Some explorers, like Jacques Cartier in 1856, learned that eating certain foods helped cure scurvy. Cartier's crew ate spruce tree needles; other crews ate oranges, lemons, limes, and berries. In 1742, British physician James Lind wrote the first real scientific discussion about the possibility that scurvy was a dietary deficiency. In his classic experiment, Lind demonstrated that patients given lemon juice recovered from scurvy. Although some explorers adopted Lind's finding by rationing citrus fruits on long voyages—Captain James Cook's crew avoided scurvy altogether in his three long voyages between 1768 and 1779—the British Navy did not adopt the use of lime juice rations for its crews until 1804, some 62 years after Lind's discovery. Today's mainstream medical community appears to have adopted the same timeline for integrating scientific information about the importance of nutrition.

Vitamin C was identified as the "antiscorbutic principle" and was first isolated by Albert Szent-Gyorgyi in 1928. Nearly 70 years later, researchers are still discovering health-promoting benefits for ascorbic acid. Although scurvy is now rare in our society, subclinical or marginal vitamin C deficiency is common, especially in the elderly. The following table illustrates the percentages of population groups with unequivocally low vitamin C levels as determined by measuring the vitamin C content of the *buffy coat* layer of blood. The buffy coat consists of all the cellular components of blood, but primarily white blood cells.[1]

Group	Percent with Scurvy	Percent with Low Vitamin C Reserves
Young, healthy	0	3
Elderly, healthy	3	20
Elderly, outpatients	20	68
Young, institutionalized	30	100
Patients with cancer	46	76
Elderly, institutionalized	50	95

Recommended Dietary Allowance

Recommended Dietary Allowance of Vitamin C

Group	Milligrams
INFANTS	
Under 6 months	30
6–12 months	35
CHILDREN	
1–3 years	40
4–10 years	45
11–14 years	50
ADOLESCENTS AND ADULTS	
15+ years	60
Pregnant females	70
Lactating females	95

Beneficial Effects

The primary function of vitamin C is the manufacture of collagen, the main protein substance of the human body. Specifically, vitamin C aids the joining of a portion of a molecule of the amino acid proline to form hydroxyproline. The result is a very stable collagen structure. Since collagen is such an important protein for the structures that hold our bodies together (connective tissue, cartilage, tendons, etcetera), vitamin C is vital for wound repair, healthy gums, and the prevention of easy bruising.[2]

In addition to its role in collagen metabolism, vitamin C is also critical to immune function, the manufacture of certain nerve transmitting substances and hormones, carnitine synthesis, and the absorption and utilization of other nutritional factors. Vitamin C is also a very important nutritional antioxidant.

Immune Function

Many people have made claims about the role of vitamin C in enhancing the immune system, particularly with regard to the prevention and treatment of the common cold. However, despite numerous positive clinical and experimental studies, for some reason this effect is still hotly debated. From a biochemical viewpoint, there is considerable evidence that vitamin C plays a vital role in many immune mechanisms. Infection rapidly depletes the normal high concentration of vitamin C in white blood cells, particularly lymphocytes, and a relative vitamin C deficiency may ensue if vitamin C is not regularly replenished.[3]

Vitamin C affects various immune functions by enhancing white blood cell function and activity and increasing interferon levels, antibody responses, antibody levels, secretion of thymic hormones, and integrity of ground substance. Vitamin C also possesses many biochemical effects similar to interferon, the body's natural antiviral and anticancer compound.[3]

During times of chemical, emotional, psychological, or physiological stress, the urinary system excretes vitamin C at a significantly increased rate, thereby elevating the body's need for vitamin C during these times.[4] Examples of chemical stressors include cigarette smoke, pollutants, and allergens. Extra vitamin C in the form of supplementation or increased intake of vitamin C–rich foods is often recommended to keep the immune system working properly during times of stress. In certain instances, vitamin C supplementation is the only way to meet the concentrations needed for many health conditions.[4] For example, cancer patients should supplement their diet with additional vitamin C and consume foods containing high levels of vitamin C, particularly vegetable juices because they are also a rich source of carotenes. Later in this chapter, the Principal Uses section lists other conditions where extra vitamin C is recommended.

As an Antioxidant

Vitamin C works as an antioxidant in aqueous (water) environments in the body—both outside and inside human cells. It is the first line of antioxidant protection in the body. In other words, it is the body's most important antioxidant. Its primary antioxidant partners are vitamin E and carotenes because these antioxidants are fat-soluble. Vitamin C also works along with antioxidant enzymes such as glutathione peroxidase, catalase, and superoxide dismutase. It is responsible for regenerating oxidized vitamin E in the body, thus potentiating the antioxidant benefits of vitamin E.[5]

Health food stores and health magazines bombard consumers with the word *antioxidant*. They often point them in the direction of some rather high-priced "super antioxidants"; but when we really compare these super antioxidants to vitamin C in terms of cost to benefit, vitamin C comes out far superior.

For example, let's compare the cost-to-benefit ratio of vitamin C versus N-acetyl-cysteine and glutathione in the ability to raise tissue glutathione levels. Along with vitamins C and E, glutathione assumes a critical role in defense against free-radical damage. Individuals with a hereditary deficiency of glutathione because of a defect in synthesis have markedly increased cell damage. The red blood cells, white blood cells, and nerve tissue are affected most. As a result, red blood cells often burst, white blood cells do not function properly, and nerve tissue degenerates.

In an effort to increase antioxidant status in individuals with impaired glutathione synthesis, a variety of antioxidants have been used including: glutathione, 2-mercaptopropionyl-glycine, vitamin E, vitamin C, and N-acetylcysteine (NAC). Of these agents, only vitamin C and NAC have offered some possible benefit. To determine the relative effectiveness of vitamin C versus NAC, researchers recently studied a 45-month-old girl with an inherited deficiency of glutathione synthesis before and during treatment with vitamin C or NAC. She took high doses of vitamin C (500 milligrams or 3 grams per day) or NAC (800 milligrams per day) for one to two weeks. Measurements of glutathione (GSH) levels indicated that 3 grams per day of vitamin C increased white blood cell GSH fourfold and plasma GSH levels eightfold . NAC also increased white blood cell numbers by 350 percent and plasma by 200 to 500 percent. Based on these results, the researchers decided that they would administer vitamin C for 1 year at the 3-grams-per-day dosage. At the end of a year glutathione levels remained elevated, the hematocrit increased from a baseline 25.4 percent to 32.6 percent, and the number of immature red blood cells (reticulocyte count) decreased from 11 percent to 4 percent. These results indicate that vitamin C can decrease cellular damage in patients with hereditary glutathione deficiency and is more effective and less expensive than NAC.[6]

The significance of these results to the general population is that vitamin C may offer the benefits attributed to NAC at only a slightly reduced cost. To put this in perspective, a daily dosage of 3 grams of vitamin C costs about $10 per month, while a dosage of 1 gram of NAC costs about $20 per month.

There is more to this story. Over the past 5 to 10 years, the use of NAC and glutathione products as antioxidants has become increasingly popular among nutritionally oriented physicians and the public, but is this use valid?

There is a biochemical rationale for this practice. Some biochemists believe that NAC acts as a precursor for glutathione and that taking extra glutathione should raise tissue glutathione levels. While supplementing the diet with high doses of NAC may be beneficial in cases of extreme oxidative stress (e.g., AIDS), it may be an unwise practice in healthy individuals. The reason? One study indicated that when NAC was given orally to 6 health volunteers at a dosage of 1.2 grams per day for 4 weeks, followed by 2.4 grams per day for an additional 2 weeks, it actually increased oxidative damage by acting as a pro-oxidant.[7]

In controlled studies, the concentration of glutathione in NAC-treated subjects was reduced by 48 percent, and the concentration of oxidized (inactive) glutathione was 80 percent higher. Oxidative stress actually increased by 83 percent in those receiving NAC—and there was no sign of antioxidant effects. From the results of this study, we can conclude that at high doses NAC may act as a pro-oxidant in healthy subjects. Unfortunately, 1.2 grams per day is not an unreasonable dosage to attain from commercially available sources of NAC.

Now let's examine the role of supplemental glutathione. First of all, a deficiency of intracellular glutathione has been identified in a number of clinical conditions including cancer, alcohol-induced liver disease, and AIDS. Intravenous glutathione shows some promise in increasing intracellular glutathione concentrations; however, the question of oral absorption remains in doubt.

To assess the feasibility of supplementing oral glutathione, seven healthy subjects ingested a single dose of up to 3,000 milligrams of glutathione. Blood values indicated that the concentration of glutathione, cysteine, and glutamate in plasma did not increase significantly, suggesting the systemic availability of a single dose of up to 3,000 milligrams of glutathione is negligible.[8]

The authors of the study concluded "Dietary glutathione is not a major determinant of circulating glutathione, and it is not feasible to increase circulating glutathione to a clinically beneficial extent by the oral administrating of a single dose of 3 grams of glutathione."[8] In contrast, in healthy individuals, a daily dosage of 500 milligrams of vitamin C may be sufficient to elevate and maintain good tissue glutathione levels. In one double-blind study, the average red blood cell glutathione concentration rose nearly 50 percent with 500 milligrams per day of vitamin C.[9] Increasing the dosage to 2,000 milligrams only raised red blood cell glutathione levels by another 5 percent. In light of these findings, consumers and physicians desiring to increase tissue levels of glutathione may want to use vitamin C instead of higher priced "super antioxidants" and save money in the process because both NAC and glutathione supplements are expensive.

Finally, many nutritionists recommend drinking red wine to improve antioxidant status. This recommendation is based on several studies showing that frequent red wine ingestion offers protection against heart disease and stroke. Because the French consume more saturated fat per capita than people in the United States or United Kingdom, yet have a lower incidence of heart disease, many suggest that red wine consumption is the reason behind the "French Paradox." Presumably this protection is the result of flavonoids in red wine protecting against oxidative damage to LDL cholesterol.

To better determine the antioxidant capacity of red wine, researchers conducted a study comparing the effects of red wine, white wine, and vitamin C on serum antioxidant capacity. They determined serum antioxidant capacity (SAOC) in 9 subjects who had consumed 300 milliliters of red wine and compared to 9 subjects consuming 300 milliliters of white wine and 4 subjects consuming 1,000 milligrams of vitamin C.[10] Here are the results:

Percent Increase in Serum Antioxidant Capacity

Item Ingested	At 1 Hour	At 2 Hours
Red wine	18	11
White wine	4	7
Vitamin C	22	29

These results appear to indicate that consuming 1,000 milligrams of vitamin C rather than 300 milliliters of red wine offers significantly better protection. What all of these studies indicate is that vitamin C supplementation offers exception antioxidant benefits at an affordable price.

Available Forms

You can find Vitamin C in a number of different forms—crystals, powders, capsules, tablets, timed-released tablets, etcetera. The actual vitamin C in these different forms varies. Ascorbic acid is the most widely used and least expensive form. Buffered vitamin C refers to the use of sodium, magnesium, calcium, or potassium ascorbate. Buffered vitamin C is used primarily because sometimes the acid content of nonbuffered ascorbic acid bothers some people's stomachs. The only real concern with buffered vitamin C products is that sodium ascorbate may be a problem for people who are sodium sensitive. The same is true for "corn-free" vitamin C. Most commercially available vitamin C is derived from corn. In people who are sensitive to corn, vitamin C derived from another commercially available source, the sago palm, is recommended.

Recently a "new form" of vitamin C called Ester-C has entered the marketplace. Its manufacturers claim that this form is composed of esters (a chain of repeating units) of vitamin C and is absorbed and utilized by the body. However, absorption studies do not indicate that the body absorbs it better. Furthermore, to justify the fact that Ester-C is three times more expensive than regular forms of C, Ester-C should be three times better. The research simply does not support this to be the case. In one study at the Foods and Nutrition Laboratory at Arizona State University, the absorption of Ester-C and regular ascorbic acid did not differ significantly (although blood levels were higher with regular vitamin C).[11]

Taking vitamin C with bioflavonoids may offer benefits in absorption, but only if the product contains bioflavonoids at a meaningful level. When the amount of citrus bioflavonoids is just window dressing, there is no real increase in absorption. However, if the level of bioflavonoids is equal to or greater than the level of vitamin C, then absorption is enhanced.[11,12] In general, the best form of vitamin C for most people is simple ascorbic acid. It is by far the most economical form, and there is substantial data on its effectiveness.

Principal Uses

Numerous experimental, clinical, and population studies show that vitamin C intake benefits the body in numerous ways, including: reducing cancer rates, boosting immunity, protecting against pollution and cigarette smoke, enhancing wound repair, increasing life expectancy, and reducing the risk for cataracts. Research indicates Vitamin C is useful in many health conditions as a result of its antioxidant and immune-enhancing properties. Because of space constraints, I am focusing my discussion on only a few health conditions because supplemental vitamin C, in my opinion, is an important part of any nutritional supplement program.

Some of the major conditions where vitamin C is of value:

- Asthma
- Atherosclerosis
- Auto-immune disorders
- Cancer
- Candidiasis
- Capillary fragility
- Cataract
- Cervical dysplasia
- Crohn's disease
- Common cold
- Coronary artery disease
- Diabetes
- Eczema
- Fatigue
- Gallbladder disease
- Gingivitis
- Glaucoma
- Hepatitis
- *Herpes simplex*
- *Herpes zoster*
- High blood pressure
- Hives
- Infections
- Infertility
- Macular degeneration
- Menopause
- Mitral valve prolapse
- Multiple sclerosis
- Osteoarthritis
- Parkinson's disease
- Periodontal disease
- Peptic ulcers
- Peripheral vascular disease
- Preeclampsia

- Rheumatoid arthritis
- Skin ulcers
- Sports injuries
- Wound healing

Asthma and Other Allergies

The number of asthma sufferers is rapidly rising in the United States, especially in children. From 1980 to 1987, the rate of physician-diagnosed asthma in people younger than 20 years of age increased 43 percent from 35 to 50 cases per 1,000. Reasons scientists often give to explain the rise in asthma include: increased stress on the immune system (because of factors such as greater chemical pollution in the air, water, and food), earlier weaning and earlier introduction of solid foods to infants, use of food additives, and genetic manipulation of plants resulting in food components with greater allergenic tendencies.

A recent study sought the answer to a very important question—could deficiencies in dietary antioxidants contribute to asthma?[13] There is substantial evidence to suggest such a correlation. Vitamin C intake in the general population appears to correlate with asthma, indicating low vitamin C (in the diet and the blood) is an independent risk factor for asthma. Children of smokers have a higher rate of asthma (cigarette smoke depletes respiratory vitamin C and E levels) than do children of nonsmokers, and symptoms of ongoing asthma in adults appear to be increased by exposure to environmental pro-oxidants and decreased by vitamin C supplementation.

For further evidence, you only need to look at the physiological roles of vitamin C in the lungs. Vitamin C is the major antioxidant substance in the airway surface area of the lungs, where it plays an important role in protecting against both endogenous- and exogenous-induced oxidative damage. Nitrogen oxides are oxidants that can arise from both endogenous and exogenous sources. Vitamin C offers significant protection against nitrogen oxide damage in the lungs in animal models.

From a clinical perspective, asthmatics have a higher need for vitamin C than do members of the general population. Since 1973 there have been 11 clinical studies of vitamin C supplementation in asthma.[14] Seven of these studies showed significant improvements in respiratory measures and asthma symptoms as a result of supplementing the diet with 1 to 2 grams of vitamin C daily. This dosage recommendation appears extremely wise based on the increasing exposure to inhaled oxidants along with the growing appreciation on the antioxidant function of vitamin C in the respiratory system.

High-dose vitamin C therapy may also help asthmatics by lowering histamine levels.[15] Of course, this effect has value in other allergic conditions as well. Vitamin C's importance as a natural antihistamine has emerged for several reasons, including concern over the safety of antihistamine medications and recently recognized immune-suppressing effects of histamine. In the initial stages of an immune response, histamine amplifies the immune response by increasing capillary permeability and smooth muscle contraction, thus enhancing the flow of immune factors to the site of infection. Subsequently, histamine exerts a suppressive effect on the accumulated white blood cells in an attempt to contain the inflammatory response.

Vitamin C exerts a number of effects against histamine. Specifically it prevents the secretion of histamine by white blood cells and increases the detoxification of histamine. A recent study examined the antihistamine effect of acute and chronic vitamin C administration and its effect on white blood cell (neutrophil) function in healthy men and women. In the chronic study, 10 subjects ingested a placebo during weeks 1,2,5, and 6, and 2 grams per day of vitamin C during weeks 3 and 4. Fasting blood samples were collected after the initial 2-week period (baseline) and at the end of weeks 4 and 6. Blood vitamin C levels rose significantly following vitamin C administration, while blood histamine levels fell by 38 percent during the weeks vitamin C was given. The ability of white blood cells to move in response to an infection (chemotaxis) increased by 19 percent during vitamin C administration and fell 30 percent after vitamin C withdrawal. However, these changes were linked to histamine concentrations. Chemotaxis was greatest when histamine levels were the lowest. In the part of the study looking at the acute effects of vitamin C, blood histamine concentrations and chemotaxis did not change 4 hours following a single dose of vitamin C. This result suggests that vitamin C lowers blood histamine only if taken over a period of time. Individuals prone to allergy or inflammation should increase their consumption of vitamin C through supplementation.[15]

Atherosclerosis, Elevated Cholesterol Levels, and High Blood Pressure

A high dietary vitamin C intake significantly reduces the risk of death from heart attacks and strokes (and other causes, including cancer) in numerous population studies.[16-18]

One of the most detailed studies analyzed the vitamin C intake of 11,348 adults over 5 years. Researchers divided them into three groups: (1) less than 50 milligrams daily dietary Vitamin C intake; (2) greater than 50 milligrams daily dietary intake with no vitamin C supplementation; and (3) greater than 50 milligrams daily dietary intake plus vitamin C supplementation (estimated at milligrams or more).[18] Analysis of standardized mortality ratio (SMR), a comparison to the average death rate, was up to 48 percent lower in the high vitamin C intake group versus the low intake group for cardiovascular disease and overall mortality. In practical terms, these differences correspond to an increase in longevity of 5 to 7 years for men and 1 to 3 years for women.

How does vitamin C lower the risk for cardiovascular disease? Apparently it does so by acting as an antioxidant, by strengthening the collagen structures of the arteries, lowering total cholesterol and blood pressure, raising HDL cholesterol levels, and inhibiting platelet aggregation.[17]

Oxidative damage to LDL cholesterol plays a major role in the initiation of atherosclerosis. Vitamin C is extremely effective in preventing LDL cholesterol from being oxidized, even in smokers.[19] In addition, because vitamin C regenerates oxidized vitamin E in the body, it potentiates the antioxidant benefits of vitamin E.

Cholesterol

Dozens of observational and clinical studies show that vitamin C levels correspond to total cholesterol and HDL cholesterol levels.[17,20–22] One of the best-designed studies indicated that the higher the vitamin C content of the blood, the lower the total cholesterol and triglycerides and the higher the HDL cholesterol.[22] The benefits on HDL were particularly impressive. For each 0.5 milligrams per deciliter increase in vitamin C content of the blood, HDL cholesterol increased 14.9 milligrams per deciliter in women and 2.1 milligrams per deciliter in men. For every 1 percent increase in HDL cholesterol, the risk for heart disease drops 4 percent. This study and others demonstrate that the association between vitamin C and HDL levels persists even when well-nourished individuals with normal levels of vitamin C in their blood supplement their diets with additional vitamin C. However, evidence suggests that there may be a threshold for the beneficial effects of vitamin C supplementation on total cholesterol and HDL cholesterol in healthy subjects. This threshold may be as low as 215 milligrams per day for women and 345 milligrams per day in men.

Results in double-blind clinical studies examining the benefit of high dosage vitamin C supplementation (usually 1,000 milligrams) on lowering total cholesterol while raising HDL cholesterol levels are inconsistent. More recent studies show that only in subjects with low or marginal vitamin C status does high dosage supplementation produce an effect.[17,20,23]

Blood Pressure

Population and clinical studies also show vitamin C levels inversely correlate with blood pressure; i.e., the higher the intake of vitamin C the lower the blood pressure. Several preliminary studies show a modest blood-pressure–lowering effect (e.g., a drop of 5 millimeters of mercury) of vitamin C supplementation in people with mild elevations of blood pressure.[17]

One of the ways in which vitamin C may help keep blood pressure in the normal range is by promoting the excretion of lead. Chronic exposure to lead from environmental sources, including drinking water, is associated with high blood pressure and increased cardiovascular mortality.[24] Areas with a soft water supply have an increased lead concentration in drinking water because of the acidity of the water, and people living in these areas may be predisposed to high blood pressure. Soft water is also, of course, low in calcium and magnesium, two minerals that protect against high blood pressure.

Coronary Bypass

Hospitals rarely employ vitamin C supplementation, despite the possible significant advantages of doing so and despite the frequently low–vitamin C status of hospitalized patients. To illustrate the apparent need for vitamin C supplementation in the hospital, let's look at a study analyzing the vitamin C status of patients undergoing coronary artery bypass. In this study, the plasma concentration of vitamin C plummeted by 70 percent 24 hours after coronary artery bypass surgery and persisted in most patients up to 2 weeks after surgery.[25] In contrast, vitamin E and carotenoid levels did not change to any significant degree, presumably because they are fat-soluble and therefore the body retains them for longer periods of time. Given the importance of vitamin C—the serious depletion of vitamin C may deteriorate defense mechanisms against free radicals, infection, and wound repair in these patients—supplementation appears to be essential in patients recovering from heart surgery, or any surgery for that matter.

Cancer Prevention

Vitamin C performs many functions that may offer protection against cancer, including acting as an antioxidant and protecting cellular structures (including DNA) from damage. Vitamin C also helps the body deal with environmental pollution and toxic chemicals, enhance immune function, and inhibit the formation of cancer-causing compounds in the body.[26,27]

The epidemiological evidence of a protective effect of vitamin C against cancer is undeniable. A high vitamin C intake reduces the risk for virtually all forms of cancer, including cancers of the lung, colon, breast, cervix, esophagus, oral cavity, and pancreas.[26,27] The bottom line from all of the research is once again that Americans need to increase the consumption of foods high in vitamin C and possibly supplement with vitamin C for added protection. While most of this evidence is based upon a high vitamin C intake from foods also rich in carotenes and other protective nutrients against cancer, a few of the studies also looked at supplementation. Let's examine the evidence in some of these cancers in closer detail.

Lung Cancer

Of the 11 investigations into the role of vitamin C against lung cancer, 9 found reduced risk with high intake of Vitamin C. In five of these studies, the results were quite significant and in four of these five studies the protection offered by vitamin C was greater than that provided by beta-carotene in several of the studies. Gladys Block, one of America's foremost authorities on the role of antioxidant intake and cancer risk, has stated that "Whereas a large body of evidence suggests an important effect for carotenoids in lung cancer prevention, the recent data suggests that there may be an independent protective effect of vitamin C intake."[26]

Stomach, Esophageal, and Oral Cancers

Seven of eight oral cancer studies found low vitamin C intake to be a major risk factor. Persons with the lowest vitamin C intake had a twofold increase in oral cancer compared to persons with the highest vitamin C intake. Similar results were seen in esophageal cancer. In stomach cancer, all 16 investigations in stomach cancer showed a substantial reduction in risk with high vitamin C intake. Stomach cancer is linked to excessive formation of cancer-causing compounds known as nitrosamines within the stomach. Nitrosamines are formed most of the time by ingesting nitrates and nitrites used in the production of cured meats (e.g., bacon). Vitamin C significantly inhibits the formation of nitrosamines.[26,27]

Breast Cancer

A meta-analysis of the role of dietary factors in breast cancer concluded "Vitamin C intake had the most consistent and statistically significant inverse association with breast cancer risk."[28] The level of vitamin C was more important than the intake of saturated fat, beta-carotene, and vitamin E.

Cervical Cancer

Cervical cancer risk is increased dramatically with low vitamin C intake. Women with intakes less than 88 milligrams have a fourfold increase compared with women with higher intakes. Women with cervical dysplasia (a precancerous condition) and carcinoma *in situ* show a significant decrease in vitamin C intake and blood levels compared with women with normal cervixes. Inadequate vitamin C intake is an independent risk factor for the development of cervical dysplasia and carcinoma *in situ*.[29,30]

Pancreatic Cancer

High vitamin C intake reduces the risk for pancreatic cancer in six out of seven studies. The risk for pancreatic cancer in someone consuming less than 70 milligrams of vitamin C per day is 2.6 times greater than for someone consuming 159 milligrams per day.[26,27]

Colon Cancer

Six out of eight studies show a high intake of vitamin C reduces the risk for colon cancer. Low vitamin C intake carries with it almost a twofold increase in risk for colon cancer.[26,27] In a study conducted by the National Cancer Institute, vitamin C reduced the formation of cancer-causing chemicals by bacteria in the colon.[31]

Cancer Treatment

Perhaps the most controversial use of vitamin C supplementation is the treatment of cancer. Mainstream medicine has difficulty accepting the possibility that vitamin C, as well as other nutrients, may offer therapeutic benefits to cancer patients. The first rule of scientific thinking is to have an open mind, yet most mainstream medical people react "unscientifically" when asked about nutritional supplements.

In 1976, Dr. Linus Pauling, one of the greatest scientists of the twentieth century and a two-time Nobel Prize winner, brought vitamin C into the limelight by reporting the results of a study he conducted along with Dr. Ewan Cameron. Pauling and Cameron gave terminally ill cancer patients 10 grams of vitamin C per day.[32] Of these 100 terminally ill patients, 16 survived more than one year. Now, this survival percentage may not seem that significant until you look at the survival rate in the control group of 1,000 subjects. Only three patients in the control group survived for more than 1 year.

Cameron followed up the original study with another and reported similarly impressive results. The study included 1,826 "incurable" patients. Of these patients,

294 received high dosage vitamin C supplementation (10 grams per day). The remaining 1,532 patients served as controls. In analyzing the data, the researchers found that "the ascorbate-supplemented patients had an overall survival time (343 days) almost double that of the controls (180 days.)[33]

As promising as these results are, critics quickly pointed out that the studies were not double-blind, indicating a placebo effect could have been responsible for the benefit noted. Double-blind studies designed to examine (some say disprove) Pauling's contentions have not shown vitamin C to produce any greater benefit than a placebo.[34] At this time it appears that vitamin C is most effective at preventing rather than curing cancer. Nonetheless, in my opinion, vitamin C supplementation is indicated in cancer patients because of the increased frequency of low or marginal vitamin C status in cancer patients and because of possible enhancement of immune function.

Cataracts

Individuals with higher dietary intakes of vitamins C and E, selenium, and carotenes have a much lower risk for developing cataracts and macular degeneration than do individuals with lower intakes.[35] In addition to preventing cataracts, these antioxidant nutrients may offer some therapeutic effects as well. Several clinical studies demonstrate that vitamin C supplementation halts cataract progression and, in some cases, significantly improves vision. For example, in one study, 450 patients with cataracts were placed on a nutritional program that included 1 gram of vitamin C per day, resulting in a significant reduction in cataract development.[36] Though similar patients had previously required surgery within 4 years, in the vitamin C treated patients only a small handful of patients required surgery—and in most patients there was no evidence that the cataract progressed over the 11-year period of the study.

The dosage of vitamin C necessary to increase the vitamin C content of the lens is 1,000 milligrams.[37] The lens of the eye and active tissues of the body require higher concentrations of vitamin C. The level of vitamin C in the blood is about 0.5 milligrams per deciliter, whereas in the adrenal and pituitary glands, the level is 100 times this concentration. In the liver, spleen, and lens of the eye it is concentrated by at least a factor of 20. In order to maintain these concentrations in these tissues, the body has to generate enormous amounts of energy to pull vitamin C out of blood against this tremendous gradient. By keeping blood vitamin C levels elevated, you help your body concentrate the vitamin C into active tissue by reducing the gradient. That is probably why dosages of at least 1,000 milligrams are required to increase the vitamin C content of the lens.

Common Cold

Many claims have been made about the role of vitamin C (ascorbic acid) in enhancing the immune system, especially with regard to the prevention and treatment of the common cold. Twenty years have passed since Linus Pauling wrote *Vitamin C and the Common Cold*.[38] Pauling based his opinion on several studies that showed vitamin C was very effective in reducing both the severity of symptoms and the duration of the common cold. Since 1970, 20 double-blind studies have tested Pauling's assertion.[39] However, despite the fact that every study demonstrated that the group receiving the vitamin C had either a decrease in duration or symptom severity, for some reason the medical community still debates the clinical effect. A recent article that appeared in the *Journal of the American College of Nutrition* sheds some light on the controversy.[40]

In 1975 Thomas Chalmers analyzed the possible effect of vitamin C on the common cold by calculating the average difference in the duration of cold episodes in vitamin C and control groups in seven placebo-controlled studies. He found that episodes were 0.11 days shorter in the vitamin C groups and concluded that there was no valid evidence to indicate that vitamin C is beneficial in the treatment of the common cold. Scientific articles and monographs extensively cite Chalmers' review. However, other reviewers have concluded that vitamin C significantly alleviates the symptoms of the common cold. A careful analysis of Chalmers' review reveals serious shortcomings. For example, Chalmers did not consider the amount of vitamin C used in the studies and included in his meta-analysis a study in which only 25 to 50 milligrams per day of vitamin C was administered to the test subjects. For some studies Chalmers used values that are inconsistent with the original published results. Using data from the same studies, the authors of the new study calculated that vitamin C at a dosage of 1 to 6 grams per day decreased the duration of the cold episodes by 0.93 days; the relative decrease in the episode duration was 21 percent. The argument in the medical literature that vitamin C has no effect on the common cold is based in large part on a faulty review written two decades ago.

The best recommendation is to supplement with vitamin C in any sort of infection, particularly in elderly patients. A recent double-blind study of 57 elderly patients admitted to St. Luke's Hospital in Huddersfield, England, for severe acute bronchitis and pneumonia demonstrates the value of this recommendation.[41] The patients were given either 200 milligrams of vitamin C per day or a placebo. Patients were assessed by clinical and laboratory methods (vitamin C levels in the plasma, white blood cells, and platelets; sedimentation rates; and white blood cell counts and differential). Patients receiving the modest dosage of vitamin C demonstrated increased vitamin C levels substantially in all tissues, even in the presence of an acute respiratory infection.

Using a clinical scoring system based on major symptoms of respiratory infections, results indicated the patients receiving the vitamin C fared significantly better than those on placebo. The benefit of vitamin C was most obvious in patients with the most severe illness, many of whom had low plasma and white blood cell vitamin C levels on admission.

These results indicate that even relatively small doses of vitamin C in a hospital setting can produce significant clinical improvement. Vitamin C supplementation is warranted in all elderly patients with acute respiratory infection, especially those who are severely ill. Pneumonia is still a major killer of the elderly.

In acute infections, intravenous administration may be appropriate. This recommendation is especially true for viral hepatitis, whether acute or chronic. According to Robert Cathcart, M.D., hepatitis is one of the easiest diseases for ascorbic acid to cure.[42,43] He recommends intravenous doses of vitamin C of 40 to 100 grams for hepatitis and AIDS. Dr. Cathcart demonstrated that vitamin C in these high doses can greatly improve acute viral hepatitis in 2 to 4 days. He showed clearing of jaundice within 6 days.[43] Other studies demonstrated similar benefits.[44–46] If you cannot find a physician to administer the vitamin C intravenously, call the American College of Advancement in Medicine (1-800-532-3688) or take enough vitamin C to bowel tolerance (see below under Dosage Ranges).

Diabetes

Because insulin facilitates the transport of vitamin C into cells, most diabetics suffer from deficient intracellular vitamin C.[47] Therefore, without high dosage vitamin C supplementation, a relative vitamin C deficiency exists in many diabetics despite an "adequate" dietary amount of vitamin C. The diabetic simply needs more vitamin C. High dosage vitamin C supplementation is absolutely essential in the treatment of diabetes.

Failure to correct a chronic, latent intracellular vitamin C deficiency leads to a number of problems for the diabetic, including an increased capillary permeability, poor wound healing, elevations in cholesterol levels, and a depressed immune system. Furthermore, diabetes is also associated with increased free-radical damage. Vitamin C is the principal modulator of free-radical activity in diabetes, improves blood sugar control, reduces the accumulation of sorbitol within cells, and inhibits the glycosylation of proteins. Sorbitol accumulation and glycosylation of proteins (both described below) are linked to many complications of diabetes, especially eye and nerve diseases.[48–50]

Vitamin C offers a significant cost-to-benefit ratio in the treatment of diabetes. Based on current available information, it appears that an effective dosage of vitamin C in diabetics is approximately 1,000 to 3,000 milligrams daily in divided dosages.

Sorbitol and Diabetic Complications

Sorbitol is a byproduct of glucose metabolism formed within the cell with the help of an enzyme—aldose reductase. In nondiabetic individuals, once sorbitol is formed it can be metabolized with the help of another enzyme (polyol-dehydrogenase) to fructose. This conversion to fructose allows the sorbitol to be excreted from the cell if concentrations increase. Unfortunately, in the diabetic with routine hyperglycemia (elevated blood sugar levels), sorbitol accumulates and plays a major role in the development of chronic complications of diabetes.

We can best understand the mechanism by which sorbitol is involved in the development of diabetic complications by considering its involvement in cataract formation. Although the lens does not have any blood vessels, it is an actively metabolizing tissue that continuously grows throughout life. Hyperglycemia results in shunting of glucose to the sorbitol pathway. Since the lens membranes are virtually impermeable to sorbitol and lack the enzyme polyol-dehydrogenase, sorbitol accumulates to high concentrations. These high concentrations persist even if glucose levels return to normal. This accumulation creates an osmotic gradient that results in water being drawn into the cells to maintain osmotic balance. As the water is pulled in, the cell must release small molecules like amino acids, inositol, glutathione, niacin, vitamin C, magnesium, and potassium to maintain osmotic balance. Since these latter compounds function to protect the lens from damage, their loss results in an increased susceptibility to damage. As a result, the delicate protein fibers within the lens become opaque, and a cataract forms.

Drugs designed to inhibit sorbitol accumulation are extremely toxic. In contrast, vitamin C supplementation has an excellent safety profile and significantly lowers sorbitol levels. Vitamin C supplementation at a dosage as low as 100 milligrams daily, but usually 1,000 milligrams, normalizes red blood cell sorbitol in type I diabetics within 30 days in well designed, double-blind controlled trials.[51,52]

Glycosylation Inhibition

The binding of glucose to proteins, a process referred to as glycosylation, leads to changes in the structure and function of many body proteins. In diabetes, excessive glycosylation also occurs with albumin (a blood protein) and the proteins of the red blood cell, lens, and myelin sheath. This glycosylation causes abnormal structures and functions of involved cells and tissues and contributes greatly to the complications of diabetes. For example, glycosylated LDL molecules (found in high levels in diabetics) do not bind to LDL receptors or shut off cholesterol synthesis in the liver. As a result, diabetics typically have elevated cholesterol levels and a significantly increased risk for atherosclerosis.

Fortunately, high dosage vitamin C supplementation (1,000 to 3,000 milligrams daily) significantly reduces glycosylated proteins, e.g., a reduction of 33 percent for glycosylated albumin.[53,54]

Low Sperm Counts

Vitamin C (ascorbic acid) plays an especially important role in protecting the sperm's genetic material (DNA) from damage. Ascorbic acid levels are much higher in seminal fluid compared to other body fluids, including the blood. When dietary vitamin C was reduced from 250 milligrams to 5 milligrams per day in healthy human subjects, the seminal fluid ascorbic acid decreased by 50 percent, and the number of sperm that had damage to their DNA increased by 91 percent.[55] These results indicated that dietary vitamin C plays a critical role in protecting against sperm damage and that low dietary vitamin C levels likely lead to infertility.

We know cigarette smoking greatly reduces vitamin C levels throughout the body. Even the Food and Nutrition Board, the organization that calculates RDAs, acknowledges that smokers require at least twice as much vitamin C as nonsmokers.[56] One of the reasons a smoker may have a reduced sperm count is vitamin C depletion. In one study, men who smoked one pack of cigarettes a day received either 0, 200, or 1,000 milligrams of vitamin C. After one month, sperm quality improved proportional to the level of vitamin C supplementation; that is to say, as the level of vitamin C increased, so did sperm quality.[57]

Nonsmokers appear to benefit as much from vitamin C as smokers. In one study, 30 infertile but otherwise healthy men received either 200 milligrams or 1,000 milligrams of vitamin C or placebo daily.[58] There were weekly measurements of sperm count, viability, motility, agglutination, abnormalities, and immaturity. After one week the 1,000-milligram group demonstrated a 140 percent increase in sperm count, the 200-milligram group 112 percent, and the placebo group no change. After three weeks both vitamin C groups continued to improve, with the 200-milligram group catching up to the improvement of the 1,000-milligram group. One of the key improvements was the number of agglutinated sperm. Sperm become agglutinated when antibodies produced by the immune system bind to the sperm. Antibodies bound to sperm are often associated with chronic genitourinary tract or prostatic infection. When more than 25 percent of the sperm are agglutinated, fertility is very unlikely. At the beginning of the study, all three groups had over 25 percent agglutinated sperm; after three weeks, only 11 percent of the sperm in the vitamin C groups were agglutinated. Although this result is impressive, the most impressive result of the study was that at the end of 60 days, all of the vitamin C group had impregnated their wives, compared to none for the placebo group. We can conclude from these results that vitamin C supplementation is very effective in treating male infertility, especially if the infertility is because of antibodies bound to sperm.

Parkinson's Disease

We don't know the cause of Parkinson's disease, but many scientists think that a neurotoxin causes oxidative damage to the basal ganglia in the brain. The basal ganglia controls muscle tension and movement. In the oxidative damage model, oxidation reactions lead to the generation of free radicals—highly reactive molecules—that are capable of destroying the cell membranes and nerve cells.

Antioxidant nutrients like vitamin C and E are quite effective in slowing down the progression of Parkinson's disease in those patients not yet on medications. These results have led to a pilot trial of high-dose vitamins C and E in early Parkinson's disease and a large study of high-dose vitamin E and the drug Deprenyl. Patients require high dosages because it is more difficult to increase antioxidant levels in brain tissue than in other body compartments.

In the vitamin C and E pilot study beginning in 1979, 21 patients with early Parkinson's disease were given 3,000 milligrams of vitamin C and 3,200 I.U. of vitamin E each day.[59] The patients were followed closely for 7 years. Although all patients eventually required drug treatment (Sinemet or Deprenyl), the progression of the disease as determined by need for medication was considerably delayed in those receiving the nutritional antioxidants. After dividing the patients in both groups into younger-onset and older-onset patients, researchers found that those patients not receiving antioxidants required medication 40 and 24 months, respectively, after the onset of the disease. In contrast, the two age groups in the pilot study were able to delay the need for drug therapy for 65.3 and 59.2 months, respectively. Thus, the patients receiving the vitamins were effectively able to delay the need for medication for up to 2 to 3 years longer. These results are quite promising and offer some hope in slowing down the progression of this dreaded disease.

Skin Ulcers and Wound Healing

Up to 10 percent of all hospital patients and 30 percent of all elderly patients suffer from pressure sores. Elderly patients with hip fractures are particularly at risk. As many as 60 percent of these patients develop sores, most of which occur within the first 5 days of hospitalization.

Analysis of vitamin C levels in 21 patients admitted to a hospital for hip fracture indicated that the patients who developed bed sores had vitamin C levels that were 50 percent lower than the patients who did not develop bed sores. Interestingly, low levels of zinc, vitamin A, and vitamin E were not associated with an increased risk of developing pressure sores.[60]

The significance of this study is tremendous. Pressure sores are extremely painful and are often difficult to heal. If pressure sores could be prevented by maintaining optimal vitamin C levels, it would be a major medical accomplishment. Of course, over 20 years ago studies showed vitamin C was extremely effective in healing existing pressure sores in a double-blind study.[61] How easy and cost effective would it be to add additional vitamin C to I.V. bags versus trying to deal with an extensive pressure sore?

Pregnancy-Related Conditions

Vitamin C supplementation appears indicated to prevent at least two complications of pregnancy—preeclampsia and premature rupture of membranes.

Preeclampsia

Preeclampsia is a serious condition of pregnancy associated with elevations in blood pressure, fluid retention, and loss of protein in the urine. Preeclampsia affects approximately 7 percent of all pregnancies. It is associated with increased infant mortality and morbidity related to intrauterine growth retardation, premature delivery, and perinatal asphyxia. In addition, the mother is at risk for abruptio placentae, intracerebral hemorrhage, and liver and kidney failure.

A number of nutritional factors play a role in preeclampsia. Most notable are low magnesium and calcium levels. Recently another nutritional cause has been suggested—low levels of antioxidants.[62] Free-radical damage to the lining of blood vessels (vascular endothelium) plays a key role in the development of preeclampsia. Antioxidants are critically involved in the protection of the vascular endothelium. Low antioxidant levels may be a predisposing factor in preeclampsia.

In a study of 30 women with preeclampsia and 44 women with uncomplicated pregnancy, the women with mild to severe preeclampsia had significantly lower levels of vitamin C. Levels of alpha-tocopherol and beta-carotene were significantly lower only in severe preeclampsia. These results indicate that increasing antioxidant intake during pregnancy may be an additional preventive measure against preeclampsia.[62]

Prevention of Premature Rupture of Fetal Membranes

Premature rupture of the fetal membranes (PROM) is one of the major contributors of perinatal morbidity and mortality. The etiology of PROM is unclear but may be because of nutritional status. In particular, low levels of vitamin C can be a risk factor. The increased rate of PROM in smokers may be due in part to the known depleting effects of smoking of vitamin C stores.

Low levels of vitamin C may lead to impaired integrity of the amniotic sac because of reduced collagen content or leave the amniotic tissue extremely susceptible to the damaging effects of free radicals.

A recent study sought to determine more fully the role of vitamin C, vitamin E, beta-carotene, and retinol in PROM.[63] Eighty pregnant women with or without PROM were analyzed for these antioxidant nutrients. There were no differences in the serum levels of retinol, vitamin E, or vitamin C among the groups. However, PROM subjects had significantly lower amniotic fluid levels of vitamin C and lower ratios of amniotic to serum ascorbic acid levels than did controls. Serum beta-carotene levels were also lower in subjects with PROM compared to controls.

These results appear to substantiate the possible role of low amniotic fluid vitamin C levels and PROM. Beta-carotene and vitamin C may work synergistically to maintain the health of the amniotic membranes. Pregnant women, especially those at high risk for PROM, may benefit from supplementation of vitamin C and beta-carotene.

Dosage Ranges

The debate over how much vitamin C humans require still goes on. At one end of the spectrum, two-time Nobel Prize winner Linus Pauling and his followers recommend an intake somewhere between 2 to 9 grams a day during periods of health and even higher doses during times of stress or illness. During these latter times, they recommend taking as high a dosage as possible without producing diarrhea, a practice commonly referred to as vitamin C dosing to "bowel tolerance."[43] At the other end of the spectrum, the RDA is 60 milligrams for adults.

My own belief is that in healthy individuals and pregnant women, a daily dosage of 500 milligrams is probably sufficient to provide exceptional antioxidant protection and health benefits. However, there are numerous instances where high-dose vitamin C therapy is indicated or required—most notably diabetes; cataracts; glaucoma; and infectious conditions including the common cold, cancer, Parkinson's disease, and many others. In these health conditions a dosage of 1,000 milligrams at the low end to bowel tolerance at the high end should be viewed as a proper dosage range.

I want to stress that you should not rely on supplements to meet all your vitamin C requirements. Vitamin C–rich foods are rich in compounds like flavonoids and carotenes, which work to enhance the effects of vitamin C as well as exert favorable effects of their own.

Safety Issues

Vitamin C is extremely safe in most people. Diarrhea and intestinal distension or gas are the most common complaints. The primary concern with high dosages often cited in the medical literature is the development of calcium oxalate kidney stones. However, numerous studies demonstrate that in persons not on hemodialysis or suffering from recurrent kidney stones, severe kidney disease, or gout, high-dosage vitamin C therapy does not cause kidney stones. Vitamin C administration of up to 10 grams per day has not shown any effect on urinary oxalate levels.[64,65]

Some researchers report that abrupt cessation of high-dosage vitamin C intake leads to "rebound scurvy" or in pregnant women the presence of rebound scurvy after birth of their babies. However, other studies do not support the existence of rebound scurvy with sudden cessation or after pregnancy. While the existence of rebound scurvy is controversial (some experts question its existence), it is better to favor the side of caution. So, if you have been taking high dosages of vitamin C (e.g., greater than 500 milligrams per day), reduce your dosage gradually. At this time a safe recommendation to pregnant women would be a daily dosage of 500 milligrams daily.

Interactions

Vitamin C is intricately involved with other nutritional antioxidants, especially vitamin E, selenium, and beta-carotene. Combination of antioxidants may provide greater benefit than any single nutrient (e.g., vitamin C). For example, in one study a mixture of beta-carotene, vitamin E, glutathione, and vitamin C was more effective than any of these antioxidants given individually in preventing the growth of experimental oral cancer in hamsters.[66] The anticancer effects noted were not merely additive; a true synergism was noted.

Vitamin C increases the absorption of iron, decreases the absorption of copper, and interferes with the blood test for vitamin B_{12}. There are no known adverse interactions with vitamin C and any drug.

8

Thiamin (Vitamin B₁)

Thiamin was the first B vitamin discovered; hence its designation as vitamin B$_1$. Severe thiamin deficiency causes a syndrome known as "beriberi." Symptoms include mental confusion, muscle wasting (dry beriberi), fluid retention (wet beriberi), high blood pressure, difficulty walking, and heart disturbances.

Beriberi was relatively common in Asia, among sailors, and in prisons. Prior to the late 1890s, no one knew what caused beriberi. Then in 1873 a Dutch naval doctor observed that European crews member had significantly fewer cases of beriberi than sailors recruited from the East Indies. By decreasing the amount of white rice the sailors ate, the rate of beriberi was decreased, but the doctor believes that the beriberi was caused by some toxin or infectious agent in the white rice. Takaki, a Japanese naval doctor, was the first to report that beriberi seemed to be a nutritional deficiency. He based his opinion on that fact that by giving Japanese sailors additional meat, dry milk, and vegetables, the incidence of beriberi dropped. However, it was a Dutch physician, Christian Eijkman, who began what are now classic experiments in the 1890s that began to clarify the role of diet in beriberi.

Eijkman noticed that feeding fowl polished white rice produced symptoms similar to beriberi. By adding rice polishings (the material removed from whole rice to produce white rice) to the feed, Eijkman was able to cure the fowl of beriberi. His associate later demonstrated that the addition of green peas, green beans, and meat prevented beriberi in fowl and deduced correctly that there was something in natural foodstuffs that prevented beriberi. In 1911, Casimir Funk, working at the Lister Institute of London, isolated from rice polishings what he considered the substance that would cure and/or prevent beriberi. Funk termed his discovery a "vitamine." What Funk actually isolated, however, turned out to be the antipellagra vitamin, or niacin (vitamin B$_3$). In Java in 1926, two Dutch scientists, Jansen and Donath, isolated pure thiamin, the true antiberiberi vitamin. Today, white rice is often enriched with thiamin and other nutrients lost during milling. However, beriberi is still prevalent in many parts of Asia where white rice supplies up to 80 percent of the total calories consumed by the people. Beriberi and many other nutrient deficiencies in Third

World countries could be prevented if the people simply ate whole grains. In regard to rice, I discuss this more fully below.

The story of beriberi and the discovery of thiamin highlights the value of whole grains over polished grains. In addition to many known nutrients, whole grains provide substantially more accessory food compounds and possibly many unknown compounds with health-promoting properties as well. Instead of removing natural nutrients from the grains and then adding back a small portion of synthetic counterparts, wouldn't it make more sense to eat whole grains?

Whole grains are a major source of complex carbohydrates, dietary fiber, minerals, and B vitamins. The protein content and quality of whole grains is greater than that of refined grains. Diets rich in whole grains are protective against the development of chronic degenerative diseases, especially cancer, heart disease, diabetes, varicose veins, and diseases of the colon including colon cancer, inflammatory bowel disease, hemorrhoids, and diverticulitis.

Food Sources

Rich plant sources of thiamin are soybeans, brown rice, sunflower seeds, and peanuts. Good sources are whole wheat and nuts (see Table 8.1). Thiamin is extremely sensitive to alcohol, tannins in coffee and in black tea, and sulfites. Any of these compounds destroy thiamin or render it useless. Thiamin is also sensitive to a factor in uncooked freshwater fish and shellfish.

TABLE 8.1   Thiamin Content of Selected Foods, in Milligrams per 3^1/$_2$-oz. (100-g.) Serving

Yeast, brewer's	15.61	Lima beans, dry	.48
Yeast, torula	14.01	Hazelnuts	.46
Wheat germ	2.01	Wild rice	.45
Sunflower seeds	1.96	Cashews	.43
Rice polishings	1.84	Rye, whole-grain	.43
Pine nuts	1.28	Mung beans	.38
Peanuts, with skins	1.14	Cornmeal, whole-ground	.38
Soybeans, dry	1.10	Lentils	.37
Peanuts, without skins	.98	Green peas	.35
Brazil nuts	.96	Macadamia nuts	.34
Pecans	.86	Brown rice	.34
Soybean flour	.85	Walnuts	.33
Beans, pinto & red	.84	Garbanzos	.31
Split peas	.74	Garlic, cloves	.25
Millet	.73	Almonds	.24
Wheat bran	.72	Lima beans, fresh	.24
Pistachio nuts	.67	Pumpkin & squash seeds	.24
Navy beans	.65	Chestnuts, fresh	.23
Buckwheat	.60	Soybean sprouts	.23
Oatmeal	.60	Peppers, red chili	.22
Whole-wheat flour	.55	Sesame seeds, hulled	.18
Whole-wheat grain	.55		

Deficiency Signs and Symptoms

Severe thiamin deficiency results in beriberi. Although severe thiamin deficiency is relatively uncommon (except in alcoholics), many Americans do not consume the RDA of 1.5 milligrams, especially elderly patients in hospitals or nursing homes. Milder deficiency usually results in fatigue, depression, pins-and-needles sensations or numbness of the legs, and constipation. In alcoholics, the combination of thiamin deficiency and alcohol can produce the Wernicke-Korsakoff syndrome, a serious brain disorder.[1]

Recommended Dietary Allowance

Recommended Dietary Allowance of Thiamin

Group	Milligrams
INFANTS	
Under 6 months	0.3
6–12 months	0.4
CHILDREN	
1–3 years	0.7
4–6 years	0.9
7–10 years	1.0
YOUNG ADULTS AND ADULTS	
Males 11–14 years	1.3
Males 15–50 years	1.5
Males 51+ years	1.2
Females 11–50 years	1.1
Females 51+ years	1.0
Pregnant females	1.5
Lactating females	1.6

Beneficial Effects

Thiamin functions as part of an enzyme (thiamin pyrophosphate, or TPP) essential for energy production, carbohydrate metabolism, and nerve cell function.

Available Forms

Thiamin is available in most nutritional supplements as thiamin hydrochloride.

Principal Uses

The principal use of thiamin is to prevent thiamin deficiency (especially in diabetes, Crohn's disease, multiple sclerosis, and other neurological diseases) and to prevent and treat impaired mental function in the elderly, in Alzheimer's patients, and in epileptics being treated with Dilantin (phenytoin).

Thiamin is essential for proper energy production in the brain. Thiamin deficiency is characterized by impaired mental function and, in severe deficiency, psychosis. Up to 30 percent of all subject who enter psychiatric wards are deficient in thiamin.[2]

In addition to its role as a nutrient, thiamin also demonstrates some pharmacological effects on the brain. Specifically, it mimics the important neurotransmitter involved in memory, acetylcholine. Patients with Alzheimer's disease exhibit a severe loss of acetylcholine action within certain key areas of the brain. Thiamin, however, potentiates and mimics the effects of acetylcholine in the brain.[3] This effect explains the positive clinical results of thiamin intake (3 to 8 grams per day) in improving mental function in Alzheimer's disease and age-related impaired mental function (senility).[4,5]

Thiamin supplementation also improves mental function in patients with epilepsy who take the drug Dilantin (phenytoin). In one study, 72 epileptic patients receiving phenytoin alone or in combination with phenobarbital for more than 4 years were divided into four groups, the first taking two placebo tablets per day, the second folic acid (5 milligrams per day) and placebo, the third placebo and thiamin (50 milligrams per day), and the fourth both vitamins.[6] The clinical trial lasted 6 months. Analysis of the results indicated thiamin improved mental functions in both verbal and nonverbal IQ testing. Folic acid therapy was ineffective. These results indicate that in epileptics chronically treated with Dilantin, thiamin supplementation (50 milligrams daily) improves mental function.

Dosage Ranges

For general supplementation and in epileptics taking Dilantin, a daily dosage of 50 to 100 milligrams appears safe and appropriate. In elderly individuals suffering from either Alzheimer's disease or age-related mental impairment, the recommended dosage for therapeutic effects is 3 to 8 grams daily.

Safety Issues

Thiamin is not associated with any toxicity.

Interactions

Thiamin is intricately involved with other B vitamins in energy metabolism. Magnesium is required in the conversion of thiamin to its active form. Alcohol, Dilantin, and possibly other drugs may inhibit thiamin.

9

Riboflavin (Vitamin B₂)

Riboflavin, or vitamin B_2, was first recognized as a yellow-green pigment in milk in 1879. Ingesting an excess of riboflavin results in an increased urine content of riboflavin, which can give urine a yellow-green fluorescent glow. Riboflavin functions in two important enzymes, FMN and FAD, involved in energy production.

Food Sources

Rich sources of riboflavin are organ meats (liver, kidney, heart). Good plant sources are almonds, mushrooms, whole grains, soybeans, and green leafy vegetables (see Table 9.1). Riboflavin is destroyed by light but is not destroyed by cooking. The RDA for riboflavin is 1.7 milligrams for males and 1.3 milligrams for females.

Deficiency Signs and Symptoms

Severe riboflavin deficiency is characterized by cracking of the lips and corner of the mouth; an inflamed tongue; visual disturbances such as sensitivity to light and loss

TABLE 9.1 Riboflavin Content of Selected Foods, in Milligrams per 3 ½-oz. (100-g.) Serving

Food	mg	Food	mg	Food	mg
Yeast, torula	5.06	Wheat bran	.35	Sunflower seeds	.23
Yeast, brewer's	4.28	Collards	.31	Navy beans	.22
Liver, calf	2.72	Soybeans, dry	.31	Beet & mustard greens	.22
Almonds	.92	Split peas	.29	Lentils	.22
Wheat germ	.68	Kale	.26	Prunes	.22
Wild rice	.63	Parsley	.26	Rye, whole grain	.22
Mushrooms	.46	Cashews	.25	Mung beans	.21
Millet	.38	Rice bran	.25	Beans, pinto & red	.21
Peppers, hot red	.36	Broccoli	.23	Blackeye peas	.21
Soy flour	.35	Pine nuts	.23		

of visual acuity; cataract formation; burning and itching of the eyes, lips, mouth, and tongue; and other signs of disorders of mucous membranes. Riboflavin deficiency can also produce anemia and seborrheic dermatitis.

While severe riboflavin deficiency is rare, low levels of riboflavin intake and blood determinations are quite common in the elderly.

Recommended Dietary Allowance

Recommended Dietary Allowance of Riboflavin

Group	Milligrams
INFANTS	
Under 6 months	0.4
6–12 months	0.5
CHILDREN	
1–3 years	0.8
4–6 years	1.1
7–10 years	1.2
YOUNG ADULTS AND ADULTS	
Males 11–14 years	1.5
Males 15–18 years	1.8
Males 19–50 years	1.7
Males 51+ years	1.4
Females 11–50 years	1.3
Females 51+ years	1.2
Pregnant females	1.6
Lactating females	1.8

Beneficial Effects

Riboflavin is crucial in the production of energy and is involved in regenerating glutathione, one of the main cellular protectors against free-radical damage. Low dietary levels of riboflavin have been linked to certain esophageal cancers.[1]

Available Forms

Riboflavin is available in supplemental form as simple riboflavin and activated riboflavin (riboflavin-5-phosphate).

Principal Uses

Although riboflavin is a very important nutrient, there are few clinical indications for its use. Its principal uses are in migraine headaches, cataracts, and sickle cell anemia.

Prevention of Migraine Headaches

One hypothesis as to the cause of migraine headaches is that they are caused by a reduction of energy production within the mitochondria (energy-producing units of cells) of cerebral blood vessels. Therefore, riboflavin, which has the potential of increasing mitochondrial energy efficiency, might have preventive effects against migraine. To test this hypothesis, researchers treated 49 patients suffering from migraine with 400 milligrams of riboflavin daily for at least 3 months. Twenty-three patients also received a daily dose of 75 milligrams of aspirin. Overall improvement after therapy was 68.2 percent in the riboflavin group as determined by the migraine severity score used in the study. With the exception of one patient in the riboflavin-plus-aspirin group who withdrew because of gastric intolerance, no drug-related side effects were reported. The results from this preliminary study suggest high-dose riboflavin could be an effective, low-cost preventive treatment of migraine.[2]

Cataracts

Some scientists believe riboflavin deficiency enhances cataract formation because of reduced regeneration of glutathione.[3,4] While riboflavin deficiency is fairly common in the geriatric population (33 percent), original studies demonstrating an association between riboflavin deficiency and cataract formation were followed by studies demonstrating no association.[3,4]

Although correction of the deficiency is warranted, individuals with cataracts should not use more than 10 milligrams per day of riboflavin. Since riboflavin is a photosensitizing substance, in experimental studies riboflavin and light have been used to induce cataracts as a result of free radicals being generated by the interaction of light, oxygen, and riboflavin. The evidence appears to suggest that excess riboflavin does more harm than good in the cataract patient.

Sickle Cell Anemia

Riboflavin supplementation (5 milligrams twice daily) is of benefit in patients with sickle cell disease. In one controlled study of 18 patients with sickle cell disease, riboflavin supplementation led to significant improvements in iron status (increased total iron-binding capacity and serum ferritin) and glutathione levels.[5]

Dosage Ranges

For general health, a daily dosage of 5 to 10 milligrams appears reasonable. For the prevention of migraine headaches, the dosage used in the preliminary study was 400 milligrams daily. However, absorption studies indicate that the capacity of the human gastrointestinal tract to absorb riboflavin may be less than 20 milligrams in a single oral dose.[6]

Safety Issues

No toxicity or side effects of riboflavin have been demonstrated.

Interactions

Riboflavin interacts quite closely with thiamin. Certain drugs, particularly anti-malarials, interfere with riboflavin metabolism.

10

Niacin (Vitamin B₃)

Because the body converts tryptophan to create niacin or vitamin B_3, many nutritionists do not consider niacin an essential nutrient as long as tryptophan intake is adequate. Niacin functions in the body as a component in the coenzymes NAD and NADP, which are involved in well over 50 different chemical reactions in the body. Niacin-containing enzymes play an important role in energy production; fat, cholesterol, and carbohydrate metabolism; and the manufacture of many body compounds including sex and adrenal hormones.

Food Sources

Rich food sources of niacin include liver and other organ meats, eggs, fish, and peanuts (see Table 10.1). All of these foods are also rich sources of tryptophan. Good sources of niacin include legumes, whole grains (except corn), milk and avocados. Although the RDA for niacin is based on caloric intake (6.6 milligrams per 1,000 calories), most authorities recommend an intake of at least 15–20 milligrams per day.

TABLE 10.1   Niacin Content of Selected Foods, in Milligrams per 3½-oz. (100-g.) Serving

Yeast, torula	44.4	Wild rice	6.2	Whole-wheat grain	4.4
Yeast, brewer's	37.9	Sesame seeds	5.4	Whole-wheat flour	4.3
Rice bran	29.8	Sunflower seeds	5.4	Wheat germ	4.2
Rice polishings	28.2	Brown rice	4.7	Barley	3.7
Wheat bran	21.0	Pine nuts	4.5	Almonds	3.5
Peanuts, with skins	17.2	Buckwheat, whole-grain	4.4	Split peas	3.0
Peanuts, without skins	15.8	Peppers, red chili	4.4		

Deficiency Signs and Symptoms

Niacin was discovered during the search for the cause of pellagra, a common disease in Spain and Italy in the eighteenth century. In Italian, pellagra means "skin that is rough." Now we know pellagra is caused by a severe deficiency of niacin and tryptophan. Pellagra is characterized by the "3-Ds" of pellagra—dermatitis, dementia, and diarrhea. The skin develops a cracked, scaly dermatitis; the brain does not function properly, leading to confusion and dementia; and diarrhea results from the impaired manufacture of the mucous lining of the gastrointestinal tract.

Recommended Dietary Allowance

Recommended Dietary Allowance of Niacin

Group	Milligrams
INFANTS	
Under 6 months	5
6–12 months	6
CHILDREN	
1–3 years	9
4–6 years	12
7–10 years	13
YOUNG ADULTS AND ADULTS	
Males 11–14 years	17
Males 15–18 years	20
Males 19–50 years	19
Males 51+ years	15
Females 11–50 years	15
Females 51+ years	13
Pregnant females	17
Lactating females	20

Beneficial Effects

Niacin is essential in the production of energy. It is also involved in the regulation of blood sugar, antioxidant mechanisms, and detoxification reactions. In addition to its nutritional effects, niacin supplementation exerts a favorable effect on several health conditions, especially high cholesterol levels.

Available Forms

Vitamin B$_3$ is available in nutritional supplements as either niacin (nicotinic acid or nicotinate) or niacinamide (nicotinamide). Each form has different applications. In its nicotinic acid form, vitamin B_3 is an effective reducer of blood cholesterol levels. While in its niacinamide form, it is useful in arthritis and early-onset type I diabetes.

Doses in excess of 50 milligrams of niacin, but not niacinamide, typically produce a transient flushing of the skin. To get around the problem of skin flushing, drug and supplement manufacturers have developed "timed released" products. However, while these preparations may effectively eliminate the problem of skin flushing, they are associated with greater liver destruction and serious side effects (discussed below under Safety Issues). A better way to eliminate the problem of skin flushing is to use inositol hexaniacinate (also known as inositol hexanicotinate and, for short, hexaniacin). This form of niacin has been used in Europe for over 30 years with an excellent safety record.

Principal Uses

The principal uses of niacin and inositol hexaniacinate are in the treatment of elevated cholesterol and triglyceride levels, Raynaud's phenomenon, and intermittent claudication. Niacinamide is used in recent-onset type I diabetes mellitus and arthritis.

Lowering Blood Lipids

Despite the fact that niacin has demonstrated better overall results in reducing the risk for coronary heart disease than other cholesterol-lowering agents, physicians are often reluctant to prescribe niacin. The reason is a widespread perception that niacin is a difficult and somewhat dangerous medicine. There is much confusion about the benefits versus the risks in patients taking niacin. In contrast, most physicians are unaware of the considerable risks and limited benefits of commonly used prescription cholesterol-lowering agents. In addition, since niacin is a widely available "generic" agent, no pharmaceutical company stands to generate the huge profits that the other lipid-lowering agents have enjoyed. As a result, niacin does not enjoy the intensive advertising that the HMG CoA reductase inhibitors and gemfibrozil enjoy. Despite the advantages of niacin over other lipid-lowering drugs, niacin accounts for only 7.9 percent of all lipid-lowering prescriptions.

Comparative Studies

The lipid-lowering activity of niacin was first described in the 1950s. we now know niacin does much more than lower total cholesterol. Specifically, niacin lowers LDL cholesterol, Lp(a) lipoprotein, triglyceride, and fibrinogen levels while simultaneously raising HDL cholesterol levels.[1]

The famed Coronary Drug Project demonstrated that niacin was the only lipid-lowering agent to actually reduce overall mortality.[2] Its effects are long-lasting as demonstrated in a 15-year follow-up study to the Coronary Drug Project, which showed that the long-term death rate for patients treated with niacin was actually 11 percent lower than the group receiving a placebo, even though the treatment had been discontinued in most patients many years earlier.[3] In contrast, patients being treated with clofibrate and/or cholestyramine actually experienced an increased mortality. Clofibrate was associated with a 36 percent higher mortality rate.[4] Presumably both clofibrate and cholestyramine lowered cholesterol and reduced the mortality rate for coronary artery disease but increased the risk of dying prematurely from cancer, complications from gallbladder surgery (clofibrate causes gallstones), and from other conditions.

The HMG CoA reductase inhibitors (the "statin" family of drugs) and gemfibrozil (a newer fibric acid derivative) have replaced clofibrate, and, to a lesser extent, bile-sequestering resins. Are these newer drugs effective in reducing mortality? The jury is still out. Preliminary studies show some benefits. For example, a 5-year safety and efficacy study with lovastatin in 745 patients with severe hypercholesterolemia (total cholesterol levels greater than 360 milligrams per deciliter) demonstrated the effectiveness of lovastatin is maintained over time, there was no increase in mortality, and it was generally well-tolerated.[5] Longer-term studies with larger patient populations are now in progress with all of the statin drugs, but these results will not be available for several years. In the meantime, millions of Americans are being placed on these drugs like human guinea pigs.

Lovastatin versus Niacin

To evaluate how niacin compares in safety and efficacy to the new lipid-lowering drugs, you need only examine the results in several recent head-to-head comparison studies. In 1994 the *Annals of Internal Medicine* published the first clinical study that compared niacin and lovastatin directly.[6] One hundred thirty-six patients with LDL cholesterol levels greater than 160 milligrams per deciliter were included in the controlled, randomized, open-label 26 week study performed at five lipid clinics. Patients were first placed on a 4-week diet run-in period, after which eligible patients were randomly assigned to receive treatment with either lovastatin (20 milligrams per day) or niacin (1.5 grams per day). On the basis of the LDL cholesterol response and patient tolerance, the doses were sequentially increased to 40 and 80 milligrams per day of lovastatin or 3 and 4.5 grams per day of niacin after 10 and 18 weeks of treatment, respectively. In the two patient groups, 66 percent of the patients treated with lovastatin and 54 percent of the patients treated with niacin took the full dosage. The following table illustrates the results.

Lovastatin versus Niacin in Cholesterol Reduction in Percentages

Group	Week 10	Week 18	Week 26
LDL CHOLESTEROL REDUCTION			
Lovastatin	26	28	32
Niacin	5	16	23
HDL CHOLESTEROL INCREASE			
Lovastatin	6	8	7
Niacin	20	29	33
LP(A) LIPOPROTEIN REDUCTION			
Lovastatin	0	0	0
Niacin	14	30	35

These results indicate that while lovastatin produced a greater effect on LDL cholesterol reduction, niacin provided better overall results despite the fact that fewer patients were able to tolerate a full dosage of niacin because of skin flushing. The percentage increase in HDL cholesterol, a more significant indicator for coronary heart disease, was dramatically in favor of niacin (33 percent versus 7 percent). Equally as impressive was the percentage decrease in Lp(a) lipoprotein for niacin. Lp(a) is a plasma lipoprotein whose structure and composition closely resemble that of low-density lipoprotein but with an additional molecule of apolipoprotein attached to apolipoprotein B by a disulfide bond. Several studies indicate that an elevated plasma level of Lp(a) is an independent risk factor for coronary heart disease, particularly in those patients with elevated LDL cholesterol levels.[7,8] While niacin produced a 35 percent reduction in Lp(a) lipoprotein levels, lovastatin did not produce any effect. Niacin's effect on Lp(a) in this study confirmed a previous study that showed niacin (4 grams per day) reduced Lp(a) levels by 38 percent.[9]

Renal Transplant Patients

Lipid abnormalities are seen frequently in renal transplant patients, and cardiovascular disease is a primary cause of morbidity and mortality in these patients. A study was designed to assess the efficacy and safety of niacin and lovastatin in these patients.[10] Twelve renal transplant patients who had persistent hyperlipidemia despite 6 weeks of dietary treatment participated in this prospective, randomized, open-labeled crossover trial. After 16 weeks of therapy with niacin (3 grams per day), total cholesterol dropped from 312 to 229 milligrams per deciliter, LDL cholesterol dropped from 218 to 142 milligrams per deciliter, triglycerides dropped from 255 to 150 milligrams per deciliter, and HDL cholesterol increased from 44 to 58 milligrams per deciliter. In contrast, lovastatin (40 milligrams per day) produced less dramatic improvement; e.g., total cholesterol dropped from 285 to 233 milligrams per deciliter, and LDL cholesterol dropped from 201 to 147 milligrams per deciliter. There were no significant changes in the triglyceride and high-density lipoprotein cholesterol levels. These results clearly show niacin is more advantageous than lovastatin in this patient group.

Niacin, Gemfibrozil, and Lovastatin

Another comparative study sought to determine the lipoprotein responses to niacin, gemfibrozil, and lovastatin in patients with normal total cholesterol levels but low levels of HDL cholesterol.[11] The first phase of the study compared lipoprotein responses to lovastatin and gemfibrozil in 61 middle-aged men with low levels of high-density lipoproteins. In the second phase, 37 patients agreed to take niacin; 27 patients finished this phase at a dose of 4.5 grams per day. In the first phase, gemfibrozil therapy increased high-density lipoprotein cholesterol levels by 10 percent and lovastatin by 6 percent. In the second phase, niacin therapy raised HDL cholesterol by 30 percent.

Inositol Hexaniacinate

Inositol hexaniacinate is a special form of niacin composed of six nicotinic acid molecules bound to and surrounding one molecule of inositol, an unofficial member of the B vitamin group. Inositol hexaniacinate exerts the benefits of niacin without flushing or other side effects. It has been used in Europe for over 30 years not only to lower cholesterol, but also to improve blood flow in the treatment of intermittent claudication (a painful cramp in the calf produced when walking as a result of decreased oxygen supply to the calf muscle) and Raynaud's phenomena (a painful response of the hands or feet to cold exposure because of constriction of blood vessels supplying the hands). Although inositol hexaniacinate yields slightly better results than standard niacin, the big advantage is that it is safer and much better tolerated.[12–15]

Recent-Onset Insulin-Dependent Diabetes

Scientists acknowledge that insulin-dependent diabetes mellitus (IDDM)is generally because of an insulin deficiency. Although the exact cause is unknown, current theory suggests it is because of a genetic predisposition coupled with some environmental factor that results in an immune-mediated destruction of the pancreatic beta-cells, which produce insulin. For example, recent studies provide strong evidence that exposure to a protein in cow's milk (bovine albumin peptide) in early infancy may trigger an autoimmune process and subsequent type I diabetes. In case-controlled studies, patients with type I diabetes were more likely to have been breast-fed for less than 3 months and to have been exposed to cow's milk or solid foods before 4 months.[16] Presumably early dietary exposure to bovine albumin peptide in predisposed children leads to the development of antibodies that cross-react with insulin-producing beta-cells of the pancreas.

Other suspected environmental factors include dietary free radicals (e.g., nitrosamines) and various viruses. Beta-cell injury caused by free-radicals or viral infection ultimately leads to an autoimmune reaction because the damage exposes normally concealed antigens to the immune system. Antibodies to pancreatic cells are present in 75 percent of all cases of IDDM compared to 0.5 to 2.0 percent of individuals without diabetes.[17]

With the discovery that IDDM may be a chronic autoimmune reaction, drugs commonly used to suppress the immune system have been used to halt or at least slow down the destruction of the beta-cells. The most widely used and accepted drug for this purpose is prednisone. However, there is a great deal of evidence to indicate that niacinamide (also known as nicotinamide) is both safer and more effective.

Prednisone in Recent-Onset IDDM

The effects of prednisone in the treatment of recent-onset IDDM are conflicting. The reason may be that while prednisone and other corticosteroids may suppress the immune system, they also substantially increase blood glucose levels in prediabetic conditions.

In one study, prednisone was administered at immunosuppressive dosage (1 milligram per kilogram bodyweight per day) during the initial 10 days and at a maintenance dosage (0.3 milligrams per kilogram body weight per day for 50 days. Thirty-two patients were enrolled within 6 weeks after diagnosis and matched in pairs for age, sex, presence of islet cell antibodies (ICA), and glucagon-stimulated C-peptide levels. All the patients who received prednisone became ICA negative during treatment, but in some (4 out of 10) this effect was only transient. No patient experienced complete remission, but in ten prednisone and four control patients the insulin requirements were below 0.3 I.U. per kilogram body weight. These results show some benefit.[18]

In another study, 25 patients with IDDM between the ages of 18 and 30 entered the trial within 8 weeks of the onset of diabetes. They were allocated to one of the following treatments: prednisone (15 milligrams per day), indomethacin (100 milligrams per day), or placebo. All treatments lasted 8 months, and all patients achieved satisfactory metabolic control with a multi-injection regimen (three injections per day) within a few weeks and maintained it throughout the entire period of observation. A lower insulin requirement was observed in the prednisone group than in other patients at 12 months (0.33 versus 0.57 units per kilogram body weight per day), 18 months (0.34 versus 0.64), and 24 months (0.38 versus 0.63). Endogenous insulin release, evaluated as urinary C-peptide, was higher in the prednisone group. Although these results indicate that prednisone administration effectively restored endogenous insulin release in IDDM patients, the overall clinical significance of this effect is not known, given the side effects of prednisone.[19]

In a study of children with newly diagnosed IDDM, 31 were given either prednisone (60 milligrams twice daily for 14 days followed by a dose of 30 milligrams and 15 milligrams daily for 7 days) or a placebo. All patients were treated with continuous subcutaneous insulin infusion for the first 15 days of treatment, and then with two daily injections of a mixture of intermediate- and fast-acting insulin. All subjects were followed for 1 year. The results of the study indicated that short-term prednisone therapy does not modify the natural course of the disease.[20]

To achieve better results, some studies have used even more powerful drugs. For example, in one study prednisone was combined with the immunosuppressive drug azathioprine.[21] Forty-six patients (mean age, 11.7 years; range, 4.5 to 32.8) with newly diagnosed insulin-dependent diabetes mellitus, within two weeks of beginning insulin, were given either corticosteroids for 10 weeks plus daily azathioprine for one year or no immunosuppressive therapy. Half the 20 immunosuppressed patients completing the one-year trial had satisfactory metabolic outcomes—hemoglobin A_{1C} less than 6.8 percent; stimulated peak C-peptide greater than 0.5 nmol (nanomole) per liter; insulin dose less than 0.4 U/kilograms body weight per day) as compared with only 15 percent of the controls. Three of 20 immunosuppressed patients, but no controls, did not have to use insulin at 1 year. Two of these continued to receive azathioprine without insulin after more than 27 months of follow-up. The response to immunosuppression correlated with older age, better initial metabolic status, and lymphopenia (less than 1,800 lymphocytes per cubic millimeter) resulting from immunosuppression. Several of those on azathioprine experienced gastrointestinal disturbances, including vomiting, and one patient had mild hair loss. The use of prednisone resulted in a transient cushingoid appearance, weight gain, and hyperglycemia. Altogether, the results of these studies and others do not appear to offer much support that the benefits of immunosuppressive therapy outweigh the risks.

Niacinamide in Recent-Onset IDDM

Niacinamide, also called nicotinamide, was first shown in the early 1950s to prevent the development of diabetes in experimental animals.[22] Additional animal studies in the 1980s confirmed these earlier studies and ultimately led to several pilot clinical studies.[23] The mechanism of action appears to be inhibition of macrophage- and interleukin-1-mediated beta cell damage and inhibition of nitric oxide production, along with niacinamide's antioxidant role.[24] Niacinamide also enhances insulin secretion and increases insulin sensitivity.[25]

In one of the first pilot studies of newly diagnosed IDDM, 7 patients ingested niacinamide daily and 9 ingested a placebo. After six months, 5 patients in the niacinamide group and 2 in the placebo group were still not taking insulin and had normal blood glucose and HgbA1c. At 12 months, 3 patients in the niacinamide group but none in the placebo group were in clinical remission.[26]

The results of this pilot study and others suggested that niacinamide can prevent type I diabetes from progressing in some patients if given soon enough at the onset of diabetes. It does so by helping restore beta cells.[27–31] As of April 1995, eight studies exist of niacinamide treatment in recent onset IDDM or IDDM of less than 5 years' duration and residual beta-cell mass. Six of these studies are double-blind, placebo-controlled studies. Out of these six, three studies show a positive effect compared to a placebo in terms of prolonged noninsulin-requiring remission, lower insulin requirements, improved metabolic control, and increased beta-cell function as determined by C-peptide secretion. Some newly diagnosed type I diabetics have experienced complete resolution of their diabetes with niacinamide supplementation. The main differences between the positive and negative studies in recent-onset IDDM occur with the older age and higher baseline fasting C-peptide in positive studies.

In the spring of 1993, researchers began a large multicenter study involving 18 European countries, Israel, and Canada to follow up these encouraging preliminary findings. Other clinical trials are also in progress or have been proposed.

The daily dose of nicotinamide is based on body weight, 25 milligrams per kilogram. The studies in children used 100 milligrams to 200 milligrams per day.

Niacinamide in the Prevention of IDDM in High-Risk Cases

In addition to studies using niacinamide in the treatment of recent-onset IDDM, there are also several studies that have examined the ability of niacinamide in preventing the development of IDDM in high-risk individuals.[32–34] These studies demonstrated that niacinamide supplementation shows promising effects in reducing the development of IDDM in these children.

These preliminary results led to the design of a larger population-based study being conducted in New Zealand. Of 32,000 five- to seven-year-old children offered screening for islet cell antibodies, 20,000 were tested and 150 were found to be eligible for treatment with 1,000 milligrams of niacinamide. Eligibility criteria was ICA values greater than 10 per milliliter. In the 20,000 children tested, including the 150 treated with niacinamide, the diabetes incidence was 8.1 per 10,000 per year, compared with an incidence of 15.1 in those 12,000 children offered a test but who declined, and 20.1 in 48,000 children not offered testing (see Figure 10.1).[35,36]

These results are quite impressive. Given the facts that IDDM is a very expensive disease to treat and niacinamide is relatively cheap, large-scale screening for islet cell antibodies and subsequent treatment with niacinamide for those at high risk may actually prove to be a good way to cut health-care costs. In 1992, diabetics accounted for only 4.5 percent of the U.S. population but accounted for one in seven health care dollars spent, or roughly 14.6 percent of the total U.S. health care expenditures ($105 billion).[37]

A large multicenter, placebo-controlled trial, the European Nicotinamide Diabetes Intervention Trial (ENDIT), is currently in progress to follow up these preliminary studies.

Niacinamide Combined with Immunosuppressive Drugs

Researchers have conducted several studies combining niacinamide with immunosuppressive drugs. One study, a 1-year, open, randomized, controlled, multicenter trial carried out on 90 patients with recent-onset IDDM (less than 4 weeks) compared the effect of niacinamide alone with the combination of niacinamide and low-dose cyclosporin on clinical remission and optimization of metabolic control during the

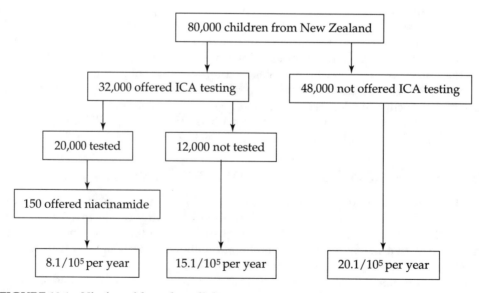

FIGURE 10.1   Niacinamide and prediabetes.

first year from date of diagnosis. Three groups of 30 patients were randomly assigned to receive for 12 months either:

- Niacinamide, 25 milligrams per kilogram of body weight per day
- Niacinamide, 25 milligrams per kilogram of body weight per day in combination with cyclosporin, 5 milligrams per kilogram of body weight per day
- No treatment

Clinical remission (i.e., suspension of insulin therapy with normal metabolic parameters for more than 2 weeks according to the International Diabetes Immunotherapy Group) was achieved at 3 months in 6 out of 30 niacinamide-treated patients and in one out of 30 niacinamide-plus-cyclosporin-treated patients. The researchers observed no remission in control patients. At 6 months the number of patients achieving remission in each group was 4 out of 29, 3 out of 27, and 1 out of 29, respectively. One year after diagnosis, the respective number of patients achieving remission was 4 out of 27, 2 out of 25, and 0 out of 28. Clinical remission lasted longer (7 months) in niacinamide-treated patients than in those also receiving cyclosporin. These results indicate that cyclosporin does not improve clinical outcome and may actually impair the effectiveness of niacinamide.[38]

Niacinamide has also been tried in combination with the corticosteroid deflazacort. Unlike prednisone, this drug does not raise blood sugar levels. Deflazacort protects animals from developing diabetes by inhibiting macrophage-derived interleukin-1 and blocking the production of many other cytokines that directly or indirectly contribute to beta-cell destruction. However, just like the study with cyclosporin, the combination of niacinamide and deflazacort did not produce results as good as the results achieved with niacinamide alone.[39]

Niacinamide in Arthritis

Drs. William Kaufman and Abram Hoffer have reported very good clinical results in the treatment of hundreds of patients with rheumatoid arthritis and osteoarthritis using high dose niacinamide (i.e., 900 to 4,000 milligrams. in divided doses daily).[40,41] Unfortunately, these promising results have never been fully evaluated in detailed clinical studies.

Dosage Ranges

You should not use sustained-release niacin. If you use pure crystalline niacin, start with a dose of 100 milligrams three times a day and carefully increase the dosage over a period of 4 to 6 weeks to the full therapeutic dose of 1.5 grams to 3 grams daily in divided dosage. If you are using inositol hexaniacinate, begin with 500 milligrams three times daily for 2 weeks and then increase to 1,000 milligrams. It is best to take either crystalline niacin or inositol hexaniacinate with meals.

How Much Proof Is Required When Human Lives Are at Stake?

In our current medical system there appears to be a unnecessary time lag between the time researchers prove a vitamin or mineral to be effective in preventing or treating a certain health condition and the time when physicians accept and recommend its use. A case in point is the time lag between the demonstration and the acceptance of the role that folic acid plays in the prevention of neural tube defects (see Chapter 14).

There are countless examples where supplementing the diet with an inexpensive vitamin or mineral can provide significant preventive or therapeutic effects, yet many physicians place an unnecessary burden of proof on researchers before they feel inclined to make the recommendation. My message to these physicians is to rethink their position.

Instead of waiting for absolute proof, physicians should ask whether there is enough "reasonable certainty" that a particular recommendation *may* be of benefit. What do I mean by *reasonable certainty?* Basically, does the recommendation make sense? Is there a good chance that the recommendation may be of value? Does it provide a favorable cost-to-benefit ratio? Is the recommendation safe?

For example, I have presented above the potential role of niacinamide in the treatment of recent-onset insulin-dependent diabetes mellitus (IDDM) as well as prevention of IDDM in high-risk children. The results indicate an excellent cost-to-benefit ratio and safety profile. Most orthodox medical doctors would look at the information and say something like, "This research is very interesting, but of course I cannot recommend niacinamide until there is more absolute proof that it may be of value."

Again, I ask—How much proof is required when human lives are at stake? The results from larger double-blind studies with niacinamide will not be available until 1998 or 1999. What if the results of these larger studies are positive? It would mean that by "playing it safe" and not supplementing niacinamide, many individuals who may have benefited did not, just like the thousands of children born with neural tube defects were denied the opportunity for folic acid supplementation.

Niacinamide does not work for all recent-onset IDDM patients, but it may work for some. It is certainly worth the effort, especially since there is no other reasonable alternative.

I read so much research where I ask myself the question, how much more proof is required before the majority of physicians begin prescribing a particular vitamin, mineral, or botanical extract to prevent or treat a particular health condition? But when children are at stake, somehow the question takes on extra meaning.

Safety Issues

The side effects of niacin are well known. The most common and bothersome side effect is the skin flushing that typically occurs 20 to 30 minutes after taking the niacin. Other occasional side effects of niacin include gastric irritation, nausea, and liver damage. In an attempt to combat the acute reaction of skin flushing, several manufacturers began marketing "sustained-released," "timed-released," or "slow-released" niacin products. These formulations allow the body to absorb the niacin gradually, thereby reducing the flushing reaction. However, although these forms of niacin reduce skin flushing, they are actually more toxic to the liver. A recent study published in the *Journal of the American Medical Association (JAMA)* strongly recommended that sustained-release niacin be restricted from use because of the high percentage (78 percent) of patient withdrawal because of side effects; 52 percent of the patients taking the sustained-release niacin developed liver damage, while none of the patients taking immediate-release niacin developed liver damage.[42]

Again, inositol hexaniacinate is the safest form of niacin currently available. Both short- and long-term studies show it is virtually free of side effects other than an occasional person experiencing mild gastric upset or mild skin irritation.

Because niacin can impair glucose tolerance, is should probably not be used in diabetics unless they are under close observation. Niacin should not be used in patients with pre-existing liver disease or elevation in liver enzymes; gout; or peptic ulcers.

Regardless of the form of niacin being used, periodic checking (minimum every 3 months) of cholesterol and liver function tests are indicated when high-dose (i.e., 2 to 6 grams per day) niacin, inositol hexaniacinate, or niacinamide therapy is being used.

Interactions

Niacin is intricately involved with other B vitamins in energy metabolism. It can be combined with other lipid-lowering drugs to potentiate the drug's effect on lowering cholesterol or triglycerides.

11

Pyridoxine (Vitamin B$_6$)

Vitamin B$_6$ (pyridoxine) is an extremely important B vitamin involved in the formation of body proteins and structural compounds, chemical transmitters in the nervous system, red blood cells, and prostaglandins. Vitamin B$_6$ is also critical in maintaining hormonal balance and proper immune function.

Food Sources

Good plant sources of vitamin B$_6$ include whole grains, legumes, bananas, seeds and nuts, potatoes, brussels sprouts, and cauliflower (see Table 11.1). Vitamin B$_6$ levels inside the body's cells are intricately linked to the magnesium content of the diet as well (see Chapter 19, Magnesium).

Deficiency Signs and Symptoms

Deficiency of vitamin B$_6$ is characterized by depression, convulsions (especially in children), glucose intolerance, anemia, impaired nerve function, cracking of the lips and tongue, and seborrhea or eczema.[1]

Although extreme deficiency of vitamin B$_6$ is quite rare, numerous clinical studies demonstrate the importance of vitamin B$_6$ in a number of health conditions that typically respond to B$_6$ supplementation, including asthma, premenstrual syndrome (PMS), carpal tunnel syndrome, depression, morning sickness, and kidney stones. The increased rate of these disorders since the 1950s parallels the increased levels of vitamin B$_6$ antagonists found in the food supply or used as drugs during the same period. These antagonists to vitamin B$_6$ include the hydrazine dyes (especially FD&C yellow #5), certain drugs (isoniazid, hydralazine, dopamine, and penicillamine), oral contraceptives, alcohol, and excessive protein intake. The intake of yellow dye #5 (tartrazine) is often greater (per capita intake of 15 grams per day) than the RDA for vitamin B$_6$ of 2.0 milligrams for males and 1.6 milligrams for females.

TABLE 11.1 Pyridoxine Content of Selected Foods, in Milligrams per 3 1/2-oz. (100-g.) Serving

Yeast, torula	3.00	Navy beans, dry	.56	Spinach	.28
Yeast, brewer's	2.50	Brown rice	.55	Turnip greens	.26
Sunflower seeds	1.25	Hazelnuts	.54	Peppers, sweet	.26
Wheat germ, toasted	1.15	Garbanzos, dry	.54	Potatoes	.25
Soybeans, dry	.81	Pinto beans, dry	.53	Prunes	.24
Walnuts	.73	Bananas	.51	Raisins	.24
Soybean flour	.63	Avocados	.42	Brussels sprouts	.23
Lentils, dry	.60	Whole-wheat flour	.34	Barley	.22
Lima beans, dry	.58	Chestnuts, fresh	.33	Sweet potatoes	.22
Buckwheat flour	.58	Kale	.30	Cauliflower	.21
Blackeye peas, dry	.56	Rye flour	.30		

Recommended Dietary Allowance

Recommended Dietary Allowance of Pyridoxine

Group	Milligrams
INFANTS	
Under 6 months	0.3
6–12 months	0.6
CHILDREN	
1–3 years	1.0
4–6 years	1.1
7–10 years	1.4
YOUNG ADULTS AND ADULTS	
Males 11–14 years	1.7
Males 15+ years	2.0
Females 11–14 years	1.5
Females 15+ years	1.6
Pregnant females	2.2
Lactating females	2.1

Beneficial Effects

The human body requires vitamin B$_6$ for the proper functioning of more than 60 different enzymes. It plays a vital role in the multiplication of all cells and is, therefore, of critical importance to a healthy pregnancy and proper functioning immune system, mucous membrane, skin, and red blood cells. These tissues have greater than average needs for vitamin B_6 because of they are composed of rapidly replicating cells. Lack of vitamin B_6 greatly affects pregnancy and the function of these tissues. Vitamin B_6 also plays a critical role in brain chemistry because it is involved in the manufacture of all amino acid neurotransmitters (e.g., serotonin, dopamine, melatonin, epinephrine, norepinephrine, etcetera).

Available Forms

Vitamin B_6 is available as pyridoxine hydrochloride and pyridoxal-5-phosphate. The latter form is the most active form. However, intestinal cells remove the phosphate molecule from most of the pyridoxal-5-phosphate ingested before it is absorbed.[2] Therefore, for most people the pyridoxine form is satisfactory as long as the necessary cofactors for conversion (riboflavin and magnesium) are available. The exception is people with liver disease. Since the activation of pyridoxine to pyridoxal-5-phosphate occurs in the liver, people with liver disease (particularly liver cirrhosis) may have difficulty in converting pyridoxine to pyridoxal-5-phosphate. In liver cirrhosis, and possibly other liver disease, supplementation with injectable pyridoxal-5-phosphate may be more advantageous than oral pyridoxine.[3]

Principal Uses

Vitamin B_6 is one of the most utilized and valued nutritional supplements. It is also one of the most intensely studied. The effect of vitamin B_6 supplementation has been evaluated in over 100 different health conditions. However, because of space constraints, my discussion focuses on the following health conditions because they are the most common conditions using vitamin B_6 supplementation:

- Asthma
- Autism
- Cardiovascular disease
- Carpal tunnel syndrome
- Chinese restaurant syndrome
- Diabetes (prevention of diabetic complications)
- Depression
- Epilepsy
- Immune enhancement
- Kidney stones
- Nausea and vomiting of pregnancy
- Osteoporosis
- Premenstrual syndrome

Asthma

In general, asthmatics have a defect in tryptophan metabolism and reduced platelet transport of serotonin possibly as a result of low vitamin B$_6$ levels. Double-blind clinical studies show that some patients benefit from vitamin B$_6$ supplementation to correct the blocked tryptophan metabolism.[4,5] In one study, oral supplementation with 50 milligrams of vitamin B$_6$ twice daily resulted in a dramatic decrease in frequency and severity of wheezing and asthmatic attacks.[5] Although all patients reported benefit, in seven of the patients supplementation failed to produce a substantial elevation of the pyridoxal-5-phosphate. This suggests that some patients may need even more vitamin B$_6$ or they may be deficient in magnesium or riboflavin.

Asthmatics undergoing treatment with the drug theophylline definitely need Vitamin B$_6$ supplementation. Theophylline significantly depresses pyridoxal-5-phosphate levels.[6] In addition, another study shows that vitamin B$_6$ supplementation significantly reduces the typical side effects of theophylline (headaches, nausea, irritability, sleep disorders, etcetera).[7]

Autism

Autism has been linked to alterations in normal brain chemistry. The basic defect appears to be a decrease in several brain neurotransmitters that require vitamin B$_6$ for synthesis. Several double-blind clinical studies have investigated Vitamin B$_6$ supplementation of autistic children.[8-11] The results indicate that there is a subgroup that improves with B$_6$ supplementation. However, on the average only about 20 percent show moderate improvement in symptom scores, while about 10 percent demonstrate dramatic clinical improvement. B$_6$ supplementation had a greater effect when used in combination with magnesium.[10,11]

A 1985 study of 60 autistic children divided them into two groups and gave each group various combinations of vitamin B$_6$, magnesium, and placebo. Therapeutic effects were measured using behavioral rating scales, urinary excretion of homovanillic acid (HVA), and brain-wave tracing (evoked potential recordings). The combination of B$_6$ and magnesium resulted in significant improvement in behavior that was closely associated with decreases in HVA excretion and a normalized brain-wave tracing. However, neither magnesium nor vitamin B$_6$ were significantly effective when used alone.[12]

Although B$_6$ may not result in a cure of autism, sufficient evidence exists to support supplementation in autistic children.

Cardiovascular Disease

Vitamin B$_6$ deficiency was first suggested as a cause of atherosclerosis in 1948. Since that time, numerous studies have further substantiated the role of pyridoxine in preventing atherosclerosis. Individuals with low pyridoxal-5-phosphate levels in their blood have a five times greater risk of having a heart attack than individuals with higher levels.[13] A deficiency of pyridoxine leads to the accumulation of homocysteine, a metabolite of the amino acid methionine. Homocysteine is very damaging to the cells that line the arteries. Damage to these cells ultimately leads to atherosclerosis. Elevated homocysteine levels are a causative factor in roughly 10 percent of all heart attacks. In addition to vitamin B_6, folic acid and vitamin B_{12} are also derived from methionine during protein catabolism and converted, via pyridoxine-dependent cystathionine beta-reductase, to cystathionine.

Vitamin B_6 may also be important in other aspects of atherosclerosis. Lysyl oxidase, a copper-dependent enzyme responsible for normal cross-linking of both collagen and elastin, is also pyridoxine-dependent. Some scientists hypothesize that since the earliest visible lesion of atherosclerosis is a focal splitting of the internal elastic lamina, this lesion may be the result of imperfect cross-linking of the arterial elastin and collagen. Such a defect could be because of impaired lysyl oxidase activity secondary to a maternal copper or pyridoxine deficiency.[14]

Vitamin B_6 also inhibits platelet aggregation.[15,16] Once platelets aggregate, they release potent compounds that cause migration and proliferation of smooth muscle cells into the middle of the artery. Atherosclerosis can be prevented by inhibition of platelet function. In a recent study, the effect of vitamin B_6 (pyridoxine HCl) supplementation on platelet aggregation, plasma lipids, and serum zinc levels was determined in 24 healthy male volunteers (19 to 24 years old) given either pyridoxine at a dosage of 5 milligrams per 2.2 pounds body weight or a placebo for 4 weeks. Results demonstrated that pyridoxine inhibited platelet aggregation by 41 percent to 48 percent, but there was no change in the control group. Pyridoxine prolonged both bleeding and coagulation time, but not over the physiological limits. It had no effect on platelet count. Pyridoxine was also shown to lower considerably total plasma lipids and cholesterol levels from a pretreatment levels. Total plasma lipids were reduced from 593 to 519 milligrams per deciliter, and total cholesterol was reduced from 156 to 116 milligrams per deciliter. HDL cholesterol increased from 37.9 to 48.6 milligrams per deciliter. Serum zinc levels increased from 96 to 138 micrograms per deciliter. These results provide further evidence of the possible role of vitamin B_6 supplementation on reducing the risk of atherosclerotic mortality.

Vitamin B_6 supplementation also lowers blood pressure. In one study, vitamin B_6 supplementation at a single oral dosage of 5 milligrams per 2.2 pounds body weight for four weeks in 20 people with high blood pressure demonstrated significant reductions in systolic and diastolic blood pressure and serum norepinephrine (noradrenalin) levels. These results indicate that B_6 influences the nervous system in a manner that leads to reduction in blood pressure. The effect on blood pressure may have tremendous clinical significance; the systolic pressure dropped from 167 to 153 mm Hg (millimeters of mercury) and the diastolic pressure dropped from 108 to 98 mm Hg in the study.[17]

Carpal Tunnel Syndrome

Carpal tunnel syndrome is a common painful disorder caused by compression of the median nerve as it passes between the bones and ligaments of the wrist. Compression of the nerve causes weakness, pain when gripping, and burning, tingling, or aching. The sensation may radiate to the forearm and shoulder. Symptoms may be occasional or constant. They usually occur most frequently at night. People who perform repetitive, strenuous work with their hands, such as grocery store checkers and carpenters, frequently suffer from carpal tunnel syndrome (CTS).

Vitamin B$_6$ deficiency is a common finding in carpal tunnel syndrome. In double-blind, placebo-controlled clinical studies, John Ellis, M.D., Karl Folkers, Ph.D., and their co-workers at the University of Texas have successfully treated hundreds of patients suffering from carpal tunnel syndrome with vitamin B$_6$.[18-20] It may take as long as 3 months to produce a benefit, but vitamin B$_6$ is effective in many cases.

The increased incidence of CTS since its initial description by George Phalen, M.D., in 1950 parallels the increased presence of pyridoxine antimetabolites in the diet and environment. Particularly incriminating is tartrazine (FD&C yellow #5).[10] Even Phalen (who pioneered its surgical treatment) agrees that in the future, pyridoxine (in doses of 100 to 200 milligrams per day) may be the treatment of choice.[21] I doubt if this will ever happen, however. I remember sharing with a friend of mine, a neurosurgeon, the clinical studies on B$_6$ supplementation in CTS. His response was, "I hope my patients don't find out about this. I make 30 to 40 percent of my income from performing surgeries for carpal tunnel syndrome."

Chinese Restaurant Syndrome

Chinese restaurant syndrome is a medically recognized syndrome typified by tingling and weakness around the face, temple, upper back, neck, and arms, accompanied by flushing of the skin and warmth. In some people, sensations of heart palpitations, intense thirst, anxiety, nausea, and vomiting may occur. Chinese restaurant syndrome occurs because of a reaction to monosodium glutamate, a food additive used to enhance the flavor of foods and stabilize foods. Approximately 500 million pounds of monosodium glutamate are added each year to the world food supply.

Chinese restaurant syndrome may be caused by a vitamin B$_6$ deficiency because the proper metabolism of monosodium glutamate requires vitamin B$_6$. Dr. Folkers has demonstrated that in many cases vitamin B$_6$ supplementation (50 milligrams daily) eliminates symptoms of Chinese restaurant syndrome in sensitive individuals.[22]

Depression

B$_6$ levels are typically quite low in depressed patients, especially women taking birth control pills or Premarin.[23-27] Considering the many functions of vitamin B$_6$ in the brain—including the fact that vitamin B$_6$ is absolutely essential in the manufacture of all brain neurotransmitters, including serotonin—it is likely that many of the millions of people who are taking Prozac may be suffering depression simply as a result of low vitamin B$_6$. Depressed patients with low B$_6$ status usually respond very well to supplementation. Rather than performing a blood test to see if pyridoxine status is low, depressed individuals (especially women on oral contraceptives) should simply supplement their diets with an additional 50 milligrams to 100 milligrams of vitamin B$_6$.

Diabetes

Vitamin B_6 supplementation appears to offer significant protection against the development of diabetic neuropathy because diabetics with neuropathy are deficient in vitamin B_6 and benefit from supplementation.[28] The neuropathy of a vitamin B_6 deficiency is indistinguishable from diabetic neuropathy. Individuals with long-standing diabetes or who are developing signs of peripheral nerve abnormalities should definitely supplement their diets with vitamin B_6. The standard dose for this application is 150 milligrams.

Vitamin B_6 may also prove to be important in preventing other diabetic complications because it inhibits glycosylation of proteins.[29] Vitamin B_6 supplementation should be tried as a safe treatment for gestational diabetes (diabetes caused by pregnancy). In one study of 14 women with gestational diabetes, taking 100 milligrams of vitamin B_6 for 2 weeks resulted in eliminating the diagnosis in 12 out of the 14 women.[30]

Epilepsy

Vitamin B_6 may be helpful in decreasing epilepsy and seizure activities in infants. There are two known types of vitamin B_6-related seizures in newborns and infants less than 18 months of age, B_6-deficient and B_6-dependent. They have similar neurological symptoms, EEG abnormalities, and a prognosis of mental retardation if not treated.[31]

Physicians should suspect a diagnosis of pyridoxine dependency in every infant with convulsions in the first 18 months of life. Certain clinical features may be especially suggestive, including:

- Seizures of unknown origin in a previously normal infant without an abnormal gestational or perinatal history
- A history of severe convulsive disorders
- The occurrence of long-lasting focal or unilateral seizures, often with partial preservation of consciousness
- Irritability, restlessness, crying, and vomiting preceding the actual seizure

Since unusual presentations of pyridoxine-responsive seizures have been reported, some physicians recommended a trial of injectable pyridoxine on any neonate or infant with long-lasting convulsions, especially when no clear-cut cause is present.[31,32] A 100- to 200-milligram intravenous dose or 20-milligram dose every 5 minutes to a total of 200 milligrams is recommended. If the seizures stop, the child probably has pyridoxine-responsive seizures. The chance to identify a pyridoxine-responsive seizure is lost if pyridoxine is given together with, or after, most anticonvulsant drugs.[32]

Although the administration of dietary amounts of pyridoxine promptly corrects B_6-deficient seizures, B_6-dependent seizures require continuous high-dose supplementation in the range of 25 to 50 milligrams per day.[31–34] Science doesn't fully understand the mechanism by which pyridoxine decreases seizure activity, but it is undoubtedly related to its role as a necessary cofactor in the metabolism of a variety of neurotransmitters whose production is dependent on vitamin B$_6$.

One proposed mechanism for pyridoxine dependency is that pyridoxal phosphate does not bind with its usual affinity to the enzyme glutamic acid decarboxylase, resulting in reduced production of the neurotransmitter GABA. These patients require levels of pyridoxine that are higher than normal for the activity of this enzyme.[31-34]

One uncontrolled study of infants and children with uncontrollable infantile spasms or seizures found improvement in 2 to 14 days using oral pyridoxal-5-phosphate (20 to 50 milligrams per 2.2 pounds body weight). Three had complete relief, six showed transient relief, and eight showed marked reduction in seizures and improvement in their brain-wave tracings (EEGs).[34] Some adverse reactions were seen—elevated liver enzymes, and nausea and vomiting.

Administration of vitamin B$_6$ to epileptics must be strictly monitored. Although some improvements have been noted, daily doses in the range of 80 to 400 milligrams interfere with commonly used anticonvulsants.[35]

Immune Enhancement

A pyridoxine deficiency results in depressed immunity, noted by a reduction in the quantity and quality of antibodies produced, shrinkage of lymphatic tissues (including the thymus gland), decreased thymic hormone activity, and a reduction in the number and activity of lymphocytes.[36]

Researchers have noted low pyridoxine in AIDS patients even though they were consuming adequate amounts in their diets, suggesting either a malabsorption problem or that perhaps drugs used in the treatment of AIDS interfere with vitamin B$_6$. The lack of vitamin B$_6$ correlated with a decrease in immune function.[37]

Kidney Stones

Calcium oxalate kidney stones can be effectively prevented in most recurrent stone formers with vitamin B$_6$ and magnesium supplementation. While supplemental magnesium alone is effective in preventing recurrences of kidney stones, magnesium used in conjunction with vitamin B$_6$ brings even better results. [38,39]

Vitamin B$_6$ reduces the production and urinary excretion of oxalates.[40-42] Patients with recurrent oxalate stones show abnormal vitamin B$_6$-dependent enzyme levels, indicating clinical insufficiency of vitamin B$_6$ and impaired glutamic acid synthesis. These levels return to normal but usually only after at least 3 months of treatment.[42] Restoration of normal vitamin B$_6$ and magnesium levels is important in preventing further kidney stones.

Depressed levels of glutamic acid (because of vitamin B$_6$ deficiency or other reasons) in individuals experiencing recurrent kidney stones are significant since an increased concentration of glutamic acid in the urine reduces calcium oxalate precipitation. Glutamic acid supplementation in rats significantly reduces the incidence of calculi, and it may do so in humans.[43,44]

Nausea and Vomiting during Pregnancy

Vitamin B_6 is often recommended in the treatment of nausea and vomiting during pregnancy. However, until recently previous studies consisted of open trials and one small double-blind trial. Based on the results of a new study, there is now good clinical data to support this recommendation.[45] In this study, 342 pregnant women (less than 17 weeks gestation) were randomized to receive either 30 milligrams of vitamin B_6 or a placebo in a double-blind fashion. Patients graded the severity of their nausea by a visual analog scale and recorded the number of vomiting episodes over the previous 24 hours before treatment and again during 5 consecutive days on treatment. Compared to the placebo group, the vitamin B_6 group experienced a statistically significant reduction in nausea scores and vomiting episodes. As a result, Vitamin B_6 was recommended as a first-line treatment of nausea and vomiting of pregnancy.

Although the researchers reported a positive effect in the trial, the results were not all that impressive. More than one-third of the patients still experienced vomiting and significant nausea. Perhaps a larger dosage would have been more effective, or perhaps ginger is a better recommendation (alone or in combination with vitamin B_6).

Ginger's antiemetic actions have been studied in hyperemesis gravidum, the most severe form of pregnancy-related nausea and vomiting. This condition usually requires hospitalization. In a double-blind, randomized, cross-over trial, ginger root powder at a dose of 250 milligrams four times a day brought about a significant reduction in both the severity of the nausea and the number of attacks of vomiting in 19 of 27 cases of early pregnancy (less than 20 weeks).[46] These clinical results—along with the safety and the relative small dose of ginger required and the problems (e.g., teratogenicity) with antiemetic drugs in pregnancy—support the use of ginger in nausea and vomiting in pregnancy. This is becoming a well-accepted prescription even in orthodox obstetrical practices. In a 1992 review of current drug therapy during pregnancy published in the medical journal *Current Opinion in Obstetrics and Gynecology* recommended ginger (as well as vitamin B_6) as an effective treatment of early nausea and vomiting of pregnancy.

Osteoporosis

Low levels of vitamin B_6 (as well as folic acid and vitamin B_{12}) may contribute to osteoporosis as a result of an increase in homocysteine. Increased homocysteine concentrations in the blood have been demonstrated in postmenopausal women and are thought to play a role in osteoporosis by interfering with collagen cross-linking leading to a defective bone matrix. Since osteoporosis is known to be a loss of both the organic and inorganic phases of bone, the homocysteine theory is valid because it is one of the few that addresses both factors. A vitamin B_6-deficient diet produces osteoporosis in rats, demonstrating vitamin B_6 plays an important role in bone health.[47]

Premenstrual Syndrome

The first use of vitamin B_6 in the management of cyclical conditions in women was in the successful treatment of depression caused by birth control pills, a condition noted in several studies in the early 1970s. These results led researchers to try to determine the effectiveness of vitamin B$_6$ in relieving PMS symptoms. Since 1975 there have been at least a dozen double-blind clinical trials.[48,49] The majority of these studies demonstrate a positive effect. For example, in one double-blind, cross-over trial, 84 percent of the subjects had a lower symptomatology score during the B$_6$ treatment period.[50] Although PMS has multiple causes, B$_6$ supplementation alone appears to benefit most patients. In another study, 72 percent of 106 affected young women taking 50 milligrams pyridoxine daily for one week prior and during their menstrual periods experienced a reduced premenstrual acne flare-up.[51]

It is important to note however, that not all double-blind studies of vitamin B$_6$ are positive.[48,49] These negative results may be caused by many factors, such as the inability of some women to convert B$_6$ to its active form because of a deficiency in another nutrient (e.g., vitamin B$_2$ or magnesium) that was not supplemented. These results suggest that supplementing pyridoxine by itself may not result in adequate clinical results for all women suffering from this disorder and that some women may have difficulty converting vitamin B$_6$ into its active form, pyridoxal-5-phosphate. To overcome this conversion difficulty, it may be necessary to use a broader-spectrum nutritional supplement or use injectable pyridoxal-5-phosphate.

Dosage Ranges

For most indications the therapeutic dosage of vitamin B$_6$ is 50 to 100 milligrams daily. This dosage level is generally regarded as being safe, even for long-term use. When using dosages greater than 50 milligrams, you should divide it into 50 milligrams dosages throughout the day. A single dosage of 100 milligrams of pyridoxine does not lead to a significant increase in pyridoxal-5-phosphate levels in the blood, indicating that a 50-milligram oral dosage of pyridoxine is about all the liver can handle at once.[52]

Safety Issues

Vitamin B$_6$ is one of the few water-soluble vitamins associated with some toxicity when taken in large doses or moderate dosages for long periods of time. Doses greater than 2,000 milligrams per day can produce symptoms of nerve toxicity (tingling sensations in the feet, loss of muscle coordination, and degeneration of nerve tissue) in some individuals. Chronic intake of dosages greater than 500 milligrams daily can be toxic if taken daily for many months or years.[53] There are also a few rare reports of toxicity occurring at chronic long-term dosages as low as 150 milligrams a day.[54-56] Researchers believe the toxicity is the result of supplemental pyridoxine overwhelming the liver's ability to add a phosphate group to form the active form of vitamin B$_6$ (pyridoxal-5-phosphate). As a result, they speculate that either pyridoxine is toxic to the nerve cells or it actually acts as an antimetabolite by binding to pyridoxal-5-phosphate receptors, thereby creating a relative deficiency of vitamin B$_6$. Again, it appears to make sense to limit dosages to 50 milligrams. If you desire more than 50 milligrams, then spread out the dosages throughout the day.

Interactions

Riboflavin and magnesium are necessary to convert pyridoxine to pyridoxal-5-phosphate. Vitamin B_6 interacts significantly with magnesium and zinc; supplementation with B_6 may increase the intracellular concentrations of these essential minerals.

There are many B_6 antagonists, including food colorings (especially FD&C yellow #5), certain drugs (isoniazid, hydralazine, dopamine, and penicillamine), oral contraceptives, alcohol, and excessive protein intake.

12

Biotin

Biotin is a B vitamin that functions in the manufacture and utilization of fats and amino acids. Without biotin, body metabolism is severely impaired. Since biotin is manufactured in the intestines by gut bacteria, it is not discussed too much. A vegetarian diet alters the intestinal bacterial flora in such a manner as to enhance the synthesis and promote the absorption of biotin.

Food Sources

The best dietary sources of biotin are cheese, organ meats, and soybeans. Good sources are cauliflower, eggs, mushrooms, nuts, peanuts, and whole wheat (see Table 12.1). Raw egg whites contain avidin, a protein that binds biotin and prevents its absorption.

Deficiency Signs and Symptoms

A biotin deficiency in adults is characterized dry, scaly skin; nausea; anorexia; and seborrhea. In infants under six months of age, the symptoms are seborrheic dermatitis and alopecia (hair loss). In fact, the underlying factor for seborrheic dermatitis (cradle cap) in infants appears to be a biotin deficiency.

TABLE 12.1   Biotin Content of Selected Foods, in Micrograms per 3½-oz. (100-g.) Serving

Yeast, brewer's	200	Peanut butter	39	Split peas	18
Liver, beef	96	Walnuts	37	Almonds	18
Soy flour	70	Peanuts, roasted	34	Cauliflower	17
Soybeans	61	Barley	31	Mushrooms	16
Rice bran	60	Pecans	27	Whole-wheat cereal	16
Rice germ	58	Oatmeal	24	Lentils	13
Rice polishings	57	Blackeye peas	21	Brown rice	12

Recommended Dietary Allowance

There is no official RDA for biotin, but the table below reflects safe and adequate recommendations.

Safe and Adequate Recommendations for Biotin

Group	Micrograms
INFANTS	
Under 6 months	10
6–12 months	15
CHILDREN AND ADULTS	
1–3 years	20
4–6 years	25
7–10 years	30
11+ years	30–300

Beneficial Effects

Biotin basically functions in the human body as an essential cofactor for four enzymes. All four of the enzymes are carboxylases, enzymes that add a carbon dioxide molecule to another molecule to form a carboxyl group. Biotin-dependent carboxylases are involved in the metabolism of sugar, fat, and amino acids. Specifically, biotin is involved in the utilization of glucose, the breakdown and utilization of fatty acids in energy metabolism, the removal of the amine group in the metabolism of amino acids, and cell growth and replication.

Available Forms

Biotin is available commercially either as an isolated biotin or as biocytin, a biotin complex from brewer's yeast composed of 65.6 percent biotin.

Principal Uses

Biotin promotes strong nails and healthy hair and aids in the treatment of seborrheic dermatitis and diabetes.

Promotion of Strong Nails and Healthy Hair

Biotin is a popular supplement for increasing the strength of nails and promoting healthy hair. As early as 1940, researchers demonstrated the possibility of an association between deficiency of B-complex vitamins and nail brittleness. More recent research has focused on the role of biotin in this common disorder.

Most of the early research on biotin comes from the veterinary literature. Biotin increases the strength and hardness of hooves in pigs and horses. Recent human studies have shown that biotin supplementation (2,500 micrograms per day) can produce a 25 percent increase in the thickness of the nail plate in patients diagnosed with brittle nails of unknown cause, and up to 91 percent of patients taking this dosage experience definite improvement.[1]

The beneficial effects of biotin on the health of hair possibly reflect an ability to improve the metabolism of scalp oils, much like it works in seborrheic dermatitis.

Seborrheic Dermatitis

Seborrheic dermatitis is a common condition that may be associated with excessive oiliness (seborrhea) and dandruff. The scale of seborrhea may be yellowish and either dry or greasy. The scaly bumps can coalesce to form large plaques or patches. Seborrheic dermatitis usually occurs either in infancy (usually between 2 and 12 weeks of age) or in the middle-aged or elderly and has a prognosis of lifelong recurrence.

In infancy, seborrheic dermatitis is known as cradle cap. As stated above, the underlying factor for cradle cap appears to be a biotin deficiency.[2] Scientists have produced a syndrome clinically similar to seborrheic dermatitis by feeding rats a diet high in raw egg whites (which are high in avidin, a protein that binds biotin, making it unavailable for absorption). Since a large portion of the human biotin supply is provided by intestinal bacteria, some researchers postulate that the absence of normal intestinal flora may be responsible for biotin deficiency in infants.[2] Several case histories demonstrate successful treatment of cradle cap with biotin by either giving it directly to the mother if she is breast-feeding the baby or directly to the infant if she is not.[2,3]

In adults with seborrheic dermatitis, treatment with biotin alone is usually of no value. Some scientists postulate that long-chain fatty acid synthesis is impaired in seborrheic lesions. B-vitamins (biotin, pyridoxine, pantothenic acid, niacin, thiamin, and the lipotropics) are vital for fatty-acid metabolism. Effective treatment of seborrheic dermatitis in adults probably requires all of these necessary B-vitamins.

Diabetes

Biotin supplementation enhances insulin sensitivity and increases the activity of the enzyme glucokinase.[4] Glucokinase is the enzyme responsible for the first step in the utilization of glucose by the liver. Glucokinase concentrations in diabetics are very low. Evidently, supplementing the diet with high doses of biotin improves glucokinase activity and glucose metabolism in diabetics. In one study, supplementation of 16 milligrams of biotin per day resulted in significant lowering of fasting blood sugar levels and improvements in blood glucose control in type I diabetics.[5] In a study in type II diabetics, similar effects were noted with 9 milligrams of biotin per day.[6] High-dose biotin is also very helpful in the treatment of severe diabetic nerve disease (diabetic neuropathy).[7]

Dosage Ranges

As stated above, there is no RDA for biotin. The estimated safe and adequate dietary intake for adults is 30 to 100 micrograms. To promote stronger nails and healthy hair, an effective dosage range would be 1,000 to 3,000 micrograms per day. In the treatment of cradle cap, the dosage to administer to nursing mothers is 3,000 micrograms twice daily. For infants not being breast-fed, an effective dosage is estimated to be 100 to 300 micrograms daily. These infants should also be given *Bifidobacterium bifidum* and fructo-oligosaccharides (FOS) to establish normal gut flora. *Bifidobacterium bifidum* in the presence of FOS is the primary source of biotin production in infants.[8] Most health food stores sell both products. In the treatment of diabetes and diabetic neuropathy, a dosage of 8 milligrams twice daily is recommended.

Safety Issues

Biotin is extremely safe, and no one has reported side effects with biotin supplementation.

Interactions

Biotin works synergistically with other B-vitamins as well as coenzyme Q_{10} and carnitine. Alcohol inhibits the absorption and utilization of biotin. Antibiotics may decrease biotin levels because of destruction of biotin-producing gut bacteria.

13

Pantothenic Acid (Vitamin B₅)
and Pantethine

Pantothenic acid, or vitamin B_5, is utilized in the manufacture of coenzyme A (CoA) and acyl carrier protein (ACP), two compounds that play critical roles in the utilization of fats and carbohydrates in energy production and in the manufacture of adrenal hormones and red blood cells.

A deficiency of pantothenic acid is quite rare in humans because a large number of foods contain pantothenic acid. In fact, its name is derived from the Greek word *pantos*, which means "everywhere." Additional pantothenic acid is often used to support adrenal and joint function while pantethine, the most active stable form of pantothenic acid, is used to lower blood cholesterol and triglyceride levels.

Food Sources

Pantothenic acid is found in highest concentrations in liver and other organ meats, milk, fish, and poultry. Good plant sources of pantothenic acid include whole grains, legumes, sweet potatoes, broccoli, cauliflower, oranges, and strawberries. There is no official RDA for pantothenic acid, but a daily intake of 4 to 7 milligrams is believed to be adequate (see Table 13.1).

TABLE 13.1 Pantothenic Acid Content of Selected Foods, in Milligrams per 3 1/2-oz. (100-g.) Serving

Yeast, brewer's	12.0	Oatmeal, dry	1.5	Hazelnuts	1.1
Yeast, torula	11.0	Buckwheat flour	1.4	Brown rice	1.1
Liver, calf	8.0	Sunflower seeds	1.4	Whole-wheat flour	1.1
Peanuts	2.8	Lentils	1.4	Peppers, red chili	1.1
Mushrooms	2.2	Rye flour, whole	1.3	Avocados	1.1
Soybean flour	2.0	Cashews	1.3	Blackeye peas, dry	1.0
Split peas	2.0	Garbanzos	1.2	Wild rice	1.0
Pecans	1.7	Wheat germ, toasted	1.2	Cauliflower	1.0
Soybeans	1.7	Broccoli	1.2	Kale	1.0

Deficiency Signs and Symptoms

In humans, severe pantothenic acid deficiency is characterized by the "burning foot syndrome." The symptoms consist of numbness and shooting pains in the feet. Perhaps the first sign of pantothenic acid deficiency is fatigue. Healthy men fed a low pantothenic acid diet developed fatigue and listlessness after 2 months.[1]

Recommended Dietary Allowance

There is no official RDA for pantothenic acid, but there is a Safe and Adequate Intakes recommendation.

Safe and Adequate Recommendations for Pantothenic Acid

Group	Milligrams
INFANTS	
Under 6 months	2
6–12 months	3
CHILDREN AND ADULTS	
1–6 years	3–4
7–10 years	4–5
11+ years	4–7

Beneficial Effects

Pantothenic acid as coenzyme A (CoA) and acyl carrier protein (ACP) exerts a beneficial effect on utilization of fats and carbohydrates in energy production and in the manufacture of adrenal hormones and red blood cells. Pantethine, the stable form of pantetheine (the active form of pantothenic acid, but not pantothenic acid) exerts significant cholesterol- and triglyceride-lowering activity.

Available Forms

Pantothenic acid is available most often as calcium pantothenate. The most active and useful form is pantethine.

Principal Uses

Pantothenic acid's principal uses are in the support of adrenal function and rheumatoid arthritis, while pantethine is used to lower blood cholesterol and triglyceride levels.

Adrenal Support

Pantothenic acid is particularly important for optimum adrenal function and has long been considered the "antistress" vitamin because of its central role in adrenal function and cellular metabolism. Nutritionally oriented physicians often recommend pantothenic acid supplementation (usual dosage of 250 milligrams twice daily) to treat allergies. Although there are anecdotal reports of this benefit, no clinical trials exist to disprove or prove this application.

Rheumatoid Arthritis

Some researchers report whole-blood pantothenic acid levels are lower in rheumatoid arthritis patients compared to normal controls.[2] In addition, disease activity was inversely correlated with pantothenic acid levels; i.e., the lower the level of pantothenic acid, the more severe the symptoms. Correction of low pantothenic acid levels to normal brings about some alleviation of symptoms. In one double-blind study, subjective improvement was noted in patients receiving 2 grams of calcium pantothenate daily. Patients noted improvements in duration of morning stiffness, degree of disability, and severity of pain.[3]

High Cholesterol and Triglycerides

For some reason, pantethine has significant lipid-lowering activity, but pantothenic acid has very little (if any) effect in lowering cholesterol and triglyceride levels. Pantethine administration (standard dose 300 milligrams three times daily) reduces significantly serum triglyceride (32 percent), total cholesterol (19 percent), and LDL cholesterol (21 percent) levels while increasing HDL cholesterol (23 percent) levels.[4–11] These effects are most impressive when the safety of pantethine is compared to conventional lipid-lowering drugs. Its mechanism of action is to inhibit cholesterol synthesis and to accelerate the utilization of fat as an energy source.[12,13] There appear to be no toxicity or side effects from pantethine.[4]

Because pantethine is expensive compared to the other natural cholesterol-lowering agents, such as inositol hexaniacinate, I reserve its use for people who have not responded to other natural measures, and diabetics. Several clinical studies show pantethine produces impressive lipid-lowering effects in diabetics with no side effects or deleterious effects on blood sugar control.[14–16]

Pantethine is particularly beneficial for lowering blood lipids in diabetic patients on dialysis. In one study, pantethine administration (900 milligrams per day for 2 months) produced a reduction of total cholesterol (275 versus 231 milligrams per deciliter), very-low-density lipoprotein (VLDL) cholesterol (66 versus 46 milligrams per deciliter), and triglycerides (332 versus 227 milligrams per deciliter at 2 months). Although HDL cholesterol did not change, the total cholesterol/HDL cholesterol ratio decreased significantly.[17]

As a bonus to the diabetic patient, pantethine also improves platelet function through correction of the derangement in cell membrane lipids, a condition characteristic of diabetes.[18–20]

Dosage Ranges

The recommended dosages for B_5 are:

- For general adrenal support and possible benefit in allergies, 250 milligrams of pantothenic acid twice daily
- For rheumatoid arthritis, 2 grams of pantothenic acid daily
- For lowering cholesterol and triglycerides, 300 milligrams of pantethine three times daily

Safety Issues

No significant side effects or adverse reactions have been reported with either pantothenic acid or pantethine.

Interactions

Pantothenic acid works together with carnitine and coenzyme Q_{10} in fatty-acid transport and utilization. There are no known interactions with pantothenic acid and any drug.

14

Folic Acid

Folic acid, also known as folate, folacin, and pteroylmonoglutamate, functions together with vitamin B_{12} in many body processes. It is critical to cellular division because it is necessary in DNA synthesis. Without folic acid, cells do not divide properly. Folic acid is critical to the development of the nervous system of the fetus. Deficiency of folic acid during pregnancy has been linked to several birth defects, including neural tube defects like spina bifida. Folic acid deficiency is also linked to depression, atherosclerosis, and osteoporosis.

Food Sources

Folic acid received its name from the Latin word *folium*, which means "foliage," because it is found in high concentrations in green leafy vegetables like kale, spinach, beet greens, and chard. Other good sources of folic acid include legumes, asparagus, broccoli, cabbage, oranges, root vegetables, and whole grains (see Table 14.1)

TABLE 14.1   Folic Acid Content of Selected Foods, in Micrograms per 3 1/2-oz. (100-g.) Serving

Food	Amount	Food	Amount	Food	Amount
Yeast, brewer's	2,022	Lentils	105	Whole-wheat flour	38
Blackeye peas	440	Walnuts	77	Oatmeal	33
Rice germ	430	Spinach, fresh	75	Cabbage	32
Soy flour	425	Kale	70	Dried figs	32
Wheat germ	305	Filbert nuts	65	Avocado	30
Liver, beef	295	Beet & mustard greens	60	Green beans	28
Soy beans	225	Peanuts, roasted	56	Corn	28
Wheat bran	195	Peanut butter	56	Coconut, fresh	28
Kidney beans	180	Broccoli	53	Pecans	27
Mung beans	145	Barley	50	Mushrooms	25
Lima beans	130	Split peas	50	Dates	25
Navy beans	125	Whole-wheat cereal	49	Blackberries	14
Garbanzos	125	Brussels sprouts	49	Orange	5
Asparagus	110	Almonds	45		

Deficiency Signs and Symptoms

Despite the wide occurrence of folic acid in food, folic acid deficiency is the most common vitamin deficiency in the world. The reason reflects food choices—animal foods, with the exception of liver, are poor sources of folic acid, while plant sources are rich sources but are not as frequently consumed. In addition, alcohol and many prescription drugs like estrogens, sulfasalazine, and barbiturates impair folic acid metabolism, and folic acid is extremely sensitive and easily destroyed by light or heat.[1]

In a folic-acid deficiency, all cells of the body are affected, but it is the rapidly dividing cells like red blood cells and cells of the gastrointestinal and genital tract that are affected the most, resulting in poor growth, diarrhea, anemia, gingivitis, and an abnormal pap smear in women. Other symptoms include depression, insomnia, irritability, forgetfulness, loss of appetite, fatigue, and shortness of breath.[1]

The anemia of either folic-acid or vitamin B_{12}-deficiency is characterized by enlarged red blood cells and is referred to as "macrocytic anemia." However, relying on anemia to demonstrate folic acid deficiency is not advisable The level of folate within the red blood cell (RBC folate) is considered the best assessment of folic acid status, but measuring the level of plasma homocysteine is quickly emerging as an easy and reliable method to determine the status of both vitamin B_{12} and folate. The reason is that in the absence of vitamin B_{12} and folic acid, homocysteine cannot be converted back to methionine. A recent study analyzed the plasma homocysteine, serum cobalamin, and blood folate in 296 consecutive patients who had been referred to a geriatric psychiatric ward in Sweden for diagnosis of mental disease (folic acid and vitamin B_{12} deficiency are common causes of reversible senility).[2] There was a significant correlation between the three tests, indicating that plasma homocysteine is a suitable marker for determining either a vitamin B_{12} or folic acid deficiency. As a side note, folic-acid and vitamin B_{12} supplementation brought down homocysteine levels even in individuals with normal homocysteine values.

Recommended Dietary Allowance

Recommended Dietary Allowance for Folic Acid

Group	Micrograms
INFANTS	
Under 6 months	25
6–12 months	35
CHILDREN	
1–3 years	50
4–6 years	75
7–10 years	100

(continues)

Group	Micrograms
YOUNG ADULTS AND ADULTS	
Males 11–14 years	150
Males 15+ years	200
Females 11–14 years	150
Females 15+ years	180
Pregnant females	400
Lactating females	280

Beneficial Effects

Folic acid, vitamin B_{12}, and a form of the amino acid methionine known as SAM (S-adenosyl-methionine; see Chapter 45) function as "methyl donors." They carry and donate methyl molecules to facilitate reactions, including the manufacture of DNA and brain neurotransmitters.

Much of the benefit of folic acid (along with vitamin B_6 and B_{12}) supplementation is a result of reducing body concentrations of homocysteine, an intermediate in the conversion of the amino acid methionine to cysteine. If a person is relatively deficient in folic acid, he or she experiences an increase in homocysteine. This compound has been implicated in a variety of conditions, including atherosclerosis and osteoporosis. Homocysteine most likely promotes atherosclerosis by directly damaging the artery and reducing the integrity of the vessel wall. In osteoporosis, elevated homocysteine levels lead to a defective bone matrix by interfering with the formation of proper collagen (the main protein in bone).

Available Forms

Folic acid is available as folic acid (folate) and folinic acid (5-methyl-tetra-hydrofolate). In order to utilize folic acid, the body must convert it first to tetrahydrofolate and then add a methyl group to form 5-methyl-tetra-hydrofolate (folinic acid). Therefore, supplying the body with folinic acid bypasses these steps. Folinic acid is the most active form of folic acid and is more efficient at raising body stores than folic acid.[1]

Principal Uses

Folic acid deficiency or supplementation is a factor in the following health conditions:

- Acne
- AIDS
- Anemia

- Atherosclerosis
- Cancer
- Candidiasis
- Canker sores (recurrent)
- Cataract
- Celiac disease
- Cerebrovascular insufficiency
- Cervical dysplasia
- Constipation
- Crohn's disease
- Diarrhea
- Epilepsy
- Fatigue
- Gout
- Hepatitis
- Infertility
- Osteoporosis
- Neural tube defects
- Parkinson's disease
- Periodontal disease
- Restless legs syndrome
- Seborrheic dermatitis
- Senility
- Ulcerative colitis

While folic acid supplementation may prove useful in all these conditions, the principal clinical uses of folic acid supplementation are in the prevention or treatment of neural tube defects, atherosclerosis, osteoporosis, cervical dysplasia, and depression.

Prevention of Neural Tube Defects

Neural tube defects refer to a developmental failure affecting the spinal cord or brain in the embryonic stage of fetal development. Very early in fetal development, there is a ridge of nerve tissue along the back of the embryo. As the fetus develops, this ridge becomes the spinal cord, body nerves, and brain. At the same time, the bones that make up the back gradually surround the spinal cord on all sides. If any part of the development process goes awry, many defects can occur. The worst is total lack of brain (anencephaly). The most common is spina bifida, a defect in which the vertebrae do not form a complete ring to protect the spinal cord. In the United States, approximately one to two babies per 1,000 births have a neural tube defect. Folic acid supplementation (400 micrograms per day) in early pregnancy is projected to reduce the incidence of neural tube defects by 48 percent to 80 percent.

The discovery that folic acid can prevent spina bifida and other neural tube defects has been referred to as one of the greatest discoveries of the last part of the twentieth century. Numerous studies have now demonstrated the benefit of folic acid supplementation beginning either preconception or very early on in the pregnancy and continued throughout.[3,4] The evidence became so overwhelming that the FDA finally had to reverse its previous position, acknowledge the association between folic and neural tube defects, and allow folic acid supplements and high folic acid–containing foods. Now the FDA claims that "Daily consumption of folic acid by women of childbearing age may reduce the risk of neural tube defects."

Concerning this discovery of the link between folic acid deficiency and neural tube defects, I have noticed how long it took for obstetricians and other medical doctors to begin making the recommendation of folic acid supplementation to pregnant women. Once it became "accepted medical practice," however, obstetricians felt they had to do everything possible to make sure that their patients were taking folic acid—presumably to prevent a malpractice suit being filed in the event that a child happened to be born with a neural tube defect.

Although obstetricians and other medical doctors claim the protective effect of folic acid was not known until 1992 (when the U.S. Public Health Service issued a recommendation that all U.S. women of childbearing age capable of becoming pregnant should consume 400 micrograms of folic acid), the fact of the matter is that folic acid deficiency has been linked to neural tube defects for over 30 years. The first double-blind studies showing a protective effect of folic acid supplementation were performed in the early 1980s.[5–8] It makes one wonder how long it will take the medical profession to accept other links of nutritional supplementation in the treatment and prevention of disease.

Atherosclerosis

Elevated homocysteine levels are an independent risk factor for developing a heart attack, stroke, or peripheral vascular disease. Elevations in homocysteine are found in approximately 20 to 40 percent of patients with heart disease.[9,10] It is estimated that folic acid supplementation (400 micrograms daily) alone would reduce the number of heart attacks suffered by Americans each year by 10 percent. Although folic acid supplementation (1 to 2.5 milligrams daily) on its own lowers homocysteine levels in many cases, given the importance of vitamin B_{12} and B_6 to proper homocysteine metabolism it simply makes more sense to use all three together.[11–13]

Osteoporosis

Increased homocysteine concentrations in the blood have been demonstrated in postmenopausal women and probably play a role in osteoporosis by interfering with collagen cross-linking, leading to a defective bone matrix.[14,15] Since osteoporosis is a loss of both the organic and inorganic phases of bone, the homocysteine theory has much validity because it is one of the few that addresses both factors. Folic acid supplementation reduces homocysteine levels in postmenopausal women even though none of the women were deficient in folic acid by standard laboratory criteria.

Cervical Dysplasia

Cervical dysplasia is an abnormal condition of the cells of the cervix. It is generally regarded as a precancerous lesion and has risk factors similar to those of cervical cancer. It is quite probable that many abnormal Pap smears reflect folate deficiency rather than true dysplasia, especially in women who are pregnant or taking oral contraceptives, because estrogens antagonize folic acid.[16–19] Although macrocytic anemia is the most commonly recognized sign of folic acid deficiency, abnormalities in the cervical cells are seen many weeks earlier.[16,17]

Some researchers hypothesize that oral contraceptives interfere with folate metabolism and, although serum levels may be increased, tissue levels of the cervix may be deficient.[18,19] This is consistent with the observation that tissue status, as measured by red blood cell folate levels, is typically decreased (especially in women with cervical dysplasia), while serum levels may be normal or even increased.[19] Oral contraceptives probably stimulate the synthesis of a molecule that inhibits folate uptake by cells.

In clinical studies, folic acid supplementation (10 milligrams per day) results in improvement or normalization of Pap smears in patients with cervical dysplasia.[18–20] The rate of normalization for women with untreated cervical dysplasia is typically 1.3 percent for mild and 0 percent for moderate dysplasia. When patients were treated with folic acid, the regression-to-normal rate was observed to be 20 percent in one study[19] and 100 percent in another[18]. Furthermore, the progression rate of cervical dysplasia in untreated patients is typically 16 percent at 4 months (a figure matched in the placebo group in one study), while none of the folate-supplemented group progressed.[19] All these figures were observed despite the fact that the women remained on the birth control pills.

The average time for progression from cervical dysplasia to carcinoma *in situ* in untreated women ranges from 86 months for patients with very mild dysplasia to 12 months for patients with severe dysplasia, and improvement is very uncommon. Therefore, I would suggest instituting a trial of folate supplementation (along with other considerations discussed) in mild-to-moderate dysplasia, with a follow-up Pap smear and coloscopy at 3 months. Vitamin B_{12} supplementation should always accompany folate supplementation.

Depression

Many psychiatric patients exhibit folic acid deficiency.[21–23] Correction of an underlying folate acid deficiency has brought about remarkable reversal of mental and psychological symptoms in some patients, especially elderly patients suffering from impaired mental function.[21,24–28] Folic acid exerts a mild antidepressant effect,[21] presumably via its function as a methyl donor and increasing the brain content of serotonin, SAM (S-adenosyl-methionine), and BH_4 (tetrahydrobiopterin). I discuss SAM in greater detail in Chapter 45. BH_4 functions as an essential coenzyme in the activation of enzymes that manufacture monoamine neurotransmitters like serotonin and dopamine from their corresponding amino acids. Patients with recurrent depression have reduced BH_4 synthesis, probably as a result of low folic acid or SAM levels. BH_4 supplementation produces dramatic results in these patients.[29,30] Unfortunately, BH_4 is not currently available commercially. However, since folic acid, vitamin B_{12}, and vitamin C stimulate BH_4 synthesis, it is possible that increasing these vitamin levels in the brain may stimulate both BH_4 formation and the synthesis of monoamines like serotonin.[31]

Folic acid supplementation increases methylation reactions in the brain, leading to an increase in the serotonin content of the brain. The serotonin-elevating effects are undoubtedly responsible for much of the antidepressive effects of folic acid and other methyl donors.[32–34] Typically, the dosages used in the clinical studies where folic acid has been used as an antidepressant have been very high—15 milligrams to 50 milligrams. Dosages of folate this high require a doctor's prescription. High-dose folic acid therapy is safe (except in patients with epilepsy) and can be as effective as antidepressant drugs.[21] However, there are other natural measures in this book that yield even better results (SAM).

Dosage Ranges

These are the condition-based dosages I recommend:

- For general health and the prevention of atherosclerosis and osteoporosis, 400 micrograms daily
- For the treatment of cervical dysplasia and depression, 10 milligrams daily.

> Since the FDA restricts the amount of folic acid available in nutritional supplements to 400 micrograms, ask your doctor for a prescription when higher levels are required.

Safety Issues

Folic acid supplementation should always include vitamin B_{12} supplementation (400 to 1,000 micrograms daily) because folic acid supplementation can mask an underlying vitamin B_{12} deficiency. The danger is that while the folic acid reverses the macrocytic anemia, it does not prevent or reverse the neurological symptoms of a vitamin B_{12} deficiency. Nerve damage can result that does not respond to vitamin B_{12} supplementation.

Folic acid is well-tolerated. In high dosages (e.g., 5 to 10 milligrams) it may cause increased flatulence, nausea, and loss of appetite. High dosage folic acid supplementation should be used with extreme caution in epileptics because occasionally it may increase seizure activity.

Interactions

Folic acid works together with vitamin B_{12}, SAM, vitamin B_6, and choline. Oral pancreatic extracts may reduce folic acid absorption, so they should be administered away from folate supplementation.[35]

Estrogens, alcohol, various chemotherapy drugs (especially methotrexate), sulfasalazine (a drug used in the treatment of Crohn's disease and ulcerative colitis), barbiturates, and anticonvulsant drugs all interfere with folic acid absorption or function.

15

Cobalamin (Vitamin B$_{12}$)

Vitamin B$_{12}$, or cobalamin, was isolated from a liver extract in 1948 and identified as the nutritional factor in liver that prevented pernicious anemia, a deadly type of anemia characterized by large, immature red blood cells. Vitamin B$_{12}$ is a bright red crystalline compound because of its high content of cobalt. Vitamin B$_{12}$ works with folic acid in many body processes, including the synthesis of DNA, red blood cells, and the insulation sheath (the myelin sheath) that surrounds nerve cells and speeds the conduction of the signals along nerve cells. In order to absorb the small amounts of vitamin B$_{12}$ found in food, the stomach secretes intrinsic factor, a special digestive secretion that increases the absorption of vitamin B$_{12}$ in the small intestine.

Food Sources

Vitamin B$_{12}$ is found in significant quantities only in animals foods. The richest sources are liver and kidney, followed by eggs, fish, cheese, and meat (see Table 15.1). Strict vegetarians (vegans) are often told that fermented foods like tempeh are excellent sources of vitamin B$_{12}$. However, in addition to tremendous variation of B$_{12}$

TABLE 15.1 Vitamin B$_{12}$ Content of Selected Foods, in Micrograms per 3^{1}/$_{2}$-oz. (100-g.) Serving

Liver, lamb	104.0	Salmon, flesh	4.0	Blue cheese	1.4
Clams	98.0	Tuna, flesh	3.0	Haddock, flesh	1.3
Liver, beef	80.0	Lamb	2.1	Flounder, flesh	1.2
Kidneys, lamb	63.0	Eggs	2.0	Scallops	1.2
Liver, calf	60.0	Whey, dried	2.0	Cheddar cheese	1.0
Kidneys, beef	31.0	Beef, lean	1.8	Cottage cheese	1.0
Liver, chicken	25.0	Edam cheese	1.8	Mozzarella cheese	1.0
Oysters	18.0	Swiss cheese	1.8	Halibut	1.0
Sardines	17.0	Brie cheese	1.6	Perch, filets	1.0
Trout	5.0	Gruyère cheese	1.6	Swordfish, flesh	1.0

content in fermented foods, some evidence indicates that the form of B_{12} in these foods is not exactly the form that meets our body requirements and is therefore useless. The same holds true of certain cooked sea vegetables. Although the vitamin B_{12} content of these foods is in the same range as beef, scientists do not know how well our bodies utilize this form. Therefore, at this time I would recommend that vegetarians supplement their diets with vitamin B_{12}.

Deficiency Signs and Symptoms

Unlike other water-soluble nutrients, vitamin B_{12} is stored in the liver, kidney, and other body tissues. As a result, signs and symptoms of vitamin B_{12} deficiency may not show themselves until 5 to 6 years of poor dietary intake or inadequate secretion of intrinsic factor. The classic deficiency symptom of vitamin B_{12} deficiency is pernicious anemia. However, a deficiency of vitamin B_{12} actually affects the brain and nervous system first.

A vitamin B_{12} deficiency results in impaired nerve function, which can cause numbness, pins-and-needles sensations, or a burning feeling. It can also cause impaired mental function that in the elderly mimics Alzheimer's disease. Vitamin B_{12} deficiency is thought to be quite common in the elderly and is a major cause of depression in this age group.

In addition to anemia and nervous system symptoms, a vitamin B_{12} deficiency can also result in a smooth, beefy red tongue and diarrhea. This occurs because rapidly reproducing cells such as those that line the mouth and entire gastrointestinal tract cannot replicate without vitamin B_{12}. Folic acid supplementation masks this deficiency symptom.

Measuring the level in the blood (serum cobalamin) or the level of methylmalonic acid in the urine is the best method to determine vitamin B_{12} deficiency. In addition, measuring the level of plasma homocysteine is emerging as a method to determine the status of both vitamin B_{12} and folate. Another test, the Schilling test, is used determine whether there is sufficient output of intrinsic factor. The test involves oral administration of radioactive vitamin B_{12} and then measuring the level excreted in the urine. Below-normal urinary excretion of the vitamin suggests impaired absorption because of lack of intrinsic factor.

Several investigators have found the level of vitamin B_{12} declines with age and that vitamin B_{12} deficiency is found in 3 to 42 percent of persons aged 65 and over. Physicians should attempt to diagnose cobalamin deficiency early in the elderly because it is easily treatable and, if left untreated, can lead to impaired neurological and cognitive function.[1,2]

Researchers recently studied 100 consecutive geriatric outpatients who were seen in office-based settings for various acute and chronic medical illnesses; none of these outpatients presented symptoms of vitamin B_{12} deficiency-related diseases like pernicious anemia. In this group, 11 patients had serum cobalamin levels at 148 pmol/L (picomole per liter) or below, 30 patients had levels between 148 and 295 pmol/L, and 59 patients had levels above 296 pmol/L. After the initial cobalamin determination, the subjects were followed for up to 3 years. The patients with cobalamin levels below 148 pmol/L were treated and were not included in the analysis of declining cobalamin levels. The average annual serum cobalamin level decline was 18 pmol/L for patients who had higher initial serum cobalamin levels (actual range, from 224 to 292 pmol/L). For patients with lower initial cobalamin levels, the average annual serum cobalamin decline was much higher at 28 pmol/L.[3]

These results indicate that in the elderly the following screen tests for vitamin B$_{12}$ have a high cost-to-benefit ratio:[4,5]

- Level of vitamin B$_{12}$ in the blood (serum cobalamin)
- Urinary excretion of methylmalonic acid
- Level of homocysteine

Of these three tests, the urinary methylmalonic acid assay is perhaps the best test because it is sensitive, noninvasive, and relatively convenient for the patient. Correction of an underlying vitamin B$_{12}$ deficiency improves mental function and quality of life in these patients quite significantly.

Recommended Dietary Allowance

Recommended Dietary Allowance of Cobalamin (Vitamin B$_{12}$)

Group	Micrograms
INFANTS	
Under 6 months	0.3
6–12 months	0.5
CHILDREN	
1–3 years	0.7
4–6 years	1.0
7–10 years	1.4
YOUNG ADULTS AND ADULTS	
11+ years	2.0
Pregnant females	2.2
Lactating females	2.1

Beneficial Effects

Vitamin B$_{12}$, like folic acid, function as a "methyl donor." A methyl donor is a compound that carries and donates methyl groups (a molecule of one carbon and three hydrogen molecules) to other molecules, including cell membrane components and neurotransmitters. As a methyl donor, vitamin B$_{12}$ is involved in homocysteine metabolism and plays a critical role in proper energy metabolism, immune function, and nerve function.

Homocysteine is a factor in the progression of both atherosclerosis and osteoporosis. In fact, elevations in homocysteine are an independent risk factor for having a heart attack. Approximately 20 to 40 percent of patients with heart disease exhibit elevations in homocysteine [6,7] In addition to vitamin B_{12} and folic acid, vitamin B_6 is also necessary in metabolizing homocysteine to nondamaging forms. Although research has focused much of its attention on folic acid supplementation as a mechanism to lower homocysteine levels, the prevalence of suboptimal levels of these nutrients in men with elevated homocysteine levels was 56.8 percent for B_{12}, 59.1 percent for folic acid, and 25 percent for B_6, indicating that folic acid supplementation alone would not lower homocysteine levels in many cases.[8] Folic acid supplementation lowers homocysteine levels only if there are adequate levels of vitamin B_{12} and B_6. Because of the interconnectedness of these three B vitamins, it is best to supplement with all three.[8] Folic acid and vitamin B_{12} supplementation lowers homocysteine levels even in individuals with normal vitamin B_{12}, folic acid, and homocysteine levels.[9]

Available Forms

Vitamin B_{12} is available in several forms. The most common form is cyanocobalamin; however, vitamin B_{12} is active in only two forms, methylcobalamin and adenosylcobalamin. Methylcobalamin is the only active form of vitamin B_{12} available commercially in tablet form in the United States. While methylcobalamin is active immediately upon absorption, cyanocobalamin must be converted to either methylcobalamin or adenosylcobalamin by the body to remove the cyanide molecule (the amount of cyanide produced in this process is extremely small) and add either a methyl or adenosyl group. Cyanocobalamin is not active in many experimental models, and neither methylcobalamin or adenosylcobalamin demonstrate exceptional activity. For example, in a model examining the ability of vitamin B_{12} to extend life in mice with cancer, methylcobalamin and adenosylcobalamin led to significant increases in survival time, but cyanocobalamin had no effect.[10] Methylcobalamin also produces better results in clinical trials than cyanocobalamin. I consider it the best available form.

Oral versus Injectable

Although it is popular to inject vitamin B_{12}, injection is not necessary. The oral administration of an appropriate dosage, even in the absence of intrinsic factor, results in effective elevations of vitamin B_{12} in the blood. Most physicians have ignored this fact. An editorial entitled "Oral Cobalamin for Pernicious Anemia, Medicine's Best Kept Secret," which appeared in the January 2, 1991, edition of *JAMA* (*Journal of the American Medical Association*) states that oral therapy produces reliable and effective treatment, even in severe cases of pernicious anemia.[11]

In the United States, physicians rarely use oral vitamin B_{12} therapy despite the fact that it is fully (100 percent) effective in the long-term treatment of pernicious anemia.

Let's first discuss the data showing effectiveness with oral administration before discussing the dogma cited for injectable administration.

Almost as soon as scientists isolated vitamin B$_{12}$ in 1948, companies introduced an injectable form. Researchers busily sought an oral alternative. They tried oral preparations containing intrinsic factor, but some patients developed antibodies against intrinsic factor and, therefore, would not respond.[12] Other studies soon documented that a small but constant proportion of an oral dose of cyanocobalamin was absorbed without intrinsic factor through the process of diffusion; therefore, by sufficiently increasing the dose, they could obtain adequate absorption.[13,14]

Early studies show that pernicious anemia could be completely controlled with doses of cyanocobalamin in the range of 300 to 1,000 micrograms daily.[15-18] The largest of these studies described 64 Swedish patients with pernicious anemia (and other vitamin B$_{12}$–deficiency states) who were treated with 1,000 micrograms oral cyanocobalamin daily.[17,18] In all patients studied over a 3 year period, the researchers observed complete normalization of serum levels and liver stores for vitamin B$_{12}$ as well as full clinical remission.

Despite this research, physicians in the United States do not use oral vitamin B$_{12}$ therapy. Why? Education and bias. Medical texts first state that oral vitamin B$_{12}$ therapy of pernicious anemia is "unpredictable," has poor patient compliance, and is more costly. Then after establishing this bias against oral therapy, they state that oral cobalamin is effective and can be used when injection therapy is problematic. In a survey of internists, 91 percent erroneously believed that vitamin B$_{12}$ could not be absorbed in sufficient quantities without intrinsic factor. Interestingly, 88 percent of these doctors also stated that an effective oral vitamin B$_{12}$ therapy would be useful in their practice and further stated that it would be their preferred method of delivery if it was effective. Let's reassure these doctors by answering the concerns regarding oral therapy.[11]

Is Oral Vitamin B$_{12}$ Therapy Unpredictable?

No, not at an effective dosage. Some of the very early studies with oral B$_{12}$ therapy used only 100 to 250 micrograms daily. These reports led to the U.S. Pharmacopeia Anti-Anemia Preparations Advisory Board in 1959 to caution against oral therapy for pernicious anemia because it was "at best, unpredictably effective."[19] However, based upon what we now know about oral vitamin B$_{12}$ pharmacokinetics, we consider the response to these low doses to be predictable. Research has now established that the mean absorption rate of oral cyanocobalamin by patients with pernicious anemia is 1.2 percent across a wide range of dosages.[17] Since the daily turnover rate is about 2 micrograms, an oral dosage of 100 to 250 micrograms daily results in a mean absorption of 1.2 to 3 micrograms, respectively—a dosage sufficient for many but not all patients. Higher dosages are necessary for most patients to benefit from oral therapy.

How high must the dosage be to produce predictable improvements? In a study of 64 patients taking 500 micrograms of oral cyanocobalamin daily, the lowest absorption rate was 1.8 micrograms.[17] Because this level is slightly less than the 2 micrograms daily turnover rate, it is an insufficient dosage in some cases. Therefore, the dosage of 1,000 micrograms daily is the most popular recommendation. However, even though 1,000 micrograms daily is effective, to rapidly replenish stores in the first month of treatment I recommend a dosage of 2,000 micrograms.

Does Oral Vitamin B_{12} Lead to Poor Patient Compliance?

No. The concern about patient compliance cited by the medical texts is irrational. Why is vitamin B_{12} singled out from any other oral therapy? It simply does not make any sense, especially since studies with oral cobalamin show excellent compliance. In many cases the compliance is higher with an oral preparation because many patients prefer taking a pill rather than getting a shot.[14,17]

Does Oral Vitamin B_{12} Cost More Than Injectable Vitamin B?

No way! The two forms, injectable and oral, do not differ that much in the cost of the vitamin B_{12} itself. The fee to administer the vitamin B_{12} injection (anywhere from $20 in a private practice to $100 in a nursing home) results in the injectable form being considerably more expensive.

Conclusions: Oral versus Injectable

There is absolutely no basis for the dogma that vitamin B_{12} must be administered by injection to produce clinical benefit. In the treatment of pernicious anemia, most medical texts recommend 1,000 milligrams weekly for 8 weeks, then once a month for life. For oral vitamin B_{12}, the recommended dosage is 2,000 micrograms daily (14,000 micrograms weekly) for at least 1 month, followed by a daily intake of 1,000 milligrams of vitamin B_{12}. Methylcobalamin is preferred over cyanocobalamin.

Principal Uses

Vitamin B_{12} supplementation is appropriate in many conditions, including AIDS, impaired mental function in the elderly, asthma and sulfite sensitivity, depression, diabetic neuropathy, low sperm counts, multiple sclerosis, and tinnitus.

AIDS

Ten to 35 percent of all patients who are seropositive for the human immunodeficiency virus (HIV) have vitamin B_{12} deficiency, presumably as a result of either decreased B_{12} intake, reduced absorption, or antagonism by the drug AZT.[20,21] As serum cobalamin levels decline, progression to AIDS increases and neurological symptoms worsen. In one study, researchers followed 59 asymptomatic HIV seropositive patients over a two-and-one-half-year period. Serum B_{12} levels, CD4 (helper T-cells) count, and clinical progression to AIDS or AIDS-related complex (ARC) were measured.[22] Twelve of the 59 patients progressed to AIDS or ARC. Nine of these patients had repeat serum B_{12} levels prior to progression. All nine patients had or developed falling serum B_{12} levels without any evidence of HIV-related bowel disorder. All patients progressing also had falling CD4 counts. This study indicates that serum vitamin B$_{12}$ levels may serve as a surrogate marker for HIV progression. Malabsorption of B$_{12}$ might be the reason for the drop in B$_{12}$ levels and also implies other nutrients are not being absorbed. Given the importance of maintaining good nutritional status to the immune system, if serum vitamin B$_{12}$ levels are low it may signify overall nutritional status is quite poor—a harbinger to further impairment of immune status and progression to AIDS.

In addition, vitamin B$_{12}$ (cyanocobalamin, methylcobalamin, and adenosylcobalamin) can inhibit HIV replication *in vitro*. Because the body is able to achieve high blood and tissue levels of vitamin B$_{12}$ without toxicity, vitamin B$_{12}$ therapy for HIV infection holds great promise.[23]

Alzheimer's Disease and Impaired Mental Function in the Elderly

Impaired mental function in the elderly (senility) is often a result of reversible nutritional factors. Unfortunately, physicians rarely seek out these nutritional solutions in the majority of the elderly who suffer from senility and other psychological disturbances. Two of the most common nutrient deficiencies in the elderly are folate and vitamin B$_{12}$. Deficiencies of either of these two nutrients can result in significant mental disturbances without evidence of anemia or other signs of deficiency. This fact highlights the mistaken reliance by many physicians on the presence of anemia to diagnose vitamin B$_{12}$ deficiency. In addition, changes in the blood cells may never occur even though a severe deficiency exists in the brain and other tissues. Despite these facts, most physicians are often reluctant to investigate vitamin B$_{12}$ and folate levels when there is no apparent anemia. However, in any case of impaired mental function or depression in the elderly, it is absolutely essential that physicians test for serum homocysteine, urinary methylmalonic acid, or serum cobalamin and red blood cell folate levels.[1,2]

A recent study in Sweden analyzed the plasma homocysteine, serum cobalamin, and blood folate in 296 consecutive patients referred to a geriatric psychiatric ward for diagnosis of mental disease This study demonstrates the importance of detailed examination in elderly patients with mental symptoms.[24] Patients who were deficient in vitamin B$_{12}$ or folic acid, or who had elevated levels of homocysteine, were given vitamin B$_{12}$ (dosage not specified) and/or folic acid (10 milligrams per day). When individuals with low cobalamin levels were supplemented with vitamin B$_{12}$, researchers noted significant clinical improvements.

In other studies, supplementation with vitamin B$_{12}$ shows tremendous benefit in reversing impaired mental function as a result of low levels of vitamin B$_{12}$.[1] In one larger study, a complete recovery was observed in 61 percent of cases of mental impairment because of low levels of vitamin B$_{12}$.[25] The reason why 39 percent did not respond is probably a result of long-term low levels of vitamin B$_{12}$. Several studies indicate the best clinical responders are those who have been showing signs of impaired mental function for less than 6 months.[1] In one study, 18 subjects with low serum cobalamin levels and evidence of mental impairment were given vitamin B$_{12}$.

Only those patients who had symptoms less than 1 year showed improvement.[26] I cannot overstate the importance of diagnosing and correcting low vitamin B_{12} levels in the elderly.

Alzheimer's disease patients have significantly low serum vitamin B_{12} levels and vitamin B_{12} deficiency.[27-29] Supplementation of B_{12} and/or folic acid may result in complete reversal in some patients, but generally there is little improvement in patients who have had Alzheimer's symptoms for greater than 6 months. Some scientists hypothesize that prolonged low levels of vitamin B_{12} may lead to irreversible changes that do not respond to supplementation.

Asthma and Sulfite Sensitivity

Jonathan Wright, M.D., states "B_{12} therapy is the mainstay in childhood asthma."[30] In one clinical trial, weekly intramuscular injections of 1,000 micrograms of vitamin B_{12} produced definite improvement in asthmatic patients. Of 20 patients, 18 showed less shortness of breath on exertion and improvement in appetite, sleep, and general condition.[31] Vitamin B_{12} appears to be especially effective in sulfite-sensitive individuals. It offers the best protection when given orally prior to challenge and demonstrates better results than several drugs, including cromolyn.[32] The mode of action is the formation of a sulfite-cobalamin complex, which blocks sulfite's effect. Oral supplementation with 1 to 3 milligrams of vitamin B_{12} daily may provide a benefit similar to that provided by the injectable form.

Depression

Vitamin B_{12} deficiency can cause depression, especially in the elderly.[33-35] Correcting an underlying vitamin B_{12} deficiency results in a dramatic improvement in mood. One of the key brain compounds necessary for methylation is tetrahydrobiopterin (BH_4). This compound functions as an essential coenzyme in the activation of enzymes that manufacture monoamine neurotransmitters like serotonin and dopamine from their corresponding amino acids. Patients with recurrent depression have reduced BH_4 synthesis, possibly as a result of low vitamin B_{12} levels. BH_4 supplementation produces dramatic results in these patients.[36,37] Unfortunately, BH_4 is not currently available commercially. However, since folic acid and vitamin B_{12} stimulate BH_4 synthesis, it is possible that increasing these vitamin levels in the brain may stimulate BH_4 formation.[38]

Diabetic Neuropathy

Physicians have used vitamin B_{12} supplementation with some success in treating diabetic neuropathy.[39-43] It is not clear if this is because of the correcting of a deficiency state or the normalization of the deranged vitamin B_{12} metabolism seen in diabetics.[44] Clinically, diabetic neuropathy is very similar to that of classical vitamin B_{12} deficiency. Although the best results have been obtained with injectable methylcobalamin, higher dosages (e.g., 1.5 to 2.0 milligrams per day) of methylcobalamin given orally may produce the same results.[41-43]

Low Sperm Counts

Since vitamin B_{12} is critically involved in cellular replication, a deficiency leads to reduced sperm counts and sperm motility. Even in the absence of a vitamin B_{12} deficiency, supplementation is worthwhile in men with sperm counts less than 20 million per milliliter or a motility rate of less than 50 percent. In one study, 27 percent of men with sperm counts less than 20 million given 1,000 micrograms per day of vitamin B_{12} achieved a total count in excess of 100 million.[45] In another study, 57 percent of men with low sperm counts given 6,000 micrograms per day demonstrated improvements.[46]

Multiple Sclerosis

Acquired deficiency of vitamin B_{12} and inborn errors of metabolism involving B_{12} are well-known causes of demyelination of nerve fibers in the central nervous system (CNS). Multiple sclerosis is another cause of demyelination within the CNS. The medical literature reports in several places that vitamin B_{12} levels in serum, red blood cells, and CNS are low in multiple sclerosis. The coexistence of a vitamin B_{12} deficiency in MS may aggravate the disease or promote another cause of progressive demyelination.[47–49]

Recently, researchers in Japan sought to clarify the state of vitamin B_{12} metabolism in 24 Japanese patients with MS and determine if vitamin B_{12} in massive doses provided any therapeutic benefit in 6 patients with chronic progressive MS.[50] The researchers first measured serum vitamin B_{12} levels and unsaturated vitamin B_{12}–binding capacities. Results indicated that the level of vitamin B_{12} in the serum was normal but that there was a significant decrease in the unsaturated vitamin B_{12}–binding capacities in the patients with MS, which indicated a defect in the transport of vitamin B_{12} into cells. In other words, the doors were locked for B_{12}.

The second phase of the study also provided some interesting results. In 6 patients with severe chronic progressive MS, the oral administration of 60 milligrams per day of vitamin B_{12} (methylcobalamin) improved both visual and brainstem auditory-evoked potentials by nearly 30 percent. Motor function did not improve, indicating that afferent pathways benefit from vitamin B_{12} while efferent pathways do not.

The results produced are on par with those produced by the combination of high-dose intravenous cyclophosphamide plus steroids. However, while this drug combination is associated with profound immunosuppression and toxicity, no side effects have been attributed to high doses of vitamin B_{12}.

The researchers in this study used the methylcobalamin form of vitamin B_{12} rather than the standard cyanocobalamin. Hydroxocobalamin was tried in an earlier MS study with no apparent benefit.[51] Methylcobalamin is the main form in the body and is directly related to the function of vitamin B_{12} in methylation reactions. Thus, methylcobalamin may be the superior form of vitamin B_{12} to use in MS.

Tinnitus

Vitamin B_{12} is involved in stabilizing neural activity. It is an essential cofactor for methylation of myelin basic protein and cell membrane phospholipids. Vitamin B_{12}

deficiency results in neurological pathology because of demyelination, axonal degeneration, and neuronal death. Because of the essential role of vitamin B_{12} in neurological function, researchers recently attempted to determine the incidence of vitamin B_{12} deficiency in three groups of noise-exposed subjects: those with chronic tinnitus and noise-induced hearing loss, those with noise-induced hearing loss only, and those with normal hearing.[52] Patients with tinnitus and noise-induced hearing loss demonstrated vitamin B_{12} deficiency in 47 percent of the cases. This hearing loss was significantly more than the group with noise-induced hearing loss only (27 percent) and the group with normal hearing (19 percent).

These results suggest a relationship between vitamin B_{12} deficiency and auditory dysfunction. The fact that vitamin B_{12} supplementation results in some improvement in tinnitus and associated complaints offers further support. Determination of vitamin B_{12} status is therefore warranted in patients with chronic tinnitus and noise-induced hearing loss.

Dosage Ranges

Vitamin B_{12} is necessary in only very small quantities—the RDA is 2 micrograms. For oral vitamin B_{12}, the recommended dosage in deficiency states is 2,000 micrograms daily for at least 1 month, followed by a daily intake of 1,000 micrograms. This dosage schedule is suitable for other clinical applications of vitamin B_{12} except high-dose therapy for MS. For vegetarians, I recommend a dosage of at least 100 micrograms per day. Methylcobalamin, the active form of vitamin B_{12}, supplied in sublingual tablets is preferred over cyanocobalamin.

Safety Issues

No one has ever reported clear toxicity from vitamin B_{12}.

Interactions

Vitamin B_{12} and folic acid are intricately involved in chemical processes. Since vitamin B_{12} works to reactivate folic acid, a deficiency of B_{12} results in a folic acid deficiency if folic acid levels are only marginal. A high intake of folic acid may mask a vitamin B_{12} deficiency because it prevents the changes in the red blood cells but does not counteract the deficiency in the brain.

Vitamin B_{12} also influences melatonin secretion.[53] The low levels of melatonin in the elderly may be a result of low vitamin B_{12} status. Vitamin B_{12} (1.5 milligrams of methylcobalamin per day) produces good results in the treatment of sleep-wake rhythm disorders, presumably as a result of improving melatonin secretion.[54]

16

Choline

Choline is essential in the manufacture of the important neurotransmitter acetylcholine and main components of our cell membranes, such as phosphatidylcholine (lecithin) and sphingomyelin. Choline is also required for the proper metabolism of fats. Without choline, fats become trapped in the liver, where they block metabolism. Although choline can be manufactured in humans from either the amino acid methionine or serine, it has recently been designated an essential nutrient.[1,2]

Food Sources

Choline is found in grains, legumes, and egg yolks primarily as lecithin (phosphatidylcholine) and as free choline in vegetables (especially cauliflower and lettuce), whole grains, liver, and soy (see Table 16.1). It is estimated that the average American consumes approximately 6 grams of phosphatidylcholine in the diet each day. However, whether or not the phosphatidylcholine is promoting health depends upon its composition of essential fatty acids. Phosphatidylcholine is composed of a phosphate group, 2 fatty acids, and choline. When phosphatidylcholine is ingested, most of it is broken down into choline, glycerol free fatty acids, and the phosphate group, rather than being incorporated intact into cellular membranes.

Deficiency Signs and Symptoms

When animals eat a choline-deficient diet, they develop liver and kidney disorders. However, no one had considered choline an essential nutrient for humans, primarily because for many years no one had tried to feed a choline-deficient diet to humans and observe the effects. A recent study demonstrates that humans fed a choline-deficient diet develop fatty infiltration of the liver and other signs of liver dysfunction. Choline is an essential nutrient for human cells in cell cultures, and humans receiving intravenous feeding with solutions low in choline develop signs of choline deficiency.[1,2] Both of these facts support the role of choline as an essential nutrient.

TABLE 16.1 Choline and Choline Phospholipid Content of Selected Foods, in Milligrams per Serving

Food	Free Choline	Lecithin	Total Choline
Apple (1 medium)	0.39	29.87	4.62
Banana (1 medium)	2.85	3.26	3.52
Beef liver (3.5 oz.)	60.64	3,362.55	532.28
Beef steak (3.5 oz.)	0.78	466.12	68.75
Butter (1 tsp.)	0.02	6.80	1.18
Cauliflower (1/2 cup)	6.79	107.06	22.15
Corn oil (1 tbsp.)	0.004	0.13	0.03
Coffee (6 oz.)	18.59	2.05	19.29
Cucumber (1/2 cup)	1.18	3.06	1.74
Egg (1 large)	0.22	2009.80	282.32
Ginger ale (12 oz.)	0.07	1.11	0.34
Grape juice (6 oz.)	8.99	2.11	9.37
Human milk (1 cup)	2.10	27.08	10.29
Iceberg lettuce (1 oz.)	8.53	2.86	9.06
Infant formula (1 oz.)	0.818	2.97	1.38
Lecithin supplement (commercial, powdered; 1 tbsp., 7.5 g.)	NA	1725	250
Margarine (1 tsp.)	0.02	1.74	0.26
Milk (whole, 1 cup)	3.81	27.91	9.64
Orange (1 medium)	2.91	53.03	10.40
Peanut butter (2 tbsp.)	12.96	97.39	26.09
Peanuts (1 oz.)	13.24	107.35	27.91
Potato (1)	5.95	25.97	9.75
Tomato (1)	5.50	4.94	6.58
Whole wheat bread (1 slice)	2.52	6.57	3.43

Beneficial Effects

Choline, like vitamin B_{12}, S-adenosylmethionine, and folic acid, acts in the human body as a "methyl donor." As a methyl donor, choline is essential for proper liver function. Specifically, it is required for the export of fat from the liver, or lipotropic effect.

Choline supplementation also increases the accumulation of acetylcholine within the brain. Acetylcholine is an important brain chemical utilized in many brain processes, including memory. There is some evidence that increasing acetylcholine content in the brain through supplemental choline results in improved memory, especially in Alzheimer's patients.[1]

Available Forms

Choline is available as a soluble salt (most commonly as either choline bitartrate, citrate, or chloride) or as phosphatidylcholine in lecithin. Most commercial lecithin contains only 10 to 20 percent phosphatidylcholine, while most "phosphatidyl-choline" supplements contain only 35 percent. There are newer preparations now available containing up to 98 percent phosphatidylcholine. Ideally these are the preparations that should be used since they are associated with fewer side effects (anorexia, nausea, abdominal bloating, gastrointestinal pain and diarrhea are associated with high doses of lecithin). Some clinical conditions require large doses of phosphatidylcholine (i.e., 15 to 30 grams); therefore, 100 grams of a preparation containing only 25 percent phosphatidylcholine would be necessary in order to be effective. However, this is not feasible because of the side effects noted above and the expense of the supplement.

Principal Uses

Choline supplementation, primarily as phosphatidylcholine, is used in the treatment of liver disorders, elevated cholesterol levels, Alzheimer's disease, and bipolar depression.

Liver Disorders

In Germany, manufacturers market phosphatidylcholine (tradename Essentiale) for treatment of the following liver disorders:

- Acute viral hepatitis
- Alcohol-induced fatty liver
- Chronic hepatitis
- Cirrhosis of the liver
- Decreased bile solubility
- Diabetic fatty liver
- Drug-induced liver damage
- Toxic liver damage

Good clinical data supports these applications, which have received proper authorization from the BGA, the German equivalent of the FDA. The phosphatidylcholine preparation used is of high quality (90 percent phosphatidylcholine with 50 percent of the molecule having the essential fatty acid, linoleic acid, bound at the proper position; i.e., the first and second carbon of the glycerol molecule). Similar products are available in United States health-food stores. The standard dosage recommendation is 350 milligrams three times daily with meals.[3]

Phosphatidylcholine supplementation also protects against alcohol-induced liver abnormalities and cirrhosis in baboons, and presumably it exerts the same effects in humans. While phosphatidylcholine may help in alcohol-induced liver disease, choline salts do not seem to be of any value in the treatment of alcohol-induced liver disease in humans but may be useful in general liver support.[4]

Elevated Cholesterol Levels

Phosphatidylcholine has many important functions in the body, including increasing the solubility of cholesterol, which decreases its ability to induce atherosclerosis. Phosphatidylcholine also aids in lowering cholesterol levels, removing cholesterol from tissue deposits, and inhibiting platelet aggregation.[5] Much of the benefit of phosphatidylcholine supplementation may be a result of its high content of linoleic acid.

In Germany, another approved high-quality phospholipid preparation (Lipostabil) is used in the treatment of high cholesterol levels and atherosclerosis. In 15 clinical trials ranging in length from 1 to 12 months, treatment with phosphatidylcholine lowered total serum cholesterol by 8.8 percent to 28.2 percent and triglyceride levels by an average of 25 percent; it increased HDL cholesterol levels by 13.4 percent to 20 percent. The typical dosage was 1.5 to 2.7 grams daily.[6]

In the most recent published study, 32 patients with elevated cholesterol and triglyceride levels were given a 70 percent phosphatidylcholine content lecithin product at a dosage of 3.5 grams three times daily before meals. After 30 days of treatment, total cholesterol dropped an average of 33 percent, triglycerides dropped 33 percent, and HDL cholesterol levels increased by 46 percent.[7]

Alzheimer's Disease

Alzheimer's disease is characterized by the general destruction of nerve cells in several key areas of the brain that are devoted to mental functions. This destruction results in neurofibrillary tangles and plaque formation. Scientists believe the disease's clinical features are related to a decrease in acetylcholine (which functions as a transmitting agent in the brain), although there is a general reduction in the concentration of all neurotransmitting substances.

Because phosphatidylcholine can increase acetylcholine levels in the brain in normal patients, and because Alzheimer's disease is characterized by a decrease in cholinergic transmission, it seems reasonable to assume that phosphatidylcholine supplementation would benefit Alzheimer patients. However, the basic defect in cholinergic transmission in Alzheimer's disease relates to impaired activity of the enzyme acetylcholine transferase. This enzyme combines choline (provided by phosphatidylcholine) with an acetyl molecule to form acetylcholine, the neurotransmitter. Since more choline does not necessarily increase the activity of this key enzyme, phosphatidylcholine supplementation is not beneficial in the majority patients with Alzheimer's disease. Not surprising, clinical trials using phosphatidylcholine are largely disappointing. Studies show inconsistent improvements in memory from choline supplementation in both normal and Alzheimer's patients.[8–10] However, some scientists have criticized the studies for small sample size, low dosage of phosphatidylcholine, and poor design.

In a patient with mild to moderate dementia, the use of a high-quality phosphatidylcholine preparation may be worth a try. A dosage of 15 to 25 grams daily of phosphatidylcholine is required. If there is no noticeable improvement within 2 weeks, supplementation should be halted.

Bipolar Depression

Bipolar depression, also referred to as "manic depression," is a disorder characterized by periods of major depression alternating with periods of elevated mood. If the elevated mood is relatively mild and lasts for 4 days or less, it is referred to as hypomania. Mania is longer and more intense.

Phosphatidylcholine supplementation (15 to 30 grams a day) brings good results in the treatment of bipolar depression.[11-13] Some researchers believe Lithium, the standard drug treatment for bipolar depression, promotes increased brain acetylcholine activity.[14] There is evidence that mania is associated with a reduced brain cholinergic activity. The use of phosphatidyl choline to increase brain choline levels may result in significant improvement or amelioration of symptoms in some patients.

Dosage Ranges

The dosage (three times daily with meals) of a lecithin product with 90 percent phosphatidylcholine is:

- For the treatment of liver disorders, 350 to 500 milligrams
- For lowering cholesterol, 500 to 900 milligrams
- For the treatment of Alzheimer's disease and bipolar depression, 5,000 to 10,000 milligrams

Safety Issues

Choline and phosphatidylcholine are generally well tolerated. At higher dosages, phosphatidylcholine preparations may cause a reduced appetite, nausea, abdominal bloating, gastrointestinal pain, and diarrhea. Choline at high dosages (e.g., 20 grams) produces a "fishy" odor. Phosphatidylcholine is not indicated in patients with depression (unipolar or clinical depression) unless under the supervision of a physician because high-dosage phosphatidylcholine supplementation can worsen depression in some cases.

Interactions

Choline works together with other methyl donors and helps the body conserve carnitine and folic acid.[15,16]

17

Inositol

Inositol, an "unofficial" member of the B vitamins, functions quite closely with choline; it too is a primary component of cell membranes. Inositol exists in cell membranes as phosphatidylinositol. Although inositol is not essential in the human diet, it exerts some beneficial effects, especially in cases of liver disorders, depression, and diabetes.

Food Sources

Inositol is present mainly as a fiber component known as phytic acid (inositol phosphate). The action of intestinal bacteria liberates inositol from phytic acid. It is available in animal foods as myo-inositol. Good plant sources include citrus fruits, whole grains, nuts, seeds, and legumes. The average daily intake of inositol by Americans is roughly 1,000 milligrams daily.

Deficiency Signs and Symptoms

No deficiency states have been assigned to inositol.

Beneficial Effects

Inositol, like choline, exerts a "lipotropic" effect. This means it promotes export of fat from the liver. This action is critical to the health of the liver because stagnation of fat and bile is associated with the development of more serious liver disorders like cirrhosis. Inositol is also necessary for proper nerve, brain, and muscle function.

Phytic acid demonstrates impressive anticancer effects and may be one of the key reasons why a high-fiber diet protects against so many cancers.[1]

Available Forms

Inositol is available commercially as inositol monophosphate.

Principal Uses

Inositol is used primarily in the treatment of liver disorders, depression and panic disorders, and diabetes.

Liver Disorders

Many practitioners of nutritional medicine use inositol as a component in lipotropic formulas in the treatment of a wide range of liver disorders. The effectiveness of inositol in this application has not been studied.

Depression and Panic Attacks

Inositol is required for the proper action of several brain neurotransmitters, including serotonin and acetylcholine. A reduction of brain inositol levels may induce depression, as evidenced by low inositol levels in the cerebrospinal fluid of patients with depression.

In a 1-month, double-blind, placebo-controlled study of 28 patients with depression, inositol or a placebo was given at a dosage of 12 grams per day.[2] The group receiving the inositol demonstrated therapeutic results (e.g., reduction in the Hamilton Depression Scale) similar to tricyclic antidepressant drugs, but without the side effects. Another double-blind study confirmed the antidepressant effects of inositol.[3] Based on the positive results of these studies, inositol therapy may prove quite useful in the clinical management of depression.

Because of inositol's effect on depression, a study was designed to test its effectiveness against panic disorder.[4] Twenty-one patients with panic disorder (with or without agoraphobia) completed a double-blind crossover treatment trial of 12 grams per day of inositol for 4 weeks. The frequency and severity of panic attacks and the severity of agoraphobia declined significantly more with inositol than with placebo administration. The authors conclude that inositol's efficacy, absence of significant side effects, and role as a natural component of the human diet make it a potentially attractive therapeutic for panic disorder.

Diabetes

Inositol shows some promise in diabetic neuropathy, a nerve disease caused by diabetes. Diabetic neuropathy is the most frequent complication of long-term diabetes. Much of the decreased nerve function is because of loss of inositol from the nerve cell. Inositol supplementation may improve nerve conduction velocities in diabetics but should not be relied upon as the sole therapy.[5]

Dosage Ranges

The daily dosages of inositol are:

- For general liver support, 100 to 500 milligrams daily
- For depression or panic disorder, 12 grams
- For the treatment of diabetes, 1,000 to 2,000 milligrams

Safety Issues

Inositol supplementation is not associated with any side effects.

Interactions

Inositol works together with other methyl donors. No other interactions are known.

PART THREE

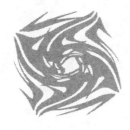

Minerals

At least 18 minerals are important in human nutrition. Along with vitamins, they function as components of body enzymes. Our bodies need minerals for proper composition of bones and blood and for maintenance of normal cell function. The minerals are classified into two categories, major and minor. On a daily basis, our bodies require more than 100 milligrams of major minerals and less than 100 milligrams of minor minerals. The major minerals are calcium, phosphorus, potassium, sodium, chloride, magnesium, and sulfur. The minor, or trace minerals, are boron, chromium, copper, iodine, iron, manganese, molybdenum, selenium, silicon, vanadium, and zinc.

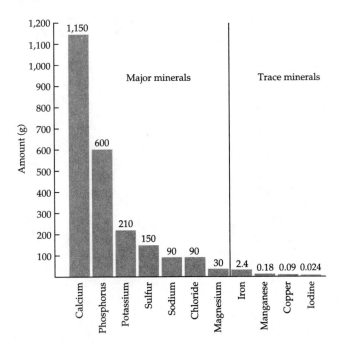

Total body mineral content.

18

Calcium

Calcium is the most abundant mineral in the body. It makes up 1.5 to 2 percent of the total body weight, and the bones contain more than 99 percent of the body's calcium. In addition to its major function in building and maintaining bone and teeth, calcium is important in much of the body's enzyme activity. The contraction of muscles, release of neurotransmitters, regulation of heart beat, and the clotting of blood all depend on calcium.

Food Sources

The primary source of calcium is dairy products. Plant foods rich in calcium include tofu, kale, spinach, turnip greens, and other green leafy vegetables (see Table 18.1). Calcium from spinach is poorly absorbed, but kale is an excellent source of absorbable calcium.[1] In fact, the rate of calcium absorption from kale is superior to that of milk. Since ounce for ounce kale is higher in calcium than milk, it is a good alternative. Other members of the cabbage family (turnip, collard, and mustard) are as beneficial as kale.

Deficiency Signs and Symptoms

Calcium deficiency in children may lead to rickets, which results in bone deformities and growth retardation. In adults, calcium deficiency may result in osteomalacia (softening of the bone). Extremely low blood levels of calcium may result in muscle spasms and leg cramps. Low calcium intake also contributes to high blood pressure, osteoporosis, and colon cancer.

TABLE 18.1   Calcium Content of Selected Foods, in Milligrams per 3 1/2-oz. (100-g.) Serving

Kelp	1,093	Yogurt	120	Black currant	60
Cheddar cheese	750	Wheat bran	119	Dates	59
Carob flour	352	Whole milk	118	Green snap beans	56
Dulse	296	Buckwheat, raw	114	Globe artichoke	51
Collard leaves	250	Sesame seeds, hulled	110	Prunes, dried	51
Kale	249	Olives, ripe	106	Pumpkin/squash seeds	51
Turnip greens	246	Broccoli	103	Beans, cooked dry	50
Almonds	234	English walnuts	99	Common cabbage	49
Yeast, brewer's	210	Cottage cheese	94	Soybean sprouts	48
Parsley	203	Soybeans, cooked	73	Wheat, hard winter	46
Dandelion greens	187	Pecans	73	Orange	41
Brazil nuts	186	Wheat germ	72	Celery	41
Watercress	151	Peanuts	69	Cashews	38
Goat's milk	129	Miso	68	Rye grain	38
Tofu	128	Romaine lettuce	68	Carrot	37
Figs, dried	126	Apricots, dried	67	Barley	34
Buttermilk	121	Rutabaga	66	Sweet potato	32
Sunflower seeds	120	Raisins	62	Brown rice	32

SOURCE: U.S.D.A., Nutritive Value of American Foods in Common Units, Agriculture Handbook No. 456.

Recommended Dietary Allowance

Recommended Dietary Allowance for Calcium

Group	Milligrams
INFANTS	
Under 6 months	400
6–12 months	600
CHILDREN	
1–3 years	800
4–6 years	800
7–10 years	800
YOUNG ADULTS AND ADULTS	
Males 11–24 years	1,200
Males 25+ years	800
Females 11–24 years	1,200
Females 24+ years	800
Pregnant females	1,200
Lactating females	1,200

Beneficial Effects

Calcium builds healthy bones and may serve as a protective factor against high blood pressure and colon cancer.

Available Forms

Several studies indicate some calcium supplements may contain substantial amounts of lead. Lead is a toxic metal that primarily affects the brain, kidney, and red blood cell manufacture. Lead toxicity is a significant problem in industrialized countries like the United States. The level of lead in the body is directly linked to IQ and criminal behavior. The higher the lead level, the lower the IQ and the greater the risk for delinquent or criminal behavior. Lead is a major problem in children. In 1988 the United States Agency for Toxic Substances and Disease Registry estimated that more than 3 million children younger than 12 (17 percent of all children in this age group) had unacceptably high-lead blood levels.

In 1981, the FDA cautioned the public to limit its intake of calcium supplements derived from dolomite or bone meal because of the potentially high lead levels in these calcium supplements. However, recent studies show that other calcium sources, such as carbonate and various chelates, may also contain high amounts of lead.

To determine the extent of the lead problem in calcium supplements, researchers measured the lead level in 70 brands of calcium supplements. The results indicated lead content is still a major concern in some calcium supplement forms. They divided 70 brands into five categories:

- Refined calcium carbonate produced in a laboratory (n=17)
- Unrefined calcium carbonate derived from limestone or oyster shells (n=25)
- Calcium bound to various organic chelates like citrate, gluconate, lactate, etcetera (n=13)
- Dolomite (n=9)
- Bone meal (n=6)[2]

Here are the results (micrograms of lead per 800 milligrams of calcium):

- Refined calcium carbonate, 0.92
- Calcium chelate, 1.64
- Dolomite, 4.17
- Unrefined calcium carbonate, 6.05
- Bone meal, 11.33

None of the dolomite and bone meal products and only 2 out of 25 of the unrefined calcium carbonate products had lead levels below the recommended level of 1 microgram per 800 milligrams of calcium. The unrefined calcium carbonate group displayed the greatest range of lead content; although two products contained very little lead, most contained higher levels, one product containing a whopping 25 micrograms of lead per 800 milligrams of calcium.

Because the total tolerable daily lead intake for children 6 years and under is less than 6 micrograms, young children should use refined calcium carbonate or chelated calcium products for supplementation. Chelated calcium, especially calcium citrate, is better absorbed than calcium carbonate; therefore, products that feature a calcium bond to citrate, gluconate, or some other organic molecule are best. The same is true for older children and adults as well.

Avoid natural oyster shell calcium, dolomite, and bone meal products unless the manufacturer provides reasonable assurance that lead levels are negligible. Although refined calcium carbonate has the lowest lead content, the body absorbs calcium chelates more efficiently.

The absorption of calcium depends somewhat on the calcium becoming ionized in the intestines. Calcium ionization is a major problem with calcium carbonate, the most widely used calcium supplement. In order for calcium carbonate to be absorbed it must first be solubilized and ionized by stomach acid.

Studies with postmenopausal women show that about 40 percent of the women studied are severely deficient in stomach acid.[3] Patients with insufficient stomach acid output can only absorb about 4 percent of a calcium carbonate oral dose, but a person with normal stomach acid can typically absorb about 22 percent.[4] Patients with low stomach acid secretion need a form of calcium already in a soluble and ionized state, like calcium citrate, calcium lactate, or calcium gluconate. Patients with reduced stomach acid absorb about 45 percent of the calcium from calcium citrate compared to 4 percent absorption for calcium carbonate.[4]

This difference in absorption clearly demonstrates that ionized soluble calcium is more beneficial than insoluble calcium salts like calcium carbonate in patients with reduced stomach acid secretion. Calcium is also more bioavailable from calcium citrate than from calcium carbonate in normal subjects.[5,6] Calcium citrate and other soluble forms (lactate, aspartate, orotate, etcetera) are the best supplements available for optimal absorption.

Some researchers express concern that increased calcium supplementation may result in increased calcium oxalate kidney stones. Calcium citrate appears to bypass this justifiable concern. Although urinary calcium rises in patients consuming calcium citrate, some of citrate's effects inhibit the formation of kidney stones. Specifically, citrate can reduce urinary saturation of calcium oxalate and calcium phosphate and retard the nucleation and crystal growth of calcium salts. In clinical studies, potassium or sodium citrate ceases recurrent calcium oxalate kidney stone formation in nearly 90 percent of the subjects.[7,8] While the use of noncitrate calcium supplements may increase the risk of developing calcium oxalate kidney stones, it greatly reduces the risk of calcium overload.

In addition to citrate, other Krebs cycle intermediates (compounds utilized in the Krebs cycle, a major energy producing cycle in cells) such as fumarate, malate, succinate, and aspartate can be used in combination with citrate. Generally, over 95 percent of the Krebs cycle intermediates citrate ingested is used in the production of energy, with the remainder being excreted in the urine. Thus the Krebs cycle intermediates fulfill all the requirements of an optimum calcium chelating agent; namely, they are:

- Easily ionized
- Almost completely degraded
- Without toxicity
- Helpful in increasing the absorption of calcium and other minerals

Principal Uses

Calcium supplementation is used primarily in the treatment of osteoporosis, high blood pressure, and pregnancy.

Osteoporosis

Osteoporosis literally means "porous bone." It affects more than 20 million people in the United States. Normally, both sexes experience a decline in bone mass after 40, but women are at much greater risk for osteoporosis. Many factors result in excessive bone loss—and different variants of osteoporosis exist—but postmenopausal osteoporosis is its most common form. Approximately one in four postmenopausal women has osteoporosis.

Although the entire skeleton may be involved in postmenopausal osteoporosis, bone loss is usually greatest in the spine, hips, and ribs. Since these bones bear a great deal of weight, they are then susceptible to pain, deformity, or fracture. At least 1.5 million fractures occur each year as a direct result of osteoporosis. Two hundred fifty thousand of these are hip fractures, which are catastrophic fractures for many sufferers. Hip fractures are fatal in 12 to 20 percent of the cases and precipitate long-term nursing care for half the survivors. Nearly one-third of all women and one-sixth of all men will fracture their hips in their lifetimes.

Major Risk Factors for Osteoporosis in Women

There are several conditions that predispose women to osteoporosis. Some of them are:

- Postmenopause
- White or Asian
- Premature menopause
- Positive family history
- Short stature and small bones
- Leanness
- Low calcium intake
- Inactivity

- Nulliparity (never pregnant)
- Gastric or small-bowel resection
- Long-term corticosteroid therapy
- Long-term use of anticonvulsants
- Hyperparathyroidism
- Hyperthyroidism
- Smoking
- Heavy alcohol use

Osteoporosis involves both the mineral (inorganic) and the nonmineral (organic matrix composed primarily of protein) components of bone. This means osteoporosis is more than a lack of dietary calcium. In fact, lack of dietary calcium in the adult results in a separate condition known as osteomalacia or "softening of the bone," where there is only a deficiency of calcium in the bone. In contrast, the bones in osteoporosis sufferers lack calcium and other minerals, and there is a decrease in the nonmineral framework (organic matrix) of bone. This organic matrix plays an important role in maintaining bone structure.

Calcium Metabolism

Bone is dynamic living tissue constantly being broken down and rebuilt, even in adults. Normal bone metabolism depends on an intricate interplay of many nutritional and hormonal factors. The liver and kidney also have a regulatory effect. Although over 24 nutrients are necessary for optimal bone health, calcium and vitamin D are the most important factors. However, in women hormones play an essential role because estrogen aids in the incorporation of calcium into bone.

Hormonal Factors

The concentration of calcium in the blood is strictly maintained within very narrow limits. If blood calcium levels start to decrease, the parathyroid glands increase the secretion of parathyroid hormone, and the thyroid and parathyroid glands decrease the secretion of calcitonin. If blood calcium levels start to increase, the secretion of parathyroid hormone and calcitonin increases. Understanding how these hormones increase (parathyroid hormone) and decrease (calcitonin) serum calcium levels is necessary in order to understand osteoporosis.

Parathyroid hormone increases serum calcium levels primarily by increasing the activity of the cells that break down bone (osteoclasts). It also decreases the excretion of calcium by the kidneys and increases the absorption of calcium in the intestines. In the kidneys, parathyroid hormone increases the conversion of $25\text{-}OHD_3$ to $1,25\text{-}(OH)_2D_3$.

Here is one of the theories that relate bone loss to estrogen deficiency. Estrogen deficiency causes the cells that break down bone (osteoclasts) to be more sensitive to parathyroid hormone. This results in increased bone breakdown, which in turn raises blood calcium levels. The elevation in blood calcium leads to a decreased parathyroid hormone level, which causes diminished levels of active vitamin D and increased calcium excretion. Evidence supports this theory as the most solid explanation.[9–11]

Dietary Considerations in Maintaining Healthy Bones

There is an incredible push to increase dietary calcium and take calcium supplements to prevent osteoporosis. While this is sound medical advice, that is not necessarily the case. Osteoporosis is more than a lack of dietary calcium. It is a complex condition involving hormonal, lifestyle, nutritional, and environmental factors. A comprehensive plan that addresses these factors offers the greatest protection against developing osteoporosis.

The primary goals of diet in the treatment and prevention of osteoporosis are:

- To preserve adequate mineral mass
- To prevent loss of the protein matrix and other structural bone components
- To assure optimal repair mechanisms for remodeling damaged areas of bone

Many general dietary factors have been suggested as a cause of osteoporosis—low calcium, high phosphorus intake; high-protein diet; high-acid/ash diet; trace mineral deficiencies to name a few. To help slow down bone loss, foods high in calcium are often recommended.

A vegetarian diet (both lacto-ovo and vegan) is associated with a lower risk of osteoporosis.[12,13] Although bone mass in vegetarians does not differ significantly from omnivores in the third, fourth, and fifth decades, there are significant differences in the later decades. The decreased incidence of osteoporosis in vegetarians is not because of increased initial bone mass, however, but rather to decreased bone loss.

Several factors may be responsible for this decrease in bone loss in vegetarians, the most probable of which is lowered protein intake. High-protein and high-phosphate diets are associated with increased excretion of calcium in the urine. Raising daily protein from 47 to 142 grams doubles the excretion of calcium in the urine.[14] A diet this high in protein is common in the United States and may be a significant factor in the increased number of people suffering from osteoporosis here.

Refined sugar is another dietary factor that increases calcium loss from the body. After sugar intake, the urinary excretion of calcium increases.[15] Each day, the average American consumes 150 grams of sucrose plus other refined simple sugars, and a glass of carbonated beverage loaded with phosphates. No wonder so many women suffer from osteoporosis in this country. When we take lifestyle factors into consideration, we understand why osteoporosis is a major medical problem.

Prevention and Treatment with Calcium Supplements

Calcium supplementation helps reduce bone loss in postmenopausal women.[16,17] Menopausal and postmenopausal women are often told that without hormone replacement therapy they will definitely develop osteoporosis. A recent study proves the inaccuracy of this commonly held view.

In the study, 118 healthy, white women who had experienced the onset of menopause within 3 to 6 years randomly received either 1,700 milligrams of calcium carbonate, a placebo, or Premarin along with 1,700 milligrams of calcium.[18] The nearly 3-year study indicated that calcium supplementation alone significantly prevented bone loss. Although the calcium alone was less effective than the Premarin-calcium combination, calcium supplementation carries with it no significant health risks; therefore, hormone replacement therapy should be reserved for women at significant risk for osteoporosis. Women who have already experienced bone loss should be placed on Fosamax, a prescription drug.[19] Using a more absorbable form of calcium like calcium citrate or calcium bound to other Krebs cycle intermediates may have provided even greater benefit than calcium carbonate because of enhanced absorption.

Most studies that document the benefits of calcium supplementation for the prevention and treatment of postmenopausal osteoporosis have been relatively short-term. This does not mean calcium supplementation produces only short-term benefits. It means continued calcium supplementation produces long-term benefits. A recent double-blind study supports this theory.

Eighty-six postmenopausal women participated in the 4-year study.[20] The women received either 1 gram of elemental calcium (from an effervescent form containing 5.24 grams calcium-lactate-gluconate and 0.8 grams calcium carbonate) or a placebo of an identical effervescent tablet containing sucrose. Clinical status, calcium intake, physical activity, and bone mineral density were assessed at baseline and every 6 months. The results of the study indicated continued calcium supplementation produces a sustained reduction in the rate of loss of total bone mineral density in healthy postmenopausal women. As a result, the incidence of bone fractures was far lower in the group taking calcium.

Many experts recommend a daily calcium intake of 1,500 milligrams to prevent osteoporosis. This amount usually requires dietary supplementation in the range of 1,000 to 1,200 milligrams daily. Calcium citrate is the best form to supplement because of better absorption and decreased risk of kidney stone development.

High Blood Pressure

Population studies suggest a link between blood pressure and dietary intake of calcium.[21] However, the association is not as strong as that for magnesium and potassium. In addition to epidemiological data, several clinical studies demonstrate calcium supplementation can lower blood pressure in hypertension. The results, however, are inconsistent.[21-29]

To clarify the effectiveness of calcium supplementation in patients with hypertension, researchers recently performed a double-blind, placebo-controlled, crossover study on 46 patients with either salt-sensitive or salt-resistant high blood pressure.[30] During the calcium supplementation phase, patients received 1.5 grams of calcium (as calcium carbonate) per day for 8 weeks. The results of the study indicate that calcium supplementation can produce effective blood pressure reduction in Blacks and salt-sensitive hypertension patients but not in salt-resistant hypertension patients. Given the safety and possible benefit of calcium supplementation in the treatment of high blood pressure, it is certainly worth a try. Another study achieved better results with calcium citrate than with calcium carbonate.[31]

Elderly hypertensives also respond to calcium supplementation. One study used 24-hour blood-pressure monitoring to evaluate the effect of calcium supplementation on mild to moderate essential hypertension in elderly hospitalized patients. The mean systolic and diastolic blood pressure over a 24-hour period declined by 13.6 millimeters of mercury and 5.0 millimeters of mercury, respectively, in patients whose diet was supplemented with 1 gram of elemental calcium.[32]

Pregnancy

Calcium might have a role in preventing the development of pregnancy-induced hypertension and preeclampsia (a serious condition of pregnancy associated with elevations in blood pressure, fluid retention, and loss of protein in the urine). Observational studies in pregnant women suggest an inverse association between calcium intake and incidence of hypertensive disorders of pregnancy; when calcium intake is high, the incidence of hypertensive disorders decreases. Results from calcium supplementation trials support this finding.[33–36]

In a study published in the *New England Journal of Medicine* in 1991, 1194 pregnant women who were in their 20th week at the study's beginning randomly received either 2 grams of elemental calcium in the form of calcium carbonate daily (593 women) or a placebo (601 women).[35] The rates of hypertensive disorders of pregnancy were lower in the calcium group than in the placebo group. The risk of these disorders was lower at all times during pregnancy, but particularly after the 28th week. The researchers concluded "Pregnant women who receive calcium supplementation after the 20th week of pregnancy have a reduced risk of hypertensive disorders of pregnancy."[35]

Calcium supplementation can lower blood pressure in pregnancy-induced blood pressure. In one double-blind study, calcium supplementation (1,000 milligrams per day) had a significant lowering effect on diastolic blood pressure in pregnant women with high blood pressure.[36]

Given the nutritional importance of calcium and its possible role in reducing pregnancy-induced hypertension and preeclampsia, calcium supplementation (along with magnesium, folic acid, and many other nutrients) during pregnancy is indicated.

Dosage Ranges

Dosage range for supplementation generally reflects the RDA. The current RDA for calcium is 1,000 milligrams daily for adults. Preadolescent, growing children may need even more than an adult—1,200 milligrams per day. During pregnancy and lactation, the RDA is also 1,200 milligrams daily.

Safety Issues

Calcium supplements are generally well tolerated at dosages less than 2,000 milligrams. Higher dosages may increase the risk for kidney stones and soft-tissue calcification;

however, neither of these conditions is linked conclusively to calcium supplementation. In general, when there is an excess influx of calcium the body reduces calcium absorption and increases both urinary excretion of calcium and calcium utilization by bone and other tissues. Patients with hyperparathyroidism and cancer should not take calcium unless under a physician's direct supervision.

Interactions

Calcium interacts with many nutrients, especially vitamin D, vitamin K, and magnesium. High dosages of magnesium, zinc, fiber, and oxalates negatively affect calcium absorption. Caffeine, alcohol, phosphates, protein, sodium, and sugar increase calcium excretion. Aluminum-containing antacids ultimately lead to an increase in bone breakdown and calcium excretion.

19

Magnesium

Magnesium is second to potassium in terms of concentration within the body's cells. Its primary function is enzyme activation. Approximately 60 percent of the magnesium in the body is in bone, 26 percent in muscle, and the remainder in soft tissue and body fluids. However, the tissues with the highest magnesium concentration are those that are the most metabolically active (brain, heart, liver, and kidney)—thus magnesium's critical role in energy production. Although calcium supplementation gets the headlines, magnesium supplementation may be far more important for many people.

The RDA for magnesium is 350 milligrams per day for adult males and 280 milligrams per day for adult females. The human body contains approximately 21 to 28 grams of magnesium, 60 percent of which is in the bone. The rest of the body's magnesium is in cells.

Food Sources

The average intake of magnesium by healthy adults in the U.S. ranges between 143 and 266 milligrams per day. This level is obviously well below the RDA. Food choices are the main reason. Since magnesium occurs abundantly in whole foods, many nutritionists and dietitians assume most Americans get enough magnesium in their diets. Most Americans, however, do not eat whole, natural foods; they consume large quantities of processed foods. Because food processing refines out a very large portion of magnesium, most Americans do not get the RDA for magnesium.

The best dietary sources of magnesium are tofu, legumes, seeds, nuts, whole grains, and green leafy vegetables (see Table 19.1). Fish, meat, milk, and most commonly eaten fruits are quite low in magnesium. Most Americans consume a low magnesium diet because their diets are high in refined foods, meat, and dairy products.

Deficiency Signs and Symptoms

Magnesium deficiency is extremely common in Americans, particularly in the geriatric population and in women during the premenstrual period. Deficiency is often

TABLE 19.1 Magnesium Content of Selected Foods, in Milligrams per 3 1/2-oz. (100-g.) Serving

Kelp	760	Soybeans, cooked	88	Potato with skin	34
Wheat bran	490	Brown rice	88	Crab	34
Wheat germ	336	Figs, dried	71	Banana	33
Almonds	270	Apricots, dried	62	Sweet potato	31
Cashews	267	Dates	58	Blackberry	30
Molasses, blackstrap	258	Collard leaves	57	Beets	25
Yeast, brewer's	231	Shrimp	51	Broccoli	24
Buckwheat	229	Corn, sweet	48	Cauliflower	24
Brazil nuts	225	Avocado	45	Carrot	23
Dulse	220	Cheddar cheese	45	Celery	22
Filberts	184	Parsley	41	Beef	21
Peanuts	175	Prunes, dried	40	Asparagus	20
Millet	162	Sunflower seeds	38	Chicken	19
Wheat grain	160	Common beans, cooked	37	Green pepper	18
Pecan	142	Barley	37	Winter squash	17
English walnuts	131	Dandelion greens	36	Cantaloupe	16
Rye	115	Garlic	36	Eggplant	16
Tofu	111	Raisins	35	Tomato	14
Coconut meat, dry	90	Green peas, fresh	35	Milk	13

secondary to factors that reduce absorption or increase secretion of magnesium, such as high calcium intake, alcohol, surgery, diuretics, liver disease, kidney disease, and oral contraceptive use.

Low levels of magnesium in the diet and in our bodies increase susceptibility to a variety of diseases, including heart disease, high blood pressure, kidney stones, cancer, insomnia, PMS, and menstrual cramps. Signs and symptoms of magnesium deficiency are fatigue, mental confusion, irritability, weakness, heart disturbances, problems in nerve conduction and muscle contraction, muscle cramps, loss of appetite, insomnia, and predisposition to stress.

Low magnesium levels are common in the elderly, but most cases go unnoticed because most physicians rely on serum magnesium levels to indicate magnesium levels. Most of the body's magnesium store lies within cells, however, not in the serum (noncellular portion of blood). A low magnesium level in the serum reflects end-stage deficiency. A more sensitive test of magnesium status is the level of magnesium within the red blood cell (erythrocyte magnesium level).

Some of the conditions associated with or causing magnesium deficiency are:

- Acute pancreatitis
- Congestive heart failure
- Dietary deficiency
- Digitalis toxicity
- Excessive sweating

- Impaired intestinal absorption
  - Chronic diarrhea
  - Ileal resection
  - Malabsorption syndromes
- Increased magnesium loss through the kidneys
  - Diuretic use
  - Diabetes
  - Antibiotics
  - Alcohol
  - Hyperthyroidism
  - Kidney disease

Recommended Dietary Allowance

Recommended Dietary Allowance for Magnesium

Group	Milligrams
INFANTS	
Under 6 months	40
6–12 months	60
CHILDREN	
1–3 years	80
4–6 years	120
7–10 years	170
YOUNG ADULTS AND ADULTS	
Males 11–14 years	270
Males 15–18 years	400
Males 19+ years	350
Females 11–14 years	280
Females 15–18 years	300
Females 19+ years	280
Pregnant females	320
Lactating females	280

Beneficial Effects

Magnesium is critical to many cellular functions, including energy production, protein formation, and cellular replication. Magnesium participates in more than 300 enzymatic reactions in the body, in particular those processes involved in energy production (i.e., production of ATP). Magnesium is also required for the activation of the sodium and potassium pump that pumps sodium out of, and potassium into, the cells. Therefore, magnesium deficiency results in decreased intracellular potassium. As a result of lower magnesium and potassium within the cell, cell function is greatly disrupted.

Magnesium has been referred to as "nature's calcium channel-blocker" because of its ability to block the entry of calcium into vascular smooth-muscle cells and heart muscle cells. As a result, magnesium supplementation can help reduce vascular resistance, lower blood pressure, and lead to more efficient heart function. Magnesium also helps regulate proper calcium metabolism through its actions on several hormones including parathyroid hormone and calcitonin.

Available Forms

Magnesium is available in several different forms. In general, all forms are equally absorbed. However, I prefer magnesium bound to aspartate or the Krebs cycle intermediates (malate, succinate, fumarate, and citrate) instead of magnesium oxide, gluconate, sulfate, and chloride. Absorption studies indicate that magnesium is easily absorbed orally, especially when bound to citrate (and presumably aspartate and other members of the Krebs cycle).[1,2] In addition, magnesium bound to aspartate or Krebs cycle intermediates may also help fight off fatigue. Aspartate feeds into the Krebs cycle, the final common pathway for the conversion of glucose, fatty acids, and amino acids into chemical energy (ATP). Citrate, fumarate, malate, and succinate are actual components of the Krebs cycle. Evidence suggests that minerals chelated to the Krebs cycle intermediates are better absorbed, utilized, and tolerated than inorganic or relatively insoluble mineral salts—including magnesium chloride, oxide, or carbonate. In addition, while inorganic magnesium salts often cause diarrhea at higher dosages, organic forms of magnesium generally do not.

> In my clinical practice, I prefer using a balanced mineral formula rather than isolated mineral chelates. When any single mineral is taken at high dosages, it can impair the absorption of other important minerals. To achieve the recommended level of magnesium, for example, I first check its value in the patient's multiple vitamin and mineral formula. If the level of magnesium is below his or her needs, I prescribe a multiple mineral formula to achieve the proper levels of magnesium rather than simply prescribe additional magnesium. However, there are some cases where I use additional magnesium or products containing primarily magnesium. Examples of these cases include angina, congestive heart failure, migraine headaches, and recurrent kidney stones. In all these conditions, I prefer using magnesium bound to Krebs cycle intermediates.

Principal Uses

Magnesium supplementation is effective treatment for a large number of health conditions. While some studies utilize injectable magnesium therapy, others demonstrate that injectable magnesium is not necessary to restore magnesium status (except in the case of an emergency situation such as an acute heart attack or acute asthma attack).[3] Oral magnesium therapy is an effective measure to raise body magnesium stores. It usually takes 6 weeks to achieve significant elevations in tissue magnesium concentrations.

These are some conditions which benefit from magnesium supplementation:

- Asthma and chronic obstructive pulmonary disease
- Cardiovascular disease
- Acute myocardial infarction
- Angina
- Cardiac arrhythmias
- Cardiomyopathy
- Congestive heart failure
- High blood pressure
- Intermittent claudication
- Low HDL-cholesterol levels
- Mitral valve prolapse
- Stroke
- Diabetes
- Eosinophilia-myalgia syndrome
- Fatigue
- Fibromyalgia
- Glaucoma
- Hearing loss
- Hypoglycemia
- Kidney stones
- Migraine
- Osteoporosis
- Pregnancy (toxemia, premature delivery, and other complications)
- Premenstrual syndrome and dysmenorrhea

Asthma and Chronic Obstructive Pulmonary Disease (COPD)

Asthma and COPD are characterized by constriction of the bronchial airways. Magnesium promotes relaxation of the bronchial smooth muscles; as a result, airways open and breathing is easier. Intravenous magnesium (2 grams of magnesium sulfate infused every hour up to a total of 24.6 grams magnesium sulfate) is a well-proven and clinically accepted measure to halt acute asthma attacks and acute exacerbations of COPD. Unfortunately long-term oral magnesium supplementation has not been fully evaluated in the treatment of asthma or COPD.[4-8]

Cardiovascular Disease

Magnesium is absolutely essential in the proper functioning of the entire cardiovascular system. Magnesium's critical role in preventing heart disease and strokes is now widely accepted. In addition, a substantial body of knowledge demonstrates that magnesium supplementation is effective in treating a wide range of cardiovascular diseases. Magnesium supplementation has been used in many of these applications for over 50 years![8-11]

Acute Myocardial Infarction

Acute myocardial infarction is the medical term for a heart attack. People dying of a heart attack have lower heart magnesium levels than people of the same age dying from other causes. Intravenous magnesium therapy is a valued treatment measure in acute myocardial infarction (MI).[12-14] The major obstacle to its acceptance as the preferred method of saving a person's life is financial interests. Magnesium is cheap compared to the new, high-tech, high-priced, genetically engineered drugs currently being promoted by drug companies. The treatment of acute myocardial infarctions is a big business in the United States. Each year in the U.S. over 1.5 million Americans experience an acute MI. Many other parts of the world now use magnesium therapy in an acute MI because of its effectiveness, low cost, safety, and ease of administration. In the U.S., however, it plays second fiddle to the high-tech drugs.

During the past decade, eight well-designed studies involving over 4,000 patients have demonstrated the benefits of intravenous magnesium supplementation during the first hour of hospital admission for acute MI. Such supplementation produces a favorable effect in reducing immediate and long-term complications and death rates.[12-14]

The beneficial effects of magnesium in an acute MI relate to its ability to:

- Improve energy production within the heart
- Dilate the coronary arteries, which results in improved delivery of oxygen to the heart
- Reduce peripheral vascular resistance, which creates reduced demand on the heart
- Inhibit platelets from aggregating and forming blood clots
- Reduce the size of the infarct (blockage)
- Improve heart rate and arrhythmias

Angina

Angina describes a squeezing or pressurelike pain in the chest. The pain radiates to the left shoulder blade, left arm, or jaw, and typically lasts for only 1 to 20 minutes. Angina is caused by an insufficient supply of oxygen to the heart muscle. Since physical exertion and stress cause an increased need for oxygen, they are often preceding factors.

Angina is usually a result of atherosclerosis, but a form of angina exists that is not related to a buildup of plaque on the coronary arteries. Known as Prinzmetal's variant angina, it is caused by spasm of a coronary artery. This form of angina is more apt to occur at rest, may occur at odd times during the day or night, and is more common in women under age 50. It usually responds to magnesium supplementation. In fact, several reports even suggest that magnesium is the treatment of choice for Prinzmetal's angina.[15,16] Magnesium supplementation (most studies have used intravenous administration) helps in angina related to atherosclerosis via the same mechanisms responsible for its effects in an acute myocardial infarction.[8-11]

Cardiac Arrhythmias

In 1935, researchers first learned magnesium is valuable in the treatment of cardiac arrhythmias. More than 60 years later, numerous clinical studies now show magnesium benefits many types of arrhythmias, including atrial fibrillation, ventricular premature contractions, ventricular tachycardia, and severe ventricular arrhythmias. The current concept is that magnesium depletion within the heart muscle also leads to potassium depletion. Given the importance of these two electrolytes for proper nerve and muscle firings, it is no wonder an arrhythmia is produced when levels are low.[8-11]

According to the results of a recent double-blind, placebo-controlled study, magnesium supplementation offers significant benefit in the treatment of new-onset atrial fibrillation (AF).[17] The drug of choice for new-onset AF is digoxin, which unfortunately offers no better treatment than a placebo to facilitate proper heart rhythm in AF. Several studies in AF patients taking magnesium caused researchers to conduct a study to determine if magnesium and digoxin were better than digoxin alone in controlling the ventricular response in AF.

Eighteen outpatients with AF of less than 7 days' duration received either digoxin plus a placebo or digoxin plus magnesium. The magnesium was given intravenously. In the initial 15 minutes, those receiving magnesium received 20 percent of a 10-gram magnesium sulfate solution in 500 milliliters of 5 percent dextrose in water. The remaining solution was infused over the next 6 hours.

The benefit of magnesium was obvious within the first 15 minutes; heart rate decreased immediately from an average of 130 to 120. After 24 hours, the group that received the magnesium had an average heart rate of roughly 80, while the group that received only digoxin had an average heart rate of 105. In the magnesium group, 6 out of 10 patients (60 percent) converted to sinus rhythm, whereas only 3 out of 8 in the other group converted. The study indicates that magnesium either greatly improves the efficacy of digoxin or exerts significant effects on its own.

Because of the lack of effectiveness of digoxin when used alone, research is focusing on newer drug therapies for new-onset AF such as esmolol and diltiazem. While these drugs are gaining greater use, side effects like symptomatic hypotension are quite common. Given the high rate of hemodynamic compromise in these patients, the fact that both drugs lower systolic blood pressure is a major concern. In one study with esmolol, almost 50 percent of the subjects had to stop treatment.

The fact that magnesium is safer and more effective is reason enough for physicians to use it alone or in combination with digoxin for new-onset AF; however, we can add one more factor to the equation—cost. Over a 24-hour period, a patient with new-onset AF requires approximately 6 grams of esmolol ($400) or 300 milligrams of diltiazem ($200)—considerably more expensive than 10 grams magnesium sulfate ($1) or 2 milligrams of digoxin ($2) or their combination.

Cardiomyopathy

Cardiomyopathy is any disease of the heart muscle that causes a reduction in the force of heart contractions. Such a reduction results in decreased efficiency of blood circulation. Cardiomyopathy may be the result of viral, metabolic, nutritional, toxic, autoimmune, degenerative, genetic, or unknown cause. Regardless of the cause, magnesium supplementation is warranted because of magnesium's importance in heart function. Several studies show magnesium supplementation produces improvements in heart function in patients with a variety of cardiomyopathies.[8–11,18]

Congestive Heart Failure

Congestive heart failure (CHF) is an inability of the heart to effectively pump blood. CHF usually occurs because of long-term effects of high blood pressure, disorder of a heart valve, or a cardiomyopathy. CHF is always characterized by an energy depletion status, and many patients with CHF have a magnesium (and a coenzyme Q_{10}) deficiency. Magnesium levels correlate directly with survival rates. In one study, CHF patients with normal levels of magnesium had 1- and 2-year survival rates of 71 percent and 61 percent, respectively, compared to rates of 45 percent and 42 percent for patients with lower magnesium levels.[19]

Magnesium supplementation also prevents the magnesium depletion caused by the conventional drug therapies for CHF—digitalis, diuretics, and vasodilators (beta-blockers, calcium channel-blockers, etcetera). It produces positive effects in CHF patients receiving conventional drug therapy even if serum magnesium levels are normal.[20]

High Blood Pressure

Population studies correlate a high magnesium intake with lower blood pressure. The principal source of magnesium in early studies was water. Water high in minerals is often referred to as "hard water." Numerous studies demonstrate that an inverse correlation between water hardness and high blood pressure exists. In other words, where magnesium content of water is high, there are fewer cases of high blood pressure and heart disease.[21]

Early studies led to more extensive dietary studies that explored the association of magnesium and high blood pressure. These dietary studies found the same results as the hard water studies—when magnesium levels are high, blood pressure is lower. In one of the most extensive studies, the Honolulu Heart Study, systolic blood pressure was 6.4 millimeters of mercury lower and diastolic blood pressure 3.1 millimeters of mercury lower in the highest magnesium intake group compared to the lowest magnesium intake group.[22]

Because of the epidemiological evidence, researchers began investigating the effect of magnesium supplementation in the treatment of high blood pressure. The results are mixed. Some of the studies show a very good blood pressure–lowering effect, others do not. Whether or not magnesium supplementation will lower blood pressure depends on several factors. First, if the individual is taking a diuretic, there is a very good chance that magnesium supplementation will lower blood pressure by overcoming the magnesium depletion the diuretic induces. Another scenario where magnesium supplementation may be valuable is when the high blood pressure is associated with a high level of renin, an enzyme released by the kidneys that eventually leads to the formation of angiotensin and release of aldosterone. These compounds cause the blood vessels to constrict and the blood pressure to increase. Finally, patients with elevated intracellular sodium or a decreased intracellular potassium (measured by red blood cell studies) respond better to magnesium supplementation than subjects with normal intracellular potassium and sodium levels. Rather than performing a blood test to measure renin or intracellular potassium and sodium, I recommend giving magnesium supplementation a 4-week trial. I also recommend consuming a high-potassium diet.

There are a number of studies that show magnesium supplementation is of value in lowering blood pressure. In one double-blind study, 91 middle-aged and elderly women with mild to moderate high blood pressure (between 140/90 and 185/105) who were not on blood pressure–lowering drugs randomly received either 480 milligrams of magnesium (as magnesium aspartate) or a placebo each day for 6 months. At the end of the study, systolic blood pressure dropped 2.7 millimeters of mercury and diastolic blood pressure dropped 2.7 millimeters of mercury more in the magnesium group than in the placebo group. The result was a near-normal average blood pressure reading of 143.8/86. Potassium supplementation did not produce any side effect, nor did the magnesium aspartate cause diarrhea.[23]

In another double-blind clinical study, 21 male patients with high blood pressure were given 600 milligrams of magnesium daily (as magnesium oxide) or a placebo. Mean blood pressure (the average between the systolic and diastolic) decreased from 111 to 102 millimeters of mercury. Several other findings are worth mentioning. The patients who responded the best were those with increased red blood cell sodium and reduced red blood cell potassium. After therapy with magnesium, the levels of intracellular sodium, potassium, and magnesium normalized, which suggests magnesium lowers blood pressure through activation of the cellular membrane pump that pumps sodium out of, and potassium into, the cell. Magnesium supplementation also lowered triglycerides from 102 to 82 milligrams per deciliter and total cholesterol from 195 to 184 milligrams per deciliter.[24]

Intermittent Claudication

Intermittent claudication is characterized by a painful leg cramp produced when walking. A lack of oxygen causes intermittent claudication, much like it causes angina in the heart. In that sense, it is a peripheral vascular disease. Atherosclerosis also causes intermittent claudication And, like coronary artery disease, peripheral vascular disease is characterized by magnesium deficiency. In one study, 120 out of 138 patients with peripheral vascular disease had low red blood cell magnesium levels. Correcting an underlying magnesium deficiency in patients with peripheral vascular disease produces good clinical results.[25]

Low HDL-Cholesterol Levels

Magnesium deficiency in animals increases in LDL cholesterol and triglycerides and lowers HDL-cholesterol levels. Evidence in studies conducted with humans indicates low magnesium levels produce similar abnormalities and magnesium supplementation can improve cholesterol and triglyceride levels. In one study, magnesium supplementation (400 milligrams daily) reduced total cholesterol from 297 milligrams per deciliter to 257 milligrams per deciliter and raised HDL-cholesterol levels from 35 milligrams per deciliter to 47 milligrams per deciliter.[26]

Mitral Valve Prolapse

Mitral valve prolapse is tone loss or slight deformity of the mitral valve that causes leakage of the valve and produces a heart murmur that can be heard by a stethoscope. Since research shows 85 percent of patients with mitral valve prolapse have chronic magnesium deficiency, magnesium supplementation is indicated. This recommendation is further supported by several studies showing oral magnesium supplementation actually improves mitral valve prolapse.[27,28]

Prevention of Strokes and Transient Ischemic Attacks (TIAs)

The blood vessels supplying the brain are extremely sensitive to magnesium status. When magnesium levels are low, vascular spasm results. This vascular spasm sometimes results in a stroke or transient ischemic attack. Conversely, with magnesium supplementation the cerebral arteries usually relax and blood flows better through the brain. Magnesium supplementation may offer significant protection against strokes (cerebral infarction), just as it may reduce the risk for myocardial infarction.[8,29]

Diabetes and Hypoglycemia

Magnesium plays a central role in the secretion and action of insulin. Without adequate magnesium levels within the body's cells, control over blood sugar levels is impossible. Several studies in patients with glucose intolerance and insulin insensitivity show magnesium is valuable in maintaining proper blood sugar levels. In one study, magnesium supplementation (400 milligrams elemental magnesium per day) given to nonobese elderly subjects demonstrated significant improvements in insulin response and action, glucose tolerance, and the fluidity of the red blood cell membrane. These improvements reflected net increases in the red blood cell magnesium concentration. The results of this study (and others) indicate supplementing the diet with magnesium when blood magnesium levels are low may allow for an improvement in blood sugar control mechanisms.[30]

Since magnesium is critically involved in glucose metabolism and can help improve insulin action, diabetics need to maintain proper magnesium levels. However, there are additional reasons that suggest magnesium supplementation is essential in diabetes—magnesium deficiency is common in diabetics, and magnesium may prevent some complications of diabetes like retinopathy and heart disease.[31] Magnesium levels are usually low in diabetics and lowest in those with severe retinopathy.[31] Insulin administration increases magnesium excretion.[32] The RDA for magnesium is 350 milligrams per day for adult males and 300 milligrams per day for adult females. The diabetic may need twice this amount. In addition to eating a diet rich in magnesium, the diabetic should supplement his or her diet with 300 to 500 milligrams of magnesium. Since the level of vitamin B_6 inside the body's cells is intricately linked to the magnesium content of the cell, diabetics should also take at least 50 milligrams of vitamin B_6 daily In other words, without vitamin B_6, magnesium does not get inside the cell and is therefore useless.

Because of the growing evidence that magnesium supplementation benefits diabetics, the American Diabetes Association sponsored a consensus panel to examine the data and come up with a recommendation. Here is the conclusion of the panel:

> In conclusion, the weight of experimental data presented to the consensus panel suggests that magnesium deficiency may play a role in insulin resistance, carbohydrate intolerance, and hypertension. Serum magnesium levels, although readily available, are relatively insensitive assessments of magnesium deficiency. The implementation of newer sensitive electrodes or phosphate NMR assays for ionized or free intracellular magnesium may extend our understanding of magnesium deficiency. However, based on available data, only diabetic patients at high risk of hypomagnesemia should have total serum magnesium assessed, and such levels should be repeated only if hypomagnesemia can be demonstrated.[33]

The "expert" panel clearly acknowledges the scientific literature supporting magnesium supplementation in diabetics and the failure of serum magnesium to reflect body magnesium stores; yet this same panel does not realize that magnesium supplementation is appropriate in diabetics. In fact, "the panel recommends that patients with diabetes at increased risk of magnesium deficiency, but in whom such deficiencies cannot be demonstrated by clinically available tests, *not* receive magnesium supplementation." The panel believes that "adequate dietary magnesium intake can generally be achieved by a nutritionally balanced meal plan as recommended by the American Diabetes Association."

This position of the panel is not logical. What the panel is saying is, Yes, we know magnesium is critical to blood glucose and blood pressure regulation and possibly the prevention of complications of diabetes. We also know that magnesium supplementation aids in the treatment of diabetes because of numerous benefits, including enhancing insulin sensitivity. We also know that current tests of magnesium status do not reflect magnesium tissue stores. Yet despite all this information, we cannot recommend magnesium supplementation unless a person has magnesium deficiency documented by a test (serum magnesium or urine magnesium) that reflects only 0.3 percent of the total body magnesium pool—a deficiency reduced only when intracellular magnesium levels are entirely depleted.

The reason for the apparent contradictions is this was a "consensus" panel. Even after Columbus returned from America, some people still argued that the world was flat. If a group of geographical experts of 1492 had been asked to make a consensus statement on the shape of the world, I am sure it would have had a similar ring of dichotomy.

Eosinophilia-Myalgia Syndrome

The eosinophilia-myalgia syndrome (EMS) is a multisystem connective tissue disease that was first recognized in 1989. In most cases it is caused by contaminated L-tryptophan. EMS is characterized by early peripheral eosinophilia, severe muscle pain, inflammation, and in some cases neural and visceral involvement. In some individuals, EMS resolved when tryptophan ingestion was discontinued, but in most symptoms became chronic. Among the most troubling late symptoms are myalgias, cramping, weakness, and paresthesias.

Utilizing magnetic resonance spectroscopy, researchers find that patients with EMS display a selective decrease in skeletal muscle ATP concentrations. One emerging hypothesis that explains this event is tissue magnesium deficiency—magnesium plays an essential role in the manufacture of ATP.

A recent case study highlights the potential of magnesium supplementation in the treatment of EMS. In the study, a 43-year-old male patient with EMS exhibited persistent myalgias, cramping, and weakness. Researchers determined he was magnesium deficient based on a magnesium-loading study (serum magnesium levels were normal). Twice-weekly intramuscular injections of 1 gram of magnesium sulfate for 8 weeks resulted in immediate disappearance of symptoms. Twelve weeks later, symptoms reappeared. A second course of intramuscular magnesium therapy once again led to immediate improvement in symptoms. Further studies on six other patients yielded similar results. A larger double-blind, placebo-controlled study is now in progress.

Although the researchers cautioned "against extrapolating these data to other EMS patients" until the results of this study are known, based on this preliminary evidence it appears magnesium supplementation may be helpful in treating this disease.

Fatigue

An underlying magnesium deficiency, even if "subclinical," can result in chronic fatigue and symptoms similar to chronic fatigue syndrome (CFS). Many patients with chronic fatigue and CFS have low red blood cell magnesium levels, a more accurate measure of magnesium status than routine blood analysis. This data alone suggests magnesium supplementation may help improve energy levels.

Recently, researchers in the United Kingdom conducted a double-blind, placebo-controlled trial to assess the effect of magnesium supplementation in CFS.[34] Thirty-two patients received either an intramuscular injection of magnesium sulfate (1 gram in 2 milliliters injectable water) or a placebo (2 milliliters injectable water) for 6 weeks. At the end of the study, 12 of the 15 patients receiving magnesium reported significantly improved energy levels, better emotional state, and less pain (based on strict criteria). In contrast, only 3 of the 17 placebo patients reported they felt better and only 1 reported improved energy levels.

This study confirms some impressive results obtained in clinical trials during the 1960s on patients suffering from chronic fatigue.[35-38] These studies used oral magnesium and potassium aspartate (1 gram each) rather than injectable magnesium. Between 75 and 91 percent of the nearly 3,000 patients studied experience relief of fatigue during treatment with the magnesium and potassium aspartate. In contrast, the number of patients responding to a placebo was between 9 and 26 percent. The beneficial effect was usually noted after only 4 to 5 days, sometimes after 10 days. Patients usually continued treatment for 4 to 6 weeks; frequently fatigue did not return later.

Fibromyalgia

Fibromyalgia is a recently recognized disorder that is a common cause of chronic musculoskeletal pain and fatigue. Symptoms of fibromyalgia include generalized aches or stiffness of at least three anatomic sites for at least 3 months; six or more reproducible tender points on muscles, generalized fatigue, chronic headache, and sleep disturbances. Magnesium deficiency within muscle cells may be a factor in the development of fibromyalgia. One study demonstrates that a daily supplement of 300 to 600 milligrams of magnesium (as magnesium malate) results in tremendous improvements in the number and severity of tender points. Although some researchers theorize that malic acid (a Krebs cycle intermediate) was also responsible for the improvements noted, I recommend magnesium chelated to the entire family of Krebs cycle intermediates.[39]

Glaucoma

Since previous studies demonstrated calcium channel-blocking drugs offer benefits for some glaucoma patients, a group of researchers at the University Eye Clinic in Basel, Switzerland, decided to evaluate the effect of supplemental magnesium that has been referred to as "nature's physiological calcium blocker." Ten glaucoma patients (six with primary open-angle glaucoma, four with normal-tension glaucoma) participated in the trial. All patients had a digital cold-induced vasospasm. Magnesium was given at a dose of 121.5 milligrams twice daily for 1 month. After 4 weeks of treatment, the visual fields improved (as noted by a decrease in the mean defect and square root of loss variance scores). All three nailfold-capillaroscopic parameters and digital temperature improved. These results demonstrate that magnesium supplementation improves the peripheral circulation and has a beneficial effect on the visual field in patients with glaucoma.[40]

Hearing Loss

Noise-induced hearing loss is a major hazard in industry, the military, and rock-oriented musicians. More than 9 million Americans are exposed to daily average occupational noise levels above 85 decibals, the level where the risk for permanent hearing loss increases exponentially. Noise-induced hearing loss results from subtle changes in the sensory cells and other structures in the Organ of Corti and cochlea. Magnesium is essential in regulating cellular membrane permeability, neuromuscular excitability, and energy production. Low magnesium and noise-induced hearing loss are associated.

To test the hypothesis that magnesium supplementation may prevent noise-induced hearing loss, researchers tested 300 young military recruits undergoing basic training for 2 months. Their training included repeated exposures to high levels of impulse noises while using ear plugs. They were given either a placebo or 167 milligrams of magnesium (aspartate) daily.[41] The study results demonstrate that the rate of noise-induced hearing loss was significantly more frequent and more severe in the placebo group. Noise-induced hearing loss correlates negatively to the magnesium content of red blood cells, but even more so with leukocyte magnesium. This study shows that supplementation with a relatively small dose of magnesium is extremely safe and effective in preventing noise-induced hearing loss.

Kidney Stones

A quick way to produce kidney stones in animals is to put them on a magnesium-deficient diet. Magnesium increases the solubility of calcium in the urine, thereby preventing stone formation. Supplementing the diet with magnesium significant prevents recurrences of kidney stones.[42-45] However, when used in conjunction with vitamin B_6 (pyridoxine), an even greater effect is noted.[46,47]

Magnesium citrate is the most beneficial form of magnesium in the treatment of kidney stones. Decreased urinary citrate is found in 20 percent to 60 percent of patients with kidney stones.[48,49] Citrate reduces urinary saturation of stone-forming calcium salts because it forms complexes with calcium. It also retards the nucleation and crystalline growth of the calcium salts. If citrate levels are low, this inhibitory activity is not present and stone formation can occur. Low citrate levels result from a variety of metabolic disturbances (acidosis, chronic diarrhea, urinary tract infection, etcetera), but in general researchers do not know the reason for low levels in many individuals who develop kidney stones. Citrate supplementation successfully prevents recurrent kidney stones; and although clinical studies have examined the effects of potassium citrate or sodium citrate in kidney stone prevention,[48,49] magnesium citrate produces the best results.

Migraine and Tension Headaches

Several researchers link low magnesium levels with both migraine and tension headaches based on their theories and clinical observations.[4,5] A magnesium deficiency sets the stage for the events that can cause a migraine attack or a tension headache. Reduced levels of magnesium are found in the serum, saliva, and red blood cells of migraine sufferers, which indicates a need for supplementation because one of magnesium's key functions is maintenance of blood vessel tone.[50,51]

The level of magnesium in the mononuclear white blood cells is probably the most reliable indicator of body magnesium stores. In a new study, mononuclear magnesium content was measured in adult migraine patients in headache-free periods and (in a number of patients) during attacks. Not surprisingly, migraine sufferers had significantly lower mononuclear magnesium levels compared to matched controls.[52]

Despite the number of clinical studies that show magnesium supplementation (as well as elimination of food allergies) is effective in many cases, most physicians choose to prescribe drugs that usually have only moderate benefits and significant side effects. Another possible benefit of magnesium in migraine sufferers may be its ability to improve mitral valve prolapse , which is linked to migraines. Mitral valve prolapse leads to changes in blood platelets, and these changes cause the platelets to release substances that ultimately cause expansion of blood vessels in the head.

Osteoporosis

Magnesium supplementation is as important as calcium supplementation in the treatment and prevention of osteoporosis. Women with osteoporosis have lower bone magnesium content and other indicators of magnesium deficiency than women without osteoporosis.[53] In magnesium deficiency of osteoporosis sufferers, there is a low serum concentration of vitamin D's most active form $(1,25\text{-}(OH)_2D_3)$.[54] This could be because the enzyme responsible for the conversion of $25\text{-}OHD_3$ to $1,25\text{-}(OH)_2D_3)$ requires adequate magnesium levels or magnesium's ability to mediate calcium metabolism.[55]

Pregnancy

Magnesium needs increase during pregnancy from 300 milligrams to 450 milligrams per day. Magnesium deficiency during pregnancy is linked to preeclampsia (a serious condition of pregnancy associated with elevations in blood pressure, fluid retention, and loss of protein in the urine), preterm delivery, and fetal growth retardation. In contrast, supplementing the diet of pregnant women with additional oral magnesium shows a significant decrease in the incidence of these complications.[56–61]

Although one double-blind study did not demonstrate a significant preventative effect of magnesium supplementation in these complications,[62] many other double-blind studies noted tremendous benefits. Therefore, considering the possibility that magnesium supplementation may help deliver a healthier baby into this world, is relatively inexpensive, and has an excellent safety profile, an additional 350 to 500 milligrams of magnesium daily is a good supplementation for pregnant women.

Premenstrual Syndrome and Dysmenorrhea

Magnesium deficiency is strongly implicated as a causative factor in premenstrual syndrome. Red blood cell magnesium levels in PMS patients are significantly lower than in normal subjects.[63,64] Because magnesium plays such an integral part in normal cell function, magnesium deficiency may account for the wide range of PMS symptoms. Furthermore, magnesium deficiency and PMS share many common features, and magnesium supplementation is an effective treatment of PMS.

A recent study attempted to understand the association even more by trying to answer two important questions: Do magnesium measures change as a function of menstrual cycle phase? Do magnesium measures change across the menstrual cycle differentially in PMS patients and controls? The researchers measured plasma, red blood cell (RBC), and mononuclear blood cell (MBC) magnesium in 26 women with confirmed PMS and in a control group of 19 women during the follicular, ovulatory, early luteal, and late luteal phases of the menstrual cycle.[65]

The principal findings of the study were:

- There were no significant differences in plasma magnesium levels in PMS patients compared with controls.

- No menstrual cycle effect on plasma magnesium was present in either group.

- PMS patients had significantly lower RBC and MBC magnesium concentrations compared to controls that were consistent across the menstrual cycle.

- Magnesium measures did not correlate with the severity of mood symptoms.

Four independent studies have confirmed the observation of low RBC magnesium concentrations in PMS patients. The low MBC magnesium concentrations are also consistent with other studies. The role that magnesium plays in PMS symptomatology is multifactorial because of magnesium's critical roles in cellular metabolism. In general, women with PMS seem to have a "vulnerability to luteal phase mood state destabilization" and chronic and enduring intracellular magnesium depletion serves as a major predisposing factor toward destabilization.[64]

In addition to emotional instability, women with PMS magnesium deficiency exhibit excessive nervous sensitivity with generalized aches and pains and a lower premenstrual pain threshold. One clinical trial of magnesium in PMS showed a reduction of nervousness in 89 percent, breast tenderness in 96 percent, and weight gain in 95 percent of the women tested after magnesium supplementation.[64] In another double-blind study, high-dosage magnesium supplementation (360 milligrams three times daily) dramatically relieved PMS-related mood changes.[66]

While magnesium is effective on its own, combining it with vitamin B_6 and other nutrients provides even better results. Several studies show that when PMS patients are given a multivitamin and mineral supplement containing high doses of magnesium and pyridoxine, they experience a tremendous reduction in PMS symptoms.[67]

Dosage Ranges

Many nutritional experts feel the ideal intake for magnesium should be based on body weight (6 milligrams per 2.2 pounds body weight). For a 110-pound person, they recommend 300 milligrams; for a 154-pound person, 420 milligrams; and for a 200-pound person, 540 milligrams. Rather than relying on dietary intake to achieve this amount of magnesium, for most people I recommend supplementing their diets with additional magnesium corresponding to the recommendation of 6 milligrams per 2.2 pounds body weight. For the conditions discussed above, I usually recommend twice this amount—12 milligrams per 2.2 pounds body weight.

Safety Issues

People with kidney disease or severe heart disease (such as high-grade atrioventricular block) should not take magnesium (or potassium) except by physician's orders. In general, magnesium is very well tolerated; however, magnesium supplementation—particularly magnesium sulfate (Epsom salts), hydroxide, or chloride—sometimes causes a looser stool.

Interactions

Magnesium, calcium, potassium, and other minerals interact extensively, and dosages of other minerals reduce the intake of magnesium and vice versa. Vitamin B_6 works together with magnesium in many enzyme systems and increases the intracellular accumulation of magnesium.[68] A high calcium intake and a high intake of dairy foods fortified with vitamin D result in decreased magnesium absorption.[69] There are many drugs that adversely effect magnesium status, particularly many diuretics, insulin, and digitalis.

20

Potassium

Potassium, sodium, and chloride are electrolytes—mineral salts that conduct electricity when dissolved in water. They are so intricately related, nutrition textbooks usually discuss them together, which I have done here. However, my primary focus is potassium. The reason why these nutrients are so intricately linked is that electrolytes are always found in pairs; a positively charged molecule like sodium or potassium is always accompanied by a negatively charged molecule like chloride.

Food Sources

The total potassium content of food is important, but so too is the proper balance of sodium and potassium consumption. Too much sodium in the diet leads to disruption of this balance. Numerous studies demonstrate that a low-potassium, high-sodium diet plays a major role in the development of cancer and cardiovascular disease (heart disease, high blood pressure, strokes, etcetera).[1,2] Conversely, a diet high in potassium and low in sodium protects against these diseases. In the case of high blood pressure, it can even be therapeutic.[3–5]

Excessive consumption of dietary sodium chloride (table salt), coupled with diminished dietary potassium, is a common cause of high blood pressure. Numerous studies show that sodium restriction alone does not improve blood pressure control in most people—it must be accompanied by a high potassium intake.[3–5] In our society only 5 percent of sodium intake comes from the natural ingredients in food. Prepared foods provide 45 percent of our sodium intake, cooking adds 45 percent, and condiments contribute another 5 percent. All the body requires in most instances is the salt supplied in food.

Most Americans have a potassium-to-sodium (K:Na) ratio of less than 1:2. This 1:2 ratio means most people ingest twice as much sodium as potassium. Researchers recommend a dietary potassium-to-sodium ratio of greater than 5:1 to maintain health. This is ten times higher than the average intake.

However, even this may not be optimal. A natural diet rich in fruits and vegetables can produce a K:Na ratio greater than 100:1 because most fruits and vegetables have a K:Na ratio of at least 50:1. Table 20.1 reflects the sodium and potassium content of certain foods, but here is a short list of the average K:Na ratios for some common fresh fruits and vegetables with high K:NA ratios:

- Apples, 90:1
- Bananas, 440:1
- Carrots, 75:1
- Oranges, 260:1.
- Potatoes, 110:1

TABLE 20.1 Potassium/Sodium Content of Selected Foods, in Milligrams per Serving

Food	Portion Size	Potassium	Sodium
FRESH VEGETABLES			
Asparagus	¹/₂ cup	165	1
Avocado	¹/₂	680	5
Carrot, raw	1	225	38
Corn	¹/₂ cup	136	trace
Lima beans, cooked	¹/₂ cup	581	1
Potato	1 medium	782	6
Spinach, cooked	¹/₂ cup	292	45
Tomato, raw	1 medium	444	5
FRESH FRUITS			
Apple	1 medium	182	2
Apricots, dried	¹/₄ cup	318	9
Banana	1 medium	440	1
Cantaloupe	¹/₄ melon	341	17
Orange	1 medium	263	1
Peach	1 medium	308	2
Plums	5	150	1
Strawberries	¹/₂ cup	122	trace
UNPROCESSED MEATS			
Chicken, light meat	3 ounces	350	54
Lamb, leg	3 ounces	241	53
Roast beef	3 ounces	224	49
Pork	3 ounces	219	48
FISH			
Cod	3 ounces	345	93
Flounder	3 ounces	498	201
Haddock	3 ounces	297	150
Salmon	3 ounces	378	99
Tuna, drained solids	3 ounces	225	38

Deficiency Signs and Symptoms

A potassium deficiency is characterized by muscle weakness, fatigue, mental confusion, irritability, weakness, heart disturbances, and problems in nerve conduction and muscle contraction. A diet low in fresh fruits and vegetables but high in sodium is the typical cause of dietary potassium deficiency. We often see dietary potassium deficiency in the elderly. However, dietary potassium deficiency is less common than deficiency caused by excessive fluid loss (sweating, diarrhea or urination) or the use of diuretics, laxatives, aspirin, and other drugs.

The amount of potassium lost in sweat is quite significant, especially with prolonged exercise in a warm environment. Athletes or people who regularly exercise have higher potassium needs. Because up to 3 grams of potassium can be lost in one day by sweating, a daily intake of at least 4 grams of potassium is recommended for these individuals.

Beneficial Effects

Potassium is an extremely important electrolyte that functions in the maintenance of:

- Water balance and distribution
- Acid-base balance
- Muscle and nerve cell function
- Heart function
- Kidney and adrenal function

Over 95 percent of the body's potassium is in cells. In contrast, most of the body's sodium is outside the cells in blood and other fluids. How does this happen? Cells actually pump sodium out and potassium in via the "sodium-potassium pump." This pump is in the membranes of all body cells, and one of its most important functions is preventing cellular swelling. If sodium is not pumped out, water accumulates in the cell, causing it to swell and ultimately burst.

The sodium-potassium pump also functions to maintain the electrical charge within the cell. This is particularly important to muscle and nerve cells. During nerve transmission and muscle contraction, potassium exits the cell and sodium enters, which results in an electrical charge change. This change causes a nerve impulse or muscle contractions, so it is not surprising that a potassium deficiency affects muscles and nerves first.

Although sodium and chloride are important, potassium is the most important dietary electrolyte. In addition to functioning as an electrolyte, potassium is essential for conversion of blood sugar into glycogen, the storage form of blood sugar in the muscles and liver. A potassium shortage results in lower levels of stored glycogen. Because exercising muscles use glycogen for energy, a potassium deficiency produces great fatigue and muscle weakness, the first signs of potassium deficiency.

Available Forms

Potassium supplements available in health food stores are either potassium salts (chloride and bicarbonate), potassium bound to various mineral chelates (aspartate, citrate, etcetera), or food-based potassium sources. The FDA restricts the amount of potassium available in non-food-based forms to only 99 milligrams per dose because of problems associated with high-dosage potassium salts; however, popular so-called salt substitutes such as NoSalt and Nu-Salt are in fact potassium chloride and provide 530 milligrams of potassium per $1/6$ teaspoon! Potassium chloride preparations are also available by prescription in a vast array of flavors and formulations (timed-release tablets, liquids, powders, and effervescent tablets). Physicians commonly prescribe potassium salts in the dosage range of 1.5 grams to 3.0 grams per day. However, potassium salts can cause nausea, vomiting, diarrhea, and ulcers when given in pill form at high-dosage levels. When potassium levels are increased through diet alone, these effects are not present. Therefore, the best course is to use foods or food-based potassium supplements to meet the human body's high potassium requirements.

Principal Uses

The principal uses of supplemental potassium are for potassium depletion (deficiency) and high blood pressure.

Potassium Depletion

Potassium depletion occurs whenever the loss rate of potassium through urinary excretion, sweat, or the gastrointestinal tract (vomiting or diarrhea) exceeds the rate of potassium intake. Severe potassium depletion usually results from the use of certain diuretics but can occur as a result of severe diarrhea or vomiting. Because severe potassium depletion can have serious consequences, consult a physician if you suspect you are suffering from potassium depletion. Most of the body's potassium stores are in cells, so low free potassium in the serum (the portion of the blood containing no blood cells) usually occurs only in extreme potassium depletion. The best test for determining the body's potassium stores is the red-blood-cell potassium level.[6]

High Blood Pressure

A diet low in potassium and high in sodium is associated with high blood pressure.[7] Many studies show that increasing dietary potassium intake can lower blood pressure.[3,8] In addition, other studies indicate that potassium supplementation alone can produce significant reductions in blood pressure in hypertensive subjects. Typically these studies use dosages ranging from 2.5 grams to 5.0 grams of potassium daily and reflect significant drops in both systolic and diastolic values. [8–13]

In one study, 37 adults with mild hypertension participated in a crossover study. Patients received either 2.5 grams of potassium per day, 2.5 grams of potassium plus 480 milligrams of magnesium, or a placebo for 8 weeks. They then crossed over to a different treatment for another 8 weeks and so on.[12] The study's results study demonstrated that potassium supplementation lowered systolic blood pressure by an average of 12 millimeters of mercury and diastolic blood pressure by an average of 16 millimeters of mercury. Interestingly the additional magnesium offered no further reduction in blood pressure.

Potassium supplementation may be especially useful in the treatment of high blood pressure in persons over the age of 65. The elderly often do not fully respond to blood-pressure–lowering drugs, which makes the use of potassium supplementation an exciting possibility. In one double-blind study, 18 untreated elderly patients (average age 75 years) with a systolic blood pressure of greater than 160 millimeters of mercury and/or a diastolic blood pressure of greater than 95 millimeters of mercury were given either potassium chloride (supplying 2.5 grams of potassium) or a placebo each day for 4 weeks.[13] After this relatively short treatment period, the group getting the potassium experienced a drop of 12 millimeters of mercury in the systolic and 7 millimeters of mercury in the diastolic. These results compare quite favorably to the blood pressure reduction produced by drug therapy in the European Working Party on High Blood Pressure in the Elderly Study.[14]

Dosage Ranges

The estimated safe and adequate daily dietary intake of potassium set by the Committee on Recommended Daily Allowances is 1.9 grams to 5.6 grams. If diet does not meet body potassium requirements, supplementation is essential to good health. This statement is particularly true for the elderly, athletes, and people with high blood pressure.

Safety Issues

Most people can handle any excess of potassium. The exception is people with kidney disease; they do not handle potassium in the normal way and may experience heart disturbances and other consequences of potassium toxicity. Individuals with kidney disorders usually need to restrict their potassium intake and follow the dietary recommendations of their physicians.

Interactions

Potassium interacts in many body systems with magnesium. Potassium supplementation (unless supervised by a physician) is contraindicated when using a number of prescription medications, including digitalis, potassium-sparing diuretics, and the angiotensin-converting enzyme inhibitor class of blood pressure–lowering drugs.

21

Zinc

Zinc is in every body cell and is a component in over 200 enzymes. In fact, zinc functions in more enzymatic reactions than any other mineral. It is also necessary for proper action of many body hormones, including thymic hormones, insulin, growth hormone, and sex hormones. The average adult body contains a total of 1.4 to 2.5 grams of zinc, where it is stored primarily in muscle (65 percent of the total) and is highly concentrated in red and white blood cells. Other tissues with high zinc concentrations include the bone, skin, kidney, liver, pancreas, retina, and prostate. The adult RDA for zinc is 15 milligrams daily.

Food Sources

The best known food source for zinc is oysters, but zinc is present in relatively high concentrations in other shellfish, fish, and red meats (see Table 21.1). Good concentrations are found in several plant foods such as whole grains, legumes, nuts, and seeds; however, the zinc in plant foods is less bioavailable because it binds to phytic acid (a fiber compound) to form an insoluble zinc-phytate complex that is not absorbed.

TABLE 21.1   Zinc Content of Selected Foods, in Milligrams per 3 1/2-oz. (100-g.) Serving

Oysters, fresh	148.7	Oats	3.2	Turnips	1.2
Pumpkin seeds	7.5	Peanuts	3.2	Parsley	0.9
Ginger root	6.8	Lima beans	3.1	Potatoes	0.9
Pecans	4.5	Almonds	3.1	Garlic	0.6
Split peas, dry	4.2	Walnuts	3.0	Carrots	0.5
Brazil nuts	4.2	Buckwheat	2.5	Whole-wheat bread	0.5
Whole wheat	3.2	Hazel nuts	2.4	Black beans	0.4
Rye	3.2	Green peas	1.6		

Deficiency Signs and Symptoms

Severe zinc deficiency is not common but is manifested by skin changes, diarrhea, hair loss, mental disturbances, and recurrent infections as a result of impaired immune function.[1] Although severe zinc deficiency is very rare in developed countries, many individuals in the United States have marginal zinc deficiency, especially the elderly.[2,3] Survey data indicate average zinc intakes range from 47 percent to 67 percent of the RDA.

Clinical conditions associated with zinc deficiency are:

- Frequent and/or severe infections
- Sleep and behavioral disturbances
- Delayed wound healing
- Psychiatric illness
- Inflammatory bowel disease
- Impaired glucose tolerance
- Malabsorption syndromes
- Reduced appetite, anorexia
- Growth retardation
- Loss of sense of smell or taste
- Delayed sexual maturation
- Night blindness
- Impotence, infertility
- All dermatological disorders
- Abnormal menstruation
- Dandruff and hair loss
- Alcohol abuse
- Connective tissue disease
- Diuretic usage
- Rheumatoid arthritis

Marginal zinc deficiency may be reflected by an increased susceptibility to infection, poor wound healing, decreased sense of taste or smell, and a number of minor skin disorders including acne, eczema, and psoriasis. Some other physical findings that often correlate with low zinc status include decreased ability to see at night or with poor lighting, growth retardation, testicular atrophy, mouth ulcers, a white coating on the tongue, and marked halitosis.[1,4,5]

White spots on the fingernails may reflect zinc status,[6] which means poor wound healing because of a zinc deficiency secondary to nail bed trauma may be responsible for the lesions in some subjects. Judgment is required to determine the significance of these lesions; i.e., do the white spots correspond to the level of trauma to the nail beds?

The best laboratory method for determining zinc status is measuring the amount of zinc inside white blood cells (the leukocyte zinc level).[1,7] Other common measurements, such as hair and blood measurements, are not reliable.

Recommended Dietary Allowance

Recommended Dietary Allowance for Zinc

Group	Milligrams
INFANTS UNDER 1 YEAR	5
CHILDREN	
1–10 years	10
YOUNG ADULTS AND ADULTS	
Males 11+ years	15
Females 11+ years	12
Pregnant females	15
Lactating females	19

Beneficial Effects

Adequate zinc levels are essential to good health. The beneficial effects of zinc are extensive because it is involved in so many enzyme and body functions. By necessity, the discussion on the beneficial effects of zinc focuses on zinc's effects on immune function, wound healing, sensory functions, sexual function, and skin health.

Adequate tissue zinc levels are necessary for proper immune system function. And zinc deficiency results in an increased susceptibility to infection. It is required for protein synthesis and cell growth, and therefore for wound healing. Zinc supplementation decreases wound-healing time, while a zinc deficiency leads to prolongation of the wound. A high zinc intake aids protein synthesis and cell growth following any sort of trauma (burns, surgery, wounds, etcetera).

Zinc is essential for the maintenance of vision, taste, and smell. A zinc deficiency results in impaired function of these special senses. Night blindness often occurs because of zinc deficiency. The loss of taste and/or smell is a common complaint in the elderly, and zinc supplementation improves taste and/or smell acuity in some individuals.

Zinc is critical to healthy male sex hormone and prostate function. A zinc deficiency may be a contributing factor in the high rate of prostate enlargement and male infertility (a zinc deficiency can result in decreased sperm count).

The importance of zinc in normal skin function is well known. Typically, serum zinc levels are lower in 13- to 14-year-old males than in any other age group. Not too surprising, then, that this group is the most susceptible to acne.

Available Forms

There are many forms of zinc to choose from. While most clinical studies have used zinc sulfate, several other forms of zinc are better absorbed and utilized. Zinc forms bound to picolinate, acetate, citrate, glycerate, or monomethionine are all excellent. Although manufacturers claim superiority for their particular zinc chelates, data indicate each of these forms is well absorbed.

Principal Uses

Zinc has many uses, but the principal ones are in zinc deficiency, pregnancy, immune function, male sexual function, rheumatoid arthritis and other inflammatory conditions, acne, macular degeneration, Alzheimer's disease, and Wilson's disease.

Zinc Deficiency

Zinc deficiency can be caused by decreased intake and/or utilization of zinc, and many health conditions are associated with zinc deficiency. Some involved with decreased intake are:

- Anorexia nervosa
- Fad diets
- Protein deficiency
- Vegetarianism
- Alcoholic cirrhosis
- Old age
- Acute infections/inflammation
- Alcoholism
- Increased Body Losses:
  - Starvation
  - Burns
  - Post-trauma

Some health conditions associated with decreased zinc absorption are:
- Diabetes mellitus
- High-fiber diet
- High dietary calcium:zinc ratio
- High dietary iron:zinc ratio
- Alcoholism
- Chelating agents
- Acrodermatitis enteropathica

- Dialysis
- Achlorhydria/hypochlorhydria
- Hepatic disease
- Celiac disease
- Inflammatory bowel disease
- Diarrhea
- Intestinal resection
- Chronic blood loss
- Short bowel syndrome
- Pancreatic insufficiency

Daily zinc dosages should be increased in the following situations:
- Old age
- Pregnancy and lactation
- Oral contraceptive use
- Growth spurts and puberty

Zinc Supplementation and Pregnancy Outcome

Because zinc is required for proper cell division, it plays a critical role in fetal development. Low zinc levels are linked to premature births, low birth weight, growth retardation, and preeclampsia—a serious condition of pregnancy associated with elevations in blood pressure, fluid retention, and loss of protein in the urine. Studies of zinc supplementation in pregnancy have produced conflicting results, largely because of methodological problems. (Small sample sizes have been the biggest shortcoming). In an effort to better understand the role of zinc and fetal development, researchers recently conducted a study of African-American women who had relatively low plasma zinc levels early in pregnancy. The women were given either a placebo or 25 milligrams of zinc in the form of zinc sulfate (a dosage higher than the 15 milligrams RDA for pregnancy) and a daily prenatal vitamin/mineral tablet that contained folic acid, iron, and other minerals but no zinc.[8]

The results of the study were remarkable. The zinc-supplemented group demonstrated greater baby body weight and head circumference than the placebo group (248-gram higher birth weight and a 0.7-centimeter larger head circumference). The data strongly indicate that zinc supplementation improves pregnancy outcomes, and support the need to include zinc in prenatal multiple vitamin/mineral supplements at a dosage higher than the RDA.

Immune Function

Zinc is involved in virtually every aspect of immunity. When zinc levels are low, the number of T cells decreases, thymic hormone levels lower, and many white blood cell functions critical to the immune response cease. Fortunately, all these effects are reversible upon adequate zinc administration.[9,10]

Zinc supplementation produces dramatic reversal of the low immune function characteristic of aging. One study assessed the effect of low-dose zinc supplementation (20 milligrams per day) on nutritional and thymic hormone status in institutionalized elderly subjects.[11] The most telling effect was zinc supplementation produced a significant restoration of serum thymulin (a hormone produced by the thymus gland). Typically, as people age, the level of thymulin and other immune-enhancing thymus hormones decreases. The reduction of these hormones leads to impaired immune function. By restoring the levels of thymulin, zinc supplementation restores immune function. This study also noted that zinc supplementation improved nutritional status. Food intake and serum albumin levels both increased with zinc supplementation. Furthermore, because zinc supplementation can depress copper levels, which leads to an increase in the ratio of LDL cholesterol to HDL cholesterol, the study also measured serum copper and lipid levels. Although copper levels decreased, there were no adverse effects on LDL-to-HDL ratios. These results indicate that low-dose zinc supplementation improves nutritional and immune status without the known disadvantages of higher doses of zinc.

Zinc, like vitamin C, also possesses direct antiviral activity, including antiviral activity against several viruses that cause the common cold. A double-blind clinical trial demonstrated zinc-containing lozenges significantly reduced the average duration of common colds by 7 days.[12] The lozenges contained 23 milligrams of elemental zinc, which the patients dissolved in their mouths every 2 waking hours after an initial double dose. After 7 days, 86 percent of the 37 zinc-treated subjects were symptom free, compared to 46 percent of the 28 placebo-treated subjects. As a result, throat lozenges containing zinc are now extremely popular in the treatment of the common cold.

The authors of the study believe the local zinc concentration was high enough to inhibit replication of cold viruses. Although this may account for some of the activity, the immune-enhancing effects of zinc also play a role. The use of zinc supplementation, particularly as a lozenge, is valuable during a cold. Because high doses of zinc can actually impair immune function, I do not recommend a daily intake of greater than 150 milligrams for more than a week.

Male Sexual Function

Zinc is perhaps the most critical trace mineral involved in male sexual function. It is used in virtually every aspect of male reproduction, including the hormone metabolism, sperm formation, and sperm motility.[13] Among other things, zinc deficiency is characterized by decreased testosterone levels and sperm counts. Zinc levels are typically much lower in infertile men with low sperm counts, indicating that a low zinc status may be the contributing factor to the infertility.

Several studies have been designed to measure the effect of zinc supplementation on sperm counts and motility.[14–16] The results from all the studies support the use of zinc supplementation in the treatment of oligospermia, especially in the presence of low testosterone levels. The effectiveness of zinc is best illustrated by examining a study in 37 men with infertility of greater than 5 years' duration whose sperm counts were less than 25 million per milliliter. Blood testosterone levels were also measured.[16] The men received a supplement of zinc sulfate (60 milligrams elemental zinc daily) for 45 to 50 days. In the 22 patients with initially low testosterone levels, mean sperm count increased significantly from 8 to 20 million. Testosterone levels also increased, and 9 out of the 22 wives became pregnant during the study. This result is quite impressive given the long-term nature of the infertility and the immediate results. In contrast, the 15 men with normal testosterone levels experienced no change in testosterone level, and no pregnancies occurred despite the slight increase in sperm count.

Rheumatoid Arthritis and Inflammatory Conditions

Zinc has antioxidant effects and functions in the antioxidant enzyme superoxide dismutase (copper-zinc SOD). Zinc levels are typically reduced in patients with rheumatoid arthritis, and several studies have used zinc in the treatment of rheumatoid arthritis. Some of the studies demonstrated a slight therapeutic effect.[17–19] Most of the studies used zinc in the form of sulfate. Better results may be produced by using a form of zinc with a higher absorption rate, such as zinc picolinate, acetate, monomethionine, or citrate.

Acne

Several double-blind studies have demonstrated the effectiveness of zinc in the treatment of acne. In fact, these studies show zinc yields results similar to tetracycline in superficial acne and superior results in deeper acne.[20–22] Although some studies of zinc in acne patients did not obtain improvements of this magnitude, the inconsistency of the results may be due to differences in dosages or the form of zinc used. For example, studies using zinc citrate or zinc gluconate show improvements similar to tetracycline, but those using plain zinc sulfate show fewer beneficial results[23,24] because zinc sulfate is poorly absorbed. There have been no studies to date using other highly absorbable forms of zinc such as zinc picolinate, zinc acetate, or zinc monomethionine.

Although some people in these studies showed dramatic improvement immediately, the majority usually required 12 weeks of supplementation before they achieved good results These forms of zinc are more effectively absorbed than the forms of zinc used in the positive studies and, therefore, may produce even better results. A safe and effective dose for zinc is 30 to 45 milligrams per day.

Macular Degeneration

Zinc is quite beneficial in the treatment of macular degeneration. The macula is the portion of the eye responsible for fine vision. Degeneration of the macula is the leading cause of severe visual loss in the United States and Europe in persons aged 55 years or older. In a study conducted at the Department of Ophthalmology at the Utah School of Medicine, 151 patients with macular degeneration received either 100 milligrams of zinc or a placebo.[25] Those receiving the zinc had significantly less loss of vision.

Alzheimer's Disease

Zinc deficiency is one of the most common nutrient deficiencies in the elderly and may be a major factor in the development of Alzheimer's disease.[26] DNA is the genetic core that serves as the blueprint for cellular functions and cell replication. Most enzymes involved in DNA replication, repair, and transcription contain zinc, and one cause of dementia may be the long-term cascading effects of error-prone or ineffective DNA-handling enzymes in nerve cells. In addition, many antioxidant enzymes, including superoxide dismutase, require zinc. The end result of zinc deficiency, then, could be the destruction of nerve cells and the formation of neurofibrillary tangles and plaques. The levels of zinc in the brain and cerebrospinal fluid in patients with Alzheimer's disease is markedly decreased.

Zinc supplementation provides good benefits in Alzheimer's disease. In one study, 10 patients with Alzheimer's disease were given 27 milligrams of zinc (as zinc aspartate) daily. Only two patients failed to show improvement in memory, understanding, communication, and social contact. In one 79-year-old-patient, the response was labeled "unbelievable" by both medical staff and family.[27] Additional studies in Germany have yielded similarly amazing results.

Wilson's Disease

Zinc is quite beneficial in the treatment of Wilson's disease—a rare, inherited disorder in which copper accumulates in the liver and is slowly released into other parts of the body, eventually leading to severe brain damage. Because zinc supplementation can interfere with copper absorption, it helps prevent the copper accumulation characteristic of Wilson's disease. In fact, a recent review of the current medical treatment of Wilson's disease concluded that "Zinc is clearly the treatment of choice" in all but the most advanced cases.[28]

Dosage Ranges

The dosage range for zinc supplementation for general health support is 15 to 20 milligrams. Since the average American consumes about 10 milligrams of zinc per day, supplementing an additional 15 to 20 milligrams results in a daily intake of 25 to 30 milligrams for most people. When zinc supplementation is used to address specific needs, the dosage range for men is 30 to 60 milligrams and for women, 30 to 45 milligrams.

Safety Issues

The principal toxic effects of zinc occur with prolonged intake at levels greater than 150 milligrams per day. These effects include copper-deficiency anemia, reduced

HDL-cholesterol levels, and depressed immune function. Acute toxicity is quite rare because the ingestion of amounts large enough to cause toxicity symptoms (2 grams per kilogram of body weight) usually provokes vomiting. The area between severe deficiency and toxicity is termed the gray area of nutrition; somewhere between these two states lies a point of optimum zinc nutriture. For zinc, the gray area is quite wide. It is probably the least toxic trace element. If taken on an empty stomach (particularly if taking zinc sulfate), zinc supplementation can result in gastrointestinal upset and nausea.

Interactions

Zinc competes with copper for absorption, and other minerals (most notably calcium and iron) can adversely effect zinc absorption if supplemented at a high dosage. Zinc supplements should be taken apart from high-fiber foods for best absorption. Zinc does not appear to interact in a negative fashion with any drug.

22

Boron

The trace mineral boron is now an interesting nutritional topic in the medical literature. Preliminary results indicate this important nutrient may be helpful in maintaining healthy bone and joint function.

Scientists have long known boron is essential in plants, however, until recently whether or not boron was critical to human health was debatable. Between 1939 and 1944, several studies unsuccessfully demonstrated a requirement for boron in rats. However, since 1980 evidence indicates that boron plays a major role in calcium and magnesium metabolism. Much of this new information comes from Forrest H. Nielsen and the United States Department of Agriculture.

Food Sources

Fruits and vegetables are the main dietary sources of boron. However, the level of boron in these foods depends on adequate levels of boron in the soil. It is estimated that the average boron intake of Americans is somewhere between 1.7 and 7 milligrams per day. Because the minimum amount required by humans to maintain health has not been determined, no one knows whether these amounts are optimal. Research suggests that they are not.

Interestingly, a diet rich in fruits and vegetables offers significant protection against osteoporosis and osteoarthritis—two conditions in which boron appears to offer benefit.[1,2] Typically, the standard American diet is severely deficient in these boron-rich foods. According to several large surveys, including the U.S. Second National Health and Nutrition Examination, fewer than 10 percent of Americans meet the minimum recommendation of two fruit servings and three vegetable servings per day, and only 51 percent eat one serving of vegetables per day.[3] The bottom line is that most Americans are probably not getting enough boron.

Deficiency Signs and Symptoms

Boron deficiency may be associated with an increased risk for postmenopausal bone loss. Boron deprivation in postmenopausal women leads to increased urinary excretion of calcium and magnesium and depressed serum concentrations of estrogen and testosterone.

Recommended Dietary Allowance

There is no RDA for boron. A daily intake of 1.5 milligrams to 3.0 milligrams is safe and probably more than adequate.

Beneficial Effects

Boron is necessary for the action of vitamin D, the vitamin that stimulates the absorption and utilization of calcium. Our bodies produce vitamin D by the action of sunlight on 7-dehydrocholesterol in the skin. The sunlight changes the 7-dehydrocholesterol into vitamin D_3 (cholecalciferol). It is then transported to the liver and converted by an enzyme into 25-hydroxycholcalciferol (25-OHD_3), which is five times more potent than cholecalciferol (D_3). An enzyme in the kidneys then converts the 25-hydroxycholecalciferol to 1,25-dihydroxycholecalciferol (1,25-$(OH)_2D_3$), which is ten times more potent than cholecalciferol and the most potent form of vitamin D_3.

Disorders of the liver or kidneys result in impaired conversion of cholecalciferol to more potent vitamin D compounds. In addition, many postmenopausal women with osteoporosis exhibit high levels of 25-OHD_3, while the level of 1,25-$(OH)_2D_3$ is quite low. This signifies an impairment of renal conversion of 25-OHD_3 to 1,25-$(OH)_2D_3$ in osteoporosis.[4,5] Scientists have proposed many theories to account for this decreased conversion, including relationships to estrogen and magnesium deficiency. However, recent evidence indicates that boron may be essential in the conversion of vitamin D to its active form.[6] In addition, boron appears to reduce body calcium loss by increasing the beneficial effects of estrogen on bone health.

Available Forms

There are several different forms of boron on the marketplace. For general health and osteoporosis, sodium borate or boron chelates are suitable. For the treatment of arthritis, look for boron as sodium tetraborate decahydrate.

Principal Uses

Boron is useful in the prevention and treatment of osteoporosis and arthritis.

Osteoporosis

Supplementing the diet of postmenopausal women with 3 milligrams of boron per day reduced urinary calcium excretion by 44 percent and dramatically increased the levels of 17 beta-estradiol, the most biologically active estrogen.[6] In addition to activating vitamin D to its most active form, boron is required to activate certain hormones, including estrogen. Subsequent studies indicate that boron supplementation can enhance as well as mimic some of the effects estrogens produce on calcium metabolism in postmenopausal women.[7] Boron deficiency may contribute greatly to the high rate of osteoporosis and menopausal symptoms in American women.

In an effort to better understand the role of boron in human nutrition, a recent study was conducted to determine the effects of boron supplementation (3 milligrams daily) on blood and urinary levels of calcium, magnesium, and phosphorus in athletic college women (ages 18 to 25) and sedentary control subjects.[8] Interestingly, results indicated boron supplementation only significantly affected blood phosphorus concentrations. The boron-supplemented group had lower serum phosphorus levels—high phosphorus levels contribute to osteoporosis. The previous effects noted on urinary calcium in post-menopausal women could not be confirmed; however, the study population was much different (young women). Regardless, the study still demonstrated a positive protective effect of boron against osteoporosis.

Arthritis

Boron may also play a role in joint health. Boron supplementation has been used in the treatment of osteoarthritis in Germany since the mid 1970s. This use was recently evaluated in a small double-blind clinical study and an open trial. In the double-blind study, of the patients given 6 milligrams of boron (as sodium tetraborate decahydrate), 71 percent improved compared to only 10 percent in the placebo group.[9] In the open trial, boron supplementation (6 to 9 milligrams daily) produced effective relief in 90 percent of arthritis patients, including patients with osteoarthritis, juvenile arthritis, and rheumatoid arthritis.[10] The preliminary indication is that boron supplements are valuable in arthritis, and many people with osteoarthritis experience complete resolution.

Dosage Range

In order to guarantee adequate boron levels, supplementing the diet with a daily dose of 3 to 9 milligrams of boron is indicated, especially in individuals at risk for osteoporosis.

Safety Issues

Orally administered boron is extremely safe when it is taken at recommended levels (3 to 9 milligrams per day). Problems such as nausea, vomiting, and diarrhea occur only at extremely high doses (greater than 500 milligrams per day).

Interactions

There are no known interactions with boron and any nutrient or drug.

23

Chromium

In 1957, researchers Walter Mertz and Kenneth Schwartz isolated a compound extracted from pork kidney they called the "glucose tolerance factor (GTF)." This pork substance restored impaired glucose tolerance in rats. Chromium was later identified as the active component of GTF in 1959. We now know chromium supplementation is useful in a number of health conditions, primarily because of its effects on blood sugar control mechanisms.[1]

Food Sources

Meats and whole grain products are the best sources of chromium. Fruits, vegetables, and dairy products have very low chromium concentrations (see Table 23.1).

Deficiency Signs and Symptoms

The primary sign of chromium deficiency is glucose intolerance characterized by elevated blood sugar and insulin levels.[1]

TABLE 23.1   Chromium Content of Selected Foods, in Micrograms per 3 1/2-oz. (100-g.) Serving

Yeast, brewer's	112	Green pepper	19	Carrots	9
Liver, calf's	55	Apple	14	Navy beans, dry	8
Whole-wheat bread	42	Butter	13	Orange	5
Wheat bran	38	Parsnips	13	Blueberries	5
Rye bread	30	Cornmeal	12	Green beans	4
Potatoes	24	Banana	10	Cabbage	4
Wheat germ	23	Spinach	10		

Recommended Dietary Allowance

There is no official RDA for chromium. Here are the safe and adequate ranges.

Safe and Adequate Dietary Range for Chromium

Group	Micrograms
INFANTS	
Under 6 months	10–40
6–12 months	20–60
CHILDREN	
1–3 years	20–80
4–6 years	30–120
CHILDREN AND ADULTS	
7+ years	50–200

Beneficial Effects

In order to appreciate how chromium works, we must review how the body controls blood sugar levels. After a meal, the body responds to the rise in blood glucose levels by secreting insulin. Insulin lowers blood glucose by increasing the rate that glucose is taken up by cells throughout the body. Declines in blood glucose, which occur during food deprivation or exercise, cause the release of glucagon—another hormone produced by the pancreas. Glucagon stimulates the release of glucose stored in body tissues (especially the liver) as glycogen. If blood sugar levels fall sharply or if a person is angry or frightened, it may result in the release of epinephrine (adrenaline) and corticosteroids (cortisol) by the adrenal glands. These hormones provide quicker breakdown of stored glucose for extra energy during a crisis or increased need.

Ideally, this is how the body works to control blood sugar levels. Unfortunately, a great deal of Americans stress these control mechanisms through poor diet and lifestyle. As a result, diabetes and hypoglycemia are common diseases. Obesity is also strongly linked to blood sugar disturbances because in obesity, there is a decreased sensitivity to insulin. Increasing the body's sensitivity to insulin, then, improves not only blood sugar control but also weight loss. The trace mineral chromium is critical to proper insulin action.

Chromium functions in the body as a key constituent of the "glucose tolerance factor." It works closely with insulin in facilitating the uptake of glucose into cells. Without chromium, insulin's action is blocked and blood sugar levels are elevated. Chromium's key benefit is helping insulin work properly.[1]

Available Forms

There are several forms of chromium available on the market. Chromium picolinate, chromium polynicotinate, chromium chloride, and chromium-enriched yeast are each touted by their respective suppliers as providing the greatest benefit. Which is the best form? There really is no firm evidence to indicate one is significantly better than another. There is one small study of 6 women and 6 men given either 400 micrograms of chromium picolinate or chromium polynicotinate. The test subjects were enrolled in an aerobics class for 3 months. Those taking the chromium picolinate increased muscle mass three times as much as those taking chromium polynicotinate (women, 4 pounds versus 1.3 pounds; men, 4.6 pounds versus 1.5 pounds).[2]

Principal Uses

The principal use for chromium supplementation is the treatment of impaired glucose tolerance (hypoglycemia and diabetes), elevated blood cholesterol and triglyceride levels, promotion of weight loss, and acne.

Impaired Glucose Tolerance

Chromium supplementation is indicated in both diabetes and hypoglycemia because of its ability to improve blood sugar control. Over 15 controlled studies demonstrate a positive effect for chromium in the treatment of impaired glucose tolerance.[1] Most of the studies were performed in patients with non-insulin-dependent diabetes mellitus (NIDDM)—a condition characterized by elevated insulin levels because of insulin resistance. Chromium deficiency is common in NIDDM patients and may contribute not only to the insulin resistance but also to the elevations in serum triglyceride and cholesterol levels.

In clinical studies in NIDDM patients, supplementing the diet with chromium decreases fasting glucose levels, improves glucose tolerance, lowers insulin levels, and decreases total cholesterol and triglyceride levels while increasing HDL-cholesterol levels.[3-6]

Obviously chromium is a critical nutrient in diabetes, but it is also very important in hypoglycemia. In one study, 8 female patients with hypoglycemia given 200 micrograms a day for 3 months demonstrated alleviation of their symptoms of hypoglycemia.[7] In addition, glucose tolerance test results improved and the number of insulin receptors on red blood cells increased.

Elevated Blood Cholesterol and Triglyceride Levels

In addition to lowering cholesterol and triglyceride levels in NIDDM patients, chromium supplementation lowers blood lipids in nondiabetic subjects.[8-13] All forms of chromium possess this effect (chromium chloride, high-chromium-content brewer's yeast, chromium picolinate, and chromium polynicotinate). However, unless initial body chromium levels are very low, chromium does not produce remarkable changes. The typical changes are small—10 percent reduction in total cholesterol and triglycerides and 2 percent increase in HDL—but still clinically relevant. Each 1 percent decrease in total cholesterol level carries a 2 percent reduction in heart attack or stroke risk, and every 1 percent increase in HDL cholesterol level carries a 4 percent decrease in risk.

Promotion of Weight Loss

Chromium has gained a great deal of attention as a weight-loss aid. One of the key methods for enhancing weight loss is to increase the sensitivity of the body's cells to the hormone insulin. Insulin plays a critical role in maintaining proper blood sugar and stimulating thermogenesis.

Chromium supplementation lowers body weight yet increases lean body mass, presumably because of increased insulin sensitivity.[14] In one study, patients were given chromium bound to picolinic acid (chromium picolinate) in one of the following three doses daily for 2 1/2 months: 0 microgram (placebo), 200 micrograms, or 400 micrograms.[15] Fifteen patients taking the 200-microgram and 400-microgram dose lost an average of 4.2 pounds of fat. The group taking the placebo lost only 0.4 pounds. Even more impressive was the chromium group's muscle gain (1.4 versus 0.2 pounds) versus that of the placebo group. The results were most striking in elderly subjects and men. The men taking chromium picolinate lost more than 7 times the body fat as those taking the placebo (7.7 versus 1 pound). The 400-microgram dose is more effective than the 200 microgram dose, as you can see below.

Effects of Chromium Picolinate Dosages Daily for 2 1/2 months

Dosage (Micrograms)	Fat Loss (Pounds)	Muscle Gain (Pounds)	Total Weight Loss (Pounds)
200	-3.3	+1.5	-1.8
400	-4.6	+1.1	-3.5

The results of these preliminary studies with chromium are very encouraging. In these initial studies, chromium picolinate promoted an increase in lean body weight percentage not because it led to fat loss but because it led to muscle gain.[16] Greater muscle mass means greater fat-burning potential.

Acne

Several dermatologists report that insulin is effective in the treatment of acne, which suggests impaired glucose tolerance and/or insulin insensitivity of the skin. The doctors gave the insulin either systemically or injected it directly into the lesion. Although oral glucose tolerance tests are normal in acne patients, repetitive skin biopsies reveal that their skin's glucose tolerance is significantly impaired.[17] One researcher describing the role of glucose tolerance in acne even coined the term "skin diabetes."[18] High-chromium yeast supplementation can produce rapid improvement in patients with acne.[19] Despite the lack of double-blind studies to document this effect of chromium, it is a safe nutritional supplement and should be considered.

Dosage Ranges

Although there is no Recommended Dietary Allowance (RDA) for chromium, it appears we need at least 200 micrograms each day in our diet. Many experts in the field of nutritional medicine currently recommend chromium dosages in impaired glucose tolerance and as a weight loss aid of 400 to 600 micrograms per day.

Safety Issues

Trivalent chromium, the form in all chromium supplements, is extremely safe. In double-blind studies, no one has reported any significant side effects or toxicity reactions with chromium supplementation. The only side effect of note is that in one double-blind study, the group receiving chromium (50 micrograms daily at 7:30 P.M.) reported increased dream activity, greater vividness and color in their dreams, and diminished sleep requirements.[20]

Interactions

Refined sugars, white flour products, and lack of exercise can deplete chromium levels,[1] and calcium carbonate and antacids may reduce chromium absorption.[21]

24

Copper

Copper is an essential trace mineral involved in several key enzymatic reactions in the human body. It is the third most abundant essential trace mineral (after iron and zinc). The highest *concentration* (amount per gram of tissue) of copper is in the brain and liver. The estimated 70 to 80 milligrams of copper in the human body are distributed among all the organs in the following percentages:

- Skeletal muscle, 24.7
- Skeleton, 19
- Skin, 15.3
- Bone marrow, 14.8
- Liver, 8 to 15
- Brain, 8

Food Sources

Copper is widely distributed in foods. The richest sources are oysters, other shellfish, and legumes (see Table 24.1). In an earlier era, the major source of copper in human nutrition was drinking water flowing through copper pipes.

Deficiency Signs and Symptoms

Since several enzyme systems require copper, copper deficiency affects several body tissues. It results in iron deficiency anemia because copper is required in proper iron absorption and utilization. Copper is necessary for the proper function of the enzyme lysyl oxidase, which is required in the crosslinking of collagen and elastin. Copper

TABLE 24.1 Copper Content of Selected Foods, in Milligrams per 3½-oz. (100-g.) Serving

Brazil nuts	2.3	Butter	0.4	Corn oil	0.2
Almonds	1.4	Rye grain	0.4	Ginger root	0.2
Hazelnuts	1.3	Barley	0.4	Molasses	0.2
Walnuts	1.3	Olive oil	0.3	Turnips	0.2
Pecans	1.3	Carrot	0.3	Green peas	0.1
Split peas, dry	1.2	Coconut	0.3	Papaya	0.1
Buckwheat	0.8	Garlic	0.3	Apple	0.1
Peanuts	0.8	Millet	0.2		
Sunflower oil	0.5	Whole wheat	0.2		

deficiency, therefore, is associated with poor collagen integrity. This poor integrity manifests itself in rupture of blood vessels, osteoporosis, and bone and joint abnormalities. Other symptoms of copper deficiency are brain disturbances, increased lipid peroxidation, elevated LDL cholesterol and reduced HDL cholesterol levels, and impaired immune function.[1]

Some clinical situations associated with copper deficiency are:

- Decreased intake
  - Low-copper infant formulas
  - Total parenteral (intravenous) nutrition without added copper
  - Malnutrition
- Decreased absorption
  - High dosage of supplemental zinc
  - High dosage of supplemental vitamin C
  - Chronic antacid intake
  - Chronic diarrhea
  - Malabsorptive states (celiac disease, Crohn's disease, etcetera)
  - Menke's kinky-hair syndrome
- Increased loss
  - Malabsorptive states
  - Nephrotic syndrome
  - Chelation therapy
  - Burns
- Increased requirement
  - Pregnancy
  - Lactation
  - Prematurity

Recommended Dietary Allowance

There is no official RDA for copper. The safe and adequate ranges are as follows.

Safe and Adequate Dietary Range for Copper

Group	Milligrams
INFANTS	
Under 6 months	0.4–0.6
6–12 months	0.6–0.7
CHILDREN	
1–3 years	0.7–1.0
4–6 years	1.0–1.5
7–10 years	1.5–2.5
ADOLESCENTS AND ADULTS	
11+ years	1.5–3.0

Beneficial Effects

Copper's beneficial effects relate to its role as the metallo portion in several enzymes (see Table 24.2). The two enzymes with the greatest clinical relevance are lysyl oxidase and superoxide dismutase (SOD).

Available Forms

Copper is available in many different forms—complexed with sulfate, picolinate, gluconate, and amino acids. However, there is little data to support a claim that one form is better than another.

TABLE 24.2 Enzymes Containing Copper

Name	Function
Superoxide dismutase	Breaks down the superoxide free radical
Lysyl oxidase	Collagen and elastin crosslinking
Cytochrome c oxidase	Electron transport involved in energy production
Dopamine hydroxylase	Converts dopamine to norepinephrine
Tyrosinase	Melanin formation
Ceruloplasmin	Antioxidant; facilitates iron absorption
Factor IV	Blood clotting
Thio oxidase	Disulfide-bond formation

Principal Uses

Copper is used principally in the prevention of cardiovascular disease and the treatment of arthritis (in the form of copper bracelets).

Cardiovascular Diseases

Copper deficiency may be a major risk factor in atherosclerotic vascular disease and aortic aneurysms (an aneurysm is a ballooning out or rupture of a blood vessel). More specifically, Dr. Leslie Klevay postulated that "Either a relative or absolute deficiency of copper characterized by a high ratio of zinc to copper results in hypocholesterolemia [elevated cholesterol levels in the blood], myocardial [heart muscle] and arterial damage and increased mortality."[2] There is evidence in the scientific literature to support this hypothesis.

Copper deficiency in animals is associated with increased blood cholesterol.[2] This effect is also seen in human studies.[2] When 24 male subjects were fed diets low in copper (0.36 milligrams per 1,000 calories) for 11 weeks, there was a significant increase in LDL-cholesterol levels (33 milligrams per deciliter) and a decrease in HDL cholesterol (18.7 milligrams per deciliter).[3]

Copper deficiency may also be a factor in the development of aortic aneurysms. The aorta is the largest blood vessel in the human body. It runs from the heart down the chest and abdomen until it splits to form the right and left iliac arteries, which ultimately deliver blood to the legs. Aneurysms of the abdominal aorta are life-threatening because they usually lead to rupture. Each time the heart beats, the blood it pushes exerts a great deal of force against the artery wall. The artery is surrounded by a strong elastic framework to keep it from becoming too distended, and the proper integrity of this elastic framework depends on the activity of the copper-containing enzyme lysyl oxidase. This enzyme is responsible for cross-linking collagen and elastin fibers. A deficiency of copper may contribute to the development of aortic aneurysms due to impaired lysyl oxidase activity.[4] There is more than enough evidence to demonstrate that Dr. Klevay may be right.

Copper Bracelets in Arthritis

The wearing of copper bracelets is a long-time folk remedy that has persisted despite most doctors telling their patients it doesn't work. However, there is some scientific support. First of all, copper as a component of ceruloplasmin and SOD performs antioxidant function. Secondly, various copper complexes exert anti-inflammatory effects. Finally, in a double-blind study performed in Australia, researchers discovered that copper bracelets do work to reduce pain and inflammation.[5] Presumably copper is absorbed through the skin and chelated to another compound that is able to exert anti-inflammatory action.[6]

Dosage Ranges

The estimated safe and adequate intake of copper for adults is 1.5 to 3 milligrams. Since nutrients like zinc and vitamin C interfere with copper absorption, a popular dosage recommendation for copper is based on zinc intake. The optimal ratio of zinc to copper is 10:1. This ratio means that if zinc is supplemented at a dosage of 30 milligrams per day, it requires a dosage of 3 milligrams of copper. However, when using zinc supplementation for specific treatment at dosages between 30 and 90 milligrams, I usually do not recommend copper at a level greater than 3 milligrams. When using long-term, high-dose zinc therapy (more than 45 milligrams per day), it is a good idea to monitor LDL- and HDL-cholesterol levels. If significant alterations occur, reduce the zinc dosage or increase the copper dosage.

Safety Issues

Copper is an emetic. As little as 10 milligrams usually produces nausea, and 60 milligrams usually produces vomiting. The lethal dose for copper may be as low as 3.5 grams. Definitely keep copper supplements away from children.

Chronic copper toxicity is rare. It is estimated that daily consumption of 10 to 35 milligrams is probably safe indefinitely. However, keep in mind that such a high dosage of copper adversely affects zinc nutriture.

Interactions

A high intake of vitamin C, zinc, iron, and other minerals may decrease the absorption of copper.[1,6]

25

Iodine

Iodine is a trace element required in the manufacture of thyroid hormone. Specifically, the thyroid gland adds iodine to the amino acid tyrosine to create the thyroid hormones.

Food Sources

Seafoods, including seaweeds like kelp, are nature's richest sources of iodine. However, in the U.S. the majority of iodine is derived from the use of iodized salt (70 micrograms of iodine per gram of salt). Sea salt in comparison has little iodine. Due to high salt intake, the average iodine intake in the U.S. is over 600 micrograms per day.

Deficiency Signs and Symptoms

A deficiency of iodine results in a wide spectrum of illnesses collectively termed iodine-deficiency disorders. Iodine deficiency can affect any age but is particularly harmful in pregnant women, the developing fetus, and the newborn.[1]

Some common iodine-deficiency disorders are:

- Goiter
- Cretinism
- Intellectual disability
- Growth retardation
- Neonatal hypothyroidism
- Neonatal hyperthyrotropinemia
- Increased early- and late-pregnancy miscarriage
- Increased infant mortality

These iodine deficiency disorders reflect the importance of proper iodine intake for normal thyroid function. Iodine deficiency most commonly leads to hypothyroidism and/or the development of an enlarged thyroid gland, commonly referred to as a goiter. When the level of iodine is low in the diet and blood, it causes the cells of the thyroid gland to become quite large. Eventually the entire gland swells at the base of the neck.

Goiters affect over 200 million people throughout the world. In all but 4 percent of these cases, the goiter is caused by an iodine deficiency. Iodine deficiency is now quite rare in the U.S. and other industrialized countries because iodine is added to table salt. Adding iodine to table salt began in Michigan, where in 1924 the goiter rate was an incredible 47 percent.

Few people in the U.S. are now considered iodine deficient, yet the rate of goiter is still relatively high (5 percent to 6 percent) in certain high-risk areas. Goiters in these areas probably result from excessive ingestion of certain foods that block iodine utilization. These foods are known as goitrogens and include such foods as turnips, cabbage, mustard, cassava root, soybean, peanuts, pine nuts, and millet. Cooking usually inactivates goitrogens.

Recommended Dietary Allowance

Recommended Dietary Allowance for Iodine

Group	Milligrams
INFANTS	
Under 6 months	40
6–12 months	50
CHILDREN	
1–3 years	70
4–6 years	90
7–10 years	120
YOUNG ADULTS AND ADULTS	
11+ years	150
Pregnant females	175
Lactating females	200

Beneficial Effects

Iodine's principal role is in the manufacture of thyroid hormones. In addition, it seems to modulate the effect of estrogen on breast tissue.

Available Forms

The term *iodine* is commonly used to describe any iodine compound. Technically speaking, only the elemental form of iodine is iodine. Iodine complexed to sodium or potassium (the most common supplement form of iodine) is more accurately referred to as an *iodide*. The body appears to handle iodide and iodine differently. Iodides exert a stronger effect on thyroid function. In contrast, elemental iodine is primarily involved in functions outside the thyroid such as the modulation of estrogen action on breast tissue. The reason for this difference is, unlike thyroid tissue, breast tissue lacks the enzymes that oxidize iodide to iodine. Thus, the breast tissue requires elemental forms of iodine. Organic sources of iodine (kelp, iodine caseinate, etcetera) are preferred to inorganic iodides (potassium iodide and sodium iodide).

Principal Uses

The primary use of iodine is in the prevention of iodine deficiency. In addition, Canadian research indicates that iodine (specifically iodine caseinate) may be effective in fibrocystic breast disease (FBD), a mildly uncomfortable to severely painful benign cystic swelling of the breasts. The theory is that an absence of iodine renders the epithelium more sensitive to estrogen stimulation. This hypersensitivity can produce excess secretions over the limit of absorption, thus distending the breast ducts to produce small cysts and later fibrosis (hardening of the tissue because of the deposition of fibrin similar to the formation of scar tissue).

In studies in rats, researchers found there is a hierarchical response to the type of iodine compound that corrects the abnormalities in mammary tissue because of iodine deprivation. While iodides correct the cystic spaces and partially correct the excessive cellular reproduction, iodine in its elemental form corrects the entire disease process. Thus, it appears that elemental iodine is the preferential form of iodine for breast metabolism.[2]

Human studies also indicate that elemental iodine may be more effective than iodides. Since 1975, three clinical trials have been performed on women with FBD:

• An uncontrolled study with sodium iodide and protein-bound iodide

• A prospective, controlled, crossover study from iodide to molecular iodine

• A prospective, controlled, double-blind study with molecular iodine[2]

Results from these studies indicate that while treatment with iodides was effective in about 70 percent of subjects, it exhibited a high rate of side effects (altered thyroid function in 4 percent, iodinism in 3 percent, and acne in 15 percent). Results with elemental iodine were about the same but without significant side effects. The most significant side effect with molecular iodine was short-term increased breast pain on examination that corresponded to a softening of the breast and disappearance of fibrous tissue plaques. The dosage of molecular iodine was 70 to 90 micrograms of iodine per kilogram (2.2 pounds) body weight. This dosage is safe and effective treatment for FBD. Unfortunately, currently the forms of iodine supplement used in the studies (iodine caseinate and liquid iodine) are not yet available on the marketplace.

Dosage Ranges

The recommended dietary allowance (RDA) for iodine in adults is quite small—150 micrograms. Too much iodine can actually inhibit thyroid gland synthesis. For this reason and because the only function of iodine in the body is thyroid hormone synthesis, my recommendation is to keep the dietary or supplementation levels of iodine (i.e., iodide) below 500 micrograms per day.

Safety Issues

Short-term oral iodide administration at dosages ranging from 1,500 micrograms to 250 milligrams per day reduces thyroid hormone secretion. In rare cases, a dosage as low as 750 micrograms per day may inhibit thyroid hormone secretion, especially in individuals with borderline hypothyroidism.[3,4] Increased dietary intake of iodine is also associated with acne-like skin eruptions.[5]

Interactions

Iodine does not interact adversely with any nutrient or drug when given at physiologic dosages (150 to 600 micrograms).

26

Iron

Iron is critical to human life. It plays the central role in the hemoglobin molecule of our red blood cells (RBC), where it functions in oxygen transportation from the lungs to the body's tissues and the carbon dioxide transportation from the tissues to the lungs. Iron also functions in several key enzymes in energy production and metabolism, including DNA synthesis.

Food Sources

The RDA for iron is 10 milligrams for males and 15 milligrams for females. There are two forms of dietary iron, *heme* and *nonheme*. Heme iron is iron bound to hemoglobin and myoglobin. It is in animal products and is the most efficiently absorbed form of iron (see Table 26.1). Nonheme iron is in plant foods and is poorly absorbed compared to heme iron.

Deficiency Signs and Symptoms

Iron deficiency is the most common nutrient deficiency in the United States. The groups at highest risk are infants under 2 years of age, teenage girls, pregnant women, and the elderly. Studies have found evidence of iron deficiency in 30 to 50 percent of the people in these groups. For example, some degree of iron deficiency occurs in 35 to 58 percent of young, healthy women. During pregnancy, the number is even higher.[1,2]

Iron deficiency may be caused by an increased iron requirement, decreased dietary intake, diminished iron absorption or utilization, blood loss, or a combination of factors. Increased requirements for iron occur during the growth spurts of infancy and adolescence and during pregnancy and lactation. Currently, the vast majority of pregnant women routinely take iron supplements because the dramatic, increased need for iron during pregnancy cannot be met through diet alone. Inadequate intake of iron is common in many parts of the world, especially areas that consume primar-

TABLE 26.1   Iron Content of Selected Foods, in Milligrams per 3 1/2-oz. (100-g.) Serving

Kelp	100.0	Cashews	3.8	Peanuts	2.1
Yeast, brewer's	17.3	Raisins	3.5	Tofu	1.9
Molasses, blackstrap	16.1	Jerusalem artichoke	3.4	Green peas	1.8
Wheat bran	14.9	Brazil nuts	3.4	Brown rice	1.6
Pumpkin & squash seeds	11.2	Beet greens	3.3	Olives, ripe	1.6
Wheat germ	9.4	Swiss chard	3.2	Artichoke	1.3
Liver, beef	8.8	Dandelion greens	3.1	Mung bean sprouts	1.3
Sunflower seeds	7.1	English walnuts	3.1	Broccoli	1.1
Millet	6.8	Dates	3.0	Currants	1.1
Parsley	6.2	Beans, cooked dry	2.7	Whole-wheat bread	1.1
Clams	6.1	Sesame seeds, hulled	2.4	Cauliflower	1.1
Almonds	4.7	Pecans	2.4		
Prunes, dried	3.9	Lentils	2.1		

ily a vegetarian diet. Typical infant diets in developed countries (high in milk and cereals) are also low in iron. The adolescent consuming a "junk food" diet is at high risk for iron deficiency.

The population at greatest risk for a diet deficient in iron, however is the low-income elderly population.[3] Unfortunately, decreased iron absorption is extremely common in the elderly as well.[4] Decreased iron absorption is often caused by a lack of hydrochloric acid secretion in the stomach.[5] This is an extremely common condition in the elderly. Other causes of decreased absorption include chronic diarrhea or malabsorption, the surgical removal of the stomach, and antacid use. Blood loss is the most common cause of iron deficiency in women of childbearing age, usually because of excessive menstrual bleeding. Interestingly enough, iron deficiency is a common cause of excessive menstrual blood loss.[6,7] Other common causes of blood loss include bleeding from peptic ulcers, hemorrhoids, and donating blood.

Consequences of Iron Deficiency

The negative effects of iron deficiency are caused by the impaired delivery of oxygen to the tissues and the impaired activity of iron-containing enzymes in various tissues. Iron deficiency can lead to anemia, excessive menstrual loss, learning disabilities, impaired immune function, and decreased energy levels and physical performance.[1,2,8]

Anemia refers to a condition in which the blood is deficient in red blood cells or the hemoglobin (iron-containing) portion of red blood cells. The primary function of the red blood cell is to transport oxygen from the lungs to the body's tissues in exchange for carbon dioxide. Symptoms of anemia, such as extreme fatigue, reflect a lack of oxygen being delivered to tissues and a buildup of carbon dioxide.

Iron deficiency is the most common cause of anemia; however, anemia is the last stage of iron deficiency. Iron-dependent enzymes involved in energy production and metabolism are the first to be affected by low iron levels. Serum ferritin is the best laboratory test for determining body iron stores.

Physical Performance

Several researchers have clearly demonstrated that even slight iron-deficiency anemia leads to a reduction in physical work capacity and productivity.[9–11] U.S. nutrition surveys indicate that iron deficiency is a major impairment of health and work capacity and, as a consequence, an economic loss to the individual and the country. Supplementation with iron shows rapid improvements in work capacity in iron-deficient individuals. Impaired physical performance because of iron deficiency does not necessarily stem from anemia. Again, the iron-dependent enzymes involved in energy production and metabolism are impaired long before anemia occurs.

Decreased absorption of iron is often because of a lack of hydrochloric acid secretion in the stomach.[5] This is an extremely common condition in the elderly. Other causes of decreased absorption include chronic diarrhea or malabsorption, the surgical removal of the stomach, and antacid use.

Recommended Dietary Allowance

Recommended Dietary Allowance for Iron

Group	Milligrams
INFANTS	
Under 6 months	6
6–12 months	10
CHILDREN	
1–10 years	10
YOUNG ADULTS AND ADULTS	
Males 11–18 years	12
Males 19+ years	10
Females 11–50 years	15
Females 51+ years	10
Pregnant females	30
Lactating females	15

Beneficial Effects

The beneficial effects of iron relate to its central role in the hemoglobin molecule of red blood cells and several key enzymes involved in energy production and metabolism including DNA synthesis.

Available Forms

As indicated earlier, here iron is the most efficiently absorbed form of iron. The absorption rate of nonheme iron supplements such as ferrous sulfate and ferrous fumarate is 2.9 percent on an empty stomach and 0.9 percent with food. The absorption rate of heme iron, however, is as high as 35 percent.[1,2] In addition, heme iron is without the side effects (nausea, flatulence, and diarrhea) associated with nonheme sources of iron.

Unbound nonheme iron is also more likely to spin off pro-oxidants and lead to the formation of free radicals than heme iron. For this reason, many practitioners elect to use heme iron over nonheme iron sources when iron supplementation is necessary.

Despite the superiority of heme iron, nonheme iron salts are the most popular iron supplements. It is easier to take higher quantities of nonheme iron salts than it is to take heme, and the net amount of iron absorbed is about equal. In other words, if you take 3 milligrams of heme iron and 50 milligrams of nonheme iron, the net absorption for each is about the same. The best form of nonheme iron is ferrous succinate.

Principal Uses

The principal use of iron is in the treatment of iron deficiency. Iron is also used prophylactically to prevent anemia and reduced iron stores associated with pregnancy. There is evidence that iron supplementation may also help the so-called "restless legs syndrome."

Routine blood analysis for the diagnosis of iron deficiency is not accurate enough to rely on. Serum ferritin is the best laboratory test for determining body iron stores. I include a serum ferritin determination in my routine analysis of women with chronic fatigue. In men, I may suspect iron deficiency is playing a role if they have a history of peptic ulcers, hemorrhoids, blood loss, or long-term use of antacids.

Restless Legs Syndrome

Low serum iron or ferritin levels have been found in psychiatric patients experiencing a condition called *akathisia*, which is derived from the Greek word meaning "can't sit down." Akathisia is a drug-induced state of agitation. The most common drugs producing akathisia are neuroleptics and Prozac. Several studies show that the level of iron depletion correlates with the severity of akathisia.

What prompted the research into iron status and akathisia was the association between low iron levels and the so-called "restless legs syndrome" (RLS) documented in clinical studies more than 30 years ago. However, while more recent studies have focused on low iron levels and akathisia, little (if any) research has been done on iron levels and RLS in the last few decades. This gap in research prompted researchers at the Department of Geriatric Medicine of the Royal Liverpool University in Liverpool, U.K., to study the relationship between iron status and RLS in 18 elderly patients and 18 controls.[12]

Serum ferritin levels were reduced in the RLS patients compared with controls; serum iron, vitamin B_{12}, folic acid, and hemoglobin levels did not differ between the two groups. A rating scale with a maximum score of 10 was used to assess the severity of RLS symptoms, and the researchers found serum ferritin levels were inversely correlated with the severity of RLS symptoms. Fifteen patients with RLS were treated with ferrous sulfate (200 milligrams three times daily) for 2 months. The RLS severity score improved by a median of 4 points in 6 patients with an initial ferritin less than 18 micrograms per liter, by 3 points in 4 patients with ferritin levels between 18 and 45 micrograms per liter, and by 1 point in five patients with ferritin levels between 45 and 100 micrograms per liter.

The conclusion of the study: "Iron deficiency, with or without anemia, is an important contributor to the development of RLS in elderly patients, and iron supplements can produce a significant reduction in symptoms."

Dosage Ranges

For iron deficiency, take 30 milligrams of iron bound to either succinate or fumarate twice daily between meals. If this recommendation results in abdominal discomfort, take 30 milligrams with meals three times daily. An alternative recommendation is to take a high-quality aqueous (hydrolyzed) liver extract at a level that provides a daily intake of 4 to 6 milligrams of heme iron.

Safety Issues

Recent news accounts highlight the possible relationship of elevated iron levels and the risk for heart attacks. The articles in the popular press are based on several scientific studies. However, the news accounts do not provide all the information. For example, let's look at the study published in the medical journal *Circulation*. [13] In this study of Finnish men, researchers demonstrated that high stored-iron levels produced by a diet of excess meat is associated with excess risk of heart attack. Although iron was singled out, the study also demonstrated an increased risk for a heart attack when LDL-cholesterol levels were elevated. In other words, the strongest link between increased stored-iron levels and risk for a heart attack was found in men with LDL-cholesterol levels greater than 193 milligrams per deciliter. Furthermore, the strongest dietary link to an increased risk for a heart attack in the study was meat intake. Meat intake was also linked to increased LDL-cholesterol levels and increased dietary intake of saturated fats.

Another way of expressing the results of the study would be to simply state that Finnish men eating more meat have an increased risk for heart attacks, elevated LDL-cholesterol levels, and elevated iron stores. Therefore, the study simply provided additional evidence that high meat intake increases the risk of heart attack. This is nothing new; it is just a different way in which high meat intake can lead to premature death.

Elevated levels of iron may lead to an increased risk of heart disease by spinning off free radicals in the blood and either damaging cholesterol or the artery walls directly. Antioxidants like vitamin C and vitamin E protect against iron-induced oxidative damage.

Other possible risks of iron overload include an increased risk for infection and even cancer.[14] For these reasons, I restrict iron supplementation to cases of iron deficiency and menstruating, pregnant, or lactating women.

Acute iron poisoning in infants can result in serious consequences. Keep all iron supplements out of the reach of children. Severe iron poisoning results in damage to the intestinal lining, liver failure, nausea and vomiting, and shock.

Interactions

High intakes of other minerals, particularly calcium, magnesium, and zinc, can interfere with iron absorption. Vitamin C enhances iron absorption. Anti-inflammatory drugs like aspirin and ibuprofen may contribute to iron loss via gastrointestinal bleeding.

27

Manganese

Manganese was first considered an essential nutrient in 1931 when researchers demonstrated poor growth and impaired reproduction in mice and rats fed a diet devoid of manganese.

Food Sources

Good dietary sources of manganese include nuts, whole grains, dried fruits, and green leafy vegetables (see Table 27.1). Meats, dairy products, poultry, and seafood are considered poor sources of manganese.

Deficiency Signs and Symptoms

Manganese deficiency in animals results in impaired growth, skeletal abnormalities, and defects in carbohydrate and fat metabolism. If manganese deficiency occurs during pregnancy, the offspring exhibit an inherited movement disorder (ataxia)

TABLE 27.1   Manganese Content of Selected Foods, in Milligrams per 3½-oz. (100-g.) Serving

Pecans	3.5	Walnuts	0.8	Brussels sprouts	0.3
Brazil nuts	2.8	Spinach, fresh	0.8	Oatmeal	0.3
Almonds	2.5	Peanuts	0.7	Cornmeal	0.2
Barley	1.8	Oats	0.6	Millet	0.2
Rye	1.3	Raisins	0.5	Carrots	0.16
Buckwheat	1.3	Turnip greens	0.5	Broccoli	0.15
Split peas, dry	1.3	Rhubarb	0.5	Brown rice	0.14
Whole wheat	1.1	Beet greens	0.4	Whole-wheat bread	0.14

characterized by incoordination, lack of balance, and retraction of the head. This condition results from impaired development of the otoliths, calcified structures of the inner ear responsible for equilibrium.[1]

Human manganese deficiency is not as well defined as in animals. Animal studies indicate that manganese deficiency could lead to significant disruption of normal growth and metabolism. In several human studies where subjects were fed a manganese-deficient diet, numerous metabolic abnormalities developed, including the appearance of a skin rash, loss of hair color, bone remodeling, reduced growth of hair and nails, and reduced HDL cholesterol.[1]

Recommended Dietary Allowance

There is no official RDA for manganese. Here are the estimated safe and adequate ranges.

Safe and Adequate Dietary Range for Manganese

Group	Milligrams
INFANTS	
Under 6 months	0.3–0.6
6–12 months	0.6–1.0
CHILDREN	
1–3 years	1.0–1.5
4–6 years	1.5–2.0
7–10 years	2.0–3.0
ADOLESCENTS AND ADULTS	
11+ years	2.5–5.0

Beneficial Effects

Manganese functions in many enzyme systems, including enzymes involved in blood sugar control, energy metabolism, and thyroid hormone function.[1] It also functions in the antioxidant enzyme superoxide dismutase, or SOD. This enzyme prevents the deleterious effects of the super oxide free radical from destroying cellular components. Without SOD, cells are susceptible to damage and inflammation. Manganese supplementation can increase SOD activity, which reflects increased antioxidant activity.[2]

Available Forms

Manganese is available commercially in various forms. Manganese salts such as manganese sulfate or chloride probably are not as well absorbed as manganese bound to picolinate, gluconate, or other chelates, although there is no data to prove this assumption.

Principal Uses

The principal uses of manganese supplementation is in the treatment of strains, sprains, inflammation, epilepsy, and diabetes.

Strains, Sprains, and Inflammation

Manganese is a popular nutritional recommendation for strains, sprains, and inflammation presumably because manganese supplementation may increase the level or activity of manganese-containing SOD.[2] The injectable form of this enzyme (available in Europe) is effective in the treatment of inflammation, including the inflammation associated with rheumatoid arthritis.[3] Although oral SOD products are available in the United States, it is not clear if any orally administered SOD can escape digestion in the intestinal tract and exert a therapeutic effect. One study indicated oral SOD did not affect tissue SOD levels.[4] In contrast, manganese supplementation can increase SOD activity, which reflects increased antioxidant activity.[2] Although no clinical studies are available that determine the effectiveness of manganese supplementation in sprains, strains, and inflammation, we can assume it is effective because it may raise tissue SOD activity. In addition, there is evidence that patients with rheumatoid arthritis and presumably other chronic inflammatory diseases have an increased need for manganese.[5]

Epilepsy

Low manganese is also linked to epilepsy. This link was first suggested in 1963 when it was observed that manganese-deficient rats were more susceptible to seizures than manganese-replete animals, and that manganese-deficient animals exhibit epileptic-like brain wave tracings.[6] This prompted researchers to look at manganese concentrations in epileptics. Low whole blood and hair manganese levels have been found in epileptics, and those with the lowest levels typically have the highest seizure activity.[7-11]

Manganese plays a significant role in cerebral function because it is a critical metal for glucose utilization within the neuron, adenylate cyclase activity, and neurotransmitter control. Obviously, for optimal central nervous system function, proper manganese levels must be maintained. A high manganese diet or manganese supplementation may be helpful in controlling seizure activity for some patients.

Diabetes

Manganese is an important cofactor in the key enzymes of glucose metabolism.[12] In guinea pigs, a deficiency of manganese results in diabetes and the frequent birth of offspring who develop pancreatic abnormalities or no pancreas at all.[13] Diabetics have only one-half the manganese of normal individuals.[14] One report in the medical literature indicates manganese supplementation (3 to 5 milligrams daily as manganese chloride) produces a positive effect in a diabetic patient who was not responding to insulin therapy.[15] Manganese supplementation appears warranted in diabetes.

Dosage Ranges

Although there is no specific RDA for manganese, most people require between 2 and 5 milligrams per day. For therapeutic purposes, the dosage ranges are as follows:

- **Sprains, Strains, Inflammation** First 2 weeks, 50 milligrams to 200 milligrams daily in divided dosages; thereafter, 15 milligrams to 30 milligrams daily
- **Epilepsy** 15 milligrams to 30 milligrams daily
- **Diabetes** 5 milligrams to 15 milligrams daily

Safety Issues

Dietary manganese and manganese-containing nutritional supplements have an extremely low level of toxicity. However, manganese toxicity as a result of environmental pollution or mining of manganese is a serious health problem. In its most severe forms, manganese toxicity can result in a syndrome called "manganese madness," which is characterized by severe psychiatric symptoms such as hallucinations, violent acts, and hyperirritability.[1]

Interactions

Manganese may inhibit the absorption of iron, copper, and zinc. Conversely, high intakes of magnesium, calcium, iron, copper, and zinc may inhibit the absorption of manganese. Antacids may also inhibit the absorption of manganese.[16]

28

Molybdenum

Molybdenum functions as a component in several enzymes, including those involved in alcohol detoxification, uric acid formation, and sulfur metabolism.[1]

Food Sources

The average diet contains between 50 and 500 micrograms of molybdenum per day. Legumes and whole grains are the richest source (see Table 28.1); however, the concentration of molybdenum in foods depends on the soil content of molybdenum.[1]

Deficiency Signs and Symptoms

Molybdenum deficiency has appeared in subjects receiving total parenteral (intravenous) nutrition. It manifests as an inability to detoxify sulfites because the enzyme that detoxifies sulfites (sulfite oxidase) is molybdenum dependent. Molybdenum

TABLE 28.1   Molybdenum Content of Selected Foods, in Milligrams per 3¹/₂-oz. (100-g.) Serving

Lentils	155	Rye bread	50	Molasses	19
Split peas	130	Corn	45	Cantaloupe	16
Cauliflower	120	Barley	42	Apricots	14
Green peas	110	Whole wheat	36	Raisins	10
Yeast, brewer's	109	Whole-wheat bread	32	Butter	10
Wheat germ	100	Potatoes	30	Strawberries	7
Spinach	100	Onions	25	Carrots	5
Brown rice	75	Peanuts	25	Cabbage	5
Garlic	70	Coconut	25		
Oats	60	Green beans	21		

supplementation brought about complete resolution of symptoms of sulfite toxicity such as increased heart rate, shortness of breath, headache, disorientation, nausea, and vomiting. Molybdenum deficiency may be a cause of sulfite sensitivities.[1]

Recommended Dietary Allowance

There is no official RDA for molybdenum. Here are the estimated safe and adequate ranges.

Safe and Adequate Dietary Range for Molybdenum

Group	Micrograms
INFANTS	
Under 6 months	15–30
6–12 months	20–40
CHILDREN	
1–3 years	25–50
4–6 years	30–75
7–10 years	50–150
ADOLESCENTS AND ADULTS	
11+ years	75–250

Beneficial Effects

Molybdenum's beneficial effects stem from its role as a necessary coenzyme in the enzymes xanthine oxidase, aldehyde oxidase, and sulfite oxidase. These enzymes are involved in uric acid formation, alcohol detoxification, and detoxification of sulfites, respectively.[1]

Available Forms

Molybdenum is available commercially as sodium molybdate. Another form, etrathiomolybdate, is used in the treatment of Wilson's disease. Molybdenum is almost completely absorbed from the intestinal tract as absorption studies show a high rate of absorption (88 to 93 percent) at dietary intakes between 22 and 1,500 micrograms per day.[2] Molybdenum is conserved at low intakes, and excess molybdenum is rapidly excreted in the urine. There is probably no advantage of one form of molybdenum over another.

Principal Uses

Molybdenum has four possible applications—sulfite sensitivity, cancer prevention, cavity prevention, and Wilson's disease.

Sulfite Sensitivity

As mentioned above, low molybdenum levels may lead to increased allergic reactions to sulfites. Sulfites are preservatives that prevent spoilage by checking the growth of microorganisms. Restaurant salad bars once used them widely on produce. Because most people were unaware of this practice and unaware they had a sensitivity to sulfites, many unsuspecting people experienced severe allergic or asthmatic reactions. For years the FDA refused to even consider a ban on sulfites, even while admitting these agents provoked attacks in an unknown number of people (5 to 10 percent of asthma victims). It was not until 1985, when sulfite sensitivity was linked to 15 deaths between 1983 and 1985, that the FDA agreed to review the matter. In 1986, the FDA finally banned sulfite use on produce and required labeling of other foods such as wine, beer, and dried fruit, which have added sulfites. The average person consumes an average of 2 to 3 milligrams of sulfites daily, while wine and beer drinkers typically consume up to 10 milligrams daily.[3]

Cancer Prevention

Population studies and experimental findings have implicated molybdenum deficiency as a factor in some forms of cancer. Specifically, population studies in China show that where soil molybdenum levels are low, the rate of esophageal cancer is higher.[4] In the United States, there is a 30 percent increase in esophageal cancer in areas where there is no molybdenum in the drinking water.[5] Animal studies indicate that the addition of molybdenum to the drinking water significantly inhibits chemically induced esophageal cancer.[6,7] Presumably the anticancer effects of molybdenum stem from its role in the detoxification of cancer-causing chemicals.

Cavity Prevention

Several population studies show that in areas where the molybdenum intake is high, there is a low rate of tooth decay.[8,9] Conversely, areas where molybdenum levels are low have higher rates of tooth decay. Molybdenum might enhance the effect of fluoride because the combined administration of molybdenum (25 or 50 parts per million) and fluoride (50 parts per million) is more effective in reducing dental cavities than water containing only fluoride (50 parts per million).[9]

Wilson's Disease

Wilson's disease is a hereditary disorder characterized by increased storage of copper. The liver fails to excrete excess copper in the bile for loss in the stool. The accumulating copper causes damage primarily to the liver and the brain. Patients typically present in the second to the fourth decades of life with liver disease, neurological disease of the movement disorder type, or a wide array of behavioral disturbances. Currently, four drugs are used as anticopper agents in Wilson's disease—zinc, which blocks intestinal absorption of copper; penicillamine and trientine, both of which are chelators that increase urinary excretion of copper; and molybdenum (as tetrathiomolybdate), which forms a complex with copper and protein and can block copper absorption from the intestine or render blood copper nontoxic. Although zinc is regarded as the clear treatment of choice, molybdenum supplementation may also be appropriate. As dietary intake of molybdenum increases, so does urinary excretion of copper.[10,11]

Dosage Ranges

The dosage range for molybdenum supplementation is 200 micrograms to 500 micrograms daily. Higher dosages, under the advice of a licensed physician, may be required in the adjunctive therapy of Wilson's disease.

Safety Issues

Molybdenum is relatively nontoxic. In order to produce toxicity, a dosage of more than 100 milligrams per kilogram body weight would have to be ingested. A daily intake of 10 to 15 milligrams may produce in some people goutlike symptoms because of enhanced production of uric acid.[1]

Interactions

Besides the interaction with copper and fluoride, there are no known interactions between molybdenum and other nutrients or drugs.

29

Selenium

The trace mineral selenium functions primarily as a component of the antioxidant enzyme glutathione peroxidase, which works with vitamin E in preventing free radical damage to cell membranes. Low levels of selenium are linked to a higher risk for cancer, cardiovascular disease, inflammatory diseases, and other conditions associated with increased free-radical damage, including premature aging and cataract formation.

Food Sources

The level of selenium in food is directly related to the level of selenium in the soil. Table 29.1 reflects estimates.

Deficiency Signs and Symptoms

Severe selenium deficiency is associated with Keshan disease, a severe heart disorder that affects primarily children and women of childbearing age. Keshan disease appears in some areas of China where selenium levels in the soil are very low. Kashin-Beck disease is an arthritic condition that is also linked to low selenium levels in China. Selenium deficiency can cause other heart disturbances and muscle weakness. However, these severe selenium-deficient states are extremely rare. More com-

TABLE 29.1 Selenium Content of Selected Foods, in Micrograms per 3 ½-oz. (100-g.) Serving

Food		Food		Food	
Wheat germ	111	Bran	63	Turnips	27
Brazil nuts	103	Red Swiss chard	57	Garlic	25
Oats	56	Barley	24	Brown rice	39
Whole-wheat bread	66	Orange juice	19		

mon is the chronically low selenium intake associated with an increased risk for cancer, heart disease, and low immune function.[1,2]

Recommended Dietary Allowance

Recommended Dietary Allowance for Selenium

Group	Micrograms
INFANTS	
Under 6 months	10
6–12 months	15
CHILDREN	
1–6 years	20
7–10 years	30
ADOLESCENTS AND ADULTS	
Males 11–14 years	40
Males 15–18 years	50
Males 19+ years	70
Females 11–14 years	45
Females 15–18 years	50
Females 19+ years	55
Pregnant females	65
Lactating females	75

Beneficial Effects

Selenium's chief beneficial effect stems from its role as an antioxidant. Specifically, selenium in the form of selenocysteine is incorporated at the four active sites of the enzyme glutathione peroxidase. This enzyme assumes a critical role in protecting against free-radical and oxidative damage. In addition to this important role, selenium appears to exert antioxidant activity on its own and is involved in the production of thyroid hormone.[3] Selenium is also antagonistic to heavy metals like lead, mercury, aluminum, and cadmium.[4]

Available Forms

Selenium is available in several different forms. Studies show inorganic salts like sodium selenite are less effectively absorbed and not as biologically active as organic forms of selenium, such as selenomethionine and selenium-rich yeast. Therefore, the preferred form of selenium supplement is either selenomethionine or high-selenium-content yeast.[5–7]

Principal Uses

Selenium supplementation is used primarily as a general antioxidant support. To appreciate the importance of selenium supplementation, let us examine the role of selenium in cancer, enhancing immune function, cardiovascular disease, inflammatory conditions, cataract formation, and pregnancy and premature infants.

Cancer

The Food and Nutrition Board develops the Recommended Dietary Allowance guidelines on the desirable amounts of essential nutrients in the diet. In 1984, it established the Committee on Diet and Health. As part of its comprehensive analysis of diet and major chronic diseases, this group of experts reviewed the studies on selenium and cancer. Their summary was "Low selenium intakes or decreased selenium concentrations in the blood are associated with increased risk of cancer in humans."[8]

A large body of scientific evidence clearly demonstrates that cancer mortality increases when dietary intake of selenium is suboptimal.[8,9] To further support this link, researchers have found consistently low levels of selenium and glutathione peroxidase in the blood of subjects suffering from many forms of cancer—including young children (age 6 months to 7 years)—compared to levels in healthy individuals.[8-10] Several of the studies were prospective; the selenium levels had been determined years before cancer developed. The anticancer effects of selenium are more significant in men than in women and are most important in the prevention of respiratory and gastrointestinal tract cancers. [8,9,11,12]

Selenium intake offers significant protection against cancer formation in a number of animal models. The National Research Council stated that "A large accumulation of evidence indicates that supplementation of the diet or drinking water with selenium protects against tumors induced by a wide variety of chemical carcinogens" in animal studies. Significant protection was demonstrated against the development breast, colon, liver, and skin cancers.[8] Taken together, this research indicates that optimal selenium levels in the diet and body offer significant anticancer effects.

Immune Function

Selenium in its vital role in glutathione peroxidase affects all components of the immune system, including the development and expression of all white blood cells. Selenium deficiency results in depressed immune function, whereas selenium supplementation results in augmentation and/or restoration of immune functions. Selenium deficiency inhibits resistance to infection as a result of impaired white blood cell and thymus function, while selenium supplementation (200 micrograms per day) stimulates white blood cell and thymus function.[13-15]

The ability of selenium supplementation to enhance immune function goes well beyond simply restoring selenium levels in selenium-deficient individuals. For example, in one study, individuals with normal selenium concentrations in their blood received selenium supplementation of 200 micrograms per day). This resulted in a 118 percent increase in the ability of lymphocytes to kill tumor cells and an 82.3 percent increase in the activity of a white blood cell known as a "natural killer cell" because of its powerful ability to kill cancer cells and microorganisms.[14] These effects apparently resulted from the ability of selenium to enhance the expression of the immune-enhancing compound interleukin-2. This in turn increased the rate of white blood cell proliferation and differentiation into forms capable of killing tumor cells and microorganisms. The supplementation regimen did not produce significant changes in the blood selenium levels of the participants. The results indicate that the immune-enhancing effects of selenium in humans require supplementation above the normal dietary intake.

Cardiovascular Disease

Selenium supplementation, like other antioxidant supplementation, appears to offer protection against heart disease and strokes. Rates for heart disease are highest where selenium intake is lowest, although the relationship between the two is not as strong as it is between cancer and selenium.[16–18] If there is an association between low selenium levels and increased risk for heart disease and strokes, it is presumably the result of decreased glutathione peroxidase activity. Other mechanisms may, however, account for the association. Selenium supplementation (97 micrograms of selenium from yeast tablets) increases the ratio of HDL to LDL cholesterol and inhibits platelet aggregation.[19,20] Selenium appears to offer protection in smokers more than any other group.[18]

Selenium supplementation should definitely be part of any post-heart attack or stroke plan. In one double-blind study, 81 heart attack patients were randomly assigned to receive 100 micrograms of selenium (from selenium-rich yeast) or a placebo. After 6 months, there were 4 fatal heart attacks and 2 nonfatal heart attacks in the placebo group compared to no deaths and 1 nonfatal heart attack in the selenium group.[21]

Inflammatory Conditions

Selenium and glutathione peroxidase levels are low in patients with rheumatoid arthritis, eczema, and psoriasis and may be low in most inflammatory conditions.[22,23] Because free radicals, oxidants, prostaglandins, and leukotrienes cause much of the damage to tissues seen in rheumatoid arthritis, a deficiency of selenium results in even more significant damage because of low levels of glutathione peroxidase. Glutathione peroxidase is especially important in reducing the production of inflammatory prostaglandins and leukotrienes.

Clinical studies have not yet clearly demonstrated that selenium supplementation alone improves the signs and symptoms of rheumatoid arthritis; however, one clinical study indicates that selenium combined with vitamin E does provide significant benefit.[24,25] Supplementing the diet with 50 to 200 micrograms of selenium and 200 to 400 I.U. of vitamin E is appropriate in inflammatory conditions because of an increased need, the low selenium levels typically seen in inflammatory conditions, and selenium and vitamin E's synergistic effects as antioxidants.

Cataracts

Cataracts are the leading cause of impaired vision and blindness in the United States. Approximately four million people have some degree of vision-impairing cataract, and at least 40,000 people in the U.S. are blind because of cataracts. Cataracts create a tremendous financial burden on our society—cataract surgery is the most common major surgical procedure done in the United States (600,000 per annum) for persons on Medicare.

The origin of cataract formation is ultimately related to free-radical damage. The lens, like many other tissues of the body, depends on adequate levels and activities of superoxide dismutase (SOD), catalase, and glutathione peroxidase, and adequate levels of the accessory antioxidants vitamins E and C and selenium.

Maintaining proper selenium levels appears to be especially important because human lens glutathione peroxidase is selenium-dependent. Low selenium levels would greatly promote cataract formation. Previous studies show the selenium content in a human lens with a cataract is only 15 percent of normal levels.[26] Recently, researchers conducted a study to better examine the role of selenium in cataract formation.

In that study, selenium levels in the serum, lens, and aqueous humour were determined in 48 patients with cataracts and compared to matched controls. The selenium levels of the serum and aqueous humour were found to be significantly less in the patients with cataracts (serum, 0.28 versus 0.32 micrograms per milliliter; aqueous humour, 0.19 versus 0.31 micrograms per milliliter). However, the selenium levels in the lens itself did not significantly differ in patients with cataracts and normal controls.[27]

The study's most important finding was the decreased level of selenium in the aqueous humour in patients with cataracts. Excess hydrogen peroxide levels, up to 25 times the normal levels, are found in the aqueous humour in patients with cataracts. An excess of hydrogen peroxide is associated with increased lipid peroxidation and altered lens permeability as a result of damage to the sodium-potassium pump. These changes ultimately leave the lens unprotected against free-radical and sun damage. As a result, a cataract forms. Since selenium-dependent glutathione peroxidase is responsible for the breaking down of hydrogen peroxide, low selenium levels appear to be a major factor in the development of a cataract.

Pregnancy and SIDS

There is substantial evidence that selenium is essential for proper fetal growth and development. Selenium requirements appear to increase during pregnancy; selenium concentrations in the blood tend to be lower during pregnancy, particular during the later stages.[28] Selenium levels also tend to be very low in low birth weight babies.[29]

Low selenium levels in the newborn have been linked to sudden infant death syndrome (SIDS).[30–32] Like heart disease and cancer, SIDS has the highest occurrence in areas of the world where the selenium content of the soil and diet is lowest. Deficiency of selenium and vitamin E in animals is associated with a condition known as "white muscle disease" (WMD) and sudden death in young animals. A condition often seen in both of these diseases (when a selenium deficiency is present) is a heart disturbance (cardiomyopathy) very similar to the heart disturbance of Keshan disease. WMD, Keshan disease, and SIDS share some common features. All are associated with the same basic underlying pathological feature—a small area of the heart becomes damaged (focal cardiac necrosis), which leads to heart failure or cardiovascular shock. While the strict definition of SIDS requires no identifiable cause of death on autopsy, according to some published reports heart damage is a common finding. In fact, in one study of 200 cases of SIDS, focal cardiac necrosis was found in all cases.[33] The hypothesis is that a selenium and/or vitamin E deficiency leaves the heart muscle susceptible to oxidative damage. The heart muscle becomes damaged, resulting in focal cardiac necrosis and subsequent fatality. Although such a theory is highly controversial, the link between folic acid deficiency and neural tube defects was controversial for over 30 years before it was accepted as an undeniable association. Surely low selenium is not a cause in every SIDS case—there are some autopsy studies showing normal selenium levels in infants dying of SIDS. However, supplementing 200 micrograms of selenium during pregnancy and lactation appears warranted given its increased need during pregnancy, possible benefit, and safety.

Dosage Ranges

Although there is no specific RDA for selenium, for adults a daily intake of 50 to 200 micrograms is often recommended. At high-intake levels (daily intake in excess of 1,000 micrograms), selenium can produce toxicity. For children, a good dosage recommendation is 1.5 micrograms per pound of body weight.

Safety Issues

The human body requires a small amount of selenium. Dosages as low as 900 micrograms daily over prolonged periods of time can produce signs of selenium toxicity in some people. Signs and symptoms related to chronic toxicity include depression, nervousness, emotional instability, nausea and vomiting, a garlic odor of the breath and sweat, and in extreme cases loss of hair and fingernails. Acute selenium toxicity from dietary sources is rare.[1]

In 1983 and 1984, 13 people in the U.S. suffered from toxic effects brought about by ingesting dietary supplement tablets containing very high levels of selenium. Because of a manufacturing error, each tablet contained 27.3 milligrams of selenium, a level 182 times greater than the label claim. The experience of one woman illustrates the severity of the problem. A 57-year-old woman had already consumed 77 tablets from a 99-tablet bottle when she learned of the recall. Her estimated cumulative dose was 2,387 milligrams of selenium in about 3 months. She had noticed pronounced hair loss about 11 days after starting the selenium supplement, loss that had progressed to almost complete baldness over a 2-month period. Later, she noticed horizontal white streaking on one fingernail, along with pain and swelling of the fingertip and signs of infection. These changes subsequently progressed to involve all fingernails. She ultimately lost the originally affected fingernail. She had also experienced periodic episodes of nausea and vomiting, a "sour-milk" breath odor, and progressive fatigue. Other persons who had consumed the mislabeled selenium product reported similar signs and symptoms.[34]

Interactions

Other antioxidant nutrients work synergistically with selenium in raising glutathione peroxidase activity. Selenium absorption is adversely affected by heavy metals (lead, mercury, cadmium, etcetera) and high dosages of vitamin C (affects sodium selenite more than organic forms of selenium). Presumably selenium absorption is reduced with high intakes of other trace minerals, particularly zinc. Various drugs, particularly chemotherapy drugs, may increase selenium requirements.

30

Silicon

Silicon is the second most abundant element on earth—oxygen is first. Crystalline silicon (quartz) is the most abundant mineral on the earth's crust. Despite the abundance of silicon on earth, until 1972 it was not regarded as an essential nutrient. Although no one has determined silicon's exact biological role, we do know it is required for proper integrity of the skin, ligaments, tendons, and bone.[1-3]

Food Sources

The richest sources of silicon are unrefined grains, such as oatmeal and brown rice, and root vegetables. The estimated average human daily intake of silicon from food is approximately 21 to 46 milligrams.

Deficiency Signs and Symptoms

Silicon deficiency in humans has not been demonstrated. In animals, silicon deficiency is characterized by abnormal ligament, tendon, and bone integrity. Chickens fed a silicon-deficient diet demonstrate bone abnormalities consistent with depressed collagen synthesis. Collagen is the major protein component in the human body essential to proper bone and connective tissue integrity.[1-3]

Recommended Dietary Allowance

There is no RDA for silicon. A daily intake between 20 and 40 milligrams is safe and probably adequate.

Beneficial Effects

Silicon is required for the proper functioning of an enzyme (prolyhydroxylase) that functions in the formation of collagen in bone, cartilage, and other connective tissues. It also may be important in bone calcification—high concentrations of silicon have been found at the calcification sites of growing bones. The highest concentrations of silicon, however, are found in the skin and hair. Interestingly, the silicon content of the aorta, thymus, and skin tends to decline with aging while in other tissues it does not.[1-3]

Available Forms

Silicon is available in several different forms: silicon-rich horsetail (the plant *Equisetum arvense*), sodium metasilicate, and colloidal silicic acid. There is no real clear-cut advantage to any of these forms, although the colloidal form may have an advantage because it can also be used topically.

Principal Uses

Despite a lack of scientific knowledge or support, silicon is a popular nutritional recommendation to strengthen the bones, connective tissue, hair, and skin. One of the few studies on silicon's benefits featured the colloidal silicic acid. A total of 50 women with signs of aging of their facial skin, thin hair, and brittle nails were enrolled in an open, uncontrolled 90-day study. The women took a daily oral dose of 10 milliliters of colloidal silicic acid and applied colloidal silicic acid twice daily to the face. Statistically significant improvements were noted in the thickness of the skin, strength of the skin, wrinkles, and health of the hair and nails. Ultrasound examination revealed that silicon supplementation increased the thickness of the dermis, the connective tissue support structure that lies just below the surface of the skin.[4]

Dosage Ranges

Until more is learned about the role and need for silicon, dosages should not exceed 50 milligrams daily. There is no RDA for silicon, but an estimated daily requirement is 5 to 20 milligrams.[1]

Safety Issues

Silicon is generally regarded as being nontoxic. However, increased levels of silicon and aluminum complexes have been detected in the neurofibrillary tangle and senile plaque in the brains of Alzheimer's disease patients.[5,6] Dietary and environmental sources of aluminum are probably the more significant factor. Aluminum is in many antacids and many processed foods and in underarm deodorants, bentonite clay, cooking pans, and drinking water.

Interactions

The interactions of silicon are not known.

31

Vanadium

Vanadium—named after the Scandinavian goddess of beauty, youth, and luster—has been receiving a great deal of attention in the marketplace and in medical literature. A recent review article published in the *Journal of the American Dietetic Association* provides evidence that vanadium is an essential nutrient in human nutrition.

Food Sources

Although Table 31.1 lists the vanadium content of some selected foods, it is not known how meaningful these figures are because some studies show that most ingested vanadium (greater than 99 percent) is not absorbed. The estimated average daily intake of vanadium for Americans is 10 to 60 micrograms. Total human body content of vanadium is about 100 micrograms. Vanadium is not concentrated to any extent in a particular organ or tissue. Good food sources of vanadium include black pepper, dill, parsley, mushrooms, and shellfish.

TABLE 31.1 Vanadium Content of Selected Foods, in Micrograms per 3 1/2-oz. (100-g.) Serving

Food	µg	Food	µg	Food	µg
Buckwheat	100	Corn	15	Onions	5
Parsley	80	Green beans	14	Whole wheat	5
Soybeans	70	Peanut oil	11	Beets	4
Safflower oil	64	Carrots	10	Apples	3
Sunflower seed oil	41	Cabbage	10	Plums	2
Oats	35	Garlic	10	Lettuce	2
Olive oil	30	Tomatoes	6	Millet	2
Sunflower seeds	15	Radishes	5		

Deficiency Signs and Symptoms

Although vanadium may function in hormone, cholesterol, and blood sugar metabolism, no specific deficiency signs or symptoms in humans have been reported. Some researchers speculate that a vanadium deficiency may contribute to elevated cholesterol levels and faulty blood sugar control manifesting as either diabetes or hypoglycemia.[1]

While the significance of vanadium in human nutrition is unknown, during the past decade there has been a growing awareness that vanadium is an essential nutrient for certain plants, animals, and microorganisms. Perhaps the most meaningful study involved placing goats on a vanadium-restricted diet (5 micrograms per kilogram dry diet). After 3 years on such a diet, female goats gave birth to kids with irreversible bone deformities in their front legs. Some kids died within 3 days; some could not stand after birth. The vanadium-deficient mothers produced significantly less milk. Thus, vanadium's necessity in the nutrition of goats has been confirmed and may relate to its role in human nutrition.[1]

Recommended Dietary Allowance

There is no RDA for vanadium. A daily intake of 10 to 60 micrograms is safe and probably adequate.

Beneficial Effects

Most research on vanadium has focused on its role in improving or mimicking insulin action. In animal studies, high dosages of vanadium (most often as vanadyl sulfate) have led to improved glucose tolerance, inhibition of cholesterol synthesis, and improved mineralization of bones and teeth.[2]

Available Forms

Vanadium exists in five different forms, with the most biologically significant being either vanadyl or vanadate. Vanadyl sulfate is the most popular form of vanadium for nutritional supplementation.

Principal Uses

Vanadyl sulfate is popular with diabetics and bodybuilders because it may improve insulin action or mimic insulin. However, there is little clinical data to support its use for that purpose. Most recent research on vanadium has focused on vanadyl's role in glucose metabolism in test tubes and animals. Studies in guinea pigs and other animals show that vanadyl can improve oral glucose tolerance. It should produce similar effects in humans.[1,2]

In one study, six non-insulin-dependent diabetes mellitus (NIDDM) patients treated with diet and/or with glucose-lowering drugs (sulfonylureas) were examined at the end of three consecutive periods: placebo for 2 weeks, vanadyl sulfate (100 milligrams daily) for 3 weeks, and placebo again for 2 weeks. Glycemic control at baseline was poor as demonstrated by an elevated fasting blood glucose level (average of 210 milligrams per deciliter) but improved after treatment to average levels of 181 milligrams per deciliter. These results indicate that 3 weeks of treatment with vanadyl sulfate improves hepatic and peripheral insulin sensitivity in insulin-resistant NIDDM humans. These preliminary results are encouraging.[3]

Dosage Ranges

A dosage of 50 to 100 micrograms per day should be a safe and sufficient amount to meet nutritional requirements.[1] Vanadium may prove to be toxic at levels commonly promoted by manufacturers of vanadyl sulfate products designed for the bodybuilding market or in patients with diabetes (dosage recommendations have ranged from 15 milligrams to 100 milligrams). At this time, based on available data, I cannot recommend high dosages of vanadyl sulfate. The preliminary data is exciting, but the dosages used (100 milligrams a day) go well beyond a nutritional effect.

Safety Issues

Toxic effects of vanadium observed in animal studies include elevation of blood pressure, reduction of coenzyme A and coenzyme Q_{10} levels, stimulation of monoamine oxidase inhibitors, and interference with cellular energy production.[1] However, the toxicity studies used vanadate, not vanadyl, and humans subjects appear to tolerate vanadium better than other species.

When 12 human subjects were fed 13.5 milligrams of vanadium daily for 2 weeks followed by 22.5 milligrams daily for 5 months, five patients exhibited cramps and diarrhea at the high dosage.[1] There were no significant side effects in the study described above in patients with non-insulin-dependent diabetes who were given 100 milligrams of vanadyl sulfate.[3]

Another concern is excessive levels of vanadium have been linked to manic depression. Increased levels of vanadium are found in hair samples from manic patients, and these values fall toward normal levels with recovery. Vanadium in vandate form is a strong inhibitor of the sodium-potassium pump. Lithium, the drug of choice for manic depression, can reduce this inhibition.[1]

Interactions

There are no known interactions with vanadium and other nutrients or with any drug other than lithium.

PART FOUR

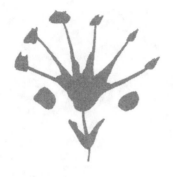

Essential Fatty Acids

The human body cannot function properly without two polyunsaturated fats—linoleic and alpha-linolenic acid. These fatty acids are referred to as "essential fatty acids" because they truly are essential to normal cell structure and body function. Both essential fatty acids function as components of nerve cells, cell membranes, and hormone-like substances known as prostaglandins. Many of the beneficial effects of a diet rich in plant foods is a result of the low levels of saturated fat and the relatively higher levels of essential fatty acids. While a diet high in saturated fat has been linked to many chronic diseases, a diet low in saturated fat but high in essential fatty acids prevents these very same diseases.

32

Understanding Fats and Oils

To understand the harmful effects of some fats and the beneficial effects of others, we need to grasp the terminology that describes fats and oils. Let's start at the beginning and define *fat*. Technically speaking, a *fat* or *lipid* describes compounds composed of carbon, hydrogen, and oxygen and that are not soluble in water. The three major classes of dietary fats are triglycerides, phospholipids, and sterols (like cholesterol).

Triglycerides

The most common dietary fats are triglycerides. They comprise approximately 95 percent of all ingested fats. A triglyceride is composed of a glycerol molecule with three fat molecules. These fat molecules are called *fatty acids*. A fatty acid molecule is composed of a long chain of carbon molecules with an acid group on one end (see Figure 32.1).

The body handles dietary triglycerides by breaking the bond between the glycerol and the fatty acid. This breaking of the chemical bond is achieved by emulsifying the triglyceride with bile so that enzymes (lipases) can add water to the glycerol molecule. When this happens, the fatty acid is liberated from the glycerol molecule. This process happens during digestion. Initially the triglyceride is converted into a diglyceride, then a monoglyceride. The body can absorb free fatty acids, glycerol, and monoglycerides much easier than the bulkier tri- and diglycerides.

Once digested, the free fatty acids and monoglycerides are absorbed into the body and transported by special protein-wrapped molecules known as *lipoproteins*. The major categories of lipoproteins are very low-density lipoprotein (VLDL), low-density lipoprotein (LDL), and high-density lipoprotein (HDL). VLDL and LDL are responsible for transporting fats (primarily triglycerides and cholesterol) from the liver to body cells, and HDL is responsible for returning fats to the liver; therefore, elevations of either LDL or VLDL are associated with an increased risk for developing atherosclerosis, the primary cause of a heart attack or stroke. In contrast, elevations of HDL are associated with a low risk of heart attacks.

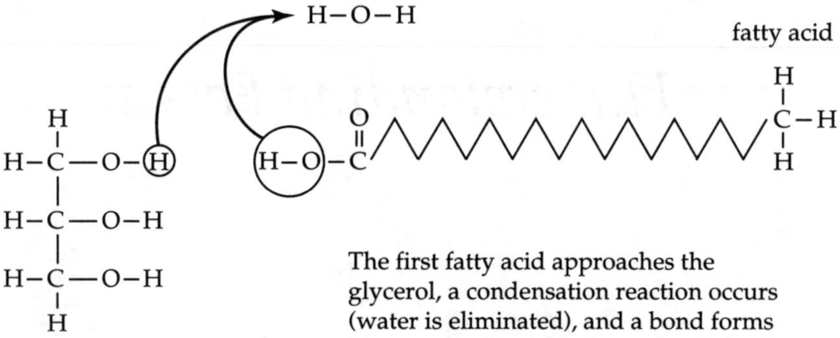

water

H−O−H

fatty acid

The first fatty acid approaches the glycerol, a condensation reaction occurs (water is eliminated), and a bond forms between an O on the glycerol and the C at the acid end of the fatty acid.

glycerol

Later, two more fatty acids attach themselves to the glycerol by the same means; the resulting structure is a triglyceride.

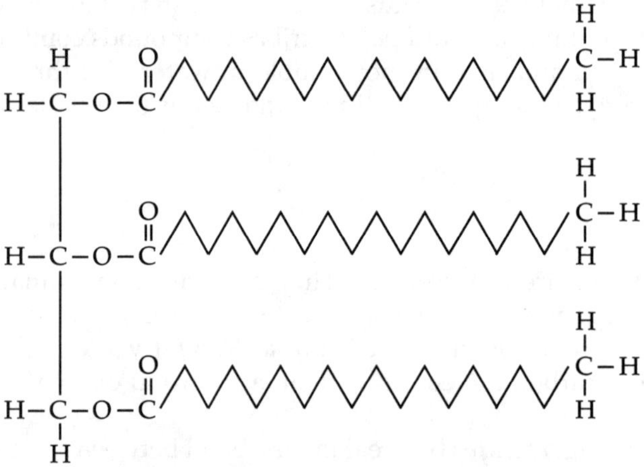

A fat (triglyceride) that might be found in butter.

FIGURE 32.1   Glycerol + fatty acid.

Saturated and Unsaturated Fats

A triglyceride is a *saturated fat* because the carbon molecules in the fatty acids are "saturated" with all the hydrogen molecules they can carry (see Figure 32.1) If some of the hydrogen molecules were removed, what remains is an *unsaturated* fatty acid and thus an *unsaturated fat*.

Saturated fats are typically animal fats like butter, lard, and tallow and are semi-solid to solid at room temperature. In contrast, unsaturated fats are typically liquid at room temperature and are therefore often referred to as *oils*. Most vegetable oils contain primarily unsaturated fats.

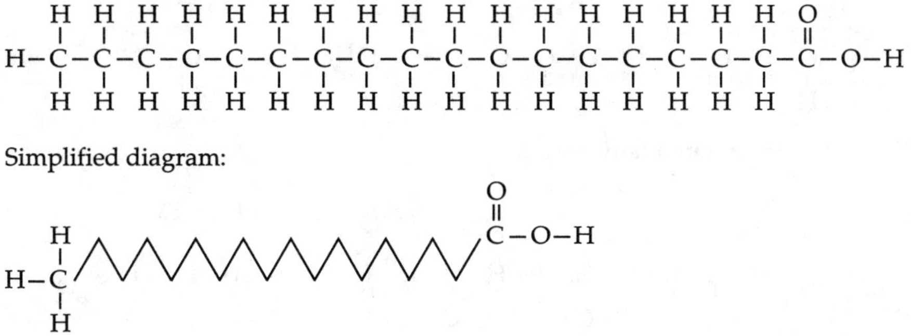

H–C–C–C–C–C–C–C–C–C–C–C–C–C–C–C–C–C–C–O–H

Simplified diagram:

FIGURE 32.2   Stearic acid.

Again, the terms *saturated* and *unsaturated* denote whether all the carbon molecules are saturated or unsaturated with hydrogen molecules. To illustrate the difference in structure, let's look at the 18-carbon family of fatty acids. Stearic acid is an 18-carbon-long saturated fatty acid (see Figure 32.2). This means that it is carrying as many hydrogen molecules as it can.

Oleic acid is an 18-carbon-long monounsaturated fatty acid. It is missing two hydrogen molecules, leaving two carbon molecules unsaturated (see Figure 32.3). This causes the carbons to bind to each other to form a "double-bond" (see Figure 32.4)

Oleic acid is a monounsaturated fatty acid; it contains one (mono) double bond, in this case at the ninth carbon molecule. In a shorthand way to illustrate this, oleic acid is C18:1w9. This means that oleic acid is a fatty acid composed of a chain of 18 carbon molecules and one double bond at the ninth carbon molecule. Oleic acid is an *omega-9* oil because its first unsaturated bond occurs at the ninth carbon molecule from the omega end (see Figure 32.5).

Linoleic acid is an 18-carbon-long *polyunsaturated* fatty acid because it contains more than one double bond; it has two (see Figure 32.6). Linoleic acid would be written C18:2w6. Linoleic acid is classified as an *omega-6* oil because the first double bond occurs at the sixth carbon from the omega end.

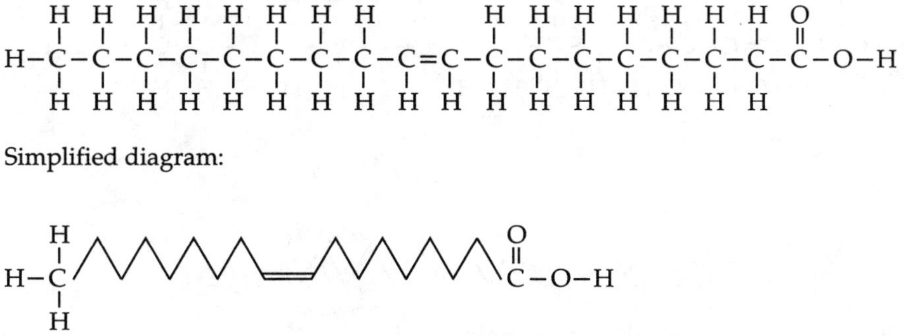

H–C–C–C–C–C–C–C–C–C=C–C–C–C–C–C–C–C–C–O–H

Simplified diagram:

FIGURE 32.3   Oleic acid.

241

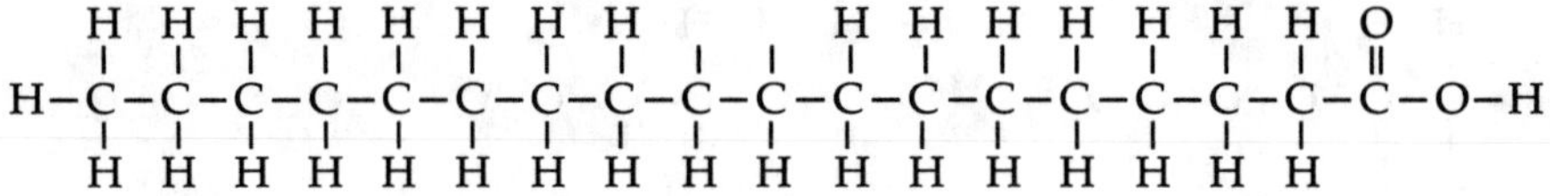

$$H-\overset{\overset{\displaystyle H}{|}}{\underset{\underset{\displaystyle H}{|}}{C}}-\overset{\overset{\displaystyle H}{|}}{\underset{\underset{\displaystyle H}{|}}{C}}-\overset{\overset{\displaystyle H}{|}}{\underset{\underset{\displaystyle H}{|}}{C}}-\overset{\overset{\displaystyle H}{|}}{\underset{\underset{\displaystyle H}{|}}{C}}-\overset{\overset{\displaystyle H}{|}}{\underset{\underset{\displaystyle H}{|}}{C}}-\overset{\overset{\displaystyle H}{|}}{\underset{\underset{\displaystyle H}{|}}{C}}-\overset{\overset{\displaystyle H}{|}}{\underset{\underset{\displaystyle H}{|}}{C}}-\overset{\overset{\displaystyle H}{|}}{\underset{\underset{\displaystyle H}{|}}{C}}-\cdots$$

FIGURE 32.4   Unsaturated fatty acid.

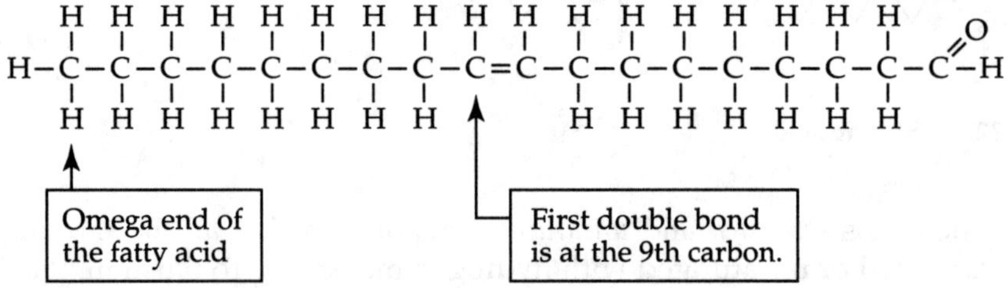

FIGURE 32.5   An omega-9 oil (oleic acid).

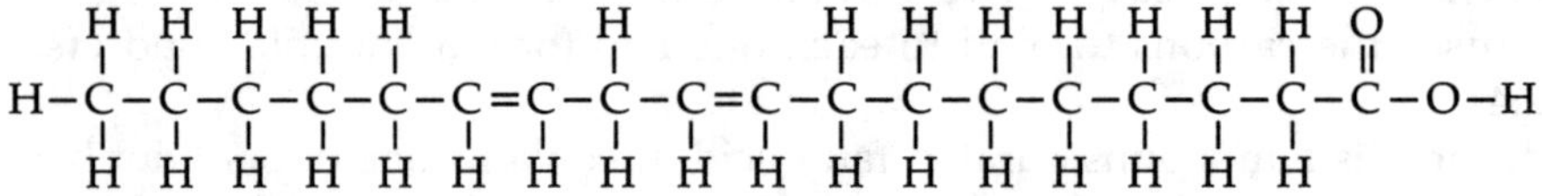

Omega end of the fatty acid

First double bond is at the 9th carbon.

Simplified diagram:

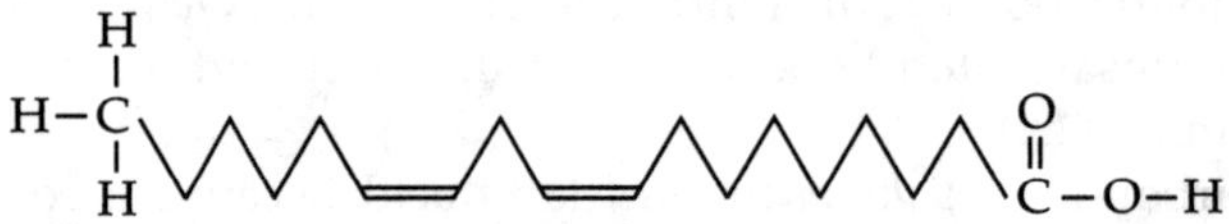

FIGURE 32.6   An omega-6 oil (linoleic acid).

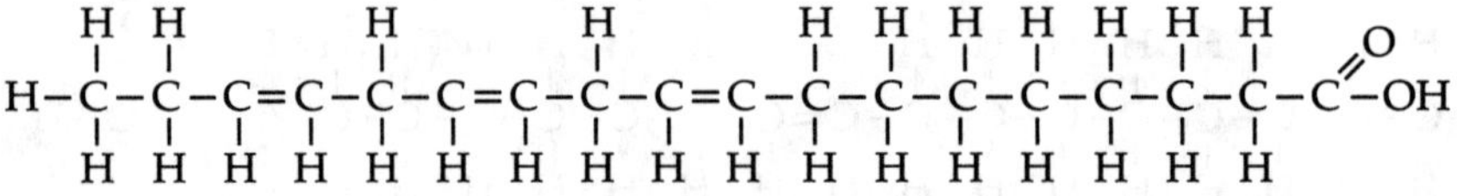

Simplified diagram:

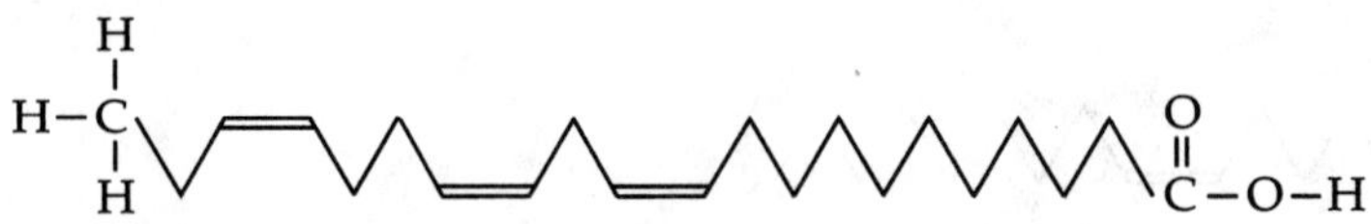

FIGURE 32.7   An omega-3 oil (alpha-linolenic acid).

242

Alpha-linolenic acid is an 18-carbon-long polyunsaturated fatty acid with three double bonds, C18:3w3 (see Figure 32.7). Alpha-linolenic acid is an *omega-3* oil because its first double-bond is at the third carbon from the omega end.

Fatty Acid Composition of Vegetable Oils

Vegetable oils can be loosely divided into two categories: *cooking oils* and *medicinal oils* (see Table 32.1). Medicinal oils contain gamma-linolenic acid (evening primrose, borage, and black currant) or alpha-linolenic acid (flaxseed). These oils are highly polyunsaturated, which means they do not hold up well when exposed to heat.

Most experts now agree the best oils for cooking are canola and olive oil. These oils are composed chiefly of oleic acid, a monounsaturated oil that is more resistant to the damaging effects of heat and light compared with highly polyunsaturated oils like corn, safflower, and soy. When the polyunsaturated oils are exposed to heat or light, the chemical structure of the essential fatty acids is changed to toxic derivatives known as lipid peroxides.

For medicinal purposes, I recommend flaxseed oil for most people. Most Americans suffer a relative insufficiency of omega-3 oils. Since flaxseed is nature's richest source of omega-3 oils, it is the obvious choice.

What about Margarine?

During the manufacture of margarine and shortening, vegetable oils are "hydrogenated." This means that a hydrogen molecule is added to the oil's natural unsaturated fatty acid molecules to make it more saturated. Hydrogenation, the adding of

TABLE 32.1 Fatty Acid Composition (Percent of Total Fat) of Selected Oils

	Saturated Fats	Oleic Acid	Linolenic Acid	Gamma-linoelic Acid (An Omega-6 Oil)	Alpha-linoleic Acid (An Omega-3 Oil)
COOKING OILS					
Canola	7	54	30	0	7
Olive	16	76	8	0	0
Soy	15	26	50	0	9
Corn	17	24	59	0	0
Safflower	7	10	80	0	0
MEDICINAL OILS					
Evening Primrose	10	9	72	9	0
Black Currant	7	9	47	17	13
Borage	14	16	35	22	0
Flaxseed	9	19	14	0	58

hydrogen molecules, results in changing the structure of the natural fatty acid to numerous "unnatural" fatty acid forms and from the cis to the trans configuration (see Figure 32.8). The result is the vegetable oil is now solid or semi-solid.

Trans fatty acids and hydrogenated oils can contribute to the following disorders:

- Low birth weight infants
- Low quality and volume of breast milk
- Abnormal sperm production
- Decreased testosterone in men
- Increased incidence of heart disease
- Increased levels of harmful cholesterol levels in humans
- Increased cancer rates
- Increased rate of prostate disease
- Increased prevalence of diabetes
- Increased incidence of obesity
- Immune suppression
- Essential fatty acid deficiencies

Many researchers and nutritionists have been concerned about the health effects of margarine since it first came on the market. Although many Americans assume they are doing their bodies good by consuming margarine versus butter and saturated fats, in truth they are actually doing more harm. Margarine and other hydrogenated vegetable oils not only raise LDL cholesterol, they also lower the protective HDL-cholesterol level, interfere with essential fatty acid metabolism, and are suspected of being causes of certain cancers.[1-4] Although butter may be better than margarine, the bottom line is that both should be restricted in a healthy diet and natural polyunsaturated oils like canola, safflower, soy, and flaxseed should be used to meet essential fatty acid requirements. The requirement for essential fatty acids is not

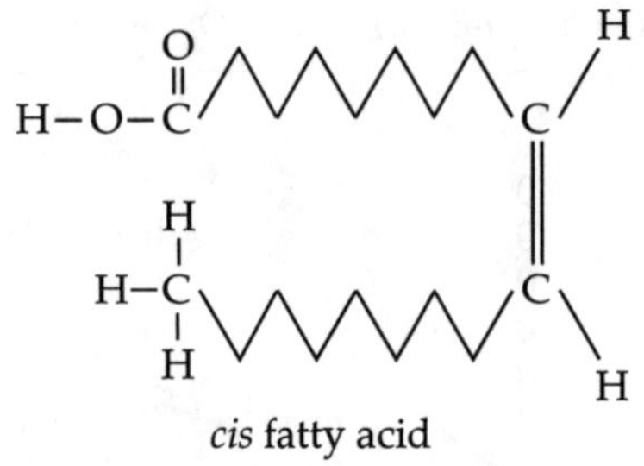

cis fatty acid

The H's are on the same side of the double bond, forcing the molecule to assume a horseshoe shape.

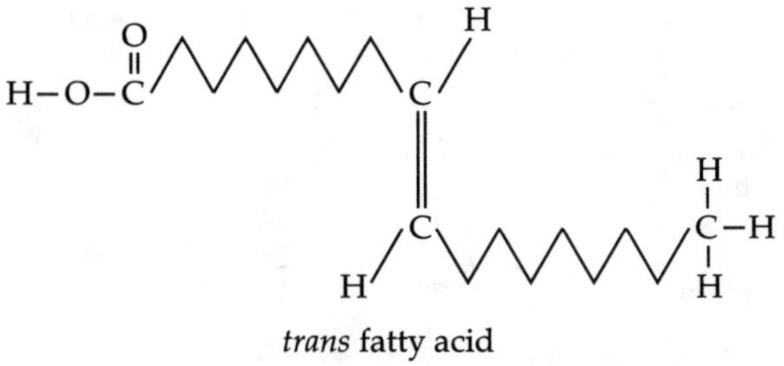

trans fatty acid

The H's are on opposite sides of the double bond, forcing the molecule into an extended position.

FIGURE 32.8 *Cis* vs. *trans* **fatty acid configuration.**

high—one tablespoon of a high-quality flaxseed oil provides more than enough in most cases.

Foods typically containing partially or totally hydrogenated vegetable oils and trans isomers are:

- Virtually all refined and processed foods
- Margarine
- Bread
- Cereals
- Salad oils

Why Saturated Fats Are "Bad" and Essential Fatty Acids Are "Good"

What makes saturated fats "bad" and essential fatty acids "good" relates to the function of essential fatty acids in the body and how saturated fats and hydrogenated oils interfere with this function. To illustrate, let's examine the role of essential fatty acids in cellular membranes.

Essential Fatty Acids in Cell Membranes

All cells throughout the human body are enveloped by a membrane composed chiefly of essential fatty acids in the form of compounds known as *phospholipids*. A phospholipid differs from a triglyceride in that instead of three fatty acids attached to the glycerol molecule, one of the fatty acids is replaced with a phosphorus-containing molecule like choline or serine. Most of the phospholipids in the cell membranes are manufactured by adding the phosphate group to a diglyceride.

Phospholipids play a major role in determining the integrity and fluidity of cell membranes. The type of fat consumed determines the type of phospholipid in the cell membrane. Although we can ingest preformed phospholipids like lecithin or phosphatidylcholine, most of these phospholipids are broken down into glycerol, free fatty acids, and the phosphate group, rather than being incorporated intact into cellular membranes.

A phospholipid composed of a saturated fat or trans fatty acid differs considerably in structure from a phospholipid composed of an essential fatty acid. In addition, there are differences between the structure of an omega-3 oil–composed membrane and an omega-6–composed membrane. The degree of difference is illustrated by the difference in fluidity among the various fatty acids.

Scientists believe the cell is programmed to selectively incorporate the different fatty acids it needs to maintain optimal function; however, because the standard American diet lacks essential fatty acids (particularly the omega-3 oils), in actuality diet primarily determines what the cell incorporates into its membranes. A diet composed largely of saturated fat, animal fatty acids (arachidonic acid), cholesterol, and trans fatty acids leads to membranes that are much less fluid than the membranes of an individual consuming optimum levels of both essential fatty acids.

A relative deficiency of essential fatty acids in cellular membranes makes it virtually impossible for the cell membrane to perform its vital function—to act as a selective barrier that regulates the passage of certain materials in and out of the cell. When the structure or function of the cell membrane is disturbed, homeostasis is interrupted. *Homeostasis* is the maintenance of static, or constant, conditions in the internal environment of the cell and, on a larger scale, the human body as a whole. In other words, with a disturbance in cellular membrane structure or function, virtually all cellular processes are disrupted.

Cell Membrane Alterations and Disease

According to modern pathology (study of disease processes), an alteration in cell membrane function is the central factor in the development of cell injury and death.[5] Without a healthy membrane, cells lose their ability to hold water, vital nutrients, and electrolytes. They also lose their ability to communicate with other cells and be controlled by regulating hormones. They simply do not function properly. For an example, let's take a look at the effect of membrane fluidity upon the action of the hormone insulin.

Insulin stimulates the uptake of blood glucose into cells. If there is insufficient insulin or the cell does not respond to insulin, blood glucose levels can be elevated—a condition known as diabetes mellitus. Diabetes is divided into two major categories: type I and type II. Type I or Insulin-Dependent Diabetes Mellitus (IDDM) occurs most often in children and adolescents. It is associated with complete destruction of the beta cells of the pancreas, which manufacture insulin. The type I diabetic requires lifelong insulin for the control of blood sugar levels. Only about 10 percent of all diabetics are type I; the rest are type II.

Type II or Non-Insulin Dependent Diabetes Mellitus (NIDDM) usually has an onset after 40 years of age. In type II diabetes, insulin levels are typically elevated, indicating a loss of sensitivity to insulin by the body's cells. Obesity and certain types of dietary fat are major contributing factors to this loss of insulin sensitivity.

The dietary fat profile linked to type II diabetes is an abundance of saturated fat and a relative insufficiency of essential fatty acids.[6,7] It appears that such a dietary pattern leads to reduced membrane fluidity, which in turn causes reduced insulin binding to receptors on cellular membranes and/or reduced insulin action.[8,9]

In contrast, omega-3 oils appear to improve insulin action.[8,9] Population studies show that frequent consumption of a small amount of omega-3 oils protects against the development of type II diabetes.[10] In addition, animal studies show that omega-3 fatty acids prevent the development of insulin resistance.[11] All this evidence indicates that altered membrane fluidity may play a critical role in the development of type II diabetes.

To better determine the role of specific fatty acids in increasing the risk of developing NIDDM, researchers recently examined the fatty acid composition of the serum cholesterol esters among 50-year-old men in a 10-year follow-up to the famous Uppsula study. The fatty acid composition of the serum cholesterol esters reflects the average quality of fat consumed over several weeks or perhaps even longer periods of time. Of the 1,828 men who did not have diabetes in 1970 to 1973, 75 developed NIDDM.[12]

The study results showed striking differences in the serum cholesterol esters. The subjects with diabetes had higher proportions of saturated fatty acids and palmitoleic acid (16:1n7), a low proportion of linoleic acid (18:2n6), and relatively high (although numerically small) increases of gamma-linolenic (18:3n6) and dihomo-gamma-linolenic acid (20:3n6). The development of NIDDM was significantly predicted by a high proportion of dihomo-gamma-linolenic acid (DHGLA). The altered fatty acid profiles preceded the development of NIDDM.

The dietary factors responsible for such a fatty acid pattern are high intakes of meat and dairy products along with a low intake of vegetable oils. A high proportion of DHGLA, a significant marker for the likelihood of developing NIIDM, can be explained by an increased consumption of arachidonic acid or, possibly, by genetic factors. DHGLA is converted into arachidonic acid by an enzyme (delta-5 desaturase). However, when arachidonic acid levels are high, the activity of this enzyme is reduced via feedback inhibition.

The results of this study indicate the following dietary recommendations related to fatty acid intake might significantly reduce the risk of developing NIDDM and improve serum cholesterol and triglyceride levels as well.

- Reduce intake of saturated fatty acids
- Increase consumption of essential fatty acids (linoleic and alpha-linolenic acids)
- Increase consumption of omega-3 oils by consuming cold-water fish and/or flaxseed oil

Determinants of Healthy Cellular Membranes

Although scientists have determined that cellular health critically depends on the health and integrity of the cellular membrane, for some reason they have been slow to clarify the factors that determine the health of the membrane itself. Existing research on this subject points to two important factors, adequacy of essential fatty acid intake (including alpha-linolenic acid) and adequate levels of antioxidants. Accumulating research demonstrates that a high intake of antioxidant nutrients can help prevent some major degenerative diseases of our society and perhaps slow down the aging process.[13-15] A high antioxidant intake is also recommended for individuals consuming higher quantities of essential fatty acids. Consuming a diet rich in fresh fruits and vegetables is the first step in achieving higher antioxidant levels. The second step is taking extra antioxidant nutrients. I recommend the following daily essential fatty acids supplements:

- Vitamin C, 1,000 to 3,000 milligrams
- Vitamin E, 400 to 800 International Units
- Selenium, 200 micrograms

Other Reasons Why Essential Fatty Acids Are "Good"

Essential fatty acids also play critical roles in other body functions and structures. They are transformed into regulatory compounds known as *prostaglandins,* and both the prostaglandins and essential fatty acids are important in a host of bodily functions. They are important because they

- Regulate steroid production and hormone synthesis
- Regulate pressure in the eye, joints, and blood vessels
- Regulate response to pain, inflammation, and swelling
- Mediate immune response
- Regulate bodily secretions and their viscosity
- Dilate or constrict blood vessels
- Regulate collateral circulation
- Direct endocrine hormones to their target cells
- Regulate smooth muscle and autonomic reflexes
- Are primary constituents of cellular membranes
- Regulate the rate at which cells divide (mitosis)
- Maintain the fluidity and rigidity of cellular membranes
- Regulate the flow of substances into and out of the cells
- Are necessary for the transport of oxygen from the red blood cell to the bodily tissues
- Are necessary in kidney function and fluid balance
- Are important in keeping saturated fats mobile in the blood stream.
- Prevent blood cells from clumping together (conglomeration), the cause of atherosclerotic plaque and blood clots, precursors of stroke
- Mediate the release of cellular pro-inflammatory substances that may trigger allergic conditions
- Regulate nerve transmission
- Stimulate steroid production
- Are the primary energy source for the heart muscle

In addition to their critical role in normal physiology, essential fatty acids may actually be protective and therapeutic against heart disease, cancer, autoimmune diseases like multiple sclerosis and rheumatoid arthritis, many skin diseases, and other health conditions. The following chapter focuses on how to achieve the greatest benefit from essential fatty acid supplements.

33

Essential Fatty Acid Supplementation

In this day and age of fat phobia and the resultant barrage of lowfat and nonfat food products lining the grocery store aisles, daily essential fatty acid supplementation may be puzzling to consumers. However, this recommendation makes perfectly good sense. While it is true Americans should consume no more than 30 percent of their daily calories as fats, a lack of dietary essential fatty acids probably plays a significant role in the development of many chronic degenerative diseases such as heart disease, cancer, and strokes.

Many experts estimate that approximately 80 percent of our population consumes an insufficient quantity of essential fatty acids. This dietary insufficiency presents a serious health threat to Americans.

Cause of Essential Fatty Acid Deficiency

Mass commercial refinement of fats, oil products, and the foods containing them has effectively eliminated the essential fatty acids from our food chain. In addition, there has been a tremendous increase in the amount of unnatural fats and oils added to the diet in the form of trans fatty acids, partially hydrogenated oils. In 1909, Americans consumed about 125 grams of fat per day. Today, they consume closer to 175 grams per day, an increase of some 40 percent (about 50 extra pounds per year). They have decreased their consumption of natural, unadulterated essential fatty acids and drastically increased their consumption of refined and adulterated fats and oils. These refined and processed compounds actually inhibit the body's ability to use the essential fatty acids it consumes.

Because "synthetic fats" have been prevalent in the diet for only the last 100 years, our body systems have not evolved to the point where they can handle these deadly compounds. The adulteration of polyunsaturated oils contributes to an overt deficiency of these life-sustaining nutrients. The essential fatty acids take on the role of Dr. Jekyll and Mr. Hyde, becoming transformed from life-sustaining and health-promoting in their natural state to life-taking and deadly when processed.

The three primary factors contributing to our current essential fatty acid deficiency are

- Unavailability of quality oils rich in essential fatty acids because of mass commercialization and refinement of fats and oils products
- Transformation of healthful omega-3 and omega-6 oils into toxic compounds (hydrogenated and trans isomers)
- Metabolic competition of hydrogenated and trans fatty acids with the essential fatty acids

Recognizing Essential Fatty Acid Deficiency

The signs and symptoms of essential fatty acid deficiency may be overt or chronically nagging and range from mild fatigue to fatal heart attack. Most orthodox health-care practitioners may never make the association between a health symptom and essential fatty acid deficiency; therefore, the underlying cause of illness continues to manifest. Most physicians are not trained in nutrition, and the laboratory analysis to measure essential fatty acid deficiency is not widely available or appreciated. In addition, the symptoms of essential fatty acid deficiency are not as obvious as those of many other nutrient deficiencies. The consequences, however, are far more deadly in this day and age. Even if an essential fatty acid deficiency were recognized, few orthodox clinicians would know how to treat it.

In general, a deficiency of essential fatty acids can be so vague and broad that symptoms are typically written off as something else. Suffice it to say, surveys suggest that Americans are up to 90 percent deficient in the essential fatty acids. This simply means we are obtaining only 10 percent of what we need for optimal health. For this reason, I strongly recommend flaxseed oil to all of my patients, regardless of their condition.

Some signs and symptoms typical but not exclusive to EFA deficiency are:

- Fatigue, malaise, lackluster energy
- Lack of endurance
- Dry skin
- Cracked nails
- Dry, lifeless hair
- Dry mucous membranes, tear ducts, mouth, vagina
- Maldigestion, gas, bloating
- Constipation
- Immune weakness
- Frequent colds and sickness
- Aching, sore joints
- Angina, chest pain
- Depression
- Lack of motivation

- Forgetfulness
- Forgetfulness, uh oh!!
- High blood pressure
- History of cardiovascular disease
- Arthritis

Importance of the Omega-6 to Omega-3 Ratio

The balance of omega-6 to omega-3 oils is critical to proper prostaglandin metabolism. *Prostaglandins* and related compounds are hormonelike molecules derived from 20-carbon chain fatty acids that contain three, four, or five double bonds. Linoleic and linolenic can be converted to prostaglandins by the addition of two carbon molecules and removal of hydrogen molecules (if necessary). Prostaglandins are important for the regulation of:

- Inflammation, pain, and swelling
- Blood pressure
- Heart function
- Gastrointestinal function and secretions
- Kidney function and fluid balance
- Blood clotting and platelet aggregation
- Allergic response
- Inflammation
- Nerve transmission
- Steroid production and hormone synthesis

Prostaglandin Nomenclature

The number of double bonds in the fatty acid determines the classification of the prostaglandin. Series 1 and 2 prostaglandins come from the omega-6 fatty acids with linoleic acid serving as the starting point. Linoleic acid is changed to gamma-linolenic acid and then dihomo-gamma-linolenic acid, which contains three double bonds and is the precursor to prostaglandins of the 1 series. Dihomo-gamma-linolenic acid (DHGLA) can also be converted to arachidonic acid, which contains four double bonds and is a precursor to the 2 series of prostaglandins. However, because delta-5 desaturase (the enzyme responsible for the conversion of DHGLA to arachidonic acid) prefers the omega-3 oils, in humans diet is the greatest source of arachidonic. Arachidonic acid (along with saturated fats) is found almost entirely in animal foods.

The omega-3 prostaglandin pathway can begin with alpha-linolenic acid that can be eventually converted to eicosapentaenoic acid (EPA), the precursor to the 3 series prostaglandins. Although EPA is found preformed in cold-water fish such as salmon, mackerel, and herring, by providing alpha-linolenic acid, certain vegetable oils like flaxseed and canola can increase body EPA and 3-series prostaglandin levels.

Prostaglandins of the 1 and 3 series are generally considered "good" prostaglandins; those of the 2 series are considered "bad." This labeling makes sense when we look at their effects on platelets. Prostaglandins of the 2 series promote platelet stickiness, a factor that leads to hardening of the arteries, heart disease, and strokes. In contrast, the 1 and 3 series prostaglandins prevent platelets from sticking together, improve blood flow, and reduce inflammation.

Manipulating Prostaglandin Metabolism

By altering the type of dietary oils consumed and stored in cell membranes, we can manipulate prostaglandin metabolism. Prostaglandin manipulation can be extremely powerful in the treatment of inflammation, allergies, high blood pressure, and many other health conditions. The basic goal in most situations is twofold: reduce the level of arachidonic acid inflammation and increase the level of DHGLA and EPA. This goal is achieved in most circumstances by reducing the intake of animal foods (with the exception of cold-water fish) and supplementing the diet with flaxseed oil.

Although several studies have shown flaxseed oil is not as effective as fish oils in increasing tissue concentrations of EPA and lowering tissue concentrations of arachidonic acid, these studies failed to address an important factor[1,2]—the subjects tested continued to consume a diet rich in omega-6 fatty acids. Desaturation and elongation enzymes prefer alpha-linolenic acid to the omega-6 oils; however, in these studies only relatively small amounts of alpha-linolenic acid were converted to EPA because of the much higher concentrations of omega-6 oils. A more recent study attempted to determine the potential of dietary flaxseed oil to increase tissue EPA concentration in healthy human subjects.[3]

Unlike the previous studies, this study incorporated a diet low in omega-6 oils by restricting the use of other vegetable oils while supplementing the diet with 13 grams (approximately 1.5 tablespoons) of flaxseed oil daily. The results of the study indicated that flaxseed oil supplementation, along with restriction of linoleic acid, raises tissue EPA levels comparable to fish oil supplementation.

Because encapsulated fish oils contain very high levels of lipid peroxides and are expensive to use at therapeutic dosages (1.8 grams EPA per day), flaxseed oil will probably emerge as the preferred source of omega-3 fatty acids in the treatment of atherosclerosis, high blood pressure, and inflammatory conditions such as psoriasis, rheumatoid arthritis, eczema, multiple sclerosis, and ulcerative colotis.

GLA Supplements

Evening primrose, black currant, and borage oil contain gamma-linolenic acid, an omega-6 fatty acid that eventually acts as a precursor to the favorable 1 series prostaglandins. Although GLA supplementation is quite popular, the results of research on GLA supplements are controversial and not as strong as the results on omega-3 oils. Studies actually show that over the long term, GLA supplementation increases tissue arachidonic acid levels while decreasing tissue levels of EPA.[4] Obviously, this effect is contrary to the treatment goal of reducing inflammation by reducing tissue levels of arachidonic acid and raising levels of EPA.

Also, because GLA can be formed from linoleic acid, it is difficult to determine to what extent the effects are caused by GLA versus linoleic acid. Most sources of GLA are much richer in linoleic acid than GLA. For example, evening primrose contains only 9 percent GLA but 72 percent linoleic acid.

In most instances, high-linoleic-acid-containing oils, like safflower and soy oil, may provide nearly as much benefit as GLA products at a fraction of the cost. The only exceptions to this generalization might be in individuals with diabetes. Diabetics

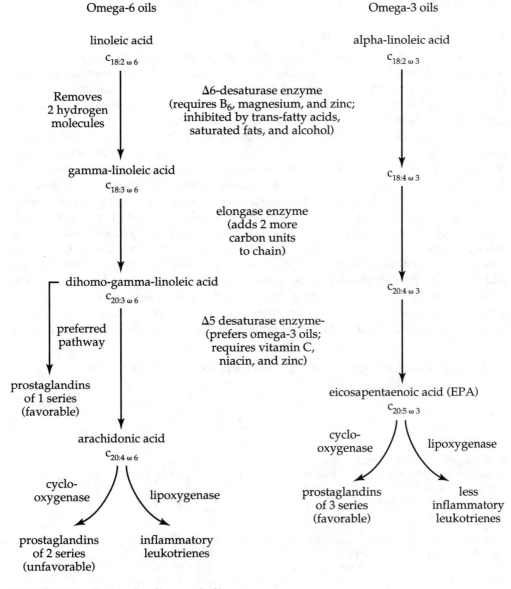

FIGURE 33.1 Prostaglandin metabolism.

cannot form GLA from linoleic acid. GLA supplementation in diabetics improves nerve function and prevents diabetic nerve disease,[5] and the dosage required is relatively small (240 to 480 milligrams of GLA per day).

Once again, it appears flaxseed oil is the better supplement. Although most of the research on omega-3 oils has featured fish oils rich in eicosapentaenoic acid (EPA), EPA can be manufactured in the body from alpha-linolenic acid. Flaxseed oil contains more than twice as much omega-3 oil as fish oil contains and is also a good source of linoleic acid. In addition, flaxseed oil may offer other benefits that fish oil and GLA products do not and at a much lower price (see Table 33.1).

Achieving Balanced Prostaglandin Synthesis

The production of the series 1,2, and 3 families of prostaglandins depends on the type and quality of fats and oils we consume. The challenge lies in consuming an approximate ratio of omega-6 to omega-3 fatty acids that produces a favorable production of "friendly" series 1 and 3 prostaglandins while at the same time managing production of the potentially volatile prostaglandin 2 series.

The optimal ratio of omega-6 to omega-3 fatty acids is 4:1, or four times the amount of omega-6 fatty acids as omega-3 fatty acids.[6] This means that to achieve optimal prostaglandin synthesis we should consume four parts omega-6 to one part omega-3. These data lead some to advocate consumption of fat and oil products that come close to achieving a 4:1 profile. Initially this recommendation appears to be prudent advice. Unfortunately, further consideration is warranted before deciding to consume a primarily omega-6–dominant product. Americans consume 10 to 20 times the amount of omega-6 fatty acids that we need. (Omega-6 fatty acids are the primary fatty acids found in low-quality grocery store oil products and are the primary oil ingredient added to most processed food stuffs). Instead of a 4:1 omega-6 to omega-3 ratio, we currently consume a ratio greater than 20:1. The last thing we should do is increase the amount of omega-6 fatty acids in an attempt to achieve an optimal omega-6 to -3 profile. Instead, a more appropriate approach is eliminating the hidden sources of

TABLE 33.1 Cost Comparison of Essential Fatty Acid Products

Source	Daily Dosage in Grams[a]	Average Cost in Dollars
OMEGA-6 OILS		
Evening primrose oil (9 percent GLA)	GLA, 1.4	90
Black currant seed oil (17 percent GLA)	GLA, 1.4	90
Borage oil capsules (22 percent GLA)	GLA, 1.4	75
Borage oil liquid (22 percent GLA)	GLA, 1.4	60
OMEGA-3 OILS		
EPA from fish oils (180 mg. EPA/1,000 mg. oil)	EPA, 1.8	70
Flaxseed oil capsules (55 percent alpha-LA)	Alpha-LA, 5.0	18
Flaxseed oil liquid (55 percent alpha-LA)	Alpha-LA, 5.0	12

[a]Estimated therapeutic dosage in rheumatoid arthritis based on clinical data.

omega-6 oils in our diets and supplementing our diets with flaxseed oil. The omega-6 to -3 ratio for flax is 1:3. This means the omega-3 fatty acids outnumber the omega-6 fatty acids three to one. The elimination of poor quality omega-6 fatty acids and the addition of high-quality flaxseed oil in our diets helps us return to the optimal ratio of omega-6 to -3 fatty acid profile while providing balanced and efficient production of prostaglandins and their health-enhancing qualities.

Principle Uses of Essential Fatty Acid Supplements

Over 60 health conditions can benefit from essential fatty acid supplementation. This chapter focuses on the use of essential fatty acids in the following situations:

- Cardiovascular disease, including high cholesterol levels and high blood pressure
- Allergic and inflammatory conditions, including psoriasis and eczema
- Autoimmune diseases like multiple sclerosis, lupus, and cancer

Some health conditions that exhibit fatty acid deficiencies and/or improvement with EFA supplementation are:

- Acne
- AIDS
- Allergies
- Alzheimer's
- Angina
- Angioplasty
- Arthritis
- Atherosclerosis
- Autoimmune diseases
- Behavioral disorders
- Breast cysts
- Breast pain
- Breast pain
- Breast tenderness
- Cancer
- Cartilage destruction
- Coronary bypass
- Cystic fibrosis
- Dementia

- Dermatitis
- Diabetes
- *E. coli* infection
- Eczema
- Heart disease
- Hyperactivity
- Hypertension
- Hypoxia
- Ichthyosia
- Immune disorders
- Infant nutrition
- Inflammatory conditions
- Intestinal disorders
- Kidney function
- Learning
- Leprosy
- Leukemia
- Lupus
- Mastaglia
- Menopause
- Mental illness
- Metastasis
- Multiple sclerosis
- Myocardial infarction
- Myopathy
- Neurological disease
- Obesity
- Osteoarthritis
- Postviral fatigue
- Pregnancy malnutrition
- Psoriasis
- Refsum's syndrome
- Reye's syndrome
- Rheumatoid arthritis
- Schizophrenia
- Sepsis
- Sjogren-Larson syndrome

- Stroke
- Vascular disease
- Vision

Cardiovascular Disease: A Brief Overview

Most cardiovascular diseases results from atherosclerosis, which is hardening of the artery walls because of a buildup of plaque containing cholesterol, fatty material, and cellular debris. Atherosclerosis and its complications are the major causes of death in the United States and have reached epidemic proportions throughout the Western world. Heart attacks, strokes, and other cardiovascular diseases related to atherosclerosis cause roughly 43 percent of all deaths in the U.S.

The first step in the prevention and treatment of heart disease and strokes is the reduction of blood cholesterol levels. Evidence overwhelmingly demonstrates that elevated cholesterol levels are deadly. However, not all cholesterol is bad; it serves many vital functions in the body, including the manufacture of sex hormones and bile acids. Without cholesterol, many body processes would not function properly. Cholesterol is transported in the blood by molecules known as lipoproteins. Cholesterol bound to low-density lipoprotein (LDL) is often called "bad" cholesterol, and cholesterol bound to high-density lipoprotein (HDL) is called "good" cholesterol. LDL cholesterol increases the risk of heart disease, strokes, and high blood pressure, while HDL cholesterol actually protects against heart disease.

LDL transports cholesterol to the tissues. HDL, on the other hand, transports cholesterol to the liver for metabolism and excretion from the body. Therefore, the LDL-to-HDL ratio (also referred to as the cardiac-risk-factor ratio) largely determines whether cholesterol is being deposited into tissues or broken down and excreted. The risk for heart disease can be reduced dramatically by lowering LDL cholesterol while simultaneously raising HDL cholesterol. Research shows that for every 1 percent drop in the LDL cholesterol level, the risk for a heart attack drops by 2 percent. Conversely, for every 1 percent increase in HDL levels, the risk for a heart attack drops 3 to 4 percent.

In addition to keeping an eye on your cholesterol level, it is also important to keep the level of triglycerides in the proper range. Here are the recommended levels of blood cholesterol and triglycerides:

- Total cholesterol—less than 200 milligrams per deciliter
- LDL cholesterol—less than 130 milligrams per deciliter
- HDL cholesterol—greater than 35 milligrams per deciliter
- LDL-to-HDL ratio—less than 4:5
- Triglycerides—50 to 150 milligrams per deciliter

Omega-3 Fatty Acids and Cholesterol Levels

Hundreds of studies indicate omega-3 fatty acids lower cholesterol and triglyceride levels.[7-11] The majority of these studies feature EPA- and DHA-rich fish oils, but flaxseed oil can produce similar benefits because it contains alpha-linolenic acid, an omega-3 oil that the body can convert to EPA. Alpha-linolenic acid produces many of the same effects as EPA and several of its own.

Furthermore, although a substantial body of evidence exists that documents the beneficial effects of increased fish oil intake in lowering blood cholesterol levels, the question remains: Should you take fish oil supplements or increase your dietary intake of fish? In an effort to resolve this question, a 5-week study of 25 men with high cholesterol levels compared the effects of eating equal amounts of fish oil from whole fish versus a fish oil supplement.[12] Although total cholesterol levels were unchanged in both groups, both fish and fish oil supplements lowered triglycerides and raised HDL cholesterol. However, dietary fish produced some additional benefits over the fish oil supplements. Another benefit of omega-3 oils in atherosclerosis prevention is their ability to reduce platelet "stickiness" and prevent clot formation. Once platelets adhere to each other (aggregate), they release potent compounds that dramatically promote the formation of the atherosclerotic plaque. Or they can form a clot that can stick in small arteries and produce a heart attack or stroke. While saturated fats and cholesterol increase platelet aggregation, omega-3 oils have the opposite effect. These effects are mediated through improved prostaglandin metabolism. In this study, dietary fish produced a much greater effect than the fish oil supplement on platelet stickiness reduction. These findings suggest that while both fish consumption and fish oil supplementation produce desirable effects on cholesterol, fish consumption is more effective in improving several other factors involved in cardiovascular disease.

Because commercially available fish oils contain very high levels of lipid peroxides and greatly stress antioxidant defense mechanisms, it makes the most sense to rely on cold-water fish and flaxseed oil for the omega-3 oils rather than fish oil capsules.[13–15]

Flaxseed oil provides a significant cost saving as well. The dosages effective in lowering cholesterol levels when using fish oil supplements range from 5 to 15 grams per day. Since most commercial products contain 500 milligrams of fish oil per capsule, this means a daily dose of 10 to 30 capsules at an average monthly cost of $40 to $100. At a similar dosage, flaxseed oil costs between $6 and $18 per month.

Diets High in Omega-3 Fatty Acids Prevent Heart Attacks

Population studies demonstrate that people who consume a diet rich in omega-3 oils from either fish or vegetable sources have a significantly reduced risk of developing heart disease.[16,17] Furthermore, results from autopsy studies show that the highest degree of coronary artery disease is found in individuals with the lowest concentration of omega-3 oils in their fat tissues. Conversely, individuals with the lowest degree of coronary artery disease had the highest concentration of omega-3 oils.[18]

What these studies indicate is people consuming a diet rich in omega-3 oils can prevent heart attacks. But what about people who already have significant heart disease? Can a diet rich in omega-3 oils prevent future heart attacks? The answer is yes!

People who experience a heart attack and live through it are extremely likely to experience another. Several studies have sought to determine whether dietary recommendations can prevent recurrence. As of 1995, only three studies have shown that dietary modifications are effective.

Diet and lifestyle are not only protective against heart disease, but they also can reverse dramatically the blockage of clogged arteries. The most famous of the three studies showing this effect is the Lifestyle Heart Trial conducted by Dr. Dean Ornish.[19] In this study, subjects with heart disease were divided into a control group and an experimental group. The control group received regular medical care, while the experimental group ate a lowfat vegetarian diet for at least 1 year. The diet included fruits, vegetables, grains, legumes, and soybean products. Subjects were allowed to consume as many calories as they wished. No animal products were allowed except egg white and one cup per day of nonfat milk or yogurt. The diet contained approximately 10 percent fat, 15 to 20 percent protein, and 70 to 75 percent carbohydrate (predominantly complex carbohydrate from whole grains, legumes, and vegetables).

The experimental group also performed stress reduction techniques such as breathing exercises, stretching exercises, meditation, imagery, and other relaxation techniques for an hour each day and exercised at least 3 hours a week. At the end of the year, the subjects in the experimental group showed significant overall regression of atherosclerosis of the coronary blood vessels. In contrast, subjects in the control group who were being treated with regular medical care and followed the standard American Heart Association diet actually showed progression of their disease—the control group actually got worse. Ornish states, "This finding suggests that conventional recommendations for patients with coronary heart disease (such as a 30 percent fat diet) are not sufficient to bring about regression in many patients."

Strict vegetarianism may not be as important as consuming a diet high in fiber and complex carbohydrates and low in saturated fat and cholesterol; but we know that vegetarians have a much lower risk of developing heart disease and their diet is effective in lowering cholesterol levels, blood pressure, and risk of atherosclerosis. Such a diet is rich in a number of protective factors such as fiber, essential fatty acids (including higher levels of alpha-linolenic acid), vitamins, and minerals, including potassium and magnesium.

Two other studies that show diet can prevent further heart attacks in patients suffering a first heart attack highlight the importance of omega-3 fatty acids and the ineffectiveness of the standard American Heart Association's dietary recommendations. In the Dietary and Reinfarction Trial (DART), only when the intake of omega-3 fatty acids (from fish) was increased were future heart attacks reduced.[20] The other study, the Lyon Diet Heart Study, determined that increasing the intake of alpha-linolenic acid offers the same degree of protection as increased fish intake.[21] The diet used in the Lyon Heart Study is often referred to as the Cretan Diet.

The two populations with the lowest rate of heart attacks have a relatively high intake of alpha-linolenic acid—the Japanese who inhabit Kohama Island and the inhabitants of Crete.[22,23] Typically Cretans have a threefold higher concentration of alpha-linolenic acid than members of other European countries because of their frequent consumption of walnuts and purslane. Another important dietary factor in both Kohamans and Cretans is their use of oleic acid–containing oils—canola and olive oil, respectively. LDL cholesterol largely composed of oleic acid is less susceptible to peroxidation. Although the oleic content of the diet offers some degree of protection, the rate of heart attacks in the Kohamans and Cretans is much lower than in populations that consume only oleic acid sources and little alpha-linolenic acid. The intake of alpha-linolenic acid is probably a more significant protective factor.

Effects of Omega-3 Fatty Acids on Fibrinogen

Elevated fibrinogen levels are a primary risk factor for cardiovascular disease. Fibrinogen is a protein involved in the clotting system. However, it plays many other important roles, including several that promote atherosclerosis—such as acting as a cofactor for platelet aggregation, determining the viscosity of blood, and stimulating the formation of the atherosclerotic plaque.

Early clinical studies stimulated further detailed epidemiological investigations of the possible link between fibrinogen and cardiovascular disease.[24] The first such study was the Northwick Park Heart Study in the U.K. This large study involved 1,510 men aged 40 to 64 years who were randomly recruited and tested for a range of clotting factors, including fibrinogen. At 4 years' follow-up there was a stronger association between cardiovascular deaths and fibrinogen levels than between cardiovascular deaths and cholesterol. Five other prospective epidemiological studies have confirmed this association.

The clinical significance of these findings is summarized as follows:

- Fibrinogen levels should be determined and monitored in patients with or at high risk for coronary heart disease or stroke.
- Natural therapies (e.g., omega-3 oils) designed to promote fibrinolysis may offer significant benefit in the prevention of heart attacks and strokes.
- While omega-3 oils lower fibrinogen levels, omega-6 oils do not.[25] This difference may explain some of the results noted in population and clinical studies such as the DART and Lyon Diet Heart Study.

Omega-3 Fatty Acids and Blood Pressure

Each time the heart beats, it sends blood coursing through the arteries. The peak reading of the pressure exerted by this contraction is the systolic pressure. Between beats, the heart relaxes and blood pressure drops. The very lowest reading is the diastolic pressure. A normal blood pressure reading for an adult is 120 (systolic)/80 (diastolic).

High blood pressure (hypertension) refers to a reading of greater than 140/90. An elevated blood pressure is one of the major risk factors for a heart attack or stroke. Since heart disease and strokes account for over 43 percent of all deaths in the U.S., it is very important to keep blood pressure in the normal range. Over 60 million Americans have high blood pressure. Again, dietary factors appear to be the primary reason.

Besides attaining ideal body weight, perhaps the most important dietary recommendation is to increase the consumption of plant foods in the diet. A primarily vegetarian diet typically contains more potassium, complex carbohydrates, essential fatty acids, fiber, calcium, magnesium, and vitamin C, and less saturated fat and refined carbohydrate, all of which exert a favorable influence on blood pressure.

Increasing the intake of omega-3 fatty acids can also lower blood pressure. Over 60 double-blind studies have demonstrated that either fish oil supplements or flaxseed oil are very effective in lowering blood pressure.[26–28] Although the fish oils have typically produced a more pronounced effect than flaxseed oil (the dosage of fish oils used was quite high, equal to 10 fish oil capsules daily), flaxseed oil is a better choice for lowering blood pressure, particularly when cost is considered.

Along with reducing the intake of saturated fat, taking one tablespoon of flaxseed oil daily should drop both the systolic and diastolic readings by up to 9 millimeters of mercury.[29] One study found that for every absolute 1 percent increase in body alpha-linolenic acid content there was a decrease of 5 millimeters of mercury in the systolic, diastolic, and mean blood pressure.[30]

Allergic and Inflammatory Conditions

Fatty acids are important mediators of allergy and inflammation because of their ability to form inflammatory prostaglandins, thromboxanes, and leukotrienes. Altering dietary oil intake can significantly increase or decrease inflammation, depending on the type of oil increased. The overall goal is to decrease tissue levels of arachidonic acid while simultaneously increasing the tissue levels of omega-3 fatty acids.

Vegetarian diets are often beneficial in the treatment of many chronic allergic and inflammatory conditions, presumably because of decreasing the availability of arachidonic acid for conversion to inflammatory prostaglandins and leukotrienes while simultaneously supplying linoleic and linolenic acids. These fatty acids lead to the formation of prostaglandins, which actually inhibit inflammation.

Numerous clinical studies have demonstrated the therapeutic effect of a diet supplemented with essential fatty acids in the treatment of many chronic allergic and inflammatory diseases, including rheumatoid arthritis, asthma, eczema, psoriasis, lupus, and ulcerative colitis. Particularly beneficial are the omega-3 fatty acids.

GLA Supplements in Rheumatoid Arthritis

To illustrate the power of fatty acid dietary changes to improve a severe chronic degenerative disease, let's examine the clinical studies of essential fatty acids in the treatment of rheumatoid arthritis.

Nutritionally oriented physicians often recommend GLA supplements (black currant, borage, and evening primrose oil) in the treatment of inflammatory conditions such as rheumatoid arthritis and eczema; however, these oils may actually produce a negative effect on tissue fatty acid patterns by raising the level of arachidonic acid and reducing the level of omega-3 fatty acids.[31]

In rheumatoid arthritis, some studies have shown benefit with GLA supplementation; others have not.[32,33] Apparently the key factor is whether or not subjects are allowed to take their anti-inflammatory drugs. These drugs inhibit the formation of inflammatory prostaglandins and mask the negative effects of the altered tissue fatty acid profile produced by GLA supplements.

Although positive results have been reported with GLA supplementation, closer examination is required. For example, in one double-blind study, 37 patients with rheumatoid arthritis were given either GLA (1.4 grams daily) or a placebo for 24 weeks. GLA supplementation reduced the number of tender joints by 36 percent, the tender joint score by 45 percent, swollen joint count by 28 percent, and the swollen joint score by 41 percent.[34] In contrast, no patients in the placebo group showed significant improvement in any measure. The superficial results of this study indicate that borage oil may be useful in reducing the inflammatory process of rheumatoid arthritis. However, in this study the subjects continued to take their anti-inflammatory drugs and probably masked the GLA's detrimental effects on tissue arachidonic acid and EPA levels.

The recommended daily dosage for GLA in the treatment of rheumatoid arthritis is 1.4 grams. Since evening primrose oil is 9 percent GLA, individuals would need to consume approximately 31 (500 milligrams each) capsules of evening primrose oil each day. This dosage would typically cost roughly $100 per month. Taking less than the recommended dosage is not likely to produce benefit for several reasons, including cost—flaxseed oil appears to be a better choice.

Fish Oil Supplements in Rheumatoid Arthritis

The studies of fish oil supplementation in rheumatoid arthritis demonstrate far better and more consistent responses than the studies with GLA supplementation. The first double-blind, placebo-controlled study of rheumatoid arthritis patients using 1.8 grams of EPA a day showed less morning stiffness and tender joints.[35] These results led to considerable scientific interest and numerous press accounts of the possible benefits of fish oil for allergic and inflammatory conditions.

Over a dozen follow-up studies consistently demonstrate positive benefits.[36–43] In addition to improving symptoms (morning stiffness and joint tenderness), fish oil supplementation produces favorable changes in suppressing the production of inflammatory compounds secreted by white blood cells.

While the results of these studies are impressive, all of these studies were relatively short-term (less than 1 year). In order to properly assess the beneficial effect of any treatment of rheumatoid arthritis, it is extremely important to evaluate patients over an extended period of time (ideally, at least 1 year) because the condition is associated with ups and downs in symptom severity. Recently, researchers completed a 1-year study of fish oil supplementation in rheumatoid arthritis. The results clearly indicate that supplementation with 2.6 grams per day of omega-3 oil (six 1-gram capsules of fish oil per day) results in significant clinical benefit and leads to significant reductions in the need for drug therapy. The results of this long-term study provide further validation of the short-term studies.

Flaxseed Oil in Rheumatoid Arthritis

Because alpha-linolenic acid, the essential omega-3 fatty acid from flaxseed oil, can be elongated to form EPA and DHA, the obvious question is Can flaxseed oil produce the same benefits as fish oil in the treatment of rheumatoid arthritis? A recent study attempted to answer this question. A small, 22-patient double-blind study over a 2-month period did not show any benefit with flaxseed oil (30 grams daily) versus the same amount of safflower oil.[44] However, upon examination of the data an obvious explanation exists. In order to provide clinical benefit, flaxseed oil needs to reduce the tissue concentration of arachidonic acid while simultaneously increasing the tissue concentration of EPA and DHA. Tissue analysis in patients involved in this study who were taking flaxseed oil did not demonstrate significant changes in tissue levels of either arachidonic acid or EPA and DHA. Previous studies have shown that it is possible to raise tissue levels of EPA and DHA and lower levels of arachidonic acid with flaxseed oils if the intake of omega-6 oils is restricted. The failure to improve tissue lipid concentrations in this study led to the ineffectiveness of flaxseed oil.

The reasons behind the failure to improve lipid concentrations is either failure to restrict the use of other vegetable oils while supplementing the diet with flaxseed oil or failure to correct an underlying zinc deficiency. Failure to restrict the intake of omega-6 oils as the reason is evidenced by the fact there was no significant change in the alpha-linolenic acid to linoleic acid ratio in test subjects.

Evidence to support failure to correct an underlying zinc deficiency as the reason comes from serum zinc analysis on test subjects. Zinc functions in delta-6 desaturase, the enzyme involved in the conversion of alpha-linolenic acid to EPA and DHA (and the conversion of linoleic acid to GLA). Zinc deficiency is common in rheumatoid arthritis. In fact, several studies have shown zinc supplementation to improve rheumatoid arthritis. The fact that tissue levels of alpha-linolenic acid increased while patients were on the flaxseed oil and EPA and DHA levels did not suggests zinc deficiency. This led researchers to measure serum zinc in the patients in the study.

The researchers concluded, "Low conversion of alpha-linolenic acid to EPA and DHA (due to a zinc deficiency), together with a low alpha-linolenic acid to linoleic acid ratio, might explain why a short-term alpha-linolenic acid supplementation did not alter the RA disease activity."

Flaxseed oil supplementation may inhibit the autoimmune reactions as well as EPA.[45] It may take a little longer, but I feel it is a better way to go and will save money. In order to provide benefit in rheumatoid arthritis, the dosage of fish oil must provide 1.8 grams of EPA each day. This dosage equates to approximately ten, 1-grams capsules daily with an approximate cost of $70 to $90 per month. Since 1.5 tablespoons of flaxseed oil can produce similar effects on tissue arachidonic acid and EPA levels, in contrast the monthly cost for flaxseed oil is $12 to $18.

Multiple Sclerosis

Multiple sclerosis (MS) is a debilitating syndrome of progressive nervous system disturbance. The early symptoms of multiple sclerosis may include:

- **Muscular Symptoms**   feeling of heaviness, weakness, leg dragging, stiffness, tendency to drop things, clumsiness
- **Sensory Symptoms**   tingling, pins-and-needles sensation, numbness, dead feeling, bandlike tightness, electrical sensations
- **Visual Symptoms**   blurring, fogginess, haziness, eyeball pain, blindness, double vision
- **Vestibular Symptoms**   light-headedness, feeling of spinning, sensation of drunkenness, nausea, vomiting
- **Genitourinary Symptoms**   incontinence, loss of bladder sensation, loss of sexual function

Despite considerable research, we still have many questions about MS. Mainstream medicine is almost obsessed with finding a viral cause for this disease, yet most current work suggests immune disturbances. In MS, the myelin sheath that surrounds the nerves is destroyed. For this reason, MS is classified as a "demyelinating" disease. Zones of demyelination (plaques) vary in size and location within the spinal cord. Symptoms correspond in a general way to the distribution of the plaques.

In about two-thirds of the cases, onset is between ages 20 and 40 (rarely is the onset after 50), and women are affected slightly more often than males (60 percent female, 40 percent male). The cause of MS remains to be definitively determined. Many causative factors have been proposed including viruses, autoimmune factors, and diet.

In regard to essential fatty acids, individuals with MS are thought to have a defect in essential fatty absorption and/or transport, which results in a functional deficiency state. In normal circumstances, because consumption of saturated fats increases the requirements of essential fatty acids, a relative deficiency state exists in many cases even if the level of essential fatty acids in the diet is adequate. Central to this defect in essential fatty acid metabolism in MS are deficiencies of the omega-3 oils. Omega-3 oils play a critical role in the structure and function of myelin. A deficiency of alpha-linolenic acid and other omega-3 fatty acids can result in permanently impairing normal myelin formation.[46,47]

Dr. Roy Swank's MS Diet

Dr. Roy Swank, Professor of Neurology, University of Oregon Medical School, has provided convincing evidence that a diet low in saturated fats and high in essential fatty acids maintained over a long period of time (one study lasted over 34 years) tends to halt the disease process.[48,49] Dr. Swank began successfully treating patients with his lowfat diet in 1948. He recommends:

- Elimination of butter and hydrogenated oils (margarine and shortening)
- Daily animal fat intake of no more than 15 grams
- Daily intake of 40 to 50 grams (3 to 4 tablespoons) of polyunsaturated vegetable oils
- At least 1 teaspoon of cod liver oil daily
- Normal allowance of protein mostly from vegetables, nuts, fish, white meat of turkey and chicken (skin removed), and lean meat
- Consumption of fish three or more times a week.[49]

The results of Dr. Swank's 34-year study (1949 to 1984) in MS patients are astounding.[48] Minimally disabled patients who followed his dietary recommendations experienced little disease progression—if any at all—and only 5 percent failed to survive the 34 years of the study. In contrast, 80 percent who failed to follow the diet recommendations did not survive the study period. The moderately and severely disabled patients who followed the dietary recommendations also did far better than the group that didn't. In addition to dramatically reducing the death rate, the diet prevented worsening of the disease and greatly reduced fatigue.

Dr. Swank's results in MS along with numerous other studies in other chronic degenerative diseases support the critical need to alter the production of prostaglandins and related compounds in these conditions by changing the source of dietary fatty acids. Dr. Swank's diet is a good one for virtually any chronic inflammatory or allergic condition. At the very least, such dietary manipulation lessens the dosage of corticosteroids required.

Currently, researchers believe the beneficial effects of Dr. Swank's diet are a result of:

- Decreasing the aggregation of blood platelets
- Decreasing an autoimmune response
- Reducing saturated fat intake
- Normalizing the decreased essential fatty acid levels found in the serum, red blood cells, platelets, and perhaps most importantly the cerebrospinal fluid in patients with MS.

Linoleic Acid Supplementation in MS

Researchers have investigated linoleic acid as a treatment for MS in three double-blind trials.[50–52] Although the results of the studies were mixed (two showed an effect and one did not), combined analysis indicated that patients supplementing with linoleic acid had a smaller increase in disability and reduced severity and duration of relapses than did controls. These studies used sunflower seed oil at dosage of slightly more than 1 tablespoon per day.

I believe they could have obtained better results in the double-blind studies if they had restricted dietary saturated fatty acids, used larger amounts of essential fatty acids (at least 2 tablespoons per day), and conducted longer studies (one study found that normalization of fatty acid levels required at least 2 years of supplementation). Furthermore, they would have achieved even better results if they had used flaxseed oil. Flaxseed oil contains not only linoleic acid but also alpha-linolenic acid. Linolenic acid has a greater effect on reducing platelet aggregation than linoleic acid and is required for normal CNS composition.

Benefits of Omega-3 Fatty Acids in MS

There is strong rationale for supplementation with omega-3 fatty acids in the treatment of MS. One of the key recommendations in Swank's diet was the regular consumption of fish and cod liver oil. Omega-3 oils are essential in the formation of normal collagen. These two facts provide ample reason to supplement with omega-3 oils in MS. There are also some interesting geographical features on the distribution of MS that seem to indicate that omega-3 oils may help prevent and treat MS.

Some of the first investigations into diet and MS centered around trying to explain why inland farming communities in Norway had a higher incidence of MS than areas near the coastline.[53] Researchers discovered that the diets of the farmers were much higher in animal and dairy products than the diets of the coastal dwellers and the latter's diet had much higher levels of cold-water fish rich in omega-3 oils. Since animal and dairy products are much higher in saturated fatty acids and lower in polyunsaturated fatty acids than fish, researchers explored this association in greater detail.

Subsequent studies have upheld a strong association between a diet rich in animal and dairy products and the incidence of MS. The most recent study examined the relationship between mortality rates from multiple sclerosis from 1983 to 1989 in 36 countries and dietary fat intake and latitude.[54] The results indicated that a diet rich in saturated fat from animal foods and low in marine lipids and unsaturated fatty acids was positively associated with mortality from multiple sclerosis. Although they also found that MS mortality rates increased in areas above a latitude of 30 degrees North, dietary factors appear to account for this increased incidence. For example, Japan and parts of China are above the latitude of 30 degrees North, yet the incidence and mortality from MS is very low in these two countries. Unfortunately, researchers and physicians are slow in accepting dietary omega-3 oils' role in reducing the risk for MS.

GLA and MS

Because of gamma-linolenic acid's (GLA) ready incorporation into brain lipids and its effect on immune function, it may be more effective in MS treatment than linoleic acid alone.[55] However, because of its cost and the relatively large amounts that would have to be consumed to exert a therapeutic effect, supplementation with GLA is not indicated at this time. One study demonstrated that daily supplementation with only 340 milligrams of gamma-linoleic and 2.92 grams of linoleic acid (the ratio found in evening primrose oil) had no effect on the clinical course in MS patients.[56] In the same study, those receiving 23 grams of linoleic acid demonstrated reduced frequency and severity of acute attacks, even though the study was only 24 months long.

Flaxseed Oil and Cancer

Dr. Johanna Budwig, considered Germany's premier biochemist and one of the world's leading experts on essential fatty acid nutrition, has built an international reputation for treating cancer and other degenerative diseases with flaxseed oil. In 1990, the National Cancer Institute (NCI) launched a 5-year, $20 million program to learn more about biologically active plant chemicals (phytochemicals) in certain foods that may help to prevent cancer. Flaxseed was the first of six foods to be studied. Preliminary results indicated that flaxseed oil can exert powerful anticancer properties if the oil is high in lignan precursors. Unfortunately, despite the incredible promise of preliminary results, the NCI canceled the project before it was completed. Nonetheless, there is substantial evidence that suggests flaxseed oil exerts significant anticancer properties.

Flax Lignans: Potent Anticancer Compounds

In addition to flaxseed's high level of omega-3 fatty acid, it is the most abundant source of lignans. One study showed it contains over 100 times the levels found in other plant foods.[57] Lignans are special compounds that demonstrate some rather impressive health benefits, including positive effects in relieving menopausal hot flashes and anticancer, antibacterial, antifungal, and antiviral activity.

Perhaps the most significant of these benefits is lignans' anticancer properties. Population studies and experimental studies in humans and animals have demon-

My Sweet Valentine,

Your Valentine gift to me was amazing... and very very hot. Giving you something as wonderful as that is a tall order.

I decided to send you something, literally, right off my body. This is the shirt I wore at every concert last summer. You wanted something you could hold. It will be too big for you, but your beautiful naked body will be wrapped in me.

Put in on, and feel me caress your skin.

strated that lignans exert significant anticancer effects.[58,59] In the animal experiments, researchers noted tremendous anticancer effects when the animals were fed flaxseed and flaxseed oil. Positive results occurred in not only mammary cancer but colon cancer and general tumor models. Typically, the animals receiving flaxseed oil or flaxseed demonstrated significant reduction (greater than 50 percent reduction) in tumor numbers and size after 1 to 2 months.[60–62]

Gut flora change plant lignans into enterolactone and enterodiol, two compounds that are believed to be protective against cancer, particularly breast cancer. Lignans are capable of binding to estrogen-receptors and interfering with the cancer-promoting effects of estrogen on breast tissue. In addition, lignans increase the production of a special sex hormone–binding compound. This compound, known as sex hormone–binding globulin, regulates estrogen levels by escorting excess estrogen from the body via eliminative pathways.

Lignans are probably one of the protective factors against breast cancer in vegetarian women.[63] Typically, women who excrete higher amounts of lignans in their urine (a sign of increased consumption) have much lower rates for breast cancer. High-lignan flaxseed oil may be the best choice for women going through menopause or women at risk for breast cancer. It is currently estimated that as many as one in nine American women will develop breast cancer.

Alpha-linolenic Acid and Breast Cancer

In addition to lignans, a high-lignan flaxseed oil also provides alpha-linolenic acid. Like lignans, alpha-linolenic acid demonstrates significant anticancer properties, especially against breast cancer. A prospective study in 121 women with initially localized breast cancer examined the association between the levels of various fatty acids in the fatty tissue of the breast and how much the cancer had spread (metastasized).[64] Breast tissue analyzed at the time of surgery indicated a low level of alpha-linoleic acid (18:3n3) was associated with the spread of the cancer into the lymph nodes of the armpit (axillary area) and tumor invasiveness. After 31 months of follow-up after initial surgery, 21 patients developed metastases of their cancer into other body tissues. A low level of alpha-linolenic acid was the first determinant of metastases in these patients. In other words, when all factors were considered, low levels of alpha-linolenic acid were the most significant contributor to the spread of cancer. Since the main cause of death in breast cancer patients is the development of cancer in other tissues, these findings are extremely important.

The results from this study suggest that supplementing the diet with flaxseed oil (approximately 58 percent alpha-linolenic acid) may help prevent breast cancer, tumor invasiveness, and metastasis. In addition to this prospective human study, animal models of mammary carcinogenesis have shown that a diet high in omega-6 fatty acids stimulates mammary tumor growth while alpha-linolenic acid enrichment of the diet inhibits tumor growth.[65]

Modulating Effects of Fatty Acids on the Immune System

It is possible that alpha-linolenic acid also exerts some of its anticancer effects via enhancement of immune function.[66] In one study, the possible interaction between intense exercise, known to suppress the immune system, and polyunsaturated fatty acids was examined in mice.[67] For 8 weeks the animals received either a natural-ingredient diet alone or a diet supplemented with flaxseed oil (50 percent alpha-linolenic acid), beef tallow, safflower oil (mostly linoleic acid), or fish oils. Each dietary group was divided into either a sedentary group or an exercised group. Exercise consisted of continuous swimming at high intensity until exhaustion. Three separate experiments indicated that the primary immune response in sheep red blood cells was affected by supplementation with polyunsaturated fatty acids in sedentary animals in the following order:

- Beef tallow
- Control diet
- Safflower oil
- Fish oil
- Flaxseed oil

In the exercised animals, the immune response was suppressed by exhaustive exercise except in the group receiving the flaxseed oil. Only the group receiving the flaxseed oil demonstrated a normal immune response.

The significance of these results may be to recommend flaxseed oil supplementation to people who place great physical demands on themselves because of work or exercise, thereby offsetting some of the negative effects of exercise on immune function.

Selecting a High-Quality Oil

Obtaining high-quality flaxseed oil and other healthful vegetable oils is a major challenge for consumers. In order to derive the benefits of these oils, you must use a high-quality preparation. How can you be sure the product you pick up off your grocer's shelf or in a health-food store has been processed and handled in a way to protect the delicate polyunsaturated bonds these oils possess? Your purchase could bring you a product that truly supports life or one that has the potential to cause cellular destruction, immune malfunction, and ultimately—if used regularly—promote cardiovascular disease and cancer.

This paradoxical effect may be confusing unless you appreciate the characteristics of highly polyunsaturated vegetable oils like flaxseed oil. The analogy of Dr. Jekyll and Mr. Hyde is appropriate. Without ingesting his laboratory-derived potion, Dr. Jekyll is a well-intended scientist. However, once he ingests the potion, he is transformed into the dangerous and evil Mr. Hyde. Such is the case with highly polyunsaturated oils. In their unrefined, unadulterated state, these nutrients are absolutely "essential" for life and optimal health; however, once refined or altered, these formerly life-imparting nutrients become potentially biologically dangerous compounds. Foods, including oils, have a natural shelf life unless they have been artificially preserved to increase their shelf life and stability.

People want foods that are fresh and oils that are not rancid. As a testament to the demand for foods that are "fresh," market surveys discovered that the single word most powerfully motivating consumers to buy was "fresh" on the label. Because highly polyunsaturated vegetable oils are considered semiperishable, the only way to extend shelf life is to artificially stabilize them to the point where they do not interact with the elements and thus become rancid. Three elements hold the greatest potential to destroy polyunsaturated oils—heat, light, and oxygen.

Several clever food technology methods are designed, however, to do just that. The results are the vegetable oils and artificial margarine spreads found at your local grocery store— your first hint where *not* to look for high-quality vegetable oils. The only retail outlets to date that address the important issues surrounding polyunsaturated vegetable oils are health-food stores. Consumer beware, however, because many of the therapeutic and culinary oils found in health food stores are also manufactured, distributed, packaged, and displayed in a fashion that seriously questions any health benefit they may have.

You need a knowledge of extraction, handling, and labeling methods of oils in order to intelligently purchase high-quality flaxseed oil and other essential fatty acid–rich oils. First, consider what elements lead to the destruction and breakdown of vegetable oils, including flaxseed oil. In addition, remember that the removal of naturally occurring antioxidant, vitamin, mineral, and other nutrient cofactors from the oils serves to accelerate the degradation of these products.

You would think producers of polyunsaturated oils would use every available method to avoid destroying the integrity of the oils, right? Wrong! In fact, doing so is the exception, not the rule. The majority of food-grade oil manufacturers purposefully expose polyunsaturated oils to excessive heat, light, and oxygen. Their goal is to achieve a uniform product with an exceptionally long shelf life in the most cost-effective manner possible. Oil manufacturers rely on the extremely high heat generated during processing (over 250 degrees Celsius) to unnaturally contort the fatty acid molecule while stabilizing the unsaturated bond with hydrogen–and they gain the extended shelf life they long for. Does this sound like something Dr. Jekyll might have concocted in his laboratory?

Instead of going into a long—and, yes, even boring—description of mass refinement of polyunsaturated oils, let me say that over 20 steps in this process lead to the complete destruction of the health potential of these products. They are destroyed to the point to were the manufacturer must add vitamin E and beta-carotene back again just to give the oil a hue of color. Perhaps we could refer to these oils as "enriched." Would you feel enriched if you were robbed at gunpoint, asked to strip naked, and then given your shoes back so you could walk home?

Manufacture of Commercial Oil Products

Several methods of manufacturing destroy polyunsaturated oils and/or the nutrient cofactors they contain. Avoid products produced in these ways if at all possible. Unfortunately, the federal government has not established laws compelling manufacturers to list the extraction and processing methods on vegetable oil labels. Needless to say, companies offering products extracted in these ways do not announce this fact on their labels. Your best bet in obtaining high-quality flaxseed and vegetable oils is to recognize the hallmarks of these products.

Mass Commercialized Oil Products

These products are usually extracted in a number of ways and in combinations of extraction methods. For example, although these oils initially may be extracted by the preferred expeller-press method, large commercial presses use extreme pressing temperatures and pressures to obtain high-oil yields. The seed meal is then placed in a chemical solution to obtain every remaining trace of oil, ultimately yielding 100 percent seed-oil recovery. Then come the remaining 20 or so refinement and stabilization steps. Hydrogenation is but one step that manufacturers might employ during the processing of oil products.

I have previously discussed many of the negative consequences of hydrogenation, but an explanation of the procedure bears repeating. The process of hydrogenation effectively transforms a previously unsaturated fatty acid molecule into a fat similar to a saturated fat and distorts the molecule from its healthful cis configuration to an unnatural, unhealthy trans configuration. Trans fatty acids occur when either the random process of hydrogenation or high heat straightens out the formerly C-shaped polyunsaturated molecule. It is difficult to get a bunch of C-shaped molecules to clump together, but once the molecules are straightened out, they clump together readily. This solidifies the previously liquid oil and raises the melting temperature significantly. This process is exactly what occurs in the manufacture of margarine. Imagine all the good margarine does clumping together in your arteries and clogging up cell respiration! The simple yet effective process of hydrogenation fulfills all the requirements set forth by the food industry. It reduces the likelihood of spoilage (now acts as a food preservative), extends shelf life, and enhances mouth feel. However, the detrimental effects of hydrogenated oils are now well known.[68]

Hexane (Chemical Extraction)

Some seeds—either because of their extremely small size, hardness, or low oil content—lend themselves to be more efficiently and economically extracted by chemical means. The seed from the evening of primrose flower, a fair source of gamma-linoleic acid (GLA), is a good example. In hexane and chemical extraction the desired seed is first cracked to expose the oil, perhaps even run through an expeller press, and then emerged in a solvent solution to render the oil. Obviously the seed oil must then be separated from the solvent solution. However, there is some question as to whether all of the solvent solution can be removed from the resultant oil.

Super Critical Fluid Extracted Oils

Super critical fluid extraction (SCFE) is the latest player in seed-oil extraction methods. This method employs an extremely highly pressurized chamber (similar to what you might visualize as a pressure cooker) to remove the oil from the seed. Similar to hexane extraction, the seed is ground to expose more seed meal surface area for oil extraction. Although SCFE is highly touted by some companies marketing so-called nutritional oils, it is even more damaging to polyunsaturated oils than chemical hexane extraction. SCFE oils have less chemical stability, higher average lipid peroxide levels (measure of rancidity), altered fatty acid profiles, decreased mineral content, and fractionated triglyceride formations; they are absent phosphatides and stripped of toco-pherols.[69–72] Uninformed product buyers for nutrition companies are romanced by SCFE because it uses low temperatures during the extraction process. Unfortunately, SCFE used singularly (with the exception of mass refined oils) renders the poorest quality oils available.

"Cold Pressed" Oils

Rarely in the food manufacturing business has there been a term so distorted as "cold pressed." By its very name it conjures up oils extracted under conditions of re-frigeration or other heat-free environments. Unfortunately, in the U.S. the only offi-cial designation given for cold pressed oils is that "no form of external heat is applied during extraction." This definition says nothing of the possible temperatures reached because of the extraction apparatus operation or heat the oils might be subjected to during further refinement after extraction! Needless to say, the term "cold pressed" displayed on a bottle of oil says absolutely nothing about the quality of the product. While this term has been well received by the general public (bringing about a false sense of security), quality manufacturers of unrefined vegetable oils have decided to drop this term from their labels because of the deception that surrounds it. Interest-ingly, Europeans use the term "cold pressed," but they have established regulations that allow use of the term only if extraction temperatures are below 104 degrees Fahrenheit. We should establish similar regulations in the U.S. if we allow the term "cold pressed" for labeling purposes.

Preferred Oil-Extraction Methods

Fortunately, there are a few manufacturers of flaxseed oil and other polyunsaturated vegetable and seed oils who realize the extreme need for unrefined oil products. These health-conscious companies are attempting to form a trade group that would establish regulations and commonly accepted terminology to aid consumers in distinguishing between "safe" and healthful nutritional and culinary oils and the refined and "dangerous" fat and oil products that so predominantly line our grocery and health-food store aisles. The interested parties continue to meet and correspond in order to achieve this monumental task. Until such time when industry regulations are established and common terminology is available, health-conscious consumers can use the information here to ensure they are purchasing quality oil products.

Expeller Pressing

Expeller presses resemble a screw/nut mechanism where the seed is titillated be-tween the threads and the body of the press head. The resulting pressure squeezes the oil from the seed All manufacturers of quality oil products use some form of expeller press. Usually high-quality manufacturers modify their expeller presses to reduce op-erating temperatures and pressure exerted on the seed. Unfortunately, expeller presses are also used by mass producers of oils (they use huge commercial presses) and operated at extreme temperatures and pressures for extended periods. In these instances, expeller presses are used only as a prerefinement step in the production of inferior oil products. Although expeller presses are a significant improvement over other extraction methods, they must be used singularly and under stringent conditions to yield truly healthful oils.

Modified Atmospheric Packing (MAP)

Modified atmospheric packing (MAP) is appearing to draw favor from manufacturers of high-quality oil products. This method employs the use of an expeller press modified by the oil producer to operate at low temperatures while excluding the damaging effects of light and oxygen. Oil manufacturers and trade associations such as the National Nutritional Foods Association are currently discussing regulations that will define the parameters wherein a manufacturer can display this designation. It may be some time before you find this terminology on labels. Oil manufacturers currently use tradenames for their proprietary methods (Modified Atmospheric Packing Methods), including Bio-Electron Process (Barlean's Organic Oils), Spectra-Vac (Spectrum Naturals), or Omegaflo (Omega Nutrition). Table 33.2 gives you an in-depth comparison of oil-extraction methods.

Features of High-Quality Products

Luckily there are telltale ways in which educated, health-conscious consumers can select high-quality flaxseed and other vegetable and seed oils. Simply follow these guidelines:

- **Products certified as organic by a reputable third party source, indicated on label or promotional material**   Manufacturers who have devoted time and expense to have their oil products third-party-certified organic usually have taken the measures necessary to provide extremely high-quality oils. They proudly proclaim this status on their labels.

- **Products extracted by modified expeller presses only and at temperatures that do not exceed 98 degrees Fahrenheit**   Again, manufacturers interested in human health do not sacrifice quality for the higher oil yields that extreme temperatures and pressures bring. These methods employ the elimination of light and oxygen during manufacture. They are currently recognized by several popular tradenames listed earlier in the section Modified Atmospheric Packing (MAP).

- **Products contained in opaque (light-resistant) plastic containers**   Total elimination of light coming in contact with the oil is mandatory to ensure against degradation of the oil. Every moment the oil is exposed to light, potentially thousands of photons interact with the oil, ultimately causing a rancid product. The light transmission of the various light frequencies combined results in a mean penetration in even pharmaceutical amber glass bottles of 114 percent! This percentage is in stark contrast to the 0 percent penetration opaque plastic bottles allow. Now multiply 114 percent times the number of hours and days exposed to light and you get a good idea of the potential impact on the oil. Only purchase flaxseed oil in totally opaque, high-density polyethylene bottles. Despite the accusations of a popular fat and oil author who is secured by a company that packages

TABLE 33.2   Comparison of Oil-Extraction Methods

Characteristic	Modified Atmospheric Packing[a]	Super Critical Fluid Extraction (SCFE)	Hexane (Chemical Extraction)
Oxidative stability	Highly stable for polyunsaturated	Highly unstable	Poor Stability
Average lipid peroxide Level (%)	0.1–0.3	1.7	1.3
Essential fatty acid profile	Normal	Altered	Normal
Mineral content	Normal	Decreased	Normal
Triglyceride formation	Normal	Fractionated	Normal
Phosphatides	Present, remain intact	Absent (refined out)	Present, remain intact
Exposure to light and oxygen	Protected from light and oxygen	Exposed to light and oxygen	Exposed to light and oxygen
Chemical residue	No	No	Yes
Color	Natural pigment intact	Pigments removed during process	Natural pigment intact
Taste	Smooth, nutty flavor	Bland, bitter aftertaste	Bland, bitter aftertaste
Shelf life	Liquid, 4 mos. (1 yr. in freezer) Capsules, 1 yr.	Questionable as indicated by lipid peroxide level	Questionable as indicated by lipid peroxide level
Commercially available form	Liquid or capsule	Capsule only	Liquid or capsule

[a]Example utilizing Barlean's Organic Oils "Bio-Electron" (MAP) process. Results may vary with other (MAP) extraction processes.

only in glass, the use of high-density polyethylene plastic is absolutely safe and is the preferred method of packaging these oils. HDPE plastic is fully approved by U.S. and Canadian governments for these purposes. This material has been used since the 1970s with an untarnished record of health and safety. Extensive laboratory analysis has been conducted to ensure absolutely no migration of HDPE plastic materials into oils and other foods. No scientific evidence exists to date to refute the extreme safety of this packaging material.

- **Products found in the refrigerated section of health-food stores**   Quality manufacturers of unrefined oil products insist that their products be stored in refrigerators to protect the oil from degradation after prolonged exposure to ambient temperatures.

- **Quality vegetable oil products come with dating codes on the label that signify the pressing date and the recommended use-by date**   Follow these dates stringently unless you decide to place your flaxseed oil in the freezer, where you can extend the expiration date significantly.

Products You Want to Avoid

Steer clear of the following products:

- Oils that are not third-party-certified organic
- Oils that are sold ONLY in gelatin capsule form
- Products where the label does not list the actual method of extraction; be wary of "cold pressed" oils
- Oils that have a bitter aftertaste, "rancid" flavor, or no flavor (heavily refined)

Using Flaxseed Oil

There is no better way to enjoy the virtues of essential fatty acid–rich flaxseed oil than including it in some of your favorite recipes. Because modern manufacturing methods very effectively remove or transform the vital and "essential" fatty acids into dangerous trans and hydrogenated fatty acids in our food chain, we must reintroduce the essential fatty acids back into our foods. Using flaxseed oil in recipes is a terrific way to ensure that you get your daily requirement of essential fatty acids.[73–74] Feel free to experiment with adding flaxseed oil to foods as an ingredient. Salad dressings render themselves especially suitable for the inclusion of flaxseed oil. Remember to consider the destruction that can come with excessively heating flaxseed oil. If at all possible, add flaxseed oil to cooked foods like soups after the fact. With that in mind, enjoy the culinary delights and health benefits a diet rich in essential fatty acids can bring. Here are some sample recipes complements of Barlean's Organic Oils.

Barlean's Basic Salad Dressing

Place all ingredients into a salad bowl and whisk together until smooth and creamy. This recipe is quick and delicious!

4 tablespoons organic flaxseed oil
1-$^1/_2$ tablespoons lemon juice
1 medium garlic clove, crushed
pinch of seasoned salt or salt-free seasoning
fresh ground pepper to taste

Jazz up this basic recipe to your own personal taste by using your favorite herbs and spices.

Fresh Mexican Salsa

A zesty traditional Mexican salsa now made even better with the addition of flaxseed oil. Great for dipping tortilla chips or as a sauce on enchiladas, burritos, and tacos.

3 tomatoes, diced
4 sprigs fresh cilantro
$^1/_2$ medium onion, diced

1 green onion
1 small jalapeno pepper
$^{1}/_{2}$ cup tomato sauce
3 tablespoons organic flaxseed oil

Combine tomatoes, cilantro, onions, and jalapeno pepper in a blender or food processor and process to desired consistency, chunky or saucy. In a separate bowl combine tomato sauce and flaxseed oil. Stir to uniform consistency. Combine all ingredients. Chill and serve.

Hummus

A fantastic-tasting Middle Eastern dish to be used as a dip or as a filler in pita pocket sandwiches; an excellent source of complete protein and now essential fatty acids.

one, 15-ounce can or 1-$^{2}/_{3}$ cups cooked garbanzo beans
    (chick-peas), drained (save the liquid)
$^{1}/_{4}$ cup tahini (sesame seed paste)
3 tablespoons lemon juice
3 tablespoons organic flaxseed oil
2 medium cloves garlic
$^{1}/_{4}$ teaspoon ground coriander
$^{1}/_{4}$ teaspoon cumin
$^{1}/_{4}$ teaspoon paprika
dash cayenne
$^{1}/_{4}$ cup minced scallions
2 tablespoons minced fresh parsley (for garnish)

In a blender or food processor, process the garbanzo beans, tahini, lemon juice, and flaxseed oil until the mixture reaches the consistency of a coarse paste. Use as much of the garbanzo liquid and/or water as needed. Add the garlic, coriander, cumin, paprika, and cayenne and process the ingredients again to combine thoroughly. Transfer the hummus to a bowl and stir in the scallions. Cover and chill, adding the parsley just before serving.

For More Recipes

For more delicious recipes using organic flaxseed oil, I highly recommend buying *Flax for Life*, by Jade Beutler. You can find it at most health-food stores, or you can call Barlean's Organic Oils at 1-800-445-FLAX.

Some Additional Practical Advice

The following four recommendations are easy to remember. Follow them to achieve better health and optimal levels of essential fatty acids in your body tissues.

- **Reduce the amount of saturated fat and total fat in your diet** There is a great deal of research linking a diet high in saturated fat to numerous cancers, heart

TABLE 33.3 Fat Content (as a Percentage of Calories) of Selected Foods

MEATS			Cauliflower	7
Sirloin steak, hipbone, lean w/fat		83	Eggplant	7
Pork sausage		83	Asparagus	6
T-bone steak, lean w/fat		82	Green beans	6
Porterhouse steak, lean w/fat		82	Celery	6
Bacon, lean		82	Cucumber	6
Rib roast, lean w/fat		81	Turnip	6
Bologna		81	Zucchini	6
Country-style sausage		81	Carrots	4
Spareribs		80	Green peas	4
Frankfurters		80	Artichokes	3
Lamb rib chops, lean w/fat		79	Onions	3
Duck meat, w/skin		76	Beets	2
Salami		76	Chives	1
Liverwurst		75	Potatoes	1
Rump roast, lean w/fat		71		
Ham, lean w/fat		69	LEGUMES	
Stewing beef, lean w/fat		66	Tofu	49
Goose meat, w/skin		65	Soybean	37
Ground beef, fairly lean		64	Soybean sprouts	28
Veal breast, lean w/fat		64	Garbanzo bean	11
Leg of lamb, lean w/fat		61	Kidney bean	4
Chicken, dark meat w/skin, roasted		56	Lima bean	4
Round steak, lean w/fat		53	Mungbean sprouts	4
Chuck rib roast, lean only		50	Lentil	3
Chuck steak, lean only		50	Broad bean	3
Sirloin steak, hipbone, lean only		47	Mung bean	3
Turkey, dark meat w/skin		47		
Lamb rib chops, lean only		45	DAIRY PRODUCTS	
Chicken, light meat w/skin, roasted		44	Butter	100
			Cream, light whipping	92
FISH			Cream cheese	90
Tuna, chunk, oil-packed		63	Cream, light or coffee	85
Herring, Pacific		59	Egg yolks	80
Anchovies		54	Half and half	79
Bass, black sea		53	Blue cheese	73
Perch, ocean		53	Brick cheese	72
Caviar, sturgeon		52	Cheddar cheese	71
Mackerel, Pacific		50	Swiss cheese	66
Sardines, Atlantic, in oil, drained		49	Ricotta cheese, whole-milk type	66
Salmon, sockeye (red)		49	Eggs, whole	65
			Ice cream	64
VEGETABLES			Mozzarella cheese, part skim type	55
Mustard greens		13	Goat's milk	54
Kale		13	Cow's milk	49
Beet greens		12	Yogurt, plain	49
Lettuce		12	Ice cream, regular	48
Turnip greens		11	Cottage cheese	35
Mushrooms		8	Lowfat milk	31
Cabbage		7	Lowfat yogurt	31

(continues)

TABLE 33.3   Fat Content (as a Percentage of Calories) of Selected Foods (continued)

Ice milk	29	Orange	4
Nonfat cottage cheese	22	Banana	4
		Cantaloupe	3
MEAT AND FISH PRODUCTS		Pineapple	3
Hormel Spam luncheon meat	77	Grapefruit	2
Mrs. Paul's Buttered Fish Filets	75	Papaya	2
Del Monte Bonito	67	Peach	2
Morton Beef Tenderloin	64	Prune	1
Mrs. Paul's Fried Shrimp	58		
Mrs. Paul's Clam Crepes	55	GRAINS	
Hormel Dinty Moore Corned Beef	53	Oatmeal	16
Swanson Salisbury Steak	52	Buckwheat, dark	7
Nabisco Chicken in a Biskit	51	Rye, dark	7
Morton House Beef Stew	49	Whole wheat	5
Mrs. Paul's Flounder	48	Brown rice	5
Swanson Veal Parmigiana	48	Corn flour	5
Swanson Fried Chicken	46	Bulgur	4
Hormel Dinty Moore Beef Stew	45	Barley	3
Morton Beef Pot Pie	45	Buckwheat, light	3
Mrs. Paul's Fish Au Gratin	43	Rye, light	2
Morton Chicken Croquettes	40	Wild rice	2
FRUITS		NUTS AND SEEDS	
Olive	91	Coconut	85
Avocado	82	Walnut	79
Grape	11	Sesame	76
Strawberry	11	Almond	76
Apple	8	Sunflower	71
Blueberry	7	Pumpkin seeds	71
Lemon	7	Cashew	70
Pear	5	Peanut	69
Apricot	4	Chestnut	7

SOURCE: U.S.D.A., Nutritive Value of American Foods in Common Units, Agriculture Handbook No. 456.

disease, and strokes. Both the American Cancer Society and the American Heart Association recommend a diet containing less than 30 percent of total calories as fat. Table 33.3 makes it clear that the easiest way for most people to achieve this goal is to eat less animal products and more plant foods. With the exception of nuts and seeds, most plant foods are very low in fat. And although nuts and seeds contain high levels of fat calories, the calories are derived largely from polyunsaturated essential fatty acids.

- **Eliminate the intake of margarine and foods containing trans fatty acids and partially hydrogenated oils**   During the process of margarine and shortening manufacture, vegetable oils are "hydrogenated." This means that a hydrogen molecule is added to the natural unsaturated fatty acid molecules of the vegetable oil to make it more saturated. Hydrogenation results in changing the structure of the natural fatty acid to many "unnatural" fatty acid forms that interfere with the body's ability to utilize essential fatty acids. Margarine and other hydrogenated vegetable oils are being linked to heart disease and certain cancers.

- **Take one or two tablespoons of flaxseed oil daily**   Many nutritionists consider organic, unrefined flaxseed oil to be the answer to restoring the proper level of essential fatty acids. Flaxseed oil is unique because it contains both essential fatty acids, alpha-linolenic (an omega-3 fatty acid) and linoleic acid (an omega-6 fatty acid), in appreciable amounts. Flaxseed oil is the world's richest source of omega-3 fatty acids. At a whopping 58 percent by weight, it contains over two times the amount of omega-3 fatty acids as fish oils.

- **Limit total dietary fat intake to 20 to 30 percent of calories consumed (400 to 600 calories a day, based on a standard 2,000-calories-a-day diet)**   Make a strong effort to incorporate "healthful" fats in the form of essential fatty acid–rich oils like flaxseed oil in place of dangerous trans, hydrogenated, and saturated fats. Watch for these "stealth fats" by reading food labels carefully before you choose.

PART FIVE

Accessory Nutrients

This section reviews a wide range of substances collectively referred to as accessory nutrients. The term *nutrient* is defined as a substance that either provides nourishment or is necessary for body functions or structures. In previous sections the focus has been on essential nutrients—signifying that these vitamins, minerals, and essential fatty acids are essential for normal body functions. While most of the accessory nutrients discussed in this section are not "essential," they do exert profound health benefits. Furthermore, there are situations in which supplementation may be absolutely essential. For this reason, many of these accessory nutrients are also referred to as "conditionally essential" or "semi essential" by many nutrition educators.

34

Carnitine

Carnitine is a vitaminlike compound responsible for the transport of long-chain fatty acids into the energy producing cell units, the mitochondria. Since carnitine can be synthesized from the essential amino acid lysine, many nutritionists and researchers argue that it should not be considered a vitamin. Others argue that if niacin can be synthesized from the essential amino acid tryptophan and labeled a vitamin, then so should carnitine.

Carnitine was originally isolated from meat extracts in 1905; its chemical structure was determined in 1932. However, despite extensive studies in the thirties, carnitine's role in human physiology remained a mystery until nearly 50 years after its discovery.[1-3]

Then in 1952, a group of researchers established carnitine as a growth factor for the mealworm, *Tenebrio molitor*. Hence, carnitine became also known as vitamin B_T.[4] When researchers discovered other species of organisms were dependent on carnitine, they began to reexamine its role in humans. They soon demonstrated that carnitine was essential in the breakdown of fats into energy.

Carnitine is essential because it is critical in the transport of fatty acids into the mitochondria. Since the carrier molecule for fatty acids, acyl-CoA, cannot penetrate the cell membrane of the mitochondria, a deficiency in carnitine results in decreased fatty acid concentrations in the mitochondria and, as a result, reduced energy production.

The fatty acid must be transferred from CoA to carnitine. The acyl-carnitine molecule can then transport the fatty acid molecule to the mitochondrial surface of the inner mitochondrial membrane. There it releases the fatty acid so that it can be converted to energy (i.e., so that the fat can be "burned").

Carnitine has several other physiological functions, including the conversion of keto-acid analogues of the branched chain amino acids valine, leucine, and isoleucine.[1-3] This function is extremely important during fasting, starvation, and exercise.

Food Sources

Meat and dairy products are the major dietary sources of carnitine. In general, the redder the meat, the higher the carnitine content. Grains, fruits, and vegetables contain little or no carnitine. Preliminary studies indicate that the typical daily diet contains 5 to 100 milligrams of carnitine.[5] However, most of the carnitine in the human body is synthesized from the essential amino acid lysine with the aid of another essential amino acid (methionine), three vitamins (vitamin C, niacin, and vitamin B$_6$), and iron. Obviously, a deficiency of any one of these nutrients results in a carnitine deficiency. The final steps of carnitine formation occur only in the liver, kidney, and brain because the enzyme required (butyrobetaine hydroxylase) in the final formation is present only in these tissues.

This final-step enzyme largely controls the synthesis of carnitine. The heart muscles, skeletal muscles, and many other tissues depend primarily on fatty acids as an energy source; and although they cannot synthesize carnitine, their normal function depends on proper transport of carnitine into these tissues.

Specific transport proteins for carnitine have been identified for the heart, skeletal muscles, epididymis, liver, and kidney. The transport proteins facilitate the transfer of carnitine from the serum into the cells via carrier-mediated transport mechanisms. This active transport mechanism allows the tissues to concentrate carnitine at levels more than 10 times the levels found in plasma.

In infancy, the activity of the final-step enzyme of carnitine synthesis is only 12 percent of the normal adult mean. By 2.5 years, the activity is 30 percent of the adult mean and does not reach full activity until 15 years. These data reflect the importance of preformed carnitine of breast milk in infant nutrition.[1–3]

Initial carnitine concentration in the newborn depends on maternal carnitine concentration. Concentrations in fetal and umbilical cord blood are higher than in maternal blood, suggesting the placenta actively works to concentrate carnitine to the fetus, whose carnitine synthesis is not fully developed.[1–3]

In women with suspected carnitine synthesis impairment, supplementation of carnitine during pregnancy may be needed to ensure adequate tissue concentrations in both the fetus and the mother. Blood carnitine levels are typically lower in pregnant women than nonpregnant women, apparently because of increased demand by the fetus.[5,6]

The newborn infant is almost entirely dependent on external sources of carnitine. Breast-fed infants have the best chance of achieving optimal carnitine concentrations. The bioavailability of carnitine from breast milk is significantly greater than that of infant formulas, which are milk-based formulas.[7] Unless fortified, soy-based infant formulas contain no detectable carnitine.

Carnitine administration to preterm infants has two important goals—weight gain and growth.[8] In preterm infants, serum values of carnitine decrease dramatically because of limited storage capacity and a decreased ability to synthesize carnitine. Administration of L-carnitine to preterm infants can produce tremendous benefit but is rarely done.

Deficiency Signs and Symptoms

The first carnitine-deficient human subjects were described in 1973.[9] It had always been assumed that an individual could synthesize adequate amounts of carnitine, ingest adequate amounts of dietary carnitine, or meet needs by a combination of both. The discovery that some individuals require supplemental carnitine to maintain normal energy metabolism means we need to consider carnitine as an essential vitamin.[10]

Carnitine-deficiency states are classified into two major groups: systemic (whole-body) carnitine deficiency and myopathic (muscle) deficiency. Diagnosis of systemic carnitine deficiency can be made using serum or 24-hour urine samples. Total, free, and esterified carnitine levels should be determined. Diagnosis of myopathic carnitine deficiency requires skeletal muscle biopsy.[11]

Here are some of the known causes of carnitine deficiency:

- Dietary deficiency of the precursor amino acids lysine and methionine
- Deficiency of any cofactor (such as iron, ascorbic acid, pyridoxine, and niacin) required by the enzymes of the lysine-to-carnitine pathway
- Genetic defect of carnitine biosynthesis
- Defective intestinal absorption of carnitine
- Liver or kidney dysfunction that impairs carnitine synthesis
- Increased metabolic losses of carnitine because of catabolism, impaired tubular resorption, or genetic defect
- Defective transport of carnitine from tissues of synthesis to tissues where it is maximally utilized
- Increased carnitine requirement because of a high-fat diet, drugs (e.g., valproic acid), metabolic stress, or disease

To date, no patients with primary systemic carnitine deficiency have been identified. The systemic deficiency is usually secondary to a factor other than a carnitine synthesis defect. The consequences of systemic carnitine deficiency are impaired lipid metabolism and lipid accumulation in the skeletal muscles, heart muscle, and liver. All patients exhibit progressive muscle weakness with a buildup of fats in the muscle cells.[11] In adults, compensation mechanisms are apparently stimulated, resulting in some degree of adaptation. This adaptation occurs in starvation, diabetes, high-fat diets, and other causes of secondary carnitine deficiency. Systemic carnitine deficiencies usually respond dramatically to orally administered supplemental L-carnitine.

Children are apparently unable to adapt to low carnitine levels as well as adults do. Several cases of carnitine deficiency in children have been reported where the children present a clinical picture resembling Reye's syndrome—acute brain swelling associated with altered liver function because of the accumulation of fats.[12–14] The clinical presentation of secondary carnitine deficiency in children includes loss of muscle tone, failure to thrive, recurrent infection, swelling of the brain, hypoglycemia, and heart disturbances. Several fatal cases of systemic carnitine deficiency have been reported.[15]

In primary myopathic carnitine deficiency, there is an inborn error of carnitine metabolism that is limited to skeletal muscle. The defect is apparently in the transport of carnitine into the skeletal muscle as serum carnitine; the carnitine levels in other tissues are normal. Severe fat accumulation within the muscle cells results.[8]

Supplemental carnitine is generally of no value in myopathic carnitine deficiency. Rather, diets high in medium-chain triglycerides and low in long-chain triglycerides bring improvement.[11]

Beneficial Effects

Carnitine supplementation may improve the utilization of fat as an energy source. Therefore, carnitine can be beneficial in the treatment of a wide variety of conditions associated with impaired fat utilization and energy production.

Available Forms

Carnitine is available in several different forms. Always use the form L-carnitine alone or bound to either acetic or propionic acid. Never use the D form of carnitine (discussed in this chapter under Safety Issues). As to which form is best, it really depends upon the objective. For Alzheimer's disease and brain effects, it appears that L-acetylcarnitine (LAC) is the best. For angina, L-propionylcarnitine (LPC) may be the best choice because the myocardium apparently prefers it to L-acetylcarnitine; L-carnitine (LC) is the second choice.[16,17] L-carnitine is, however, the most widely available, least expensive, and best studied form of carnitine.

Principal Uses

Many disease states may benefit from carnitine administration. Most clinical research, however, has revolved around its use in various cardiovascular diseases, enhancing physical performance, Alzheimer's disease and age-related senility, kidney disease, and hemodialysis.

Some conditions that may benefit from carnitine supplementation are:

- Cardiovascular diseases
- Angina pectoris
- Acute myocardial infarction
- Myocardial necrosis
- Arrhythmias and cardiotoxicity induced by drugs
- Familial endocardial fibroelastosis
- Cardiac myopathy
- Idiopathic mitral valve prolapse
- Elevated cholesterol levels
- Elevated triglyceride levels
- Poor physical performance

- Alzheimer's disease, senile depression, and age-related memory defects
- Kidney disease and hemodialysis
- Diabetes
- Liver diseases
- Alcohol-induced fatty liver disease
- Liver cirrhosis
- Muscular dystrophies
- Low sperm counts and decreased sperm motility
- Chronic obstructive pulmonary disease (COPD)
- AIDS
- Inborn errors of amino acid metabolism
- Organic acidurias
- Glutaric aciduria
- Isovaleric acidemia
- Propionic acidemia
- Methylmalonic aciduria

Cardiovascular Disease

Normal heart function depends on adequate concentrations of carnitine. A deficiency of carnitine in the heart would be similar to driving an automobile without a fuel pump. There may be plenty of fuel, but there is no way to get it to the engine. While the normal heart stores more carnitine than it needs, if the heart does not have a good supply of oxygen, carnitine levels quickly decrease. This lack of oxygen leads to decreased energy production in the heart and increased risk for angina and heart disease.

Carnitine is useful in angina because of its ability to improve oxygen utilization and energy metabolism by the myocardium. As a result of improving fatty acid utilization and energy production, carnitine also prevents the production of toxic fatty acid metabolites.[18] These compounds are extremely damaging because they disrupt cellular membranes. Changes in cell membrane properties throughout the heart probably contribute to impaired contraction of the heart muscle and increased susceptibility to irregular beats—and eventual heart tissue death. Supplementing the diet with carnitine increases heart carnitine levels and prevents the production of these fatty acid metabolites. All these properties make carnitine beneficial not only in angina but also in recovery from a heart attack, arrhythmias, and congestive heart failure.[19]

Carnitine benefits blood lipids by lowering triglycerides and total cholesterol levels while raising HDL cholesterol. After 4 months of therapy with L-carnitine, patients with elevated blood lipids typically experience a 20 percent reduction in total cholesterol, a 28 percent decrease in triglycerides, and a 12 percent increase in HDL levels.[20,21] Because carnitine is more expensive than other natural agents (inositol hexaniacinate, garlic, and gugulipid) its use should be reserved for cases unresponsive to these more cost-effective measures.

Carnitine aids in the treatment of intermittent claudication, a condition much like angina but where the pain usually occurs in the calf muscle. Like angina, the pain is a cramp or tightness. The pain is caused by reduced oxygen delivery along with an increased production of toxic metabolites and cellular free radicals. Carnitine's benefits in peripheral vascular disease stem from improved energy production during ischemia rather than any effect on blood flow. Nonetheless, it has produced good results in intermittent claudication and other peripheral vascular diseases.

Angina

Numerous clinical trials using all three commercial forms of carnitine demonstrate that it improves angina and heart disease.[19,22-28] Carnitine supplementation normalizes heart carnitine levels and allows the heart muscle to use its limited oxygen supply more efficiently. This translates to improvements in angina such as exercise tolerance and heart function. The results indicate that for angina, carnitine is an effective alternative to drugs.

L-propionylcarnitine (LPC) may offer the greatest benefit in angina and other cardiovascular diseases. Myocardial cells absorb LPC more rapidly than other forms of carnitine.[16] In one study, LPC (15 milligrams per kilogram of body weight intravenously) significantly diminished myocardial ischemia. Patients experienced a significant 12 percent and 50 percent reduction in ST-segment depression and left ventricular end-diastolic pressure, respectively, during the atrial pacing test.[29] Left ventricular ejection fraction increased by 18 percent. Recovery of heart function after exercise occurred much quicker in the LPC group compared to the placebo group.

L-carnitine and LAC also exhibit very good results. In one of the larger studies, 200 patients with exercise-induced stable angina received either standard therapy alone (nitroglycerin, calcium channel blockers, beta-blockers, antihypertensives, diuretics, digitalis, antiarrhythmics, anticoagulants, and hypolipidemics) or in combination with 2,000 milligrams a day of L-carnitine over a 6-month period.[30] Compared with the control group, the patients on L-carnitine exhibited a significant reduction in premature ventricular contractions at rest and an increased tolerance to exercise. They experienced an increased maximal cardiac frequency, maximal systolic blood pressure, and cardiac output and reduced ST-segment depression (70 percent reduction in the L-carnitine group versus no change in the control group). Reductions in LDL-cholesterol (8 percent) and triglycerides (12 percent) were also noted. These results are highly significant and provide a strong rationale for the inclusion of carnitine in patients using standard medical therapy.

Recovery from Myocardial Infarction

In addition to benefiting angina patients, carnitine is useful in helping individuals recover more quickly from a heart attack.[19] In one double-blind study of 160 patients released from a hospital after a heart attack, the group receiving 4 grams of L-carnitine daily showed significant improvements in heart rate, blood pressure, angina attacks, rhythm disturbances, and clinical signs of impaired heart function compared to the control group.[31]

In Italy, a larger study involving 472 patients showed additional benefits.[32] The study was performed to evaluate the effects of L-carnitine administration on long-term, left ventricular dilation in patients with acute anterior myocardial infarction. Patients received a placebo or L-carnitine intravenously at a daily dose of 9 grams for the first 5 days and then orally 6 grams daily for the next 12 months. Left ventricular volumes and ejection fraction were evaluated on admission, at discharge from the hospital, and at 3, 6, and 12 months after acute myocardial infarction. A significant attenuation of left ventricular dilation in the first year after acute myocardial infarction was observed in patients treated with L-carnitine compared with those receiving a placebo. The percent increase in both end-diastolic and end-systolic volumes from admission to 3-, 6-, and 12-month evaluation was significantly reduced in the L-carnitine group.

Arrhythmias

In double-blind trials, angina patients who received carnitine experienced reductions in their use of conventional antiarrhythmic drugs.[19]

Congestive Heart Failure

Several double-blind clinical studies indicate carnitine (again, LPC is apparently more effective than LC or LAC) improves cardiac function in patients with congestive heart failure.[19] In one double-blind study of LPC versus placebo in a group of 60 patients with mild to moderate (II and III NYHA class) congestive heart failure, LPC produced demonstrable benefit.[33] The group was made up of men and women aged between 48 and 73 years in chronic treatment with digitalis and diuretics for at least 3 months and still displaying symptoms. Thirty of these patients were chosen randomly and for 180 days received 500 milligrams of LPC three times daily in addition to their usual treatment. At basal conditions and after 30, 90, and 180 days researchers evaluated maximum exercise time using an exercise tolerance test performed on an ergometer bicycle; they tested left ventricular ejection fraction with echocardiography. After 1 month of treatment, the patients treated with LPC showed significant increases in the values of both tests, increases that became even more evident after 90 and 180 days. At the stated times, the increases in the maximum exercise time were 16.4 percent, 22.9 percent, and 25.9 percent, respectively. The ventricular ejection fraction increased by 8.4 percent, 11.6 percent, and 13.6 percent, respectively.

In another double-blind study in similar patients, after 6 months of treatment, maximum exercise time on the treadmill increased 16.4 percent and the ejection fraction increased by 12.1 percent in the group treated with 1 gram of PLC twice daily.[34]

Peripheral Vascular Disease

All three forms of carnitine (2 to 4 grams daily) improve walking distance without pain in patients with intermittent claudication. Presumably this improvement results from improved energy metabolism within the muscle because carnitine did not improve blood flow to the calf. LPC appears to be more beneficial than either L-carnitine or LAC.[35,36] However, in one double-blind study L-carnitine at a dosage of 2 grams twice daily demonstrated a 75 percent increase in walking distance after only 3 weeks of therapy.[37]

Enhancing Physical Performance

The ability to enhance exercise tolerance and physical performance with carnitine may not be limited to patients with cardiovascular disease; carnitine supplementation benefits healthy subjects and athletes as well. Like the myocardium, skeletal muscle depends on an adequate supply of carnitine for efficient utilization of fatty acids

Carnitine supplementation (usually 2 grams two to three times daily) resulted in significant improvements in cardiovascular function after exercise in several double-blind studies in both athletes and normal subjects.[38–40] Compared to control groups, subjects on carnitine have shown improvements not only in exercise intensity or time but also in improved energy metabolism within the muscle (lowered blood lactic acid and free fatty acid levels). Obviously, the improved production of energy by the exercising muscle and the improved heart function could be responsible for carnitine's ability to enhance physical performance.

Although at least three studies showed the benefits of carnitine on exercise performance to be of no more value than a placebo, carnitine supplementation should still be viewed as beneficial, especially in endurance-related events.[41–43] Studies have also demonstrated carnitine improves energy-producing enzyme levels in long-distance runners.[44] These athletes received either a placebo or 2 grams of L-carnitine twice daily for 4 weeks. Runners receiving the L-carnitine showed a significant increase in enzymes involved in energy production (cytochrome c reductase and cytochrome oxidase). In contrast, there were no changes in the placebo group.

Also of note, normal subjects taking carnitine have improved cardiovascular function and a more rapid return of heart rate to the resting rate after exercise.[45] Apparently carnitine can mimic the benefits in heart and vascular function produced by regular exercise training without working up a sweat.

Alzheimer's Disease, Senile Depression, and Age-Related Memory Defect

A great deal of research has been conducted over the last decade with L-acetylcarnitine (LAC) in the treatment of Alzheimer's disease, senile depression, and age-related memory defects. LAC is a molecule composed of acetic acid and L-carnitine bound together. This reaction occurs naturally in the human brain; therefore, no one knows whether LAC, L-carnitine, or LPC has the greatest effect. However, LAC may be substantially more active than these other forms of carnitine in conditions involving the brain.[46,47]

LAC is structurally related to acetylcholine, a major neurotransmitter responsible for memory and proper brain function. In Alzheimer's disease—and to a lesser extent in the normal aging human brain—there is a defect in acetylcholine utilization. The close structural similarity between LAC and acetylcholine led researchers to begin testing LAC in Alzheimer's disease. The results have been incredibly encouraging.

Researchers have now shown that LAC does indeed mimic acetylcholine and benefits not only patients with early-stage Alzheimer's disease, but also elderly patients who are depressed or who have impaired memory.[47] It acts as a powerful antioxidant within the brain cell, stabilizes cell membranes, improves energy production within the brain cell, and enhances or mimics the function of acetylcholine.[48]

The results in using it to delay the progression of Alzheimer's disease are outstanding. The studies have been well controlled and extremely thorough.[46,49–51] For example, in one study Alzheimer's patients received LAC (2 grams twice daily) or a placebo over the course of 1 year.[51] The patients were evaluated by 14 different outcome measures such as assessment scales, cognitive function tests, memory tests, and physician evaluations. The group receiving the LAC scored better on all outcome scores.

The memory impairment need not be as severe as in Alzheimer's disease in order for LAC to be of benefit.[52–54] In one double-blind study of 236 elderly subjects with mild mental deterioration evidenced by detailed clinical assessment, the group receiving 1,500 milligrams of (LAC) daily demonstrated significant improvement in mental function, particularly in memory and constructional thinking.[54]

Many elderly suffer from depression not only as a result of a great deal of loss in their lives, but also because of the biochemical changes in the brain associated with aging. (LAC) has improved depression in elderly subjects in double-blind studies using assessment scales standard for scientific research of antidepressant drugs (Hamilton Depression Scale, Clinical Global Impression, Sandoz Clinical Assessment, etcetera). The usual dosage was 500 milligrams three times daily. Those elderly subjects with the highest depression scores are usually the ones who benefited the most from acetyl-L-carnitine.[55,56]

Down's Syndrome

Because both Down's syndrome and Alzheimer's disease are characterized by a deficit in cholinergic transmission, researchers conducted a study to assess the effect of a 90-day treatment with L-acetylcarnitine (LAC) in individuals with Down's syndrome.[57] Findings were evaluated statistically and compared to three further groups of subjects: untreated Down's syndrome, mental deficiency because of other causes either treated or not treated with LAC. Treated Down's syndrome patients showed statistically significant improvements of visual memory and attention both in absolute terms and in comparison with the other groups. No improvement was found in mentally deficient non-Down's subjects, so the favorable effect of LAC is apparently specific for Down's patients. An effective dosage is 20 milligrams of LAC for every 2 pounds of body weight. The action of LAC in these pathologies is probably related to its direct and indirect cholinomimetic effect.

Kidney Disease and Hemodialysis

The kidney is a major site of carnitine synthesis; therefore, carnitine supplementation is indicated in kidney diseases. Damage to the kidney or reduced kidney function has a profound effect on carnitine metabolism. Patients undergoing hemodialysis suffer from carnitine deficiency because they lose considerable quantities of carnitine during dialysis and carnitine synthesis decreases. Serum carnitine levels drop nearly 80 percent during hemodialysis.[1–3]

Researchers have studied carnitine supplementation in patients undergoing hemodialysis because of their chronic renal failure. These studies indicate that L-carnitine supplementation is effective in reducing triglyceride levels while raising HDL-cholesterol levels and thus helps to decrease the risk of heart disease in dialysis patients.[58–61] Carnitine-treated dialyzed patients show additional benefits, including disappearance of angina pectoris and arrhythmias occurring during dialysis, reduction of muscle symptoms including muscle cramps, increased muscle mass, and significant improvement of the chronic anemia seen in these patients (demonstrated by an increased hematocrit, hemoglobin, and red blood cell count).[62–64]

Over the last decade, recombinant human erythropoietic (EPO) therapy has been a major advancement in the treatment of anemia associated with hemodialysis. However, this therapy is expensive and not without side effects. In a recent study published in the *American Journal of Kidney Diseases*, L-carnitine (1 gram intravenously after every dialysis session) administered for 6 months led to a significant reduction in dosage of EPO and improvements in membrane fragility and the body's natural EPO secretion.[65] Given the high cost of EPO, if doctors are unwilling to follow this procedure, perhaps insurance companies can get involved and enable dialysis units to employ L-carnitine.

Diabetes

Patients with diabetes have reduced serum carnitine concentrations but normal skeletal muscle carnitine levels.[66] Because of the increased risk of atherosclerotic cardiovascular disease and reduced kidney and liver function in diabetic patients, supplementation with L-carnitine appears warranted. Carnitine (especially LPC) also greatly improves peripheral vascular function and nerve function in patients with diabetes.[67]

Liver Disease

Carnitine plays an extremely important role in the utilization and metabolization of fatty acids in the liver. There is some evidence that carnitine deficiency within the liver promotes fatty infiltration (also known as steatosis or liver congestion).[68]

Alcohol ingestion is a common cause of fatty infiltration of the liver. Some researchers suggest that chronic alcohol consumption results in a functional deficiency of carnitine, which means there is plenty of carnitine around but its function is inhibited as if there were a deficiency. Many commonly used agents for fatty infiltration, such as choline, niacin, and cysteine, appear to have little value in relieving alcohol-induced fatty liver. However, carnitine significantly inhibits and reverses alcohol-induced fatty liver disease.[69]

Since carnitine normally facilitates fatty acid transport and oxidation in the mitochondria, a high liver-carnitine level may be necessary to handle the increased fatty acid load produced by alcohol consumption or other liver injury.[70] Supplemental carnitine can reduce free fatty acid levels in patients with liver cirrhosis and reduce serum triglycerides and liver enzyme levels while elevating HDL cholesterol in alcohol-induced fatty liver disease.[68–70]

Carnitine's use in liver disorders associated with fatty infiltration appears warranted, especially when these changes happen because of the ingestion of alcohol or exposure to xenobiotics (man-made chemicals such as pesticides and herbicides that are toxic to biological processes).

Muscular Dystrophies

Patients with various muscular dystrophies have reduced levels of carnitine in their skeletal muscles.[71–73] Although these levels are not as low as observed in patients with classical myopathic carnitine deficiency, the low carnitine levels probably contribute to the muscular weakness experienced by these patients. Unfortunately, for some reason no one has determined if supplemental carnitine would be of any value in patients with muscular dystrophy.

Low Sperm Counts and Decreased Sperm Motility

In the human sperm, high carnitine concentrations are critical to sperm energy metabolism. Several studies have shown that the level of free carnitine in the seminal fluid is inversely correlated with sperm count and motility.[74,75] The lower the carnitine content, the lower the sperm count and the more likely a man is to be infertile. Therefore, a recent study assessed the therapeutic effect of carnitine in men with low sperm counts and depressed sperm motility.[76] One hundred men selected from infertility clinics participated in this "Italian Study Group on Carnitine and Male Infertility." Each subject was given 3,000 milligrams of L-carnitine daily for 4 months.

The results of the study indicated that L-carnitine increased sperm counts and sperm motility, both in a qualitative and quantitative manner. The number of ejaculated sperm increased from 142 billion to 163 billion, the percentage of motile sperm increased from 26.9 percent to 37.7 percent, the percentage of sperm with rapid linear progression increased from 10.8 percent to 18 percent, and the mean sperm velocity increased from 28.4 percent to 32.5 percent. The results are even more impressive in patients with the poorest sperm motility. This subgroup saw even more significant gains on all parameters. For example, the percentage of motile sperm increased from 19.3 percent to 40.9 percent, and the percentage of sperm with rapid linear progression increased from 3.1 percent to 20.3 percent.

Chronic Obstructive Pulmonary Disease

Patients with chronic respiratory insufficiency are often severely affected by even the simplest physical activity. Treatment with L-carnitine (2 grams, three times a day) resulted in significant improvements in exercise capability.[77]

AIDS

Several reports indicate that systemic carnitine deficiency may be a problem in patients with AIDS. Reduced levels of serum carnitine are most often found in AIDS patients. However, more important is the carnitine depletion in peripheral blood mononuclear cells (PBMC). In fact, even AIDS patients with normal serum carnitine levels demonstrate low levels of carnitine in white blood cells.[78] Increasing the carnitine content of the PWBC strongly improved lymphocyte function and thus highlights the importance of carnitine to immune function.

L-Carnitine can prevent the toxicity of the drug AZT on the mitochondria of the muscle cells.[79] AZT poisons the muscles' mitochondria, leading to abnormal energy production within the muscle. This then manifests clinically as muscle fatigue and pain. If L-carnitine can prevent this negative effect of AZT in human AIDS patients, it would be a major improvement in the clinical management of AIDS.

Preliminary studies indicate that L-carnitine supplementation can improve immune function and reduce the level of HIV-induced immune suppression. When AIDS patients treated with AZT were given 6 grams of L-carnitine per day, it led to significantly increased PMBC proliferation and reduced blood levels of triglycerides and circulating tumor necrosis factor.[80] Given AIDS' suspected systemic carnitine deficiency and carnitine's safety, carnitine supplementation appears warranted in AIDS.

Inborn Errors of Amino Acid Metabolism

The use of carnitine in the treatment of inborn errors of metabolism involving the urea acid cycle is apparently well justified. Preliminary studies have shown impressive therapeutic response to L-carnitine supplementation in cases of glutaric aciduria, isovaleric acidemia, propionic acidemia, and methylmalonic aciduria.[81–84]

Protection against Drug Toxicity

Carnitine can protect against the damaging effects on the heart produced by the chemotherapy drug adriamycin.[85] Carnitine can also improve the symptoms attributed to anticonvulsant medications such as valproic acid (tradenames Depa, Depakene, Depakote, and Deproic) and carbamazepine (tradenames Epitol and Tegretol).[86,87] However, the most recent study challenges the need to administer carnitine prophylactically because no significant differences were noted in well-being scores of the carnitine group and the placebo group.[88]

Dosage Ranges

The daily dosage of L-carnitine in all its forms is usually between 1,500 and 4,000 milligrams in divided doses. Patients undergoing hemodialysis should avoid higher doses because a paradoxical effect on triglyceride levels and platelet aggregation in patients on hemodialysis has been reported.[89] Slightly higher doses were used

(3 grams per day) compared to other studies of supplementation in chronic renal failure (typical dose 20 milligrams per kilogram of body weight or 2 grams per day). In addition, the study size was extremely small, and the results are in conflict with other studies using similar doses. However, it appears physicians should heed this risk by using lower doses and carefully monitoring patients with impaired renal function.

Safety Issues

L-Carnitine is extremely safe with no significant side effects reported in any human clinical studies. Again, only L-carnitine should be used. The D form, the mirror image of the L form, has produced side effects, indicating it interferes with the natural L form of carnitine. Patients undergoing hemodialysis given a mixture containing D,L-carnitine for 45 days experienced muscle pain and loss of muscle function, presumably because of lack of energy.[90] The symptoms disappeared upon cessation of D,L-carnitine supplementation. Subsequent studies showed that D-carnitine produces an L-carnitine deficiency in cardiac and skeletal muscle.[91] While L-carnitine results in significant improvement in exercise tolerance in angina patients, D,L-carnitine dangerously reduces exercise tolerance in these patients.[92]

Interactions

There are no known adverse interactions between carnitine and any drug or nutrient. Carnitine and coenzyme Q_{10} appear to work synergistically when combined.[93] The same is true for pantethine.[94]

Perhaps the most important interaction is that with choline. In young adult women, daily choline supplementation (20 milligrams per kilogram of body weight) resulted in a 75 percent lower urinary carnitine excretion than in controls without significantly altering plasma carnitine concentrations. Studies in guinea pigs demonstrated that choline supplementation resulted in a significantly lower urinary excretion and higher skeletal muscle carnitine concentrations. These studies indicate that choline supplementation results in a conservation of carnitine and may increase intracellular carnitine levels.[95]

35

Coenzyme Q₁₀

Coenzyme Q_{10} (CoQ_{10}), also known as ubiquinone, is an essential component of the mitochondria—the energy producing unit of the cells of our body. CoQ_{10} is involved in the manufacture of ATP, which is the energy currency of all body processes. A good analogy for CoQ_{10}'s role is similar to the role of a spark plug in a car engine. Just as the car cannot function without that initial spark, the human body cannot function without CoQ_{10}.

Professor F. L. Crane and his colleagues at the University of Wisconsin first discovered CoQ_{10} in 1957. Since then, the person most responsible for the ongoing research on CoQ_{10} is Dr. Karl Folkers of the University of Texas. Research now indicates that CoQ_{10} supplementation can provide significant benefit as an antioxidant and in the treatment of a number of health disorders. CoQ_{10} is quite popular in Japan, where it is currently one of the top six pharmaceutical agents used.

Food Sources

CoQ_{10} is also known as ubiquinone because it is in every plant and animal cell. However, the amount of CoQ_{10} from dietary sources is probably insufficient to produce the clinical effects noted for high-dosage CoQ_{10}. The plasma level of CoQ_{10} is considerably higher (more than double) in vegetarians than in omnivores, which indicates that a high intake of plant foods may preserve high CoQ_{10} levels.

Deficiency Signs and Symptoms

Although the body can synthesize CoQ_{10}, deficiency states can exist. Because the heart is one of the most metabolically active tissues in the body, a CoQ_{10} deficiency mostly affects the heart and leads to heart failure. Deficiency could be a result of impaired CoQ_{10} synthesis because of nutritional deficiencies, a genetic or acquired defect in CoQ_{10} synthesis, or increased tissue needs. Examples of diseases that require increased tissue levels of CoQ_{10} are primarily cardiovascular diseases such as angina, high blood pressure, mitral valve prolapse, and congestive heart failure. In addition, the elderly in general may have increased CoQ$_{10}$ requirements because CoQ$_{10}$ levels can decline with advancing age.

Beneficial Effects

The beneficial effects of CoQ$_{10}$ revolve around its ability to improve energy production and act as an antioxidant. These effects are most beneficial in the prevention and treatment of cardiovascular disease and cancer.

The antioxidant activity of CoQ$_{10}$ is limited to protection against lipid peroxidation. It exerts a sparing effect on vitamin E and works together with vitamin E in preventing damage to lipid membranes and plasma lipids. CoQ$_{10}$ supplementation, like other antioxidants, may offer significant protection against atherosclerosis by preventing lipid peroxide formation and oxidation of LDL cholesterol (see Chapter 5).[1-5]

Available Forms

Coenzyme Q$_{10}$ is primarily available in tablet or capsules. Based on bioavailability studies, the best preparations are soft-gelatin capsules that contain CoQ$_{10}$ in an oil base (soybean oil).[6]

Principal Uses

The primary clinical applications of CoQ$_{10}$ are cardiovascular diseases such as congestive heart failure, high blood pressure, cardiomyopathy, mitral valve prolapse, coronary artery bypass surgery, and angina; diabetes; periodontal disease; immune deficiency; cancer; as a weight-loss aid; muscular dystrophy; and as a "performance-enhancing" agent in athletes. Since the response of CoQ$_{10}$ can take time, a clinical response might not occur until 8 or more weeks after therapy begins.

Cardiovascular Disease

An important yet frequently overlooked component in the overall treatment of cardiovascular disease is the promotion of a better functioning heart. Degenerative lesions of the heart are found in most types of cardiovascular disease, including angina, high blood pressure, and congestive heart failure. They result from repeated insults to the heart such as low oxygen supply, inflammation, and other factors. CoQ$_{10}$ can reverse or prevent the degenerative lesions of the heart associated with these diseases and enhance the mechanical function of a failing heart. It does so by providing optimal nutrition at the cellular level.

The potential therapeutic use of CoQ$_{10}$ in cardiovascular disease has been clearly documented in both animal studies and human trials. CoQ$_{10}$ deficiency is common in cardiac patients. Biopsy results from heart tissue in patients with various cardiovascular diseases showed a CoQ_{10} deficiency in 50 to 75 percent of cases.[7-10] Correcting a CoQ_{10} deficiency can produce dramatic clinical results.

To highlight the effectiveness of CoQ_{10} for a wide variety of cardiovascular disease, let's examine the results from a clinical cardiology unit that utilized CoQ_{10} in 424 patients with various forms of cardiovascular disease over an 8-year period (1985–1993). Doses of CoQ_{10} ranged from 75 to 600 milligrams per day by mouth (average, 242 milligrams). Treatment was guided primarily by the patient's clinical response. In many instances, CoQ_{10} levels were employed with the aim of producing a whole blood level greater than or equal to 2.10 micrograms per milliliter. Patients were followed for an average of 17.8 months, with a total accumulation of 632 patient years. Eleven patients were omitted from this study, ten because of noncompliance and one who experienced nausea. Eighteen deaths occurred during the study period with 10 attributable to cardiac causes. Patients were divided into six diagnostic categories: ischemic cardiomyopathy, dilated cardiomyopathy, primary diastolic dysfunction, high blood pressure, mitral valve prolapse, and heart disease because of heart valve disorders. For the entire group and for each diagnostic category, clinical response was evaluated according to the New York Heart Association (NYHA) functional scale. Of 424 patients, 58 percent improved by one NYHA class, 28 percent by two classes, and 1.2 percent by three classes. A statistically significant improvement in heart function was documented using the following echocardiographic parameters: left ventricular wall thickness, mitral valve inflow slope, and fractional shortening. Before treatment with CoQ_{10}, most patients were taking from one to five cardiac medications. During this study, overall medication requirements dropped considerably—43 percent stopped between one and three drugs. Only 6 percent of the patients required the addition of one drug. No apparent side effects from CoQ_{10} treatment were noted other than a single case of transient nausea. The cardiologists concluded, "CoQ_{10} is a safe and effective adjunctive treatment for a broad range of cardiovascular diseases, producing gratifying clinical responses while easing the medical and financial burden of multidrug therapy."[11]

Congestive Heart Failure

Congestive heart failure (CHF) is an inability of the heart to pump blood effectively. CHF occurs most often because of long-term effects of high blood pressure, disorder of a heart valve, or a cardiomyopathy. Conventional drug therapy for CHF involves the use of digitalis, diuretics, and vasodilators (beta-blockers, calcium channel-blockers, etcetera). Treatment is tailored according to the severity of the syndrome and the patient profile. CHF is always characterized by an energy depletion status, as indicated by low ATP and coenzyme Q_{10} levels within the heart muscle. The main clinical problems in patients with CHF are the frequent need of hospitalization and the high incidence of life-threatening arrhythmias, pulmonary edema, and other serious complications.

Numerous studies show CoQ_{10} supplementation is extremely effective in the treatment of CHF. Most of these studies utilized CoQ_{10} along with conventional drug therapy. In other words, CoQ_{10} was used as an adjunct. In one of the early studies, 17 patients with mild congestive heart failure received 30 milligrams of CoQ_{10} per day. All patients improved and 9 (53 percent) became asymptomatic after 4 weeks.[12] In another early study, 20 patients with congestive heart failure due to either atherosclerosis or high blood pressure were treated with CoQ_{10} at a dosage of 30 milligrams per day for 1 to 2 months.[13] Fifty-five percent of the patients reported subjective improvement, 50 percent showed a decrease in New York Heart Association (NYHA) classification, and 30 percent showed a "remarkable" decrease in chest congestion as seen on chest X-ray. Patients with mild disease tended to improve more often than those with more severe disease. Subjective improvements in these patients were confirmed by various objective tests, including increased cardiac output, stroke volume, cardiac index, and ejection fraction. These results were consistent with CoQ_{10} producing an increased force of heart muscle contraction (a positive inotropic effect) similar to, but less potent than, digitalis.[14] In addition, CoQ_{10} prevented the negative inotropic effect of beta-blocker therapy apparently without reducing the beneficial effect of the beta-blockers on myocardial oxygen consumption.[15]

Three more recent studies also show CoQ_{10} is effective in significantly improving heart function in patients with CHF. Results from a Scandinavian study in 80 patients with CHF were presented in 1992 at the meeting of the American College of Cardiology.[16] In this double-blind study, patients were given either CoQ_{10} (100 milligrams per day) or a placebo for 3 months and then crossed over (those taking CoQ_{10} were then given the placebo and vice versa). The improvements noted with CoQ_{10} were significant because the results were more positive than those obtained from conventional drug therapy alone.

In another double-blind study, 641 patients with CHF, received either CoQ_{10} (2 milligrams per kilogram of body weight) or a placebo for 1 year.[17] The number of patients requiring hospitalization or experiencing serious consequences because of CHF was significantly reduced in the CoQ_{10} group compared to the placebo group.

In the most recent and largest study to date, a total of 2,664 patients in New York Heart Association (NYHA) classes II and III were enrolled in an open study in Italy.[18] The daily dosage of CoQ_{10} was 50 to 150 milligrams orally for 90 days, with the majority of patients (78 percent) receiving 100 milligrams per day. After 3 months of CoQ_{10} treatment, the percentages of patients with improvement in clinical signs and symptoms were as follows:

- Cyanosis (purple hue of skin), 78.1
- Edema (fluid retention), 78.6
- Pulmonary edema, 77.8
- Enlargement of liver area, 49.3
- Venous congestion, 71.81
- Shortness of breath, 52.7
- Heart palpitations, 75.4
- Sweating, 79.8
- Subjective arrhythmia, 63.4

- Insomnia, 62.8
- Vertigo, 73.1
- Nighttime urination, 53.6

Improvement of at least three symptoms occurred in 54 percent of the patients, indicating a significantly improved quality of life with CoQ_{10} supplementation. The results also showed a low incidence of side effects; only 36 patients (1.5 percent) reported mild side effects attributed to CoQ_{10}.

All together, the effectiveness and safety of CoQ_{10} in these studies suggest that it might be the treatment of choice for mild CHF and can effectively reduce hospitalization and serious consequences when used along with conventional drug therapy in moderate to severe CHF.

High Blood Pressure

CoQ_{10} deficiency is present in 39 percent of patients with high blood pressure. This finding alone suggests a need for CoQ_{10} supplementation. However, CoQ_{10} appears to provide benefits beyond correction of a deficiency. In several studies, CoQ_{10} actually lowered blood pressure in patients with hypertension.[19–21] However, the effect of CoQ_{10} on blood pressure is usually not seen until after 4 to 12 weeks of therapy. Thus, CoQ_{10} is not a typical antihypertensive drug; rather, it apparently corrects some metabolic abnormality that in turn has a favorable influence in blood pressure. Typical reductions in both systolic and diastolic blood pressure with CoQ_{10} therapy in patients with high blood pressure are in the 10 percent range.

While the mechanism of CoQ_{10} in heart condition is well understood, how CoQ_{10} lowers blood pressure is a mystery. Blood pressure is similar to water pressure as water passes through a garden hose. If the arteries (hose) are constricted, pressure increases. Several physiological factors are associated with increased resistance to blood flow, namely, elevated renin, sodium, or aldosterone levels. When ten patients with high blood pressure were given 100 milligrams of CoQ_{10} daily for 10 weeks, systolic blood pressure in the group dropped from 161.5 to 142 millimeters of mercury and diastolic pressure dropped from 98.5 to 83 millimeters of mercury, but there were no changes in renin, sodium, or aldosterone levels.[19] Cholesterol levels dropped from 227 milligrams per deciliter to 204 milligrams per deciliter, and a sophisticated test for peripheral resistance revealed significant improvements. These results indicate that CoQ_{10} lowers blood pressure by unusual mechanisms of action: lowering cholesterol levels and stabilizing the vascular membrane via its antioxidant properties. As a result of these actions, peripheral resistance to blood flow is reduced. An analogy is that CoQ_{10} acts in a manner similar to opening up the diameter of a garden hose sprayer.

Cardiomyopathy

Cardiomyopathy is any disease of heart muscle that reduces force of heart contractions, thus decreasing the efficiency of blood circulation. Cardiomyopathy may be the result of a viral, metabolic, nutritional, toxic, autoimmune, degenerative, genetic, or unknown cause. Regardless of cause, a deficiency of CoQ$_{10}$ is found in the blood and myocardial tissue of most patients with cardiomyopathy.[10] CoQ$_{10}$ supplementation can raise CoQ$_{10}$ levels and produce improvements in heart function as a result of improved energy production by heart muscle.

Several double-blind studies in patients with various cardiomyopathies show significant benefit with CoQ$_{10}$ supplementation. In one double-blind trial, daily administration of 100 milligrams of CoQ$_{10}$ for 12 weeks increased cardiac ejection fraction significantly, reduced shortness of breath, and increased muscle strength.[22] These improvements lasted as long as the patients were continuously treated (3 years in this study). However, cardiac function deteriorated when CoQ$_{10}$ was discontinued, indicating that individuals with cardiomyopathy need to be on CoQ$_{10}$ indefinitely. Of the 80 patients treated, 89 percent improved while on CoQ$_{10}$.

In an open trial, 100 milligrams of CoQ$_{10}$ was given daily to 34 patients with severe (NYHA Class IV) congestive cardiomyopathy.[14] Eighty-two percent of the patients improved, as evidenced by increased stroke volume and cardiac index. Mean ejection fraction increased from about 25 percent to about 40 percent, and 2-year survival rate was 62 percent compared with less than 25 percent for a similar series of patients treated by conventional methods alone.

These studies and others indicate that CoQ$_{10}$ supplementation is a critical therapeutic measure in cardiomyopathy that can result in improved quality and increased life span.

Mitral Valve Prolapse

Mitral valve prolapse is a common, slight deformity of the mitral valve, which is the heart valve that separates the left atrium (upper chamber) from the left ventricle (lower chamber). Mitral valve prolapse is also referred to as "floppy valve syndrome" and is associated with a heart murmur. Usually there are no symptoms of mitral valve prolapse; occasionally, however, it may produce chest pain, arrhythmia, or leakage of the valve sufficient to lead to congestive heart failure.

CoQ$_{10}$ is quite helpful in cases of symptomatic mitral valve prolapse. In one study, 8 children received CoQ$_{10}$ (2 milligrams per kilogram of body weight) each day for 8 weeks, and 8 received a placebo. Heart function became normal in 7 of the CoQ$_{10}$-treated patients and none of the placebo-treated patients. Relapse frequently occurred in patients who stopped the medication within 12 to 17 months but rarely occurred in those who took CoQ$_{10}$ for 18 months or more.[23]

Coronary Artery Bypass Surgery

Return of blood flow (reperfusion) after coronary artery bypass surgery results in oxidative damage to the vascular endothelium and myocardium, and thus greatly increases the risk for subsequent coronary artery disease. A recent study was designed to evaluate the effectiveness of coenzyme Q$_{10}$ in preventing oxygen-induced reperfusion injury in patents undergoing coronary artery surgery.[24] Forty patients undergoing elective surgery received either 150 milligrams of coenzyme Q_{10} each day for 7 days before the surgery or served in the control group. Concentrations of malondialdehyde, lipid peroxides, and cardiac isoenzymes were measured 5 minutes after heparin administration, at 10 and 30 minutes after aortic cross-clamp removal, and 5 minutes after protamine administration. The concentrations of malondialdehyde, lipid peroxides, and creatine kinase in patients receiving coenzyme Q_{10} were significantly lower than the control group. The treatment group also showed a statistically significant lower incidence of ventricular arrhythmias during the recovery period. These results indicate that by reducing oxidative damage, pretreatment with coenzyme Q_{10} can play a protective role during routine bypass surgery.

Angina

Angina describes a squeezing or pressurelike pain in the chest. It is caused by an insufficient supply of oxygen to heart muscle. Since physical exertion and stress cause an increased need for oxygen by the heart, symptoms of angina are often preceded by these factors. The pain may radiate to the left shoulder blade, left arm, or jaw. The pain typically lasts for only 1 to 20 minutes.

Angina is almost always caused by atherosclerosis, which is the buildup of cholesterol-containing plaque that progressively narrow and ultimately block the blood vessels supplying the heart, the coronary arteries. This blockage results in a decreased blood and oxygen supply to the heart tissue. When the flow of oxygen to the heart muscle is substantially reduced, or when there is an increased need by the heart, angina results.

CoQ_{10} is effective in several small studies in angina patients. In one of the first studies, 12 patients with stable angina pectoris were treated with CoQ_{10} (150 milligrams per day for 4 weeks) in a double-blind, crossover format.[25] Compared to a placebo, CoQ_{10} reduced the frequency of anginal episodes by 53 percent and the need for nitroglycerin There was also a significant increase in treadmill exercise tolerance (time to onset of chest pain and time to development of EKG disturbances; i.e., ST-segment depression) during CoQ_{10} treatment. The results of this study and others suggest that CoQ_{10} may offer a safe and effective treatment for angina pectoris. However, these results need to be confirmed in larger studies.

Diabetes Mellitus

CoQ_{10} apparently is beneficial in patients with diabetes. In a study of 120 diabetic patients, 8.3 percent were found deficient in CoQ_{10}, compared with 1.9 percent of a group of healthy controls. The incidence of CoQ_{10} deficiency was higher (around 20 percent) in patients receiving oral hypoglycemic drugs, probably because these drugs interfere with CoQ_{10} metabolism.[26]

CoQ_7, a molecule similar to CoQ_{10}, was given to 39 stable diabetics at a dosage of 120 milligrams per day for periods ranging from 2 to 18 weeks.[27] This treatment reduced fasting blood sugar by at least 20 percent in 14 of 39 patients (36 percent) and by at least 30 percent in 12 of 39 patients (31 percent). Ketone bodies fell by at least 30 percent in 13 of 22 patients (59 percent). In some cases, termination of CoQ_7 treatment resulted in increased blood sugar or blood ketone bodies. One patient who was poorly controlled on 60 units of insulin showed a marked fall in fasting blood sugar and ketone bodies after CoQ_7 was added. This study with CoQ_7 was done in 1966 before CoQ_{10} was commercially available. Since CoQ_7 and CoQ_{10} are interchangeable in the body, similar results might be expected from CoQ_{10}.

The mechanism by which CoQ_{10} improves diabetic control is not known. Something more than simple correction of a deficiency is probably involved because the incidence of positive responses is far greater (36 to 59 percent) than the incidence of CoQ_{10} deficiency (8.3 percent). Perhaps CoQ_{10} administration induces synthesis of increased amounts of CoQ_{10}-dependent enzymes, which in turn enhance carbohydrate metabolism.[26]

Periodontal Disease

Periodontal disease affects 60 percent of young adults and 90 percent of individuals over age 65. Although proper oral hygiene is helpful, many suffer from intractable gingivitis, which often requires surgery and results in eventual loss of teeth. Healing and repair of periodontal tissue requires efficient energy production, a metabolic function dependent on an adequate supply of CoQ_{10}.

CoQ_{10} deficiency has been reported in gingival tissue of patients with periodontal disease.[28-31] The frequency of CoQ_{10} deficiency in several studies ranged from 60 to 96 percent. Periodontitis may itself lead to localized CoQ_{10} deficiency. However, 86 percent of the patients also had a low level of CoQ_{10} in leukocytes, indicating the presence of systemic imbalance.[29] Oral treatment with CoQ_{10} reversed the deficiency in gingival tissue.

Eighteen patients with periodontal disease received either 50 milligrams per day of CoQ_{10} or a placebo in a 3-week, double-blind study.[32] Results of therapy were evaluated according to a "periodontal score," which included gingival pocket depth, swelling, bleeding, redness, pain, exudate, and looseness of teeth. All 8 patients receiving CoQ_{10}, but only 3 of 10 receiving the placebo, improved. A group of 8 dentists who were unaware a study was being conducted consistently remarked upon the "very impressive" acceleration of healing. One prosthodontist commented that the degree of healing seen in 3 weeks usually took about 6 months.

In an open trial, CoQ_{10} administration produced "extraordinary" postsurgical healing (two to three times faster than usual) in seven patients with advanced periodontal disease.[33] The beneficial effect of CoQ_{10} has been confirmed in dogs, whose experimentally induced periodontal disease was significantly reduced by CoQ_{10} supplementation.[34]

The effect of CoQ_{10} in periodontal disease may be mediated by an improvement in the energy-dependent processes of healing and tissue repair. CoQ_{10} also helps correct abnormal citrate metabolism, which is present in many patients with periodontitis and which appears to contribute to the development of the disease.[35]

Topical application of CoQ_{10} may also be of benefit. A recent study evaluated the effect of topical CoQ_{10} applied to the periodontal pocket and concluded that "CoQ_{10} improves adult periodontitis not only as a sole treatment but also in combination with traditional nonsurgical periodontal therapy."[36]

Immune Deficiency

Many chronic illnesses are associated with abnormalities of the immune system. Numerous studies document impairments of immunity in cancer, heart disease, hypertension, allergies, thyroiditis, pernicious anemia, and recurrent infections. Attempts to improve immune function are a key component of the treatment of cancer and certain chronic infections, including candidiasis and acquired immune deficiency syndrome (AIDS).

Tissues and cells involved with immune function are highly energy-dependent and therefore require an adequate supply of CoQ_{10} for optimal function. Several studies document an immune-enhancing effect of CoQ.[37–45]

Immune function tends to decline with advancing age. In one study, elderly mice had thymic atrophy, marked CoQ deficiency in thymic tissue, and pronounced suppression of the immune response. This immune suppression was partially reversed by treatment with CoQ_{10}.[43,44] Thus, CoQ_{10} supplementation may help prevent or reverse age-related immunosuppression.

In human studies, 8 patients with cardiovascular disease, diabetes, or cancer were treated for long periods of time with coenzyme Q_{10} (60 milligrams per day). The level of immunoglobulin G (IgG) in the serum of these patients significantly increased after 27 to 98 days of CoQ_{10} treatment.[45] According to the authors of the report, this increase in serum IgG within the normal range could represent a correction of immunodeficiency or an increase in immune function.

Cancer

CoQ_{10} supplementation is used in cancer because of its immune-enhancing and antioxidant effects. Also, CoQ_{10} should definitely be used by cancer patients taking any chemotherapy drug that is associated with heart toxicity (adriamycin, athralines, etcetera).

In one of the few studies of CoQ_{10} in cancer therapy, 32 women with breast cancer, aged 32 to 81 years and classified "high risk" because of tumor spread to the lymph nodes in the axilla (armpit), were studied for 18 months following an Adjuvant Nutritional Intervention in Cancer protocol (ANICA protocol) that included CoQ_{10}.[46] The nutritional protocol was added to the surgical and therapeutic treatment of breast cancer as required by Danish regulations. The added daily treatment was a combination of:

- Nutritional antioxidants: vitamin C, 2,850 milligrams; vitamin E, 2,500 International Units; beta-carotene, 32.5 International Units; selenium, 387 micrograms; plus secondary vitamins and minerals

- Essential fatty acids: gamma linolenic acid,1.2 grams; n-3 fatty acids, 3.5 grams
- Coenzyme Q_{10}: 90 milligrams

The ANICA protocol is based on the concept of testing the synergistic effect of nutritional supplements, including vitamin Q_{10}, that previously exhibited deficiency and/or therapeutic value as single elements in diverse forms of cancer because cancer may be synergistically related to diverse biochemical dysfunctions and vitamin deficiencies. Biochemical markers, clinical condition, tumor spread, quality of life parameters, and survival were followed during the trial. The main observations were:

- None of the patients died during the study period (the expected number was four).
- None of the patients showed signs of further distant metastases.
- Quality of life improved (no weight loss, reduced use of pain killers).
- Six patients showed apparent partial remission.

In one of the six cases showing partial remission, the dosage of CoQ_{10} was increased to 390 milligrams. In 1 month, the tumor was no longer palpable, and in another month mammography confirmed the absence of tumor. Encouraged, the researchers then treated another case—a patient who had had a verified breast tumor, after nonradical surgery and with verified residual tumor in the tumor bed—with 300 milligrams of CoQ_{10}. After 3 months, the patient was in excellent clinical condition and there was no residual tumor tissue. Although these results could not be based solely upon the CoQ_{10} supplement, nonetheless CoQ_{10} should be included in the treatment of breast cancer while more research is forthcoming.

Most of the studies in cancer patients given CoQ_{10} have focused on CoQ_{10}'s ability to prevent damage to the heart caused by a chemotherapy drug. Many potent chemotherapy drugs like adriamycin are often of limited value because of the development of serious toxicity to heart muscle after long-term treatment and because of CoQ_{10} deficiency. CoQ_{10} supplementation can reverse the deficiency state and may help prevent toxicity to the heart muscle as well.

In animals, administration of CoQ_{10} reduced the cardiotoxicity of adriamycin and increased the survival rate in acute adriamycin toxicity.[47] In a human clinical trial, CoQ_{10} (100 milligrams per day) was given by mouth to seven patients beginning 3 to 5 days before adriamycin treatment.[48] An additional seven patients received adriamycin without CoQ_{10}. Administration of CoQ_{10} prevented the decrease in heart function (stroke index, cardiac index, and ejection fraction) that occurred in patients given adriamycin alone, even though the CoQ_{10} group received a cumulative adriamycin dosage that was about 50 percent greater. Similar results were noted in children with acute lymphoblastic leukemia or non-Hodgkin lymphoma treated with adriamycin who were given CoQ_{10} compared to those given a placebo.[49]

Weight Loss

The tendency to become overweight may be associated in some cases with a metabolic makeup that results in decreased thermogenesis (heat production). Human

305

subjects with a family history of obesity have a 50 percent reduction in their thermogenic response to meals, suggesting the existence of an hereditary defect in energy production. Since CoQ_{10} is an essential cofactor for energy production, it is possible that CoQ_{10} deficiency is a contributing cause of some cases of obesity.

In one study, serum coenzyme Q_{10} levels were found to be low in 52 percent (14 of 27) of the obese subjects tested.[50] Nine subjects (five with low CoQ_{10} levels) were given 100 milligrams per day of CoQ_{10} along with a 650-kilocalorie diet. After 8 to 9 weeks, mean weight loss in the CoQ_{10}-deficient group was 13.5 kilograms, compared with 5.8 kilograms in those with initially normal levels of CoQ_{10}. This study suggests that about 50 percent of obese individuals may be deficient in CoQ_{10} and that treatment with this coenzyme may accelerate weight loss resulting from a low-calorie diet.

The effect of CoQ_{10} is most likely because of improvement in cellular respiration and a consequent increase in caloric output. It is possible, however, that CoQ_{10} treatment had nothing to do with the increased weight loss. Those with low serum CoQ levels may merely respond differently to a low-calorie diet. A controlled trial of CoQ_{10} supplementation would be useful in determining how beneficial it might be in promoting weight loss.

Muscular Dystrophy

Deficiency of CoQ_{10} has been found in muscle mitochondria of humans with muscular dystrophy.[51] This deficiency may be involved in the development of heart disease that is associated with virtually every form of muscular dystrophy and myopathy.

Two double-blind studies have been performed in patients with progressive muscular dystrophy (Duchenne, Becker, and the limb-girdle dystrophies, myotonic dystrophy, Charcot-Marie-Tooth disease, and the Welander disease). In the first study, the 12 patients given 100 milligrams of CoQ_{10} daily for 3 months demonstrated significant improvement in cardiac output, stroke volume, and increased physical well-being. Subjective improvements included increased exercise tolerance, reduced leg pain, better control of leg function, and less fatigue. The second double-blind trial was similar with 15 patients having the same categories of disease. Definitely improved physical performance was recorded.[52]

Patients suffering from these muscle dystrophies should be treated with vitamin Q_{10} indefinitely. The mechanism of action of CoQ_{10} is probably related to improved energy production in muscle cells. The enhancement of cardiac function and physical well-being is an important advance in management of muscle diseases for which no other effective therapy currently exists.

Performance-Enhancing Agent in Athletes

Because CoQ_{10} is involved in energy production, supplementation might enhance aerobic capacity and muscle performance. In one study, six healthy sedentary men (mean age 21.5 years) performed a bicycle ergometer test before and after taking coenzyme Q_{10} (60 milligrams per day) for 4 to 8 weeks.[53] CoQ_{10} treatment improved certain performance parameters, including work capacity at submaximal heart rate, maximal work load, maximal oxygen consumption, and oxygen transport. These improvements ranged from 3 to 12 percent and were evident after about 4 weeks of therapy.

This study suggests that CoQ_{10} supplements improve physical performance in sedentary individuals. CoQ_{10} might also improve the performance of trained athletes or relieve some cases of chronic fatigue, but no one has yet investigated these possibilities.

Dosage Ranges

The usual dosage of CoQ_{10} is 50 to 150 milligrams per day. Although most studies used a dosage of 100 milligrams per day, larger doses (up to 300 milligrams per day) may be needed in cases of severe heart disease. Perhaps a more accurate dosage recommendation is based upon a person's weight. Some of the studies used a dosage of 2 milligrams CoQ_{10} for each kilogram (2.2 pounds) body weight.

Safety Issues

Coenzyme Q_{10} is generally well tolerated, and no serious adverse effects have been reported with long-term use. Because safety during pregnancy and lactation has not been proven, CoQ_{10} should not be used during these times unless the potential clinical benefit (as determined by a physician) outweighs the risks.

Interactions

There are no known adverse interactions between CoQ_{10} and any drug or nutrient. CoQ_{10} works synergistically with carnitine and pantethine.

While there are no adverse drug interactions, many drugs adversely affect CoQ_{10} levels, or CoQ_{10} can mitigate the side effects of the drug. In addition to the adverse effects of adriamycin (discussed earlier), CoQ_{10} supplementation can counteract some adverse effects of certain cholesterol-lowering, beta-blocker, and psychotropic drugs.

The drugs lovastatin (Mevacor), pravastin (Pravachol), and simvastatine (Zocor) are widely used to lower blood-cholesterol levels. They work by inhibiting the enzyme (HMG CoA reductase) that is required in the manufacture of cholesterol in the liver. Unfortunately, in doing so these drugs also block the manufacture of other substances necessary for body functions, including CoQ_{10}. Supplementing CoQ_{10} (100 milligrams per day) is necessary to prevent the depletion of CoQ_{10} in body tissues while on these drugs.[54]

CoQ_{10} can also help prevent some of the side effects of beta-blockers. These drugs are frequently prescribed for high blood pressure, angina, congestive heart failure, and certain arrhythmias. Beta-blockers can inhibit CoQ_{10}-dependent enzymes.[55] The antihypertensive effect of these drugs may therefore be compromised in the long run by the development of CoQ_{10} deficiency. In fact, it is well known that long-term therapy with beta-blockers leads to congestive heart failure in some cases. This development could be a result of CoQ_{10} deficiency. In one study, CoQ_{10} (60 milligrams per day) prevented the cardiac contractility decrease produced by the beta-blocker propranolol in normal volunteers and increased contractility in patients with hypertensive heart disease. Three of five volunteers treated with propranolol complained of general malaise, while none of seven individuals given propranolol plus CoQ_{10} reported side effects.[56]

CoQ_{10} may also help reduce the cardiac side effects from the use of certain psychotropic drugs, including phenothiazines and tricyclic antidepressants. EKG abnormalities (ST segment depression, prolonged QT interval, widened QRS complex, and flattened T waves) occur commonly in patients taking these drugs. Arrhythmia, heart failure, myocardial infarction, and sudden death have also been associated with the use of these psychotropic medications. Tissue studies suggest that the mechanism of cardiac side effects may be related to inhibition of CoQ_{10} function. In one experiment, all phenothiazines and tricyclic antidepressants studied inhibited CoQ_{10}-dependent enzymes. This inhibition could be reversed by addition of CoQ_{10}. It seems likely, therefore, that the cardiotoxicity of these psychotropic drugs is caused by inhibition of CoQ_{10}-dependent enzymes, which results in impaired energy production in myocardial cells. In two clinical studies, CoQ_{10} supplementation prevented electrocardiographic changes in patients on psychotropic drugs. CoQ_{10} supplementation may, therefore, be useful for the prevention of cardiotoxicity because of phenothiazines and tricyclic antidepressants.[57]

36

Fiber Supplements

Dietary fiber used to mean the sum of plant compounds that are indigestible by the secretions of the human digestive tract. This definition is vague because it depends on an exact understanding of what exactly is indigestible. For our purposes, the term *dietary fiber* refers to the components of plant cell walls *and* the indigestible residues.

Food Sources

The composition of the plant cell walls varies according to the species of plant. In general, most plant cell walls contain 35 percent insoluble fiber, 45 percent soluble fiber, 17 percent miscellaneous fiber compounds, 3 percent protein, and 2 percent ash (see Table 36.1). Dietary fiber is a complex of these constituents; supplementation of a single component does not substitute for a diet rich in high-fiber foods.

Insoluble Fibers

The best example of an insoluble fiber is wheat bran. Wheat bran is rich in cellulose and is relatively insoluble in water, but it has an ability to bind water. This ability accounts for its effect of increasing fecal size and weight, thus promoting regular bowel movements. Although cellulose cannot be digested by humans, it is partially digested by the microflora of the gut. This natural fermentation process that occurs in the colon results in the degradation of about 50 percent of the cellulose and is an important source of the short-chain fatty acids that nourish our intestinal cells.

Soluble Fibers

The majority of the fiber in most plant cell walls is water-soluble compounds. Included in this class are hemicelluloses, mucilages, gums, and pectin substances. This group of fiber compounds is the most beneficial. For example, hemicelluloses like those found in oat bran also promote regular bowel movements and provide short-chain fatty acids; but unlike cellulose, they can also lower cholesterol levels.

TABLE 36.1   Classification of Dietary Fiber

Fiber Class	Chemical Structure	Sources	Physiological Effect
Cellulose	Unbranched 1-4-beta-D-glucose polymer	Principal plant wall component; wheat bran	Increases fecal weight and size
Noncellulose polysaccharides: Hemicellulose	Mixture of pentose and hexose molecules in branching chains	Plant cell walls; oat bran	Same as above; binds bile acids; lowers cholesterol
Gums	Branched-chain uronic acid containing polymers	Karaya; gum arabic	Same as above
Mucilages	Similar to hemicelluloses	Found in endosperm of plant seeds; guar; legumes; psyllium	Hydrocolloids that bind steroids and delay gastric emptying; heavy metal chelation
Pectins	Mixture of methylesterified galacturan, galactan, and arabinose in varying proportions	Citrus rind; apple; onion skin	Same as above
Algal polysaccharides	Polymerized D-mannuronic and L-glucuronic acids	Algin; carrageenan	Same as above

Mucilages

Structurally, mucilages resemble the hemicelluloses, but they are not classified as such because of their unique location in the seed portion of the plant. They are generally found within the inner layer (endosperm) of grains, legumes, nuts, and seeds. Guar gum, found in most legumes (beans), is the most widely studied plant mucilage. Commercially, guar gum is used as a stabilizer and as a thickening and film-forming agent in the production of cheese, salad dressing, ice cream, soups, toothpaste, pharmaceutical jelly, lotion, skin cream, and tablets. Guar gum is also used as a laxative.

Guar gum and other mucilages, including psyllium seed husk and glucomannan, are perhaps the most potent cholesterol-lowering agents of the gel-forming fibers. In addition, mucilage fibers can reduce fasting and after-meal glucose and insulin levels in both healthy and diabetic subjects. They also can decreased body weight and hunger ratings when taken with meals by obese subjects.[1]

Pectin and Pectinlike Substances

Pectins are found in all plant cell walls and in the outer skin and rind of fruits and vegetables. For example, the rind of an orange contains 30 percent pectin, an apple peel 15 percent, and onion skins 12 percent. The gel-forming properties of pectin are well known to anyone who makes jelly or jam. These same gel-forming qualities are responsible for the cholesterol-lowering effects of pectins. Pectins lower cholesterol by binding the cholesterol and bile acids in the gut and promoting their excretion.

Miscellaneous Fiber Compounds

One of the most important miscellaneous fiber compounds is the lignan precursor, which is changed by the gut flora into the animal lignans enterolactone and enterodiol. Lignans exhibit important properties such as anticancer, antibacterial, antifungal, and antiviral activity. Flaxseeds and flaxseed oil are the most abundant sources of lignan precursors. Additional good sources of lignans are other seeds, grains, and legumes (see Table 36.2.)[1]

Deficiency Signs and Symptoms

The evidence supporting diet's role in chronic degenerative diseases is substantial. Two facts support this link: A diet rich in plant foods (whole grains, legumes, fruits, and vegetables) protects against many diseases that are extremely common in so-called "Western" society; a diet low in plant food intake results in the development of these diseases and provides conditions under which other causative factors become more active.[2–5]

Much of the link between diet, dietary fiber, and chronic disease originated from the work of two medical pioneers, Denis Burkitt, M.D., and Hugh Trowell, M.D., authors of *Western Diseases: Their Emergence and Prevention*, first published in 1981.[2,3] Although now extremely well recognized, the work of Burkitt and Trowell is actually a continuation of the landmark work of Weston A. Price, a dentist and author of *Nutrition and Physical Degeneration*.[6] In the early 1900s, Dr. Price traveled the world observing changes in teeth and palate (orthodontic) structure as various cultures discarded traditional dietary practices in favor of a more "civilized" diet. Price followed individuals and cultures over periods of 20 to 40 years and carefully documented the onset of degenerative diseases as their diets changed. Based on extensive studies that examined the rate of diseases in various populations (epidemiological data) and his own observations of primitive cultures, Burkitt formulated the sequence of events that follows.

First Stage The primal diet of plant eaters contains large amounts of unprocessed starch staples; there are few examples of chronic degenerative diseases like osteoarthritis, heart disease, diabetes, and cancer.

Second Stage Commencing westernization of diet, obesity and diabetes commonly appear in privileged groups.

Third Stage With moderate westernization of the diet, constipation, hemorrhoids, varicose veins, and appendicitis become common complaints.

Fourth Stage Finally, with full westernization of the diet, chronic degenerative diseases like osteoarthritis, rheumatoid arthritis, gout, heart disease, cancer, etc., are extremely common.

TABLE 36.2   Dietary Fiber Content of Selected Foods

Food	Serving	Calories	Grams of Fiber
FRUITS			
Apple (with skin)	1 medium	81	3.5
Banana	1 medium	105	2.4
Cantaloupe	1/4 melon	30	1.0
Cherries, sweet	10	49	1.2
Grapefruit	1/2 medium	38	1.6
Orange	1 medium	62	2.6
Peach (with skin)	1	37	1.9
Pear (with skin)	1/2 large	61	3.1
Prunes	3	60	3.0
Raisins	1/4 cup	106	3.1
Raspberries	1/2 cup	35	3.1
Strawberries	1 cup	45	3.0
VEGETABLES, RAW			
Bean sprouts	1/2 cup	13	1.5
Celery, diced	1/2 cup	10	1.1
Cucumber	1/2 cup	8	0.4
Lettuce	1 cup	10	0.9
Mushrooms	1/2 cup	10	1.5
Pepper, green	1/2 cup	9	0.5
Spinach	1 cup	8	1.2
Tomato	1 medium	20	1.5
VEGETABLES, COOKED			
Asparagus, cut	1 cup	30	2.0
Beans, green	1 cup	32	3.2
Broccoli	1 cup	40	4.4
Brussels sprouts	1 cup	56	4.6
Cabbage, red	1 cup	30	2.8
Carrots	1 cup	48	4.6
Cauliflower	1 cup	28	2.2
Corn	1/2 cup	87	2.9
Kale	1 cup	44	2.8
Parsnip	1 cup	102	5.4
Potato (with skin)	1 medium	106	2.5
Potato (without skin)	1 medium	97	1.4
Spinach	1 cup	42	4.2
Sweet potatoes	1 medium	160	3.4
Zucchini	1 cup	22	3.6
LEGUMES			
Baked beans	1/2 cup	155	8.8
Dried peas, cooked	1/2 cup	115	4.7
Kidney beans, cooked	1/2 cup	110	7.3
Lima beans, cooked	1/2 cup	64	4.5
Lentils, cooked	1/2 cup	97	3.7
Navy beans, cooked	1/2 cup	112	6.0

(continues)

Dietary Fiber Content of Selected Foods *(continued)*

Food	Serving	Calories	Grams of Fiber
RICE, BREADS, PASTAS, AND FLOUR			
Bran muffins	1 muffin	104	2.5
Bread, white	1 slice	78	0.4
Bread, whole wheat	1 slice	61	1.4
Crisp bread, rye	2 crackers	50	2.0
Rice, brown, cooked	½ cup	97	1.0
Rice, white, cooked	½ cup	82	0.2
Spaghetti, reg. cooked	½ cup	155	1.1
Spaghetti, whole wheat, cooked	½ cup	155	3.9
BREAKFAST CEREALS			
All-Bran	⅓ cup	71	8.5
Bran Chex	⅔ cup	91	4.6
Corn Bran	⅔ cup	98	5.4
Cornflakes	1¼ cup	110	0.3
Grape-Nuts	¼ cup	101	1.4
Oatmeal	¾ cup	108	1.6
Raisin Bran-type	⅔ cup	115	4.0
Shredded Wheat	⅔ cup	102	2.6
NUTS			
Almonds	10 nuts	79	1.1
Filberts	10 nuts	54	0.8
Peanuts	10 nuts	105	1.4

Population studies and clinical and experimental data have linked the so-called "Western Diet" to a number of now common diseases. In 1984, the National Research Council's Food and Nutrition Board established the Committee on Diet and Health to undertake a comprehensive analysis on diet and major chronic diseases.[5] It is the Food and Nutrition Board that develops the Recommended Dietary Allowance guidelines on the desirable amounts of essential nutrients in the diet. Their findings, and those of the U.S. Surgeon General and other highly respected medical groups, have brought to the forefront the need for Americans to change their eating habits to reduce their risk for chronic disease. Table 36.3 lists diseases with convincing links to a diet low in plant foods and dietary fiber. Many of these now common diseases were extremely rare before the twentieth century.

Beneficial Effects

It is beyond the scope of this chapter to detail all known effects of dietary fiber on humans. Instead, I concentrate on the effects of greatest clinical significance (stool

TABLE 36.3 Diseases Highly Associated with a Diet Low in Plant Foods

Disease Category	Specific Ailment
Metabolic	Obesity, gout, diabetes, kidney stones, gall stones
Cardiovascular	Heart disease, high blood pressure, strokes, varicose veins, deep-vein thrombosis, pulmonary embolism
Colonic	Constipation, appendicitis, diverticulitis, diverticulosis, hemorrhoids, colon cancer, irritable bowel syndrome, ulcerative colitis, Crohn's disease
Other	Dental caries, autoimmune disorders, pernicious anemia, multiple sclerosis, thyrotoxicosis, various skin conditions

weight, transit time, digestion, lipid metabolism, short-chain fatty acids, and colon flora). Some of the beneficial effects of dietary fiber are:

- Decreased intestinal transit time
- Delayed gastric emptying, resulting in reduced after-meal elevations of blood sugar
- Increased satiety
- Increased pancreatic secretion
- Increased stool weight
- More advantageous intestinal microflora
- Increased production of short-chain fatty acids
- Decreased serum lipids
- More soluble bile

Stool Weight and Transit Time

Fiber has long been used in the treatment of constipation. Dietary fiber, particularly the water-insoluble fibers such as cellulose (e.g., wheat bran) increase stool weight because of their water-holding properties. Transit time, the time material takes to pass from the mouth to the anus, is greatly reduced on a high-fiber diet.[1]

People in cultures that consume high-fiber diets (100 to 170 grams per day) usually have a transit time of 30 hours and a fecal weight of 500 grams. In contrast, Europeans and Americans who typically eat a low-fiber diet (20 grams per day) have a transit time of greater than 48 hours and a fecal weight of only 100 grams.[2,3] The increased intestinal transit time associated with the Western diet allows prolonged exposure of various cancer-causing compounds within the intestines.

Fiber should be used not only in the treatment of constipation, but also in the treatment of chronic diarrhea. When fiber is added to the diet of subjects with abnormally rapid transit times (less than 24 hours), it causes slowing of the transit time. Dietary fiber acts to normalize bowel movements.

Dietary fiber's effect on transit time apparently is directly related to its effect on stool weight and size. A larger, bulkier stool passes through the colon more easily and requires less pressure production during defecation, which means less straining. This results in less stress on the colon wall and fewer episodes of the ballooning effect that happens in diverticuli. It also prevents the formation of hemorrhoids and varicose veins.[2,3]

Digestion

Although dietary fiber increases the rate of transit through the gastrointestinal tract, it slows gastric emptying. This results a more gradual release of food into the small intestine; as a result, blood glucose levels rise more gradually. Pancreatic enzyme secretion and activity also increase in response to fiber.

Lipid Metabolism

The water-soluble gels and mucilagenous fibers like oat bran, guar gum, and pectin can lower serum lipid (cholesterol and triglyceride) levels by greatly increasing their fecal excretion and preventing their manufacture in the liver. The water-insoluble fibers like wheat bran have a much smaller effect in reducing serum lipid levels.[7,8]

Short-Chain Fatty Acids (SCFA)

The fermentation of dietary fiber by the intestinal flora produces three main end products: short-chain fatty acids, various gases, and energy. The SCFAs—acetic, proprionic, and butyric acids—have many important physiological functions.

Propionate and acetate are transported directly to the liver and used for energy production, while butyrate provides an important energy source for the cells that line the colon. In fact, butyrate is the preferred source for energy metabolism in the colon. Butyrate production may also be responsible for the anticancer properties of dietary fiber. Butyrate possesses impressive anticancer activity and is being used in enemas for ulcerative colitis.[1]

Certain fibers are more effective than others in increasing the levels of SCFAs in the colon. Pectins (both apple and citrus), guar gum, and other legume fibers produce more SCFAs than beet fiber, corn fiber, or oat bran.[1]

Intestinal Bacterial Flora

Dietary fiber improves all aspects of colon function. Of central importance is its role in maintaining a suitable bacterial flora in the colon. A low-fiber intake is associated with both an overgrowth of endotoxin-producing bacteria (bad guys) and a lower percentage of *Lactobacillus* (good guys) and other acid-loving bacteria. A diet high in dietary fiber promotes the growth of acid-loving bacteria through the increased synthesis of short-chain fatty acids, which reduce the colon pH.

Available Forms

The best fiber sources for nonlaxative effects are psyllium, guar gum, glucomannan, gum karaya, and pectin because they are rich in water-soluble fibers. There are many fiber supplements to choose from in health-food stores, but make sure you select a product rich in water-soluble fiber and avoid products that add a lot of sugar or other sweeteners to camouflage the taste.

Principal Uses

In addition to its role as a laxative, supplementary dietary fiber is used in the treatment of irritable bowel syndrome and other functional disturbances of the colon, elevated cholesterol levels, and obesity.

Irritable Bowel Syndrome

The irritable bowel syndrome (IBS) is a very common condition in which the large intestine (colon) fails to function properly. It has numerous names—nervous indigestion, spastic colitis, mucous colitis, and intestinal neurosis. IBS has characteristic symptoms that can include a combination of:

- Abdominal pain and distention
- More frequent bowel movements with pain or relief of pain with bowel movements
- Constipation
- Diarrhea
- Excessive production of mucus in the colon
- Symptoms of indigestion such as flatulence, nausea, or anorexia
- Varying degrees of anxiety or depression

Irritable bowel syndrome (IBS) is extremely common. Estimates suggest that approximately 15 percent of the population have suffered from IBS at one time or another. Increasing dietary fiber as a treatment of irritable bowel syndrome has a long yet irregular history. In general, eating a diet rich in complex carbohydrates and dietary fiber while avoiding sugar and refined foods is effective in many cases. Again the best fiber supplements choices are the water-soluble forms—nevertheless, the type of fiber often used in both research and clinical practice is wheat bran (an *insoluble* fiber).[1] However, wheat is commonly implicated in malabsorptive and allergic conditions; therefore, wheat bran is usually not indicated in individuals with symptoms of IBS since food allergy is a significant causative factor in this condition. In addition, while patients with constipation are much more likely to respond to wheat bran, those with diarrhea may actually worsen their symptoms.

Elevated Cholesterol Levels

A 1994 review article in the *Journal of the American Dietetic Association* concluded that soluble-fiber supplementation was very effective in lowering cholesterol levels.[7] Specifically, a significant reduction in the level of serum total cholesterol was found in 68 of the 77 (88 percent) of the studies reviewed. The effect of soluble fiber supplementation is clearly dose-dependent. In other words, the higher the intake of soluble fiber the greater the reduction in serum cholesterol (see Table 36.4).

Many of the studies featured oat preparations containing either oat bran or oatmeal. The overwhelming majority of these studies demonstrated individuals with high cholesterol levels see significant reductions with frequent oatmeal or oat bran consumption. In contrast, individuals with normal or low cholesterol levels see little change. In individuals with high cholesterol levels (above 220 milligrams per deciliter) the consumption of the equivalent of 3 grams of soluble oat fiber typically lowers total cholesterol by 8 to 23 percent. This is highly significant because with each 1 percent drop in serum cholesterol level there is a 2 percent decrease in the risk of developing heart disease. One bowl of ready-to-eat oat bran cereal or oatmeal provides approximately 3 grams of fiber. Polyunsaturated fatty acids contribute as much to the cholesterol-lowering effects of oats as does the fiber content; and although oatmeal's fiber content (7 percent) is less than that of oat bran (15 to 26 percent), it is higher in polyunsaturated fatty acids. In practical terms, the dosage level for dry oat bran is 1/3 to 1 cup and for dry oatmeal, 1 to 1 2/3 cups.[7,8]

Obesity

When taken with water before meals, water-soluble fiber binds to water in the stomach and forms a gelatinous mass that makes an individual full. As a result, he or she is less likely to overeat. However, the benefits of fiber go well beyond this mechanical effect. Fiber supplements enhance blood sugar control and insulin effects and actually reduce the number of calories the body absorbs.[1] In some of the clinical studies demonstrating weight loss, fiber supplements reduced the number of calories absorbed by 30 to 180 calories per day (see Table 36.5).[9-20] This reduction in calories may not seem like much, but over the course of a year it would add up to 3 to 18 pounds.

Weight-loss studies using guar gum, a water-soluble fiber obtained from the Indian cluster bean (*Cyamopsis tetragonoloba*), have produced the most impressive results. In

TABLE 36.4 Average Doses of Soluble Fiber and Total Cholesterol Reductions

Fiber	Dosage (in grams)	Reduction (in percent)
Oat bran (dry)	50–100	20
Guar gum	9–15	10
Pectin	6–10	5
Psyllium	10–20	10–20
Vegetable fiber	27	10

TABLE 36.5 Clinical Studies with Dietary Fiber Supplements

Fiber	Number of Subjects	Length of Study	Dosage (g./day)	Calorie Restriction	Average Loss w/Fiber (Pounds)	Average Loss w/Placebo (Pounds)	Reference
Guar	9	2 months	20	None	9.4	No placebo group	9
Guar	7	1 year	20	None	61.9	No placebo group	10
Guar	21	2.5 months	20.00	None	15.60	No placebo group	11
Guar	33	2.5 months	15.00	None	5.50	0.9 in placebo group	12
Glucomannan	20	2 months	3.00	None	5.50	Weight gain, 1.5	13
Glucomannan	20	2 months	3.00	None	8.14	0.44 in placebo group	14
Citrus Pectin	14	4 weeks	5.56	Yes	12.80	No placebo group	15
Mixture A[a]	60	12 weeks	5.00	Yes	18.70	14.70 in placebo group	16
Mixture A	89	11 weeks	10.00	Yes	13.90	9.20 in placebo group	17
Mixture B[b]	45	3 months	7.00	Yes	13.60	9.00 in placebo group	18
Mixture B	97	3 months	7.00	Yes	10.80	7.3 in placebo group	19
Mixture B	52	6 months	7.00	Yes	12.10	6.1 in placebo group	20

[a]Mixture A 80 percent fiber from grains, 20 percent fiber from citrus.

[b]Mixture B 90 percent insoluble and 10 percent soluble fiber from beet, barley, and citrus fibers.

one study, nine women weighing between 160 and 242 pounds were given 10 grams of guar gum immediately before lunch and dinner. They were told not to consciously alter their eating habits. After 2 months, the women reported an average weight loss of 9.4 pounds—over 1 pound per week. Their cholesterol and triglyceride levels also dropped.[9] A person can lose 50 to 100 percent more weight by supplementing his or her diet with fiber than by simply restricting calories.

Dosage Ranges

Start out with a small dosage and increase gradually. Water-soluble fibers are fermented by intestinal bacteria. As a result, their ingestion can produce a great deal of gas. If you are not used to a high-fiber diet, an increase in dietary fiber can lead to increased flatulence and abdominal discomfort. Start out with a dosage between 1 and 2 grams before meals and at bedtime and gradually increase the dosage to 5 grams.

Safety Issues

If you have a disorder of the esophagus, do not take fiber supplements in pill form because they may expand in the esophagus and lead to obstruction of the intestinal tract, a very serious disorder.[21] Fiber supplements in capsules appear to be slightly better tolerated than tablets but still should be used with caution. The difference is the manner in which the tablets and capsules interact with water. One study showed that fiber (glucomannan) tablets swelled seven times their original size within 1 minute after coming in contact with water.[22] In contrast, fiber-filled gelatin capsules took 6 minutes before they began to swell. One very important recommendation: Be sure to drink adequate amounts of water when taking any fiber supplement, especially if it is in pill form.

Interactions

A number of research studies have examined the effects of fiber on mineral absorption. Although the results have been somewhat contradictory, it now appears that large amounts of dietary fiber may result in impaired absorption and/or negative balance of some minerals. Fiber as a dietary component does not appear to interfere with the minerals in other foods; however, supplemental fiber, especially wheat bran, may result in a mineral deficiencies. Fiber supplements may also inhibit the absorption of certain drugs, so it is a good idea to take the fiber supplement hours apart from any medication.

37

Flavonoids

Flavonoids are a group of plant pigments that are largely responsible for the colors of many fruits and flowers. Recent research suggests that flavonoids may be useful in the treatment and prevention of many health conditions. In fact, we now know many of the medicinal actions of foods, juices, herbs, and bee pollen are directly related to their flavonoid content. Over 4,000 flavonoid compounds have been characterized and classified according to chemical structure. For simplicity's sake, I have divided the discussions in this chapter into four categories: PCO, quercetin, citrus bioflavonoids, and green tea polyphenols.

PCO

One of the most beneficial groups of plant flavonoids is the proanthocyanidins (also called procyanidins). These flavonoids provide many health-promoting benefits. The most potent proanthocyanidins are those bound to other proanthocyanidins. Collectively, mixtures of proanthocyanidin dimers, trimers, tetramers, and larger molecules are referred to procyanidolic oligomers, or PCO for short. Although PCO exists in many plants and red wine, commercially available sources of PCO include extracts from grape seeds and the bark of the maritime (Landes) pine.

Quercetin

Quercetin is a flavonoid that serves as the backbone for many other flavonoids, including the citrus flavonoids rutin, quercitrin, and hesperidin. These derivatives differ from quercetin in that they have sugar molecules attached to the quercetin backbone. Quercetin is consistently the most active of the flavonoids in experimental studies, and many medicinal plants owe much of their activity to their high quercetin content.

Citrus Bioflavonoids

Citrus bioflavonoid preparations can include rutin, hesperidin, quercitrin, and naringin. Most of the clinical research on rutin and crude bioflavonoid complexes occurred before 1970. Since that time, most of the clinical research has used a standardized mixture of rutinosides known as hydroxyethylrutosides (HER). Impressive clinical results have been obtained in the treatment of capillary permeability, easy bruising, hemorrhoids, and varicose veins with HER. Citrus bioflavonoids provide similar, but probably not as potent, effects as HER or quercetin.

Green Tea Polyphenols

Both green tea and black tea are derived from the same plant, the tea plant (*Camellia sinensis*). Green tea is produced by lightly steaming the fresh-cut leaf, while to produce black tea the leaves are allowed to oxidize. During oxidation, enzymes present in the tea convert many "polyphenol" substances that possess outstanding therapeutic action to compounds with much less activity. With green tea, oxidation is not allowed to take place because the steaming process inactivates these enzymes. The term *polyphenol* denotes the presence of a phenolic ring in the chemical structure. The major polyphenols in green tea are flavonoids (catechin, epicatechin, epicatechin gallate, epigallocatechin gallate, and proanthocyanidins). Epigallocatechin gallate is viewed as the most significant active component.

Food Sources

Good dietary sources of flavonoids include citrus fruits, berries, onions, parsley, legumes, green tea, and red wine (see Table 37.1). The average daily intake in the United States for flavonoids is somewhere between 150 and 200 milligrams.

Deficiency Signs and Symptoms

Flavonoids (as well as vitamin C) were discovered by Albert Szent-Gyorgyi (1893–1986), one of the most respected and honored biochemists of the twentieth century. Szent-Gyorgyi received the Nobel Prize in 1937 for his discovery of some of the properties of vitamin C and flavonoids.

It was in the course of isolating vitamin C that Szent-Gyorgyi discovered the flavonoids. A friend with bleeding gums had stopped the bleeding by taking a crude vitamin C preparation isolated from lemon. When the problem reappeared, Szent-Gyorgyi gave his friend a purer form of vitamin C. He expected to observe an even more impressive result, but the purer form of vitamin C did not work. Szent-Gyorgyi then isolated the flavonoid fraction from the original crude vitamin C preparation, gave it to his friend, and observed complete healing.

Szent-Gyorgyi termed his discovery "vitamin P" because of its ability reduce vascular permeability, one of the hallmark features of scurvy. He later showed that the clinical symptoms of scurvy stem from a combined deficiency of vitamin C and flavonoids. However, because flavonoids could not fulfill all the requirements of a vitamin, the designation as vitamin P was abandoned. Although flavonoids are often referred to as "semi-essential" nutrients, apparently they are as important in human nutrition as essential vitamins and minerals.

TABLE 37.1 Flavonoid Content of Selected Foods, in Milligrams per 3¹/₂-oz. (100g.) Serving

Foods	4-Oxo-flavonoids[a]	Anthocyanins	Catechins[b]	Biflavans
FRUITS				
Grapefruit	50			
Grapefruit juice	20			
Oranges, Valencia	50–100			
Orange juice	20–40			
Apples	3–16	1–2	20–75	50–90
Apple juice				15
Apricots	10–18		25	
Pears	1–5		5–20	1–3
Peaches	1–12	10–20	90–120	
Tomatoes	85–130			
Blueberry		130–250		10–20
Cherries, sour		45		25
Cherries, sweet			6–7	15
Cranberries	5	60–200	20	100
Cowberries		100	25	100–150
Currants, black	20–400	130–400	15	50
Currant juice		75–100		
Grapes, red		65–140	5–30	50
Plums, yellow		2–10		
Plums, blue		10–25	200	
Raspberries, black		300–400		
Raspberries, red		30–35		
Strawberries	20–100	15–35	30–40	
Hawthorn berries			200–800	
VEGETABLES				
Cabbage, red		25		
Onions	100–2,000	0–25		
Parsley	1,400			
Rhubarb		200		
MISCELLANEOUS				
Beans, dry		10–1,000		
Sage	1,000–1,500			
Tea	5–50		10–500	100–200
Wine, red	2–4	50–120	100–150	100–250

[a]4-Oxo-flavonoids: The sum of flavanones, flavones, and flavanols (including quercetin).
[b]Catechins include proanthocyanins.
SOURCE: J. Kuhnau, The Flavonoids: A Class of Semi-essential Food Components: Their role in Human Nutrition. *World Review of Nutrition and Diet* 24, 117–91, 1976.

Beneficial Effects

As a class of compounds, flavonoids have been referred to as "nature's biological response modifiers" because of their ability to modify the body's reaction to other compounds such as allergens, viruses, and carcinogens. This is evidenced by their anti-inflammatory, anti-allergic, antiviral, and anticarcinogenic properties. In addition, flavonoids act as powerful antioxidants by providing remarkable protection against oxidative and free-radical damage. The practical aspect of this antioxidant activity is highlighted by the results of a an 805-man study designed to determine the effect of dietary flavonoids on protecting against heart disease. The results of the study demonstrate an inverse correlation between flavonoid intake and death from a heart attack. That is to say, when flavonoid intake was high, the risk of heart attack was quite low. Conversely, if flavonoid intake was low, the risk of heart attack was quite high.[1] This effect is probably a result of the potent antioxidant effects of the flavonoids that prevent the formation of oxidized cholesterol—similar to the antioxidant effects of vitamins C and E. However, the antioxidant activity of flavonoids is generally more potent and exerts a broader range of activity than antioxidant nutrients like vitamins C and E, selenium, and zinc.[2,3] Different flavonoids tend to provide different benefits, as I discuss below. However, there is significant overlap among them as you will see.

PCO

Proanthocyanidins and PCO extracts demonstrate a wide range of pharmacological activity. Their effects include an ability to increase intracellular vitamin C levels, decrease capillary permeability and fragility, scavenge oxidants and free radicals, and inhibit destruction of collagen.[4,5] Collagen, the most abundant protein of the body, is responsible for maintaining the integrity of "ground substance," tendons, ligaments, and cartilage. Collagen also is the support structure of the skin and blood vessels. PCO extracts are remarkable in their ability to support collagen structures and prevent collagen destruction. They affect collagen metabolism in several ways. They have the unique ability to cross-link collagen fibers, resulting in reinforcement of the natural cross-linking of collagen that forms the so-called collagen matrix of connective tissue.[6,7] They also prevent free-radical damage with their potent antioxidant and free-radical scavenging action. Further, they inhibit enzymatic cleavage of collagen by enzymes secreted by leukocytes during inflammation and microbes during infection.[8,9] PCO extracts also prevent the release and synthesis of compounds that promote inflammation and allergies, such as histamine, serine proteases, prostaglandins, and leukotrienes.[4]

In the United States, perhaps the most celebrated effects of PCO are their potent antioxidant and free-radical scavenging effects. Antioxidants and free-radical scavengers prevent against free-radical or oxidative damage. Free-radical damage has been linked to the aging process and virtually every chronic degenerative disease, including heart disease, arthritis, and cancer. Fats and cholesterol are particularly susceptible to free-radical damage. When damaged, fats and cholesterol form toxic derivatives known as lipid peroxides and cholesterol epoxides, respectively. These antioxidant and free-radical scavenging effects of PCO were discovered by Jacques Masquelier in 1986.[4]

A recent study has shed more light on the antioxidant activities and exact mechanisms underlying the primary clinical applications of PCO (varicose veins, capillary fragility, easy bruising, etcetera).[9] The study featured two primary goals: to determine the free-radical scavenging activity of PCO and to discover the inhibitory effects of

PCO on both xanthine oxidase (the primary generator of oxygen-derived free radicals) and the lysosomal enzyme system (which governs the release of enzymes that can damage the connective tissue framework acting as a protective sheath surrounding capillary walls).

The results of some very sophisticated tests provide a detailed explanation of the vascular protective action of PCO and a strong rationale for their use in vascular disease. In these studies, PCO demonstrated an ability to:

- Trap hydroxyl free radicals
- Trap lipid peroxides and free radicals
- Markedly delay the onset of lipid peroxidation
- Chelate to free iron molecules, thereby preventing iron-induced lipid peroxidation
- Inhibit production of free radicals by noncompetively inhibiting xanthine oxidase
- Inhibit the damaging effects of the enzymes (hyaluronidase, elastase, collagenase, etcetera) that can degrade connective tissue structures.

The antioxidant activity of PCO is much greater (approximately 50 times) than that of vitamin C and vitamin E. From a cellular perspective, one of the most advantageous features of PCO free-radical scavenging activity is that because of its chemical structure, it is incorporated within cell membranes. This physical characteristic, along with its ability to protect against both water- and fat-soluble free radicals, provides incredible protection to the cells against free-radical damage.

The researchers concluded their discussion with the following comment: "These findings, together (with) those of other investigators, provide a strong rationale for using these compounds in the therapeutic management of microvascular disorders."[9]

Quercetin

Quercetin has demonstrated significant anti-inflammatory activity because of direct inhibition of several initial processes of inflammation. For example, it inhibits both the manufacture and release of histamine and other allergic/inflammatory mediators. In addition, it exerts potent antioxidant activity and vitamin C-sparing action.[2,3,10–16]

Quercetin is also a strong inhibitor of aldose reductase, the enzyme responsible for the conversion of blood sugar (glucose) to sorbitol a compound strongly implicated in the development of diabetic complications (diabetic cataracts, neuropathy, and retinopathy).[17] We can best understand the mechanism by which sorbitol is involved in the development of diabetic complications by considering its involvement in cataract formation. Although the lens does not have any blood vessels, it is an actively metabolizing tissue that continuously grows throughout life. Elevated blood sugar levels result in shunting of glucose to the sorbitol pathway. Since the lens membranes are virtually impermeable to sorbitol and lack the enzyme required to break down sorbitol (polyol dehydrogenase), sorbitol accumulates to high concentrations. These high concentrations persist even if glucose levels return to normal. This accumulation creates an osmotic gradient that results in water being drawn into the cells to maintain osmotic balance. As the water is pulled in, the cell must release small molecules like amino acids, inositol, glutathione, niacin, vitamin C, magnesium, and potassium to maintain osmotic balance. Since these latter compounds function to protect the lens from damage, their loss results in an increased susceptibility to damage. As a result, the delicate protein fibers within the lens become opaque, and a cataract forms.

Quercetrin, a flavonoid converted to quercetin by gut bacteria, can significantly decrease the accumulation of sorbitol in the lens of diabetic animals, effectively delaying the onset of cataracts.[18] In addition to its effect on aldose reductase, quercetin is also indicated in diabetes for its ability to enhance insulin secretion, protect the pancreatic beta-cells from the damaging effects of free radicals, and inhibit platelet aggregation.[2,3]

Flavonoids as a group possess significant antiviral activity, with quercetin having the greatest antiviral activity against *herpes* virus type I, para-influenzae 3, polio virus type I, and respiratory syncytial virus.[19–21] *In vitro* it seems to inhibit both viral replication and infectivity. *In vivo* studies in animals have also shown quercetin to inhibit viral infection.[21,22] This would suggest quercetin may be of some benefit in viral infections, including the common cold.

Many flavonoids inhibit tumor formation, but again quercetin has consistently been the most effective. In experimental models, quercetin has demonstrated significant antitumor activity against a wide range of cancers, including squamous cell carcinoma; leukemia; and cancers of the breast, ovaries, colon, rectum, and brain. Unfortunately, there are no human studies to support the impressive results noted in animal and *in vitro* studies.[23–26]

Citrus Flavonoids

In addition to possessing antioxidant activity and an ability to increase intracellular levels of vitamin C, rutin, hesperidin, and HER exert many beneficial effects on capillary permeability and blood flow via mechanisms described for PCO. They also exhibit some of the anti-allergy and anti-inflammatory benefits of quercetin.

Green Tea Polyphenols

Most of the population and experimental studies on tea have focused on the cancer-causing and cancer-protective aspects. Green tea polyphenols are potent antioxidant compounds that have demonstrated greater antioxidant protection than vitamins C and E in experimental studies.[27]

In addition to exerting antioxidant activity on its own, green tea may increase the activity of antioxidant enzymes. In mice, after 30 days of oral feeding of a polyphenolic fraction isolated from green tea in drinking water, there were significant increases in the activities of antioxidant and detoxifying enzymes (glutathione peroxidase, glutathione reductase, glutathione S-transferase, catalase, and quinone reductase) in the small intestine, liver, lungs, and small bowel.[28]

A number of *in vitro* and experimental models of cancer show that green tea polyphenols may offer significant protection.[29–32] Specifically, green tea polyphenols inhibit cancer by blocking the formation of cancer-causing compounds like nitrosamines; suppressing the activation of carcinogens, and effectively detoxifying or trapping cancer-causing agents. In addition to these studies, human studies support the concept that green tea consumption can prevent some forms of cancer.[33] The forms of cancer that green tea prevents the best are cancers of the gastrointestinal tract, including cancers of the stomach, small intestine, pancreas, and colon; lungs; and estrogen-related cancers, including most breast cancers.[33]

In vitro studies regarding breast cancer show that green tea extracts have inhibitory effects on the growth of mammary cancer cell lines with similar potencies.[32] The main anticancer action is inhibition of the estrogen interaction with its receptors. Polyphenol compounds in green tea extracts block the interaction of tumor promoters, hormones, and growth factors with their receptors—a kind of sealing-off effect. The sealing-off effect would account for the reversible growth arrest noted in the *in vitro* studies.

Green tea consumption with meals may inhibit the formation of nitrosamines.[34,35] Nitrosamines are formed when nitrites, such as those used in the curing of bacon and ham, bind to amino acids. Numerous studies show that green tea (including green tea polyphenols and extracts) exert significant inhibitory effects on the formation of nitrosamines in various animal and human models. For example, when human volunteers ingested green tea along with 300 milligrams sodium nitrate and 300 milligrams proline, nitrosoproline formation was strongly inhibited.[34]

The popular custom of drinking green tea with meals in Japan may be a major reason for the low cancer rates there. With the cancer rate in the United States rising, more Americans might want to start drinking green tea with their meals.

Principal Uses

There is much overlap in the clinical use of flavonoid preparations. Most of the clinical research has focused on PCO-containing extracts and HER products.

PCO

The primary use of PCO extracts is the treatment of venous and capillary disorders, including venous insufficiency, varicose veins, capillary fragility, and disorders of the retina such as diabetic retinopathy and macular degeneration. Good clinical studies show positive results in the treatment of these conditions.[36–41]

It appears that most individuals can benefit from an increased intake of PCO. This suggestion is perhaps best illustrated by studies looking at the ability of grape seed PCO extract in improving visual function in healthy subjects.[42,43] In the studies, 100 normal volunteers with no retinal disorder received 200 milligrams per day of PCO or a placebo for 5 or 6 weeks; a control group received no treatment. The group receiving PCOs demonstrated significant improvement in visual performance in dark and after-glare tests compared to the placebo group. The improvement is related to improved retinal function. Based on the relatively recent demonstration of PCO's potent antioxidant activity and vasculoprotective effects, the clinical uses of PCO extracts will surely increase. Perhaps the most significant use will eventually be in the prevention of heart disease and strokes. Since PCO has a greater antioxidant effect than vitamins C and E, it is only natural to assume it could offer greater protective effects. In addition to preventing damage to cholesterol and the lining of the artery, in animal studies PCO extracts have lowered blood cholesterol levels and shrunk the size of cholesterol deposits in the artery.[1,20,44] Additional mechanisms of PCO useful in preventing atherosclerosis include inhibition of platelet aggregation and vascular constriction.[45,46] Presumably PCO extracts may exert similar benefits in humans. We should think of PCO extracts, although in a supplement form, as a necessary food in the prevention and treatment of heart disease and strokes.

Quercetin

Based on largely *in vitro* studies, quercetin appears indicated in virtually all inflammatory and allergic conditions (including asthma, hay fever, rheumatoid arthritis, and lupus) and in diabetes and cancer. However, the main shortcoming with quercetin is the lack of clinical studies and the questionable absorption. Pharmacokinetic studies in animals and humans indicate that very little quercetin is absorbed intact, with the majority of the oral dose (53 percent) being excreted in the feces.[47,48] One of the main problems in studying the absorption of quercetin and other flavonoids is their degradation by microorganisms in the colon. To sidestep this issue, a recent study examined the absorption of quercetin in healthy ileostomy patients with complete small intestines.[49]

The study examined the absorption of quercetin from fried onions (a rich source of quercetin glycosides), rutin, or 100 milligrams of pure quercetin. Absorption was defined as oral intake minus ileostomy excretion and corrected for degradation within the ileostomy bag. Absorption results were as follows: 52 percent from onions, 17 percent from quercetin rutinoside, and 24 percent from pure quercetin. These results indicate that humans do absorb appreciable amounts of quercetin and that absorption (but not necessarily pharmacological activity) may be enhanced when quercetin is bound to glucose.

Citrus Bioflavonoids

Early studies of citrus bioflavonoids featured rutin. In these studies, rutin was useful in reducing capillary fragility, easy bruising, swelling and bruising after sports injuries, and nosebleeds.[50–53] More recent and much more extensive studies have been performed with HER. Positive double-blind clinical studies exist in the treatment of venous insufficiency (varicose veins, hemorrhoids, diabetic vascular disease, and diabetic retinopathy).[54]

In double-blind studies in patients with chronic venous insufficiency, HER improves microvascular blood flow and clinical symptoms (pain, tired legs, night cramps, and restless legs) in 73 to 100 percent of patients.[54–60] Several of the studies were performed in pregnant women where HER was of great benefit in improving venous function and helping to relieve hemorrhoidal signs and symptoms. In one study, 90 percent of the women given HER (1,000 milligrams daily for 4 weeks) had improved symptoms compared to only 12 percent in the placebo group.[61] Similar results in hemorrhoids not associated with pregnancy have been reported.[54,62]

Flavonoids appear to be quite important in the long-term care of diabetes. A hallmark feature of diabetes is a significant disturbance of blood flow through small blood vessels. HER appear to significantly improve blood flow in diabetics and can be useful in the treatment of diabetic microvascular disease and retinopathy. However, PCO (or bilberry) extracts may be better than citrus flavonoids and HER in diabetics.[63,64]

Green Tea Polyphenols

Green tea polyphenols are used principally in the prevention of cancer. Population studies demonstrate that green tea consumption may actually be one of the major reasons why the cancer rate is lower in Japan.[9] In contrast to green tea's protective effects, black tea consumption may increase risk for certain cancers (cancer of the rectum, gallbladder, and endometrium).[65,66]

For example, in one study the relationship between black tea consumption and cancer risk was analyzed using data from an integrated series of case-control studies conducted in northern Italy between 1983 and 1990.[65] The data set included 119 biopsy-confirmed cancers of the oral cavity and throat, 294 of the esophagus, 564 of the stomach, 673 of the colon, 406 of the rectum, 258 of the liver, 41 of the gallbladder, 303 of the pancreas, 149 of the larynx, 2,860 of the breast, 567 of the endometrium, 742 of the ovary, 107 of the prostate, 365 of the bladder, 147 of the kidney, 120 of the thyroid, and a total of 6,147 controls admitted to the hospital for acute noncancerous conditions. The risks of developing cancer because of tea consumption were derived after allowance for age, sex, area of residence, education, smoking, and coffee consumption. Results indicated an increased risk with tea consumption for cancers of the rectum, gallbladder, and endometrium. There was no association with cancers of the oral cavity, esophagus, stomach, bladder, kidney, prostate, or any other site considered

In another study, men of Japanese ancestry were clinically examined from 1965 to 1968.[66] For 7,833 of these men, data on black tea consumption habits were recorded. Since 1965, newly diagnosed cancer incidence cases have been identified: 152 colon, 151 lung, 149 prostate, 136 stomach, 76 rectum, 57 bladder, 30 pancreas, 25 liver, 12 kidney and 163 at other (miscellaneous) sites. Compared to men who rarely drank black tea, those who habitually drank it more than once a day had a fourfold greater chance of developing rectal cancer.

Available Forms

Because each flavonoid category is available in many varieties, let me break them down for ease of understanding.

PCO

Grape seed and pine bark PCO extracts are well defined chemically. Grape seed extracts are available that contain a total of 92 percent or 95 percent PCO, while the pine bark extracts can vary from 80 to 85 percent. PCO from both grape seeds and pine bark have been marketed in France for decades. Sales for the grape seed extract in France are roughly 400 times greater than those for the pine bark. Due to aggressive advertising and some misinformation, in the United States the pine bark extract currently outsells the grape seed extract considerably.

Although both sources can be used interchangeably, for several valid reasons PCO extracted from grape seeds has emerged as the preferred source. First of all, the overwhelming majority of the published clinical and experimental studies over the past twenty years have been performed on the grape seed extract, not the extract of pine bark.[4,67]

With regard to the free-radical scavenging activities of PCO, studies demonstrate that the grape seed extract may be more potent and effective than the extract of pine bark. The reason? Only the grape seed extract contains the gallic esters of proanthocyanidins (in particular, proanthocyanidin B2-3'-0-gallate).[4,67] These compounds are the most active free-radical scavenging PCO. They are not present in the pine bark extract, but they are found in the PCO extract from the grape seed. In addition, it is far more economical to extract PCO from grape seeds than from pine bark. As a result, the grape seed extract provides greater value at a lower price.

Quercetin

Quercetin is available alone in powder and capsule form. However, if the quercetin is used for its anti-inflammatory properties, products that provide a combination of the pineapple enzyme bromelain may provide additional benefit. Bromelain exerts anti-allergy and anti-inflammatory activity on its own and may also enhance the absorption of quercetin. Combination preparations of protein-digesting enzymes (like bromelain) and flavonoids potentiate each other's anti-inflammatory activity.[68] The amount of bromelain (1,800 milk clotting units) should be equal to the amount of quercetin.

Citrus Bioflavonoids

Mixed preparations of citrus bioflavonoids are the most widely used and least expensive flavonoid sources. However, as with most things in life, you get what you pay for. Mixed citrus flavonoids are the least active and generally the least quantified source of flavonoids—most commercially available sources are only 50 percent flavonoids. Preparations containing pure rutin and hesperidin or those that clearly state the levels of rutin and hesperidin are a better buy than products that do not quantify individual flavonoid amounts. HER are probably the better choice when opting for the benefits in this class of flavonoids.

Green Tea Polyphenols

You can find commercial preparations of green tea polyphenols that have been decaffeinated and concentrated for polyphenols—anywhere from 60 to 80 percent total polyphenols. However, keep in mind that one cup of green tea may contain as much as 300 to 400 milligrams of polyphenols. The downside of simply drinking green tea as a source for the polyphenols is that it also contains 50 to 100 milligrams of caffeine.

Dosage Ranges

The dosages ranges for each of these compounds vary. Here they are by category.

PCO

As a preventive measure and as antioxidant support, a daily dose of 50 milligrams of either the grape seed or pine bark extract is suitable. When being used for therapeutic purposes, the daily dosage should be increased to 150 to 300 milligrams.

Quercetin

The recommended dosage range for quercetin is 200 to 400 milligrams 20 minutes before meals (three times per day).

Citrus Bioflavonoids

The dosage of HER in the double-blind clinical studies in the treatment of venous insufficiency and hemorrhoids ranges from 1,000 to 3,000 milligrams daily. To translate this dosage to citrus bioflavonoids, rutin, and hesperidin, multiply by 2 (2,000 to 6,000 milligrams daily).

Green Tea Polyphenols

The normal amount of green tea consumed by Japanese and other green tea–drinking cultures is about 3 cups daily, or about 3 grams of soluble components providing roughly 240 to 320 milligrams of polyphenols. In order to achieve some degree of protection, you need to consume an amount of green tea or green tea polyphenols equal to the amount consumed in the positive population studies. For a green tea extract standardized for 80 percent total polyphenol and 55 percent epigallocatechin gallate content, this means a daily dose of 300 to 400 milligrams.

When selecting commercial green tea extract, look for the level of epigallocatechin gallate and total polyphenol content.

Safety Issues

The safety of flavonoids varies according to the category of flavonoid. The remainder of this section addresses safety issues, side effects, and toxicity separately for each variety.

PCO

PCO extracts are extremely safe, and no side effects have been reported.

Quercetin

Quercetin is apparently well tolerated in humans. Carcinogenic and teratogenic studies in rats and rabbits shown that quercetin is without apparent side effects even when consumed in very large quantities (2,000 milligrams per kilogram of body weight and 5 to 10 percent of total diet) for long periods of time (up to 2 years).[69–74] In addition, quercetin administration (up to 2,000 milligrams per kilogram of body weight) to pregnant rats had no teratogenic effects.[75] As is true of any other compound, allergic reactions may occur. Although they are uncommon, discontinue use if they occur.

Citrus Bioflavonoids

Citrus bioflavonoids, rutin, hesperidin, and HER appear to be extremely safe and without side effects even during pregnancy.[54]

Green Tea Polyphenols

Green tea is not associated with any significant side effects or toxicity. If preparations contain caffeine, overconsumption may produce a stimulant effect (nervousness, anxiety, insomnia, irritability, etcetera); however, green tea usually does not produce these symptoms even in some people who are usually quite sensitive to caffeine—myself included.

Interactions

Interactions with vitamin C have been described above. As far as drug interactions, PCO, quercetin, rutin, hesperidin, HER, and green tea polyphenols do not interact with any drug. Citrus bioflavonoid preparations, however, may interact with drugs if they contain naringin. This flavonoid is in grapefruit juice but not orange juice. Studies in humans show grapefruit juice (naringin) increases the oral bioavailability of drugs like nifedipine, felodipine, verapramil, and terfenadine and inhibits the breakdown of various drugs, particularly caffeine, coumarin, and estrogens.[76] Avoid grapefruit juice and flavonoid preparations containing naringin when taking any of these drugs.

38

Gamma-oryzanol

Gamma-oryzanol (esters of ferulic acid) is a growth-promoting substance in grains and is isolated from rice bran oil. The Japanese have been using it as a medicine since 1962. Initially used in the treatment of minor anxiety, it later became approved in the treatment of menopause (1970) and elevated cholesterol and triglyceride levels (1986). Each year the Japanese process approximately 150,00 tons of rice bran to generate 7,500 tons of gamma-oryzanol.

Food Sources

Ferulic acid compounds are widely distributed in nature, and ferulic acid esters are present in rice, wheat, barley, oats, tomatoes, asparagus, olives, berries, peas, vegetables, citrus fruits, and many other foods. It is in the bran portion of grains, which means whole-grain products contain significantly higher levels than processed grains like white rice and white flour. The concentration of ferulic acid is ten times higher in whole-wheat flour than in white flour (500 micrograms per gram versus 50 micrograms per gram).[1]

Deficiency Signs and Symptoms

No deficiency signs or symptoms have been reported.

Beneficial Effects

Gamma-oryzanol and ferulic acid are important antioxidants within plant cells. Both substances have exerted significant antioxidant effects in experimental models.[2-4] Because of gamma-oryzanol's potent antioxidant effects, it may be a possible aid in preventing the damaging effects of radiation exposure and/or chemotherapy[2] —anticancer effects have been noted in several animal studies.[5,6]

Gamma-oryzanol appears to act on the hypothalamus and pituitary gland. Many bodybuilders believe that gamma-oryzanol increases growth hormone secretion. In actuality, studies in animals show gamma-oryzanol inhibits the secretion of growth hormone.[7] Other pituitary and hypothalamic hormones that appear to be inhibited by gamma-oryzanol include thyroid-stimulating hormone (TSH), prolactin, and leutinizing hormone.[7–10] The overall significance of these effects has not been fully determined. It is interesting to note that gamma-oryzanol produces these effects on these control hormones yet does not appear to alter the level of the hormones they control. For example, while gamma-oryzanol (300 milligrams per day) lowered elevated TSH levels in hypothyroid patients, it did not affect thyroid hormone levels.[8] Gamma-oryzanol and ferulic acid have also displayed mild anti-inflammatory effects and anti-anxiety effects in animal models.[11,12]

Available Forms

Gamma-oryzanol is available in capsules and tablets and is used as an antioxidant in cosmetic preparations. Orally administered gamma-oryzanol is converted to free ferulic acid.[13] The cycloartenol ferulic acid fraction of gamma-oryzanol is apparently the most useful.[12]

Principal Uses

Gamma-oryzanol is used primarily in the treatment of menopause, elevated cholesterol levels, and various gastrointestinal complaints. Bodybuilders also use it for reasons outlined later in this chapter.

Menopause

Gamma-oryzanol was first shown to be effective in menopausal symptoms, including hot flashes, in the early 1960s.[14] Subsequent studies have further documented its effectiveness in menopause.[15] Its primary action is to reduce the secretion of leutinizing hormone (LH) by the pituitary and promote endorphin release by the hypothalamus.

In one of the earlier studies, 8 menopausal women and 13 women who had had their ovaries surgically removed were given 300 milligrams of gamma-oryzanol daily. At the end of the 38-day trial, over 67 percent of the women had a 50 percent or greater reduction in their menopausal symptoms.[14] In a more recent study, the benefits of a daily 300-milligram dose of gamma-oryzanol was even more effective—85 percent of the women reported improvement in their symptoms.[15]

Elevated Cholesterol Levels

Several studies indicate gamma-oryzanol is quite effective in lowering blood cholesterol and triglyceride levels.[16–18] In one study, 300 milligrams was given to 67 subjects with elevated cholesterol and/or triglyceride levels.[16] After 4 weeks, cholesterol levels declined by 8 to 12 percent, and the mean triglyceride level dropped from an average of 222 milligrams per deciliter to 190 milligrams per deciliter. Mild elevations in HDL were also reported.

Gamma-oryzanol's cholesterol-lowering action appears to involve a combination of effects. It increases the conversion of cholesterol to bile acids, increases bile acid excretion, and inhibits the absorption of cholesterol.[19,20]

Gastrointestinal Complaints

Clinical studies conducted in Japan demonstrate gamma-oryzanol is effective in the treatment of a broad range of gastrointestinal disorders, including peptic ulcers, gastritis, the irritable bowel syndrome, and nonspecific gastrointestinal complaints. Over 23 clinical studies have been conducted with gamma-oryzanol in the treatment of these conditions. Its mechanism of action is apparently normalization of nervous system control of digestive secretions.[21–27]

Bodybuilding

A number of small, poorly controlled studies found gamma-oryzanol increases lean body mass, increases strength, improves recovery from workouts, and reduces body fat and postexercise soreness. These studies spurred researchers to conduct studies under better controls to substantiate these effects of gamma-oryzanol. Two double-blind, well-controlled studies upheld the results from the previous studies.[28–30]

In the first double-blind study, weight lifters took either 30 milligrams of ferulic acid esters or a placebo daily for 8 weeks.[29] Body weight increased significantly for supplemented subjects (1.9 kilograms) but not for the placebo subjects. Strength as measured by one repetition of a shoulder press, chest press, and leg press increased in the supplemented group compared to the control group.

In the other double-blind study, stress hormone levels in the blood were measured before and after strenuous exercise in six well-trained male endurance runners when given either ferulic acid esters (50 milligrams daily) or a placebo.[30] When taking the ferulic acid, the subjects demonstrated significant increases in beta endorphin levels, which indicates that gamma-oryzanol appears to act on the hypothalamus. This effect is supported by animal research showing an effect on the hypothalamus.[7–9]

Dosage Ranges

The usual dosage of gamma-oryzanol for therapeutic purposes is 100 milligrams three times daily.

Safety Issues

Gamma-oryzanol is an extremely safe natural substance. No significant side effects have ever been produced in experimental and clinical studies. Animal studies have shown it to be very safe.[31,32]

Interactions

There are no known interactions with gamma-oryzanol and any nutrient or drug.

39

Glucosamine

The body manufactures glucosamine, a simple molecule composed of glucose and an amine (nitrogen and two molecules of hydrogen). Its physiological function on joints is to stimulate the manufacture of glycosaminoglycans, which are key structural components of cartilage. Glucosamine also promotes the incorporation of sulfur into cartilage. Because of this effect, glucosamine sulfate may be the best source of glucosamine.

The inability to manufacture glucosamine may be the major factor leading to osteoarthritis, the most common form of arthritis (also known as degenerative joint disease). This link led researchers in Europe to ask an important question: What would happen if individuals with osteoarthritis took glucosamine? The results are astonishing.

Food Sources

There are no food sources of glucosamine. Commercially available sources of glucosamine are derived from chitin, the specially processed exoskeleton of shrimp, lobsters, and crabs.

Deficiency Signs and Symptoms

It appears that as some people age, they lose the ability to manufacture sufficient levels of glucosamine. The result is that cartilage loses its ability to act as a shock absorber. The weight-bearing joints, like the knees, hips, and joints of the hands are those most often affected with osteoarthritis. In affected joints, there is much cartilage destruction followed by hardening and the formation of large bone spurs in the joint margins. Pain, deformity, and limitation of motion in the joint results.

The onset of osteoarthritis can be very subtle—morning joint stiffness is often the first symptom. As the disease progresses, there is pain on motion of the involved joint that is worsened by prolonged activity and relieved by rest.

Beneficial Effects

Glucosamine sulfate's beneficial effects are straightforward—it stimulates the manufacture of substances necessary for proper joint function and is responsible for stimulating joint repair.

Available Forms

Glucosamine is available as glucosamine sulfate, glucosamine hydrochloride, and N-acetyl-glucosamine. Glucosamine sulfate is the preferred form. Consumers should be aware that many companies marketing N-acetyl-glucosamine, commonly referred to as "NAG," try to mislead people into believing that NAG is better absorbed, more stable, and better utilized than glucosamine sulfate. These contentions are without support in the scientific literature; in fact, the literature indicates just the opposite. Glucosamine sulfate is clearly the preferred form.

Detailed human studies on the absorption, distribution, and elimination of orally administered glucosamine sulfate show an absorption rate as high as 98 percent. Once absorbed, it then travels primarily to joint tissues, where it is incorporated into the connective tissue matrix of cartilage, ligaments, and tendons.[1,2] In addition, there are impressive clinical studies on thousands of patients. In contrast, there has never been a double-blind study using NAG for any application, nor have there ever been any detailed absorption studies on NAG in humans.

Studies in laboratory animals offer further evidence of the superiority of glucosamine sulfate over NAG. Over the years, numerous researchers have repeatedly demonstrated that glucosamine is superior to NAG in terms of absorption and utilization by at least a factor of two to one.[3-14] These researchers have concluded that "glucosamine is a more efficient precursor of macromolecular hexosamine (glycosaminoglycans) than N-acetylglucosamine. It is possible that N-acetylglucosamine does not penetrate the cell membranes and, as a result, is not available for incorporation into glycoproteins and mucopolysaccharides."[5]

The absorption of NAG is questionable in humans for several reasons:

- NAG is quickly digested by intestinal bacteria.
- NAG is a known binder of dietary lectins in the gut with the resultant lectin-NAG complex being excreted in the feces.
- A large percentage of NAG is broken down by intestinal cells.

NAG differs from glucosamine sulfate in that instead of a sulfur molecule, NAG has a portion of an acetic acid molecule attached to it. Glucosamine sulfate and NAG are entirely different molecules and appear to be handled by the body differently. The body preferentially uses glucosamine sulfate instead of NAG. This preference is exhibited by the fact that the absorption of glucosamine sulfate is an active process.[15] In other words, there are mechanisms in the body that are designed specifically for the absorption and utilization of glucosamine sulfate. No such mechanisms exist for NAG.

It is highly unlikely that NAG possesses the same kind of antiarthritic and anti-inflammatory properties that glucosamine sulfate possesses.[16,17] In addition to the question of absorption, several studies have shown that the articular tissue is not able to utilize NAG as well as it does glucosamine sulfate. [4,5]

The marketing information on NAG often uses the term "slow acetylators" to describe a very small group of individuals with Crohn's disease and ulcerative colitis who are unable to convert glucosamine to NAG as fast as individuals without these diseases can. Glucosamine and NAG are necessary in the manufacture of mucin, the glycoprotein lining of the intestinal tract. Distributors of NAG mention only one study as evidence that NAG is better. The study demonstrated that when intestinal cells from patients with Crohn's disease or ulcerative colitis were bathed in a solution with a ratio of radioactive NAG to glucosamine of 10:1, the cells incorporated more NAG than the cells from individuals without these diseases.[18] These results are expected because the higher concentrations of NAG in the solution artificially promoted passive accumulation to a greater extent than the active accumulation of glucosamine. How distributors of NAG can then use this information to claim that NAG is better than glucosamine sulfate is puzzling. The significance of this "test tube" study is unclear, especially because other studies demonstrate an increased utilization of glucosamine in these patients.[19] The problem of acetylation of glucosamine is not a factor for most people because it is not a rate-limiting step in the manufacture of glycosaminoglycans (GAGs).

The other form of glucosamine on the market is glucosamine hydrochloride. As with NAG, the research simply does not support the use of glucosamine hydrochloride. It appears that the sulfur component of glucosamine sulfate may be critical to the beneficial effects noted. Sulfur is an essential nutrient for joint tissue, where it functions in the stabilization of the connective tissue matrix of cartilage, tendons, and ligaments. As far back as the 1930s, researchers demonstrated that individuals with arthritis are commonly deficient in this essential nutrient.[20] Restoring sulfur levels brought about significant benefit to these patients.[21] Therefore, it appears the sulfur portion of glucosamine sulfate is extremely important and is another reason why glucosamine sulfate is the preferred form of glucosamine. Table 39.1 gives you a summary of the properties of all three glucosamine forms.

TABLE 39.1   Comparison of Glucosamine Preparations

Activity	Glucosamine Sulfate	NAG	Glucosamine Hydrochloride
Active intestinal transport	Yes	No	Yes
Detailed absorption studies	Yes	No	No
Detailed clinical studies	Yes	No	No
Contains sulfur molecule	Yes	No	No
Long history of use	Yes	No	No

Principal Uses

The primary use for glucosamine sulfate is treatment of osteoarthritis. Osteoarthritis, or degenerative joint disease, is the most common form of arthritis. It is seen primarily, but not exclusively, in the elderly. Surveys indicate that over 40 million Americans have osteoarthritis, including 80 percent of persons over 50. Under 45, osteoarthritis is much more common in men; after 45, it is ten times more common in women than men.

The weight-bearing joints and joints of the hands are the joints most often affected by the degenerative changes associated with osteoarthritis. Specifically, there is much cartilage destruction followed by hardening and the formation of large bone spurs in the joint margins. Pain, deformity, and limitation of motion in the joint results. Inflammation is usually minimal.

The onset of osteoarthritis can be very subtle; morning joint stiffness is often the first symptom. As the disease progresses, there is pain on motion of the involved joint that is made worse by prolonged activity and relieved by rest. There are usually no signs of inflammation.

Glucosamine is a safe and effective natural alternative to aspirin and other non-steroidal anti-inflammatory drugs. Clinical and experimental research indicates that current drugs used in osteoarthritis treatment may be producing short-term benefit but are actually accelerating the progression of joint destruction. The first drug generally used in the treatment of osteoarthritis is aspirin. It is often quite effective in relieving both the pain and inflammation and is relatively inexpensive. However, since the therapeutic dose required is relatively high (2 to 4 grams per day), toxicity often occurs. Tinnitus (ringing in the ears) and gastric irritation are early manifestations of toxicity.

Other nonsteroidal anti-inflammatory drugs (NSAIDs) are often used, especially when aspirin is ineffective or intolerable. Representative of this class of drugs are buprofen (Motrin), fenoprofen (Nalfon), indomethacin (Indocin), naproxen (Naprosyn), tolmetin (Tolectin), and sulindac (Clinoril). These drugs are also associated with side effects that include gastrointestinal upset, headaches, and dizziness, and are therefore recommended for only short periods of time.

One side effect of aspirin and other NSAIDs often not mentioned is their inhibition of cartilage repair and acceleration of cartilage destruction.[22-24] Since osteoarthritis is caused by a degeneration of cartilage, NSAIDs possibly worsen the condition by inhibiting cartilage formation and accelerating cartilage destruction even though they are fairly effective in suppressing the symptoms. This has been upheld in clinical studies that show NSAIDs use is associated with acceleration of osteoarthritis and increased joint destruction.[25-27] Simply stated, aspirin and other NSAIDs appear to suppress the symptoms but accelerate the progression of osteoarthritis. Their use should be avoided.

Clinical Trials with Glucosamine Sulfate

Numerous double-blind studies have shown glucosamine sulfate produces much better results than NSAIDs and placebos in relieving the pain and inflammation of osteoarthritis despite the fact that it exhibits very little direct anti-inflammatory effect and no direct analgesic or pain-relieving effects.[28-34] While NSAIDs offer purely symptomatic relief and may actually promote the disease process, glucosamine sulfate appears to address the cause of osteoarthritis. By getting at the root of the problem, glucosamine sulfate not only improves the symptoms—including pain—but also helps the body repair damaged joints. This effect is outstanding, especially in light of glucosamine's safety and lack of side effects.

The beneficial results with glucosamine are more obvious the longer it is used. Because it is not an anti-inflammatory or pain-relieving drug *per se*, it takes a while longer than NSAIDs to produce results. But once it starts working, it produces much better results. For example, in one study that compared glucosamine sulfate to ibuprofen (the active ingredient of Motrin, Advil, and Nuprin), pain scores decreased faster in the first 2 weeks in the ibuprofen group; however, by week 4 the group receiving the glucosamine sulfate was doing significantly better than the ibuprofen group (see Figure 39.1).[32] Physicians rating the overall response as good or fair rated 44 percent of the glucosamine sulfate-treated patients as good compared to only 15 percent of the ibuprofen group.

In addition to showing benefit in double-blind studies, oral glucosamine sulfate offered significant benefit in an open trial involving 252 doctors and 1,506 patients in Portugal.[35] This large study provides valuable clinical information on the appropriate use of glucosamine sulfate. The patients received 500 milligrams of glucosamine sulfate three times daily over a mean period of 50 days. The results were analyzed and showed that the symptoms of pain at rest, on standing, on exercise, and on limited active and passive movements improved steadily throughout the treatment period. Objective therapeutic efficacy was rated by doctors as "good' in 59 percent of the patients and "sufficient" in a further 36 percent. Therefore, a total of 95 percent of the patients achieved benefit from glucosamine sulfate. The results with glucosamine sulfate were rated by both doctors and patients as being significantly better than those obtained with previous treatment, including NSAIDs, vitamin therapy, and cartilage extracts. Glucosamine sulfate produced good benefit in a significant portion of patients who had not responded to any other medical treatment.

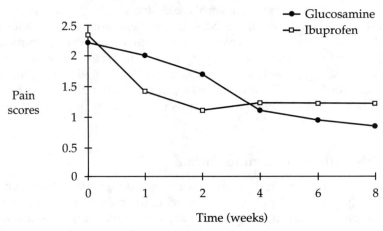

FIGURE 39.1   Glucosamine Sulfate versus Ibuprofen.

In the study, obesity was associated with a significant shift from good to fair. This finding may indicate that higher dosages may be required for obese individuals or that oral glucosamine is not enough to counteract the stress of obesity on the joints. Patients with peptic ulcers and individuals taking diuretics were also associated with a shift from good to sufficient in efficacy and tolerance. Individuals with current peptic ulcers should try and take glucosamine sulfate with foods. Individuals taking diuretics may need to increase the dosage to compensate for the reduced effectiveness.

The improvement with glucosamine lasted for a period of 6 to 12 weeks after the end of treatment. This result indicates that glucosamine may have to be taken for long periods of time or in repeated short-term courses. Given the safety and excellent tolerability of glucosamine, it is suitable for long-term, continuous use.

Glucosamine Sulfate versus Cartilage Extracts

Cartilage extracts, including purified chondroitin sulfate, sea cucumber, green-lipped mussel, and shark cartilage, are popular nutritional supplements that may also help osteoarthritis by improving cartilage function. However, these compounds differ in their degree of purity and in their effectiveness in osteoarthritis, particularly when compared to glucosamine sulfate.

Shark cartilage, sea cucumber, and green-lipped mussel contain a mixture of glycosaminoglycans (GAGs). One of the key GAGs is chondroitin sulfate. Chondroitin sulfate is composed of repeating units of glucosamine with attached sugar molecules. The difference between glucosamine sulfate, cartilage extracts, and chondroitin sulfate products is similar to the difference between crude ore (shark cartilage or chondroitin sulfate) and pure gold (glucosamine). While there is gold in crude ore, it is better to use the pure gold if you are trying to make jewelry. If you are trying to restore cartilage and joint structures, it is best to use glucosamine sulfate rather than chondroitin sulfate or shark cartilage.

This is the case because of the improved absorption and utilization of glucosamine sulfate. Cartilage extracts, shark cartilage, green-lipped mussel, sea cucumber, and chondroitin sulfate products are composed of large molecules that are extremely difficult to absorb. The absorption rate for chondroitin sulfate, the smallest molecule in these products, is estimated to be between 0 and 8 percent.[36] In contrast, detailed pharmacokinetic studies in animals and humans show up to 98 percent of orally administered glucosamine sulfate is absorbed.[1,2]

These pharmacokinetic studies indicate that after glucosamine sulfate is absorbed, it is preferentially taken up by cartilage and other joint structures where it simulates the manufacture of chondroitin sulfate and other mucopolysaccharides. One of its key effects is to also stimulate the incorporation of sulfur into cartilage.

While the effectiveness of oral glucosamine sulfate is highly documented, that of oral cartilage extracts, chondroitin sulfate, green-lipped mussel, sea cucumber, and shark cartilage in osteoarthritis is a subject of considerable debate. The positive clinical studies with glycosaminoglycan preparations used injectable forms. The use of pharmaceutical-grade cartilage preparations and chondroitin sulfate injections, according to established protocols, has well-documented benefit but fewer benefits than those attributed to glucosamine sulfate. All things considered, it is easy to see why glucosamine sulfate is preferred to cartilage extracts in the treatment of osteoarthritis.

Dosage Ranges

The standard dosage for glucosamine sulfate is 500 milligrams three times per day. Obese individuals may need higher dosages based on body weight (20 milligrams per kilogram body weight daily).

Safety Issues

Glucosamine sulfate has an excellent safety record in animal and human studies. Based on these studies, many experts recommend that glucosamine sulfate "be considered as a drug of choice for prolonged oral treatment of rheumatic disorders."[16] Side effects, when they do appear, are generally limited to light to moderate gastrointestinal symptoms, including stomach upset, heartburn, diarrhea, nausea, and indigestion. If these symptoms occur, try taking the glucosamine sulfate during a meal.

One question that often comes up when I am speaking to an audience is: I am allergic to sulfur; can I take glucosamine sulfate? When people say they are allergic to sulfur, what they really mean is they are allergic to the so-called sulfa drugs or sulfite-containing food additives. It is impossible to be allergic to sulfur because sulfur is an essential mineral. The sulfate form of sulfur is present in relatively high concentrations in human blood. In short, glucosamine sulfate is extremely well tolerated, and no allergic reactions have been reported.

Interactions

Individuals taking diuretics may need to take higher dosages (20 milligrams per kilogram body weight daily).

40

Lipoic Acid

Lipoic acid (also known thioctic acid) is a sulfur-containing, vitaminlike substance. It plays an important role as the necessary cofactor in two vital, energy-producing reactions in the production of cellular energy (ATP). Lipoic acid is not considered a vitamin because presumably either the body can usually manufacture sufficient levels or it is acquired in sufficient quantities from food. However, like many of the other compounds described in this section, a relative deficiency can occur in certain situations and its supplementation exerts benefits beyond its role in normal metabolism. Lipoic acid is an effective antioxidant. It is unique in that it is effective against both water- and fat-soluble free radicals.[1–5]

Food Sources

Liver and yeast are often listed as foods that are high in lipoic acid.

Deficiency Signs and Symptoms

Experimental studies in animals show that a deficiency of lipoic acid results in reduced muscle mass, failure to thrive, brain atrophy, and increased lactic acid accumulation. These studies provide a clue as to what would happen in human lipoic acid deficiency since such a deficiency state has not been demonstrated in humans. However, there are a number of conditions such as diabetes, cirrhosis, and heart disease where levels of lipoic acid are lower than normal.[1]

Beneficial Effects

Lipoic acid is involved in the conversion of carbohydrates to energy. When sugar is metabolized in the production of energy, it is converted to pyruvic acid. When there is plenty of oxygen available to the cell, the pyruvate is broken down by an enzyme complex that contains lipoic acid, thiamin, and niacin. When oxygen supply is low, the cell converts the pyruvic acid to lactic acid. During exercise, lactic acid tends to accumulate, especially if the activity is anaerobic (high intensity) versus aerobic (lower intensity). The accumulation of lactic acid leads to muscle fatigue.

Lipoic acid supplementation may help improve energy metabolism, especially in individuals with lower than normal levels (individuals with diabetes, liver cirrhosis, or heart disease). Lipoic acid supplementation may also help diabetics by facilitating better conversion of sugar into energy.

Lipoic acid is also a good antioxidant.[1] It possesses several unique features. First, because lipoic acid is both water- and fat-soluble, it is effective against a broader range of free radicals than vitamin C (water-soluble) and vitamin E (fat-soluble). At first it was thought that lipoic acid supplementation may be able to protect or help recycle other natural antioxidants such as vitamins C or E. However, a recent study in mice disputes this effect and now points out that lipoic acid itself can mimic the antioxidant effects of these nutrients. At 5 weeks on a vitamin E-deficient diet, mice exhibited similar decreases in tissue vitamin E levels whether supplemented or not supplemented with lipoic acid. However, while the mice not given lipoic acid displayed obvious symptoms of vitamin E deficiency, the mice given lipoic acid (1.65 grams per kilogram of body weight) did not demonstrate any signs or symptoms of vitamin E deficiency. These results indicate that although supplemental lipoic acid could not spare or regenerate tissue vitamin E levels, it could exert a vitamin E–like effect and relieve symptoms of vitamin E deficiency in mice.[6]

Available Forms

Lipoic acid is available in tablets and capsules. Because of its unique chemical properties, it is especially easy to absorb and assimilate.

Principal Uses

The principal uses of lipoic acid are in the treatment of diabetes and AIDS. Other possible uses include liver cirrhosis, heart disease, cataracts, heavy-metal toxicity, and detoxification support.

There are still many questions about lipoic acid supplementation, such as, How does the antioxidant protection offered by lipoic acid supplementation compare to other (less expensive) antioxidants? Until these questions are answered, I am reluctant to recommend lipoic acid supplementation except in patients with AIDS and in diabetics who have not fully responded to other nutritional support or who are exhibiting signs of diabetic neuropathy.

Diabetes

Lipoic acid is an approved drug in Germany for the treatment of diabetic neuropathy. Although several studies show high-dose lipoic acid supplementation (600 milligrams daily) improves diabetic neuropathy, it is not known how much better lipoic acid supplementation is than less expensive options.[7] Results from a recent study indicate that it may not be any more effective.[8]

In that study, 80 patients affected with diabetic neuropathy were randomized and arranged into four groups. Each day for 3 months patients either received a placebo (a control group), 600 milligrams of lipoic acid, 100 micrograms of selenium (sodium selenite), or 1,200 International Units of vitamin E (D-alpha-tocopherol). In comparison with the control group, all other groups treated with antioxidants showed significantly diminished serum concentrations of free-radical byproducts and urinary albumin excretion rates (indicating improved kidney function). The symptoms of diabetic neuropathy also improved in a highly significant manner in all treated groups. The results prove that oxidative stress plays a promoting role in development of long-term diabetic late complications and that a therapy with adjuvant antioxidants may lead to a regression of diabetic late complications. However, the study failed to justify the high cost of lipoic acid over the less expensive and equally effective nutritional antioxidants.

Lipoic acid's primary effect in improving diabetic neuropathy is a result of its antioxidant effects. However, studies show it also leads to an improvement in blood sugar metabolism, reduces glycosylation of proteins, improves blood flow to peripheral nerves, and actually stimulates the regeneration of nerve fibers.[9–12] Its ability to improve blood sugar metabolism is a result of its effects on glucose metabolism and an ability to increase insulin sensitivity. Diabetics taking insulin or blood sugar–lowering drugs are cautioned that lipoic acid supplementation can result in changes in dosage requirements. Close monitoring of blood sugar levels is required.

AIDS

Several studies show that individuals infected with the human immunodeficiency virus (HIV) have a compromised antioxidant defense system. Blood antioxidants are decreased and peroxidation products of lipids and proteins are increased in these patients. This blood profile may contribute to the progression of AIDS because antioxidants such as glutathione prevent viral replication while reactive oxidants tend to stimulate the virus. Consequently, it was suggested that HIV-infected patients may benefit from antioxidant supplementation therapy involving lipoic acid.

To test this hypothesis, a small pilot study was designed to determine the short-term effect of lipoic acid supplementation (150 milligrams three times daily) in HIV-positive patients.[13] Lipoic acid supplementation increased plasma ascorbate in nine of ten patients, total glutathione in seven of seven patients, total plasma sulfur groups in eight of nine patients, and T helper lymphocytes and T helper/suppressor cell ratio in six of ten patients. The lipid peroxidation product malondialdehyde decreased in eight of nine patients. The results of this pilot study indicated that lipoic supplementation led to significant beneficial changes in the blood of HIV-infected patients. Hopefully, larger double-blind studies will support these encouraging results.

Studies indicate lipoic acid also significantly inhibits the replication of HIV by reducing the activity of reverse transcriptase (the enzyme responsible for manufacturing the virus from the DNA of lymphocytes) and inhibits the activator in HIV that leads to viral replication.[14,15]

Dosage Ranges

For general antioxidant support, the recommended dosage is 20 to 50 milligrams daily. In the treatment of diabetes, the recommended dosage is 300 to 600 milligrams daily. In the treatment of AIDS, the recommended dosage is 150 milligrams three times daily.

Safety Issues

Lipoic acid supplementation is apparently very safe. There are no reports of adverse effects in over three decades of use in the treatment of diabetic neuropathy. In addition, animal studies show it has very low toxicity.

Interactions

Lipoic acid supplementation may spare vitamins C and E and other antioxidants. Lipoic acid works synergistically with thiamin and niacin in cellular energy production. As mentioned above, lipoic acid supplementation may improve blood sugar control in diabetes and thus allow a reduction in the dosage of insulin or oral blood sugar–lowering drugs.

41

Medium-Chain Triglycerides

Medium-chain triglycerides (MCTs) are special types of saturated fats prepared from coconut oil and range in length from 6 to 12 carbon chains. MCTs are used by the body differently than the long-chain triglycerides (LCTs), which are the most abundant fats found in nature. LCTs are the storage fat for both humans and plants and range in length from 18 to 24 carbons. This difference in length makes all the difference in how MCTs and LCTs are absorbed and utilized.

Food Sources

There are no significant food sources of MCTs.

Deficiency Signs and Symptoms

MCTs are not associated with any deficiency signs or symptoms.

Beneficial Effects

MCTs are an easily absorbed energy source and are a popular aid for weight loss.[1] Unlike regular fats, MCTs do not appear to cause weight gain—they actually promote weight loss by increasing the rate at which calories burn (thermogenesis). In contrast, the LCTs are usually stored in fat deposits; and since their energy is conserved, a high-fat diet actually decreases the metabolic rate. The reason for the difference in how the body handles MCTs and LCTs is size. The larger LCTs are difficult for the body to metabolize, so the body wants to store these fats. MCTs, on the other hand, are rapidly burned as energy and actually promote the burning of LCTs.[2]

A friend of mine, Dr. Julian Whitaker, has an interesting analogy: "LCTs are like heavy wet logs that you put on a small campfire. Keep adding the logs, and soon you have more logs than fire. MCTs are like rolled-up newspaper soaked in gasoline. They not only burn brightly, but will burn up the wet logs as well." Scientific studies appear to support Dr. Whitaker's view.

Available Forms

Your health-food store carries MCTs. Several companies add an orange flavor, and typically, these products cost approximately $11 to $12 for a 16-ounce bottle. Sound Nutrition, Inc., a company based in Dover, Idaho, has developed a patent-pending method of flavoring MCTs. Their product, Thin Oil, is available in Original, Buttery Flavored, Olive Oil Flavored, and Garlic Flavored flavors. Thin Oil can be used in salad dressings, as a bread spread, over pasta and popcorn, and in baked goods. Thin Oil is available in some health-food stores and directly from the company (1-800-844-6645).

Principal Uses

In addition to its use as a weight-loss aid, MCTs are used in the treatment of epilepsy and provide an easily absorbed energy source for people with malabsorption syndromes.

Weight Loss

Again, MCTs promote thermogenesis. One study compared the thermogenic effect of a high-calorie diet containing 40 percent fat as MCTs with one containing 40 percent fat as LCTs.[3] The thermogenic effect (calories wasted 6 hours after a meal) of the MCTs was almost twice as high as the LCTs—120 calories versus 66 calories. The researchers concluded that the excess energy provided by fats in the form of medium-chain triglycerides is not efficiently stored as fat and is therefore burned. A follow-up study demonstrated that MCT oil given over a 6-day period can increase diet-induced thermogenesis by 50 percent.[4]

In another study, researchers compared single meals of 400 calories composed entirely of MCTs or LTCs.[5] The thermogenic effect of MCTs over 6 hours was three times greater than that of LCTs. In addition, while the LCTs elevated blood fat levels by 68 percent, MCTs had no effect on the blood fat level. Researchers concluded that substituting MCTs for LCTs produces weight loss as long as the calorie level remains the same.

Malabsorption Syndromes

For almost 50 years, MCTs have been used in the treatment of malabsorption syndromes.[1] Unlike LCTs, MCTs do not require pancreatic enzymes and bile acids to be absorbed. Conditions associated with malabsorption where MCTs have been used with success in adults, children, and newborns are:

- **Disorders of Fat Digestion**   Major or total surgical resection of the esophagus or of the stomach, biliary atresia, obstructive jaundice, primary biliary cirrhosis, blind-loop syndrome, pancreatitis, cystic fibrosis, and pancreatomy
- **Disorders of Lipid Absorption**   Massive surgical resection of the small bowel, celiac disease, Whipple's disease, Crohn's disease, enteritis, tropical sprue, and malabsorption in neonates
- **Disorders of Lipid Transport**   Congenital beta-lipoprotein synthesis and lymphatic disorders because of engorgement or leakage

If you have a condition associated with malabsorption, please ask your doctor about the appropriateness of MCTs as an energy source.

Epilepsy

The ketogenic diet has been used in the treatment of epilepsy since the 1920s.[6,7] A ketogenic diet consists of large amounts of fat and minimal amounts of protein and carbohydrate. The low carbohydrate intake inhibits fat metabolism and results in the production of excessive levels of ketone bodies (acetone, acetoacetic acid, and beta-hydroxybutyric acid), the intermediary oxidation products. Presumably the beneficial effects of such a diet result from its induction of metabolic acidosis, which corrects an underlying tendency of epileptics toward spontaneous development of alkalosis. This acidification is thought to normalize nerve conductivity, irritability, and membrane permeability.

Although the ketogenic diet is effective, it is not without side effects. The long-term risks of a high-fat diet are well known, and a ketogenic diet is unhealthy for a growing child. However, the ketogenic does have its place in the treatment of intractable (unresponsive to treatment) epilepsy. MCTs can be substituted for LCTs in the ketogenic diet.[8]

Dosage Ranges

A good dosage recommendation for MCTs as a weight-loss aid is 1 to 2 tablespoons per day. MCTs can be used as an oil for salad dressing, a bread spread, or simply taken as a supplement. They can be used in cooking as long as the temperature is not greater than 160 degrees. For other medicinal effects of MCTs, please consult a physician for dosage recommendations.

Safety Issues

MCTs are generally regarded as safe and have a good safety record in clinical studies. However, diabetics and individuals with liver disease should not use MCTs unless under a doctor's supervision because a high intake of MCTs may lead to acidosis in these cases.

Interactions

No interactions are known for MCTs with any nutrient or drug.

42

Melatonin

Melatonin became an overnight sensation after it was featured as the cover story in the August 7, 1995, issue of *Newsweek*. The article discussed the potential of melatonin to relieve insomnia, jet lag, stress, and depression; fight cancer; boost the immune system; prevent heart disease; and act as an antioxidant. The *Newsweek* article was followed by a mad rush to health-food stores to buy this "wonder pill." However, some caution appears warranted.

Melatonin (not to be confused with melanin, the compound responsible for skin pigment) is a hormone manufactured from serotonin and secreted by the pineal gland. The pineal gland, a small pea-sized gland at the base of the brain, has been a source of curiosity since antiquity. The ancient Greeks considered the pineal gland the seat of the soul, a concept that was extended by the philosopher Descartes. In the seventeenth and eighteenth centuries physicians associated "madness" with the pineal gland. Physicians in the early 1900s believed the pineal gland was somehow involved with the endocrine system. The identification of melatonin in 1958 provided the first solid scientific evidence of an essential role of the pineal gland. Scientists now believe that the sole function of the pineal gland is to manufacture and secrete melatonin.

Although the exact function of melatonin is still poorly understood, we do know it is critically involved in the synchronization of hormone secretion. The natural biorhythm of hormone secretion is referred to as the "circadian" rhythm. The human body is governed by an internal clock that signals the secretion of various hormones at different times to regulate body functions. Melatonin plays a key role as the biological timekeeper of hormone secretion. It also helps control periods of sleepiness and wakefulness. Release of melatonin is stimulated by darkness and suppressed by light.

The antidepressant effect of light therapy in the treatment of seasonal affective disorder is probably a result of balancing the altered circadian rhythm by restoring proper melatonin synthesis and secretion by the pineal gland. Disruption of pineal function may be a major reason for seasonal affective disorder and jet lag.[1,2]

Beneficial Effects

In addition to its role in synchronizing hormone secretion, melatonin can possess antioxidant effects.[3] This action may explain the studies in rats that show melatonin supplementation leads to longer lives (31 months versus 25 months). However, the clinical significance of melatonin's antioxidant effects has not been fully determined. It is hard to imagine that its antioxidant effects are greater than vitamin C, vitamin E, and a host of other antioxidants that can be delivered at much higher concentrations. Studies indicate melatonin also exerts some anticancer effects.

Available Forms

Melatonin is available in tablet, capsule, and sublingual tablet forms. There is no definitive evidence that any of these forms is substantially superior to another, although an argument could be made in favor of the sublingual form.

Principal Uses

The primary uses of melatonin are in the treatment of jet lag and insomnia, and as an adjunct in cancer therapy. It also plays a role in depression.

Jet Lag

Several double-blind studies show melatonin is very effective in relieving jet lag.[4-7] Researchers have recommended different dosages. Some have recommended that people begin taking melatonin a few days before departure (especially when traveling eastward) at the beginning of the sleep period. Others have recommended taking melatonin just one time on the first evening upon arrival at the new destination. The latter recommendation avoids the extreme drowsiness problem sometimes produced by melatonin when it is taken at an unwanted time.

A recent study examined the question of optimal timing of melatonin supplementation.[8] In the study, 52 members of an airline cabin crew flying an international route were randomly assigned to three groups: early melatonin (5 milligrams started 3 days prior to arrival until 5 days after the return home), late melatonin (a placebo for 3 days then 5 milligrams of melatonin for 5 days at the new destination), and placebo. Daily ratings in jet lag, mood, and sleepiness measures demonstrated the best recovery in the late melatonin group. The early melatonin group actually demonstrated worse recovery than the placebo group. This study suggests the best way to use melatonin for jet lag is 5 milligrams in the evening at the new destination for 5 days.

Insomnia

Melatonin plays an important role in the induction of sleep. Low melatonin secretion at night can be a cause of insomnia. Several double-blind trials show melatonin supplementation is very effective in promoting sleep.[9–13] However, it appears the sleep-promoting effects of melatonin supplementation are most apparent if melatonin levels are low.[14] In other words, melatonin supplementation is not like taking a sleeping pill. It produces its effects only when melatonin levels are low. When melatonin is given just before going to bed in normal subjects or in patients with insomnia that have normal melatonin levels, it produces no sedative effect. That is because normally just prior to going to bed there is a rise in melatonin secretion. Melatonin supplementation is only effective as a sedative when the pineal gland's own production of melatonin is very low. However, low melatonin levels are an extremely common cause of insomnia in the elderly.[15]

Cancer

Melatonin can inhibit several types of cancers, particularly hormonally related cancers like breast cancer and prostate cancer.[16] It can inhibit both the initiation and promotion of cancer. It has been theorized that the increased cancer incidence reported in individuals living and/or working in an environment where they are exposed to higher-than-normal artificial electromagnetic fields may be caused by suppression of melatonin synthesis.[17] The exposure of humans or animals to light (visible electromagnetic radiation) at night rapidly depresses pineal melatonin production and blood melatonin levels. Likewise, the exposure of animals to various pulsed static and extremely low-frequency magnetic fields also reduces melatonin levels. Reduction of melatonin by artificial electromagnetic field exposure may be a significant risk factor for cancer.

Clinical trials in cancer patients indicate melatonin also exerts anticancer effects. In these studies, melatonin was given at moderate dosage (10 milligrams daily) to extremely high dosage (greater than 40 milligrams daily). Melatonin has most often been used in combination with other anticancer agents, including interleukin 2 and interferon. The results are extremely promising.

While interferon and interleukin 2 (IL-2) are often ineffective when used alone, in combination with melatonin they exhibit very good results. For example, in one study in patients with advanced solid neoplasms 80 patients received either IL-2 alone (3 million International Units per day 6 days a week for 4 weeks) or in combination with melatonin (40 milligrams per day orally at 8:00 P.M.).[18] A complete response was obtained in 3 out of 41 patients treated with IL-2 plus melatonin and in none of the patients receiving IL-2 alone. A partial response was achieved in 8 out of 41 patients treated with IL-2 and melatonin compared to only 1 in the IL-2-only group. The survival rate after 1 year was 19 out of 41 in the IL-2 and melatonin group compared to only 6 out of 30 in the IL-2 group. In another study of 100 patients with metastatic solid tumors, for whom no standard therapy was available, the percentage of survival at 1 year was significantly higher in patients treated with IL-2 and melatonin than in those receiving the supportive care alone (21 out of 52 versus 5 out of 48).[19]

Similar results have been shown with melatonin in combination with interferon, tumor necrosis factor, and tamoxifen, and when melatonin was used alone.[20–25] These preliminary results are quite encouraging because approximately 30 percent of the patients taking anywhere from 10 to 50 milligrams daily (at 8:00 P.M.) experienced improvements in survival time and quality-of-life assessments.

However, although melatonin can increase survival time in these studies, the results are good but not earth-shattering. For example, in one study of patients with solid tumors with brain metastasis, 15 out of 24 patients (63 percent) died within 1 year in the melatonin group compared to 21 out of 26 (88 percent) in the group receiving supportive care only. These studies, although randomized, are not double-blind; therefore, a placebo response may be partially responsible for some of the improvements noted.

Depression

Initial studies performed in the 1980s demonstrated that melatonin levels are typically below normal in patients with clinical depression.[26–28] However, in all these studies it turned out that antidepressant drugs or other factors were responsible for the depressed melatonin levels. More recent studies do not support the association of low melatonin levels and clinical depression.[29] These studies measured melatonin levels in drug-free, depressed patients and were careful to match these subjects with a control group. In addition, other studies demonstrate that normal subjects secreting no melatonin do not frequently suffer from depression.[1]

Initially it was thought that melatonin may affect mood as a result of reduced cortisol levels. The melatonin would inhibit the secretion of the pituitary hormone ACTH, which would then signal the adrenal glands to secrete cortisol. With melatonin deficiency, cortisol levels would be expected to be increased. This is apparently the case in many depressed patients because both decreased melatonin and increased cortisol concentrations are frequently found.[29–31] However, it is unlikely that melatonin supplementation can significantly reduce cortisol levels; research shows melatonin supplementation does not suppress either ACTH or cortisol secretion.[32]

What all this data indicates is that melatonin is unlikely to produce any significant positive effects in the treatment of depression in most patients. Clinical research seems to bear this out. In fact, one double-blind study conducted in 1973 demonstrated that melatonin supplementation actually dramatically worsened clinical depression in some cases.[33] Obviously, worsening of depression is quite serious because it increases the risk for suicide. A possible explanation for the worsening is the melatonin was given two to four times during the day—a time when melatonin levels are typically low. Another study in nondepressed subjects demonstrated that when melatonin was given during the day, it tended to cause fatigue, confusion, and sleepiness.[34]

Dosage Ranges

Melatonin is appropriate for supplementation when low melatonin levels are suspected, as occurs in some cases of insomnia and jet lag. The amount of melatonin necessary to produce benefit in these cases is largely unknown. A dosage of 3 milligrams at bedtime is more than enough—dosages as low as 0.1 milligrams and 0.3 milligrams can produce a sedative effect when melatonin levels are low.[35] Higher dosages may be required to produce the anticancer benefits noted above.

Safety Issues

Although there appear to be no serious side effects at recommended dosages, conceivably melatonin supplementation could disrupt the normal circadian rhythm. The dosages recommended are much greater than the 24-hour urinary excretion rate for melatonin (approximately 0.03 milligrams).[36] In one study, a daily dosage of 8 milligrams a day for only 4 days resulted in significant alteration in circadian rhythm.[32] No one knows what sort of effect occurs at commonly recommended dosages (3 milligrams). In addition, in some cases of depression the patients got much worse when they were given melatonin during the day.

Interactions

Vitamin B_{12} can influence melatonin secretion.[37] The low levels of melatonin in the elderly may be a result of low vitamin B_{12} status. Vitamin B_{12} (1.5 milligrams of methylcobalamin per day) can produce good results in the treatment of sleep-wake rhythm disorders presumably because of improved melatonin secretion.[38]

43

Phosphatidylserine

Phosphatidylserine is the major phospholipid in the brain that plays a major role in determining the integrity and fluidity of cell membranes. Normally the brain can manufacture sufficient levels of phosphatidylserine; however, if there is a deficiency of methyl donors like SAM, folic acid, and vitamin B_{12}, or essential fatty acids, the brain may not be able to make sufficient phosphatidylserine.

Food Sources

There are trace amounts of phosphatidylserine in soy lecithin.

Deficiency Signs and Symptoms

Low levels of phosphatidylserine in the brain are associated with impaired mental function and depression in the elderly.

Beneficial Effects

Phosphatidylserine supplementation in animal studies and human clinical trials has significantly improved acetylcholine release, memory, and age-related brain changes.[1-3]

Available Forms

In the United States, phosphatidylserine is available in a complex containing the following: phosphatidylserine, 100 milligrams; phosphatidylcholine, 45 milligrams; phosphatidylethanolamine, 25 milligrams; phosphatidylinositol, 5 milligrams. Commercially available phosphatidylserine is a semi-synthetic product manufactured from soy lecithin. Originally, phosphatidylserine was isolated from bovine (beef) brain.

Principal Uses

The primary use of phosphatidylserine is in the treatment of depression and/or impaired mental function in the elderly. Very good results have been obtained in numerous double-blind studies.[4–9] In the largest double-blind study, a total of 494 elderly patients (between 65 and 93 years of age), with moderate to severe senility were given either phosphatidylserine or a placebo for 6 months.[4] The patients were assessed for mental performance, behavior, and mood at the beginning and the end of the study. Statistically significant improvements were noted in the phosphatidylserine-treated group in mental function, mood, and behavior.

In a double-blind study of depressed elderly patients, phosphatidylserine improved depressive symptoms, memory, and behavior.[9] Unlike typical antidepressant drugs, phosphatidylserine promoted this improvement without influencing the levels of serotonin and other monoamine neurotransmitters, suggesting another mechanism of action. Improved brain cell membrane fluidity may be one explanation. Another is the fact that phosphatidylserine can reduce cortisol secretion in response to stress.[10–12] Typically cortisol levels are elevated in depressed patients.

Despite these impressive results, rarely do I recommend phosphatidylserine supplementation. The reason? The price. A month's dose of 100 milligrams phosphatidylserine three times per day costs about $75 per month. As phosphatidylserine develops greater popularity, I hope this price comes down. In the meantime, what I recommend to my elderly patients who are depressed or have impaired mental function is to take *Ginkgo biloba* extract and supplement the diet with the necessary nutrients their brains need to manufacture phosphatidylserine—essential fatty acid (particularly the omega-3 oils; I recommend flaxseed oil), folic acid (minimum 800 micrograms daily), vitamin B_{12} (minimum 800 micrograms daily), and vitamin C (minimum 1,000 milligrams daily).

The extract of *Ginkgo biloba* leaves, standardized to contain 24 percent ginkgo flavone glycosides and 6 percent terpenoids, demonstrates remarkable effects in improving many symptoms associated with aging. It can help delay and in some cases reverse the mental deterioration in the early stages of Alzheimer's disease. For a while, *Ginkgo biloba* extract may help enable the patient maintain a normal life and stay away from being put in a nursing home. In one study, 40 patients with a preliminary diagnosis of senile dementia of the Alzheimer's type received either 80 milligrams of *Ginkgo biloba* extract or placebo three times daily for 3 months. Patients were assessed by standard tests and brain wave studies (EEG tracings) at baseline and at 1, 2, and 3 months. Results indicated that *Ginkgo biloba* extract improved all parameters, usually in the first month, compared to the placebo. Consistent with other studies with *Ginkgo biloba* extract, the longer *Ginkgo biloba* extract is used, the more obvious the benefits become. *Ginkgo biloba* extract was well tolerated, and no side effects were noted in the trial.[13]

Dosage Ranges

The standard dosage recommendation for phosphatidylserine is 100 milligrams three times daily.

Safety Issues

No side effects or adverse interactions have been noted.

44

Probiotics

Probiotics, literally meaning "for life," is a term used to signify the health-promoting effects of "friendly bacteria." There are at least 400 different species of microflora in the human gastrointestinal tract. The most important friendly bacteria are *Lactobacillus acidophilus* and *Bifidobacterium bifidum*. Therefore, this chapter focuses on the principal uses of commercial probiotic supplements containing either or both *L. acidophilus* and *B. bifidum* as well as fructo-oligosaccharides.

Foods fermented with *Lactobacilli* have been, and still are, of great importance to the diets of most of the world's people. Most cultures use some form of fermented food in their diet such as yogurt, cheese, miso, and tempeh. The symbiotic relationship between humankind and *Lactobacilli* has a long history of important nutritional and therapeutic benefits for humans.

At the turn of the century, noted Russian scientist Elie Metchnikoff believed that yogurt was the elixir of life.[1] His theory was that putrefactive bacteria in the large intestine produce toxins that invite disease and shorten life. He believed that the eating of yogurt would cause the lactobacilli to become dominant in the colon and displace the putrefactive bacteria. For years, these claims of healthful effects from fermented foods were considered unscientific folklore. However, a substantial and growing body of scientific evidence demonstrates that *Lactobacilli* and fermented foods play a significant role in human health.

Humans are not born with *Lactobacilli* in their gastrointestinal tract. Colonization of gram-positive *Lactobacilli* begins after birth, when there is a dramatic increase in their concentration. *B. bifidum* is first introduced through breast feeding to the sterile gut of the infant, and large numbers are soon observed in the feces. Later, other bacteria (including such beneficial strains as *L. casei, L. fermentum, L. salivores, L. brevis,* etc.) become established in the gut through contact with the world. Unfortunately, potentially toxic bacteria also eventually cultivate the colon.[2] The *Lactobacilli* in the human intestine are:

- *L. acidophilus*
- *L. bifidus (Bifidobacterium bifidum)*

- *L. brevis*
- *L. casei*
- *L. cellobiosus*
- *L. fermenti*
- *L. leichmannii*
- *L. plantarum*
- *L. salivaroes*

Available Forms

In order to provide benefit, products containing *L. acidophilus* and *B. bifidum* must provide these organisms in a manner in which they can survive the hostile environment of the gastrointestinal tract. Several factors such as species, strain, adherence, growth media, and diet are involved in successful colonization.[3,4] Typically, a high-quality commercial preparation produces greater colonization than simply eating yogurt. One of the key reasons is that yogurt is usually made with *L. bulgaricus* or *Streptococcus thermophilus*. While these two bacteria are friendly and possess some health benefits, they are only transient visitors to the gastrointestinal tract and do not colonize the colon.

Proper manufacturing, packaging, and storing of the product is necessary to ensure viability, the right amount of moisture, and freedom from contamination. *Lactobacilli* are easily damaged by freeze-drying (lyophilization), spray drying, or conventional frozen storage. Excessive temperature during packaging or storage can dramatically reduce viability. Also, unless the product is stable, refrigeration is necessary. Some products do not have to be refrigerated until after the bottle has been opened.

While there are a number of excellent companies that provide high-quality probiotic products, it is difficult to sort through all the manufacturers' claims of superiority—and some products contain no active *L. acidophilus*. In fact, one study conducted at the University of Washington concluded "Most of the *Lactobacilli*-containing products currently available (1990) either do not contain the *Lactobacillus* species advertised and/or contain other bacteria of questionable benefit."[5]

I feel most confident when I recommend products that have been developed by Professor Khem M. Shahani, Ph.D., of the University of Nebraska. Dr. Shahani is considered the world's foremost expert on probiotics and is the developer of the DDS-1 strain of *L. acidophilus*—often referred to as the "super-strain" because it exerts benefits far greater than the more than 200 strains of *L. acidophilus*. Dr. Shahani has authored over 190 scientific studies on the role of *Lactobacilli* in human health and has personally endorsed several products available in health-food stores.

Principal Uses

The intestinal flora plays a major role in the host's health.[2-4,6] The intestinal flora is intimately involved in the host's nutritional status and affects immune system function, cholesterol metabolism, carcinogenesis, and aging. Due to the importance of *L. acidophilus and B. bifidum* to human health, probiotic supplements can be used to promote overall good health. There are several specific uses for probiotics, however. The five primary areas of use discussed here are promotion of proper intestinal environment, postantibiotic therapy, vaginal yeast infections, urinary tract infections, and cancer prevention.

Promotion of Proper Intestinal Environment

Lactobacilli have long been noted for the role they play in the prevention of and defense against diseases, particularly those of the gastrointestinal tract and vagina. As part of the "normal flora," they inhibit the growth of other organisms through competition for nutrients, alteration of pH and oxygen tension to levels less favorable to pathogens (disease-causing organisms), prevention of attachment of pathogens by physically covering attachment sites, and production of limiting factors such as antimicrobial factors.[2–4,6]

Lactobacilli produce a variety of substances that inhibit or antagonize other bacteria. These include metabolic end products such as organic acids (lactic and acetic acid), hydrogen peroxide, and compounds known as bacteriocins.[7–18] Although some researchers have isolated substances from *Lactobacilli* that they labeled antibiotics, these are probably more accurately described as bacteriocins. Bacteriocins, proteins that are produced by certain bacteria, exert a lethal effect on closely related bacteria. In general, bacteriocins have a narrower range of activity than antibiotics but are often more lethal.

Some of the antimicrobial activity of *L. acidophilus* happens because of hydrogen peroxide.[17,18] However, this reaction requires folic acid and riboflavin, which, if in short supply, reduces hydrogen peroxide (H_2O_2) production. Some researchers believe the antimicrobial activity also occurs because of immune-system stimulation.[19–24]

Bacteria inhibited by *L. acidophilus* are:

- *Bacillus subtilis*
- *B. cereus*
- *B. stearothermophilus*
- *Candida albicans*
- *Clostridium perfringens*
- *Escherichia coli*
- *Klebsiella pneumoniae*
- *L. bulgaricus*
- *L. fermenti*
- *L. helveticus*
- *L. lactis*
- *L. leichmannii*
- *L. plantarum*
- *Proteus vulgaris*

- *Pseudomonas aeruginosa*
- *P. flourescens*
- *Salmonella typhosa*
- *S. schottmuelleri*
- *Shigella dysenteriae*
- *S. paradysenteriae*
- *Sarcina lutea*
- *Serratia marcescens*
- *Staphylococcus aureus*
- *Streptococcus faecalis*
- *S. lactis*
- *Vibrio comma*

The earliest reported therapeutic uses of *L. acidophilus* in the 1920s suggested that their proliferation was associated with a concomitant decrease in potentially harmful coliform bacteria. This effect has since been confirmed.[25–27] However, because of inappropriate strains and problems in production, storage, and distribution to consumers, many of the earlier commercial products were less reliable than those used in later published clinical trials.[28]

Fructo-oligosaccharides

Food components that may help promote the growth of friendly bacteria include fructo-oligosaccharides (FOS). These short-chain polysaccharides are just now entering the U.S. market. However, in Japan the number of consumer products containing purified FOS reached 450 in 1991. In 1990, the Japanese market for FOS exceeded $46 million.[29]

FOS is not digested by humans. Instead, it feeds the friendly bacteria. Human studies show FOS increases *Bifidobacteria* and *Lactobacilli* while simultaneously reducing the colonies of detrimental bacteria. Other benefits noted with FOS supplementation: increased production of beneficial short-chain fatty acids like butyrate; improved liver function; reduction of serum cholesterol and blood pressure; and improved elimination of toxic compounds.[29,30]

The dosage recommendation for pure FOS is 2,000 to 3,000 milligrams daily. Natural food sources of FOS include Jerusalem artichokes, onions, asparagus, and garlic. However, the estimated average daily ingestion of FOS from food sources is estimated to be 800 milligrams. Thus, the supplementation of FOS may help boost FOS intake and promote the growth of friendly bacteria, especially *Bifidobacteria*.[30]

Postantibiotic Therapy

Acidophilus supplementation is particularly important for preventing and treating antibiotic-induced diarrhea, *Candida* overgrowth, and urinary tract infections. *L. acidophilus* can correct the increase of gram-negative bacteria observed following the administration of broad-spectrum antibiotics or that occurs with any acute or chronic diarrhea.[2–4,31–33] Similarly, a mixture of *Bifidobacterium bifidum* and *L. acidophilus* inhibits the lowering of fecal flora induced by ampicillin and maintains the equilibrium of the intestinal ecosystem.[31]

Although it is commonly believed that acidophilus supplements are not effective if taken during antibiotic therapy, research actually supports the use of *L. acidophilus* during antibiotic administration.[31,32] Reductions of friendly bacteria and/or superinfection with antibiotic-resistant flora may be prevented by administering *L. acidophilus* products during antibiotic therapy. A dosage of at least 15 to 20 billion organisms is required. I recommend taking the probiotic supplement as long after taking the antibiotic as possible.

Yeast Infections

L. acidophilus can retard the growth of *Candida albicans*, the major yeast involved in vaginal yeast infections.[34] Clinical studies suggest that the introduction of yogurt or *Lactobacilli* to the vagina can assist in clearing up and preventing recurrent vaginal yeast infections and bacterial vaginosis.[35]

L. acidophilus is a normal constituent of the vaginal flora, where it contributes to the maintenance of the acid pH by fermenting vaginal glycogen to lactic acid.[36–39] Research shows that suppression of *L. acidophilus* by broad-spectrum antibiotics leads to the overgrowth of yeast and other bacteria.[40]

Reestablishment of normal vaginal *Lactobacilli* can be accomplished by douching twice a day with an *acidophilus*-containing solution. The solution is best prepared by using a high-quality *acidophilus* supplement or active-culture yogurt. Dissolve enough of either choice in 10 milliliters of water to provide 10^8 live organisms per milliliter. Use a syringe to douche the material into the vagina. Since *Lactobacilli* are normal inhabitants of the vaginal flora, the douche can be retained in the vagina as long as desired.

Urinary Tract Infection

One of the problems with antibiotic therapy for urinary tract infections (bladder infections) is that the disturbance in the bacterial flora that protects against urinary tract infections leads to recurrent infections. The insertion of *Lactobacilli* suppositories into the vagina of women after they have been treated with antibiotics can significantly reduce the recurrence rate.[41] Women given antibiotics should routinely re-establish proper vaginal flora by following the guidelines given above for vaginal infections or insert active cultures of *L. acidophilus* into the vagina. Oral therapy is also a good idea.

Cancer

A series of population studies has suggested that the consumption of high levels of cultured milk products may reduce the risk of colon cancer.[42] *L. bulgaricus*, the primary *Lactobacilli* used for yogurt, has demonstrated potent antitumor activity.[43] In animal studies, feeding milk and colostrum fermented with *L. acidophilus* DDS1 has resulted in a 16 to 41 percent reduction in tumor proliferation.[44] In human studies, ingestion of *L. acidophilus* resulted in reduced activity of bacterial enzymes associated with the formation of cancer-causing compounds in the gut.[45]

The beneficial effects of *Lactobacilli* against cancer appear to extend well beyond the colon. In a double-blind trial conducted with 138 patients surgically treated for bladder cancer, patients were stratified into three groups: subgroup A, those with primary multiple tumors; subgroup B, those with recurrent single tumors; and subgroup C, those with recurrent multiple tumors.[46] In each group, patients were randomly allocated to receive the oral *Lactobacillus casei* preparation (LCP) or a placebo. LCP showed a better effect than the placebo in preventing cancer recurrences in subgroups A and B. However, no significant effect was noted in group C. These results indicate that *Lactobacillus* preparations are safe and effective in preventing recurrence of superficial bladder cancers as long as they are not recurring multiple tumors.

L. acidophilus preparations are also of value in cancer patients receiving chemotherapy drugs or radiation therapy involving the gastrointestinal tract. In one study, 24 patients scheduled for internal and external irradiation of the pelvic area for gynecological cancers were selected for a controlled study to test the prevention of intestinal side effects by administration of *L. acidophilus*.[47] The test group received 150 milliliters per day of a fermented milk product that supplied them with live *L. acidophilus* bacteria in a 6.5 percent lactulose substrate. The administration of this resulted in prevention of radiotherapy-associated diarrhea.

Dosage Ranges

The dosage of a commercial probiotic supplement is based upon the number of live organisms. The ingestion of 1 to 10 billion viable *L. acidophilus* or *B. bifidum* cells daily is a sufficient dosage for most people. Amounts exceeding this may induce mild gastrointestinal disturbances, while smaller amounts may not be able to colonize the gastrointestinal tract.

Safety Issues

Probiotics are extremely safe and are not associated with any side effects.

Interactions

L. acidophilus and *B. bifidum* are negatively affected by alcohol and antibiotics.[48] Although there is no evidence that the organism interferes with the activity of most antibiotics, the metabolism of sulfasalazine, chloramphenicol palmitate, and phthalylsulfathiazole is affected by *L. acidophilus*.[49]

45

S-Adenosylmethionine (SAM)

S-Adenosylmethionine (SAM) is an important physiological agent formed in the body by combining the essential amino acid methionine with adenosyl-triphosphate (ATP). SAM was discovered in Italy in 1952—not surprisingly, most of the research on SAM has been conducted in the country of its discovery.

Food Sources

Because SAM is manufactured from methionine, you might think that dietary sources of methionine provide the same benefits as SAM. However, high doses of methionine do not increase levels of SAM, nor do they provide the same pharmacological activity as SAM. On the contrary, high dosages of methionine are associated with some degree of toxicity.[1,2]

Deficiency Signs and Symptoms

Normally the body manufactures all the SAM it needs from the amino acid methionine. However, a deficiency of methionine, vitamin B_{12}, or folic acid can result in decreased SAM synthesis. In addition, tissue levels of SAM are typically low in the elderly and in patients suffering from osteoarthritis, depression, and various liver disorders.

Beneficial Effects

SAM is involved in over 40 biochemical reactions in the body. It functions closely with folic acid and vitamin B_{12} in "methylation" reactions—the process of adding a single carbon unit (a methyl group) to another molecule. SAM is many times more effective in transferring methyl groups than other methyl donors. Methylation reactions are critical in the manufacture of many body components—especially brain chemicals—and in detoxification reactions.

SAM is also required in the manufacture of all sulfur-containing compounds in the human body, including glutathione and various sulfur-containing cartilage components. The beneficial effects of SAM supplementation are far-reaching because of its central role in so many metabolic processes.

Available Forms

SAM has been available commercially in Europe since 1975. Unfortunately, as of April 1996 it was still not available in the United States. I discuss it here because I believe it will be introduced into U.S. health-food stores as a nutritional supplement in the very near future. The commercial form of SAM is a stabilized salt produced under U.S. patent numbers 3,954,726 (1976) and 4,057,686 (1977).

Principal Uses

There are five principal conditions where SAM is used: depression, osteoarthritis, fibromyalgia, liver disorders, and migraine headaches.

Depression

SAM is necessary in the manufacture of important brain compounds such as neurotransmitters and phospholipids like phosphatidylcholine and phosphatidylserine. Supplementing the diet with SAM in depressed patients results in increased levels of serotonin, dopamine, and phosphatidylserine. It improves binding of neurotransmitters to receptor sites, which causes increased serotonin and dopamine activity and improved brain cell membrane fluidity, all resulting in significant clinical improvement.[3–5]

The antidepressive effects of folic acid discussed in Chapter 14 are mild compared to the effects noted in clinical trials using SAM. Based on results from a number of clinical studies, it appears that SAM is perhaps the most effective natural antidepressant (although a strong argument could be made for the extract of St.-John's-wort standardized to contain 0.3 percent hypericin).[6–9] Tables 45.1 and 45.2 summarize double-blind studies comparing SAM to either a placebo or an antidepressant drug.

Most of the studies cited in Tables 45.1 and 45.2 used injectable SAM. However, more recent studies using a new oral preparation at a dosage of 400 milligrams four times daily (1,600 milligrams total) demonstrate that SAM is just as effective orally as it is intravenously.[10–13] SAM is better tolerated and has a quicker onset of antidepressant action than tricyclic antidepressants.

The most recent study compared SAM to the tricyclic desipramine. In addition to clinical response, the blood level of SAM was determined in both groups. At the end of the 4-week trial, 62 percent of the patients treated with SAM and 50 percent of the patients treated with desipramine had significantly improved. Regardless of the type of treatment, patients with a 50 percent decrease in their Hamilton Depression Scale

TABLE 45.1   Double-Blind Clinical Studies with SAM versus Placebo in Depression

Authors	SAM Responders	Placebo Responders	Conclusion
Fazio et al. (1973)	Not quantified*		SAM superior to placebo based on Hamilton Depression Scale
Agnoli et al. (1976)	20/20	1/10	SAM superior to placebo (100 percent response in SAM group, 10 percent in placebo)
Muscettola et al. (1982)	4/10	0/10	SAM superior to placebo
Janicak (1982)	5/7	0/5	SAM superior to placebo
Caruso et al. (1984)	Not quantified		SAM superior to placebo based on Hamilton Depression Scale
Carney et al. (1986)	Not quantified		SAM superior to placebo based on Hamilton Depression Scale & Beck Scale
De Leo (1987)	Not quantified		SAM superior to placebo based on Clinical Global Impression Scale
Total	29/37	1/25	SAM dramatically more effective than placebo (78% compared to 4%)

TABLE 45.2   Double-Blind Clinical Studies with SAM versus Antidepressant Drugs in Depression

Authors	SAM Responders	Drug Responders	Conclusion
Mantero et al. (1975)	11/16	9/15	SAM comparable to imipramine (75 mg. per day)
Barberi et al. (1978)	10/10	8/10	SAM more effective than amitryptaline (100 mg. per day)
Del Vecchio et al. (1978)	5/14	4/10	SAM comparable to clomipramine (100 mg. per day)
Miccoli et al. (1978)	35/45	30/41	SAM comparable to clomipramine (100 mg. per day)
Scarzella et al. (1978)	9/10	9/10	SAM comparable to clomipramine (100 mg. per day)
Scaggion et al. (1982)	18/22	10/18	SAM more effective than nomifensine (200 mg. per day)
Kufferle et al. (1982)	7/9	6/9	SAM comparable to clomipramine (50 mg. per day)
Plotkin (1988)	9/9	2/9	SAM more effective than imipramine (150 mg. per day)
Janicak (1988)	5/7	2/3	SAM comparable to imipramine (150 mg. per day)
Total	109/142	80/124	SAM is significantly more effective than antidepressant drugs (76% compared to 61%)

FROM: Janicak PG, et al.: Parenteral S-adenosylmethionine in depression. A literature review and preliminary report. *Psychopharmacology Bulletin* **25**:238–41, 1989.

(HAM-D) score showed a significant increase in plasma SAM concentration. These results suggest that one of the ways tricyclic drugs exert antidepressive effects is by raising SAM levels.[14]

In addition to generalized depression, there are two conditions associated with depression where SAM produces significant effects: the postpartum (after pregnancy) period and drug rehabilitation. SAM's benefits in these conditions probably stem from a combination of its effect on brain chemistry and liver function. In the study in postpartum depression (after-pregnancy "blues"), the administration of SAM (1,600 milligrams per day) produced significantly better mood scores than a placebo group.[15] As for the use of SAM in drug detoxification, SAM (1,200 milligrams daily) significantly reduced psychological distress (chiefly anxiety and depression) in the detoxification and rehabilitation of opiate abusers.[16]

Osteoarthritis

SAM has also demonstrated impressive results in the treatment of osteoarthritis. A deficiency of SAM in the joint tissue, just like a deficiency of glucosamine, leads to loss of the gel-like nature and shock-absorbing qualities of cartilage. As a result, osteoarthritis can develop. Current drugs used in osteoarthritis (aspirin and other nonsteroidal anti-inflammatory agents) not only produce significant side effects, but they also can promote the disease process by inhibiting cartilage repair and accelerating bone loss.[17–21] Natural compounds like SAM and glucosamine sulfate offer significant advantages over these popular drugs.

SAM can exert a number of effects that are highly relevant in the treatment of osteoarthritis. First of all, SAM is very important in the manufacture of cartilage components.[22] This effect has been demonstrated very well in humans. In one double-blind study conducted in Germany, the 14 patients with osteoarthritis of the hands who were given SAM demonstrated increased cartilage formation as determined by magnetic resonance imaging (MRI).[23] These results indicate SAM is capable of producing improvements in the structure and function of cartilage in joints affected by osteoarthritis. In addition, SAM has also demonstrated some mild pain-relieving and anti-inflammatory effects in animal studies.[1] All of these effects combine to produce exceptional clinical benefits.

A total of 21,524 patients with osteoarthritis have utilized SAM in detailed clinical trials. In double-blind trials, SAM has demonstrated reductions in pain scores and clinical symptoms similar to NSAIDS like ibuprofen, indomethacin, naproxen, and piroxicam. Let's examine some of these studies.

In one double-blind study, SAM was compared to the popular drug ibuprofen (Advil, Motrin, Nuprin, etcetera).[24] The 36 subjects with osteoarthritis of the knee, hip, and/or spine received a daily oral dose of 1,200 milligrams of SAM or 1,200 milligrams of ibuprofen for 4 weeks. Morning stiffness, pain at rest, pain on motion, crepitus (crackling noise upon movement of joint), swelling, and limitation of motion of the affected joints were assessed before and after treatment. The total score obtained after evaluation of all the individual clinical parameters improved to the same extent in patients treated with SAM or ibuprofen. In two other studies, SAM actually produced slightly better results.[25,26]

SAM has been compared to naproxen (Naprosyn) in several studies. In one double-blind study, 20 patients with osteoarthritis of the knee were given either SAM or naproxen for 6 weeks.[27] During the first week, SAM was administered at a dose of 400 milligrams three times daily and later at a dose of 400 milligrams twice daily; the dose of naproxen during the first week was 250 milligrams three times daily and subsequently 250 milligrams twice daily. During the first 2 weeks, the patients were allowed to take the drug paracetamol as an additional analgesic if the pain was severe. The patients were examined at the beginning of the study and after 2, 4, and 6 weeks. The parameters tested were pain, crepitus, joint swelling, circumference of joint, extent of motility, and walking time over 10 meters. At the end of the sixth week, the researchers found no statistically significant difference between the two patient groups—both groups exhibited a marked improvement on all parameters.

Another double-blind study compared SAM to both naproxen and a placebo in the treatment of osteoarthritis of the hip, knee, spine, and hand.[28] The study involved 33 rheumatologic and orthopedic medical centers and a total of 734 subjects. SAM administered orally at a dose of 1,200 milligrams daily exerted the same analgesic (pain-relieving) activity as naproxen at a dose of 750 milligrams daily. However, SAM was significantly better than naproxen in terms of both physicians' and patients' judgments and in terms of the number of patients with side effects. In fact, SAM was better tolerated than the placebo. Ten patients in the SAM group and 13 in the placebo group withdrew from the study because of intolerance to the drug.

Other double-blind studies indicate SAM offers the pain-relieving and anti-inflammatory benefit of drugs like indomethacin (Indocin and Indometh) and piroxicam (Feldene) but is generally tolerated much better than these potent NSAIDs.[29,30]

Perhaps the most meaningful study of SAM in osteoarthritis treatment is a long-term, multicenter, open, 2-year trial of 97 patients with osteoarthritis of the knee, hip, and spine.[31] The patients received 600 milligrams of SAM daily (equivalent to three tablets of 200 milligrams each) for the first 2 weeks and thereafter 400 milligrams daily (equivalent to two tablets of 200 milligrams each) until the end of the 24th month of treatment. Separate evaluations were made for osteoarthritis of the knee, hip, cervical spine, and dorsal/lumbar spine. The severity of the clinical symptoms (morning stiffness, pain at rest, and pain on movement) was assessed using scoring before the start of treatment, at the end of the first and second week of treatment, and then monthly until the end of the 24-month period. SAM administration showed good clinical effectiveness and was well tolerated. The improvement of the clinical symptoms during therapy with SAM was already evident after the first weeks of treatment and continued up to the end of the 24th month. Nonspecific side effects occurred in 20 patients, but in no case did therapy need to be discontinued. Most side effects disappeared during the course of therapy. Moreover, during the last 6 months of treatment, no adverse effect was recorded. Detailed laboratory tests carried out at the start and after 6, 12, 18, and 24 months of treatment showed no pathologic changes. SAM administration also improved the depressive feelings often associated with osteoarthritis.

Finally, in the largest study, 20,641 patients with osteoarthritis of the knee, hip, and spine and osteoarthritic polyarthritis of the fingers were studied over an 8-week period.[32] The patients received 400 milligrams of SAM three times daily for the first week, 400 milligrams twice daily for the second week, and 200 milligrams twice daily from the third week on. No additional analgesic/anti-inflammatory treatment was allowed. The efficacy of SAM was comparable to results achieved with NSAID—very good or good in 71 percent of the cases, moderate in 21 percent, and poor in 9 percent. The tolerance was assessed as very good or good in 87 percent of the cases, moderate in 8 percent, and poor in 5 percent.

All these studies indicate SAM can offer significant advantages over NSAIDs. While these drugs are associated with significant risk of toxicity, side effects, and actual promotion of the disease process in osteoarthritis, SAM offers considerable benefits without risk or side effects.

Fibromyalgia

Fibromyalgia is a recently recognized disorder which is regarded as a common cause of chronic musculoskeletal pain and fatigue. Fibromyalgia shares many common features with another recently termed syndrome, the chronic fatigue syndrome (CFS). The only difference in diagnostic criteria for fibromyalgia and CFS is the requirement of musculoskeletal pain in fibromyalgia and fatigue in CFS. The likelihood of being diagnosed as having fibromyalgia or CFS depends on the type of physician consulted. Specifically, if the patient consults a rheumatologist or orthopedic specialist, he or she is much more likely to be diagnosed with fibromyalgia than CFS. Depression is often an underlying finding in both fibromyalgia and CFS.

Diagnosis requires fulfillment of all the following major criteria and four or more minor criteria. The major criteria are:

• Generalized aches or stiffness of at least three anatomic sites for at least three months

• Six or more typical, reproducible tender points

• Exclusion of other disorders that can cause similar symptoms

The minor criteria are:

• Generalized fatigue

• Chronic headache

• Sleep disturbance

• Neurological and psychological complaints

• Joint swelling

• Numbing or tingling sensations

• Irritable bowel syndrome

• Variation of symptoms in relation to activity, stress, and weather changes

Three clinical studies show SAM produces excellent benefits in patients suffering from fibromyalgia.[33-35] The first study was a double-blind, crossover study of 17 patients with fibromyalgia.[33] During treatment with SAM (200 milligrams daily by injection for 21 days), subjects demonstrated significant reduction in the number of trigger points and painful areas and improvements in mood.

In another double-blind study, orally administered SAM (800 milligrams daily) was compared to a placebo for 6 weeks in 44 patients with fibromyalgia.[34] Researchers evaluated tender point score, muscle strength, disease activity, subjective symptoms, mood parameters, and side effects. Patients given SAM demonstrated improvements in clinical disease activity, pain experienced during the last week, fatigue, morning stiffness, and mood; however, the tender point score and muscle strength did not differ in the two treatment groups. SAM was without side effects.

The most recent study compared SAM to transcutaneous electrical nerve stimulation (TENS)—a popular treatment for fibromyalgia—in 30 patients with fibromyalgia.[35] Patients receiving SAM (200 milligrams by injection and 400 milligrams orally daily) demonstrated significantly greater clinical benefits—decreased number of tender points, subjective feelings of pain and fatigue, and improved mood. TENS offered little benefit on most symptoms while SAM was deemed "effective in relieving the signs and symptoms of primary fibromyalgia."[35]

Liver Disorders

SAM is quite beneficial in several liver disorders, including cirrhosis, Gilbert's syndrome, and oral contraceptive–induced liver damage. Its benefits are related to its function as the major methyl donor in the liver and its lipotropic activity (see Chapter 16). SAM is apparently the perfect supplement to relieve a condition naturopathic physicians often refer to as the "sluggish liver."

This term is used to denote altered or impaired liver function. Because of the liver's important role in numerous metabolic processes, even minor impairment of liver function could have profound effects. One of the leading contributors to impaired liver function is diminished bile flow or cholestasis. SAM is beneficial for a variety of liver disorders because of its ability to promote bile flow and relieve cholestasis.[36-38]

Cholestasis can be caused by a great number of factors, including obstruction of the bile ducts and impairment of bile flow within the liver. The most common cause of bile duct obstruction is the presence of gallstones. A variety of agents and conditions can cause impairment of bile flow within the liver, conditions typically associated with alterations in laboratory tests of liver function (serum bilirubin, alkaline phosphatase, SGOT, LDH, GGTP, etcetera), signifying cellular damage. However, relying on these tests alone to evaluate hepatic function may not be adequate; many of these conditions in the initial or "subclinical" stages can present normal laboratory values, but liver dysfunction may be measurable only by expensive and/or invasive tests.

At present, clinical judgment based on medical history remains the major diagnostic tool for the "sluggish liver." Fatigue, general malaise, digestive disturbances, allergies and chemical sensitivities, premenstrual syndrome, and constipation are among the symptoms people with this condition may exhibit. Causes of cholestasis are:

- Presence of gallstones
- Alcohol
- Endotoxins
- Hereditary disorders such as Gilbert's syndrome

- Pregnancy
- Natural and synthetic steroidal hormones
  - Anabolic steroids
  - Estrogens
  - Oral contraceptives

- Certain chemicals or drugs
  - Aminosalicylic acid
  - Chlorothiazide
  - Erythromycin estolate
  - Mepazine
  - Phenylbutazone
  - Sulphadiazine
  - Thiouracil

- Hyperthyroidism or thyroxine supplementation
- Viral hepatitis

A key function of SAM in the liver is inactivation of estrogens. Clinical studies show SAM is quite useful in protecting the liver from damage and improving liver function in conditions associated with estrogen excess—namely, oral contraceptive use, pregnancy, and premenstrual syndrome.[39-41]

SAM is also beneficial in the treatment of Gilbert's syndrome—a common syndrome characterized by a chronically elevated serum bilirubin level (1.2 to 3.0 milligrams per deciliter). Previously considered rare, this disorder is now known to affect as much as 5 percent of the general population. It usually presents no symptoms, although some patients do complain about loss of appetite, malaise, and fatigue (typical symptoms of impaired liver function). SAM at a dosage of 400 milligrams three times daily has resulted in a significant decrease in serum bilirubin in patients with Gilbert's syndrome.[42]

In addition to these relative minor disturbances in liver function, SAM can offer benefits in the treatment of more severe liver disorders including cirrhosis, where apparently it overcomes the SAM depletion characterized by this disorder. Since SAM is involved in so many liver processes, depleted levels of SAM within the liver have serious consequences. Supplementation with SAM to patients with liver cirrhosis results in not only improved bile flow but also improved membrane function and increased levels of glutathione.[43-45] Glutathione assumes a critical role in detoxification and defense against a variety of injurious agents by combining directly with these toxic substances to eventually form water-soluble compounds. Because many of the toxic compounds are fat soluble, conversion to water-soluble compounds results in more efficient excretion via the kidneys. When increased levels of toxic compounds are present or when the liver function is impaired, higher glutathione levels are required.

One of the greatest risks of chronic liver diseases such as chronic hepatitis is liver cancer. Supplementation with SAM is very much indicated in patients with these diseases in order to reduce the risk for liver cancer. Animal studies show a significant protective effect for supplemental SAM against liver cancer in animals exposed to liver carcinogens.[46]

Migraine

SAM is beneficial in the treatment of migraine headaches. The benefits manifest gradually and require long-term treatment for therapeutic effectiveness.[47]

Dosage Ranges

In general, the longer SAM is used, the more beneficial the results. It is perfectly suited for long-term use because of its excellent safety profile. Here are the dosage ranges for the various clinical indications:

- **Depression**   Four hundred milligrams three to four times daily. Because SAM can cause nausea and gastrointestinal disturbances in some people, it should be started at a dosage of 200 milligrams twice daily for the first day, increased to 400 milligrams twice daily on day three, 400 milligrams three times daily on day ten, and finally to the full dosage of 400 milligrams four times daily after 20 days if needed.

- **Osteoarthritis**   Start out as above for depression. After 21 days at a dosage of 1,200 milligrams daily, reduce dosage to the maintenance dosage of 200 milligrams twice daily.

- **Fibromyalgia**   Two hundred milligrams to 400 milligrams two times daily.

- **Liver Disorders**   Two hundred milligrams to 400 milligrams two to three times daily.

- **Migraine Headaches**   Two hundred milligrams to 400 milligrams two times daily.

Safety Issues

No significant side effects have been reported with oral SAM other than the occasional nausea and gastrointestinal disturbances. However, individuals with bipolar (manic) depression should not take SAM unless under strict medical supervision—SAM's antidepressant activity may lead to the manic phase in these individuals. This effect is exclusive to some individuals with bipolar depression.

Interactions

SAM functions very closely with vitamin B_{12}, folic acid, vitamin B_6 and choline in methylation reactions. Because of SAM's effects on the liver, it may enhance the elimination of various drugs from the body.[48] The clinical significance of this particular effect has not been fully determined.

PART SIX

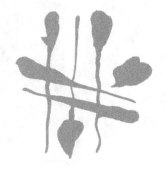

Glandular Products

For almost as long as mankind has been keeping records, glandular therapy has been an important form of medicine. The basic concept underlying the medicinal use of glandular substances from animals is "like heals like." For example, if your liver needs support or you are suffering from liver disease, then you may benefit from eating beef liver. Modern glandular therapy, however, primarily involves the use of concentrated glandular extracts.

Glands

A gland is a secretory organ. The body's internal secretory organs are called endocrine glands. These ductless glands secrete hormones directly into the blood stream. The glands that have endocrine function include the pineal, pituitary, thyroid, parathyroid, thymus, adrenal, pancreas, and gonads (testes or ovaries). Although other organs of the body are not technically glands, it is common to refer them as glandulars when they are used in glandular therapy. For example, tissue extracts of heart, spleen, prostate, uterus, brain, and other tissues are often used in glandular or organotherapy.

Effectiveness

Science has confirmed that certain glandular preparations and hormones are quite effective when taken orally because of active hormone or enzyme content—thyroid, adrenal cortex, and pancreatin preparations. There is also a good deal of literature support for pharmaceutical grade liver, aorta, and thymus extracts, and some support for pituitary, spleen, orchic (testes), and ovarian extracts as well. However, despite this scientific support, many people still question the effectiveness of glandular products on human health.

The question, however, should not be "Are glandulars effective?" but rather "Are the glandulars currently available in the health-food stores in the United States effective?" Manufacturers of glandular products ballyhoo that their method of glandular extract production is the most ideal. However, they base most of their contentions on theoretical or philosophical grounds, not on firm scientific evidence or clinical results. There are no quality-control procedures or standards enforced in the glandular industry. It is left up to each individual company to adopt quality control and good manufacturing procedures.

Nonetheless, I believe that many glandular preparations available in the United States marketplace are extremely effective. There are several companies that manufacture high-quality glandular products.

Glandular Preparations

Wise consumers purchase glandular products from well-known, reputable companies—improperly processed glandular material does not produce results. The biologically active material such as enzymes, soluble proteins, natural lipid factors, vitamins, minerals, and hormone precursors are destroyed or eliminated if the product is not prepared properly.

Most glandular products are derived from beef (bovine) sources with the exception of pancreatic extracts, which are most often derived from pork (porcine). The four most widely-known methods of processing are the azeotrophic method, salt precipitation, freeze-drying, and predigesting.

The azeotrophic method begins by quick freezing the material at well below zero degrees Fahrenheit and then washing it with a powerful solvent (ethylene dichloride) to remove the fatty tissue. The solvent is then distilled out, and the material is dried and ground into a powder to be placed in tablets or capsules. Although the azeotrophic method eliminates the problem of fat-stored toxins like pesticides and heavy metals, unfortunately it also removes fat-soluble hormones, enzymes, essential fatty acids, and other potentially beneficial materials—and traces of the solvent remain.

The salt precipitation method involves the maceration of fresh glandular material in a salt and water solution. Because the salt increases the density of the water-soluble material, when the mixture is centrifuged the lighter fat-soluble material can be separated out. The material is then dried and powdered. This method is beneficial because no toxic solvents are used to separate the fatty material. The downside is most people do not need the remaining salt in the product.

The freeze-drying process involves quickly freezing the glandular material at temperatures 40 to 60 degrees below zero degrees Fahrenheit and then placing the material into a vacuum chamber that removes the water by direct vaporization from its frozen state—hence the term freeze-drying. The benefit of freeze-drying is it contains a higher concentration of unaltered protein and enzymes as well as all of fat-soluble components. Since the fat is not removed, the glands must be derived from livestock that has grazed on open ranges not sprayed with pesticides or herbicides. The animals must also be free from antibiotics, synthetic hormones, and infection.

Finally, the predigestion method employs the aid of plant and animal enzymes to partially digest or hydrolyze the glandular material. The partially digested material is then passed through a series of filtrations to separate out fat-soluble and large molecules. The purified material is then freeze-dried. This method of extraction is ideal for glandulars (such as the liver and thymus) where the polypeptide (small proteins) and other water-soluble fractions are desired.

In general, I believe "predigested soluble concentrates" are the most effective. Like any other foods, glandulars must be digested to extract their nutrients. Because predigested glandulars need little or no further digestion, the body can assimilate their natural factors quickly and easily. Although my belief is based in part on theory and philosophy, clinical evidence supports it.

Intact Protein Absorption

Contrary to long-held theories that the healthy intestinal lining (mucosa) is an essentially impermeable barrier to proteins and large polypeptides, there is now irrefutable evidence that large macromolecules can and do pass intact from the human gut into the bloodstream under normal conditions. In some instances, the body appears to recognize which molecules it needs to absorb intact and which molecules it needs to break down into smaller units. This phenomenon may help to explain the effectiveness of glandular therapy.

Human and animal studies show that numerous whole proteins, including plant and animal enzymes, can be absorbed intact into the bloodstream following oral administration.[1-7] These include human albumin and lactalbumin, bovine albumin, ovalbumin, lactoglobulin, ferritin (molecular weight 500,000), chymotrypsinogen, elastase, and other large molecules.

Furthermore, proteins, polypeptides (small proteins), and various hormones that are absorbed intact from the gut exert effects in target tissues. For example, in addition to thyroxine (thyroid hormone) and cortisone, several peptide hormones are biologically active when administered orally, including luteinizing hormone–releasing factor and thytropin-releasing hormone.[8,9] Even insulin can be absorbed orally under certain circumstances (in the presence of protease inhibitors or hypertonic solutions in the intestines).[10,11]

What these data indicate is there may be larger molecules in glandular products that are absorbed intact and that exert beneficial effects—particularly polypeptides, which exert hormone or hormonelike action. Detractors of glandular therapy often claim that when a glandular is consumed it is immediately broken down by the body into smaller building blocks like amino acids. However, these detractors are not up to date with current understanding of normal physiology.

46

Adrenal Extracts

The adrenal glands lie just above the kidneys and are composed of two distinct parts, the adrenal medulla and the adrenal cortex. The adrenal medulla is functionally related to the sympathetic nervous system and secretes the hormones epinephrine (adrenaline) and norepinephrine (noradrenalin). These hormones stimulate many body processes related to the fight-or-flight response. They also serve to maintain normal nervous control over many involuntary bodily functions such as heart rate, respiration, digestion.

The adrenal cortex secretes an entirely different group of hormones called corticosteroids. These hormones are all formed from cholesterol. Although all corticosteroids have similar chemical formulas, they differ in function. The three major types of corticosteroids are mineralocorticoids, glucocorticoids, and 17-ketosteroids (sex hormones).

The glucocorticoids, mainly cortisol, corticosterone, and cortisone, exert a profound effect upon the metabolism of glucose. These hormones increase serum glucose. In addition, glucocorticoids reduce inflammation and the allergic response.

The mineralocorticoids, of which aldosterone is the most important, have profound effect on minerals. Specifically, aldosterone increases the retention of sodium and the excretion of potassium by the body.

The 17-ketosteroids (sex hormones) are also secreted by the adrenals. The primary sex hormone produced by the adrenal is the androgen (male hormone) dehydroepiandrosterone (DHEA).

Stress

Some basic control mechanisms are geared toward counteracting the everyday stresses of life. However, if stress is extreme, unusual, or long-lasting, these control mechanisms can be quite harmful. Stress triggers a number of biological changes known collectively as the "general adaptation syndrome." The three phases of the general adaptation syndrome are alarm, resistance, and finally exhaustion.[1] These phases are controlled and regulated by the adrenal glands.

Alarm

The initial response to stress is the alarm reaction or "flight-or-fight" response.[1-3] It is triggered by reactions in the brain that ultimately cause the adrenal medulla to secrete adrenaline and other stress-related hormones. The fight-or-flight response is designed to counteract danger by mobilizing the body's resources for immediate physical activity. This is what happens:

- The heart rate and force of contraction of the heart increases to provide blood to areas necessary for response to the stressful situation.
- Blood is shunted away from the skin and internal organs, except the heart and lung, while at the same time the amount of blood supplying needed oxygen and glucose to the muscles and brain is increased.
- The rate of breathing increases to supply necessary oxygen to the heart, brain, and exercising muscles.
- Sweat production increases to eliminate toxic compounds produced by the body and to lower body temperature.
- Production of digestive secretions is severely reduced since digestive activity is not critical for counteracting stress.
- Blood sugar levels are increased dramatically as the liver dumps stored glucose into the blood stream.

Resistance

While the fight-or-flight response is usually short-lived, the resistance reaction allows the body to continue fighting a stressor long after the effects of the fight-or-flight response have worn off. Corticosteroids secreted by the adrenal cortex are largely responsible for the resistance reaction. For example, the glucocorticoids stimulate the conversion of protein to energy so that the body has a large supply of energy long after glucose stores are depleted; the mineralocorticoids retain sodium to maintain an elevated blood pressure.

In addition to providing the necessary energy and circulatory changes required to deal effectively with stress, the resistance reaction provides those changes required for meeting emotional crisis, performing strenuous tasks, and fighting infection. However, while the effects of adrenal cortex hormones are quite necessary when the body is faced with danger, prolongation of the resistance reaction or continued stress increases the risk of significant disease and results in the final stage of the general adaptation syndrome—exhaustion.

Exhaustion

Exhaustion may manifest by a total collapse of body function or a collapse of specific organs. Two of the major causes of exhaustion are losses of potassium ions and depletion of adrenal glucocorticoid hormones like cortisone.[1] When the cells of the body lose potassium, they function less effectively and eventually die. When adrenal glucocorticoid stores become depleted, hypoglycemia results and cells of the body do not receive enough glucose or other nutrients.

Another cause of exhaustion is weakening of the organs. Prolonged stress places a tremendous load on many organ systems, especially the heart, blood vessels, adrenals, and immune system. Exhaustion usually manifests itself in the organ system that is inherently weak. Conditions strongly linked to stress are:

- Angina
- Asthma
- Autoimmune disease
- Cancer
- Cardiovascular disease
- Common cold
- Diabetes (adult onset, type II)
- Depression
- Headaches
- Hypertension
- Immune suppression
- Irritable bowel syndrome
- Menstrual irregularities
- Premenstrual tension syndrome
- Rheumatoid arthritis
- Ulcerative colitis
- Ulcers

Healthy Adrenal Function

An abnormal adrenal response, either deficient or excessive hormone release, significantly alters an individual's response to stress. Often the adrenals become "exhausted" as a result of constant demands placed upon them. An individual with adrenal exhaustion may feel "stressed out," tired, and have a reduced resistance to allergies and infection.

Atrophy (shrinking) of the adrenal cortex is a common side effect of continual stress and cortisone administration. Because of the importance of the adrenal gland, optimum health depends on optimum adrenal function. Adrenal extracts, along with supportive nutrients like vitamin C, potassium, and pantothenic acid, are often used by individuals who have been exposed to tremendous stress or who have been taking corticosteroid drugs like prednisone for long periods of time.

Available Forms

Medicine has used oral adrenal extracts since 1931.[2] Adrenal extracts may be made from the whole adrenal or just from the adrenal cortex. Whole adrenal extracts (usually in combination with essential nutrients for the adrenal gland) are most often used in cases of low adrenal function presenting as fatigue, inability to cope with stress, and reduced resistance. Because extracts made from the adrenal cortex contain small amounts of corticosteroids, they are typically used as a "natural" cortisone in severe cases of allergy and inflammation (asthma, eczema, psoriasis, rheumatoid arthritis, etcetera).

Dosage

The dosage of adrenal extract depends on the quality and potency of the product. The best measure of an effective dose for either preparation may be the level of stimulation experienced. If a high-quality preparation is used at higher dosages (for example, twice the label recommendation), individuals notice a general stimulatory effect, including irritability, restlessness, and insomnia. I suggest starting at one-third the recommended dosage on the label and slowly increasing your dosage every 2 days until you notice the stimulatory effect. Once you notice this effect, simply reduce your dosage to a level just below the level that produces stimulation.

Dealing with Stress

One of the best ways to support the adrenal glands is by dealing with stress effectively. Dealing with stress involves the use of techniques designed to reduce the amount of stress. Exercise and relaxation techniques such as meditation, prayer, biofeedback, and self-hypnosis are vital components of a stress management program. Exercise is itself a physical stressor; however, it is the beneficial way to incorporate the fight-or-flight response into your daily routine. Regular exercise leads to an increased ability to cope with stress and reduces the risk of stress-related diseases.

Relaxation techniques seek to counteract the results of stress by inducing its opposite reaction, relaxation. Although an individual may relax by simply sleeping, watching television, or reading a book, relaxation techniques are designed specifically to produce the "relaxation response."

(continues)

The physiological effects of the relaxation response are opposite to those seen with stress. With the stress response, the sympathetic nervous system dominates. With the relaxation response, the parasympathetic nervous system dominates. The parasympathetic nervous system controls bodily functions such as digestion, breathing, and heart rate during periods of rest, relaxation, visualization, meditation, and sleep. While the sympathetic nervous system is designed to protect us against immediate danger, the parasympathetic system is designed for repair, maintenance, and restoration of the body.

To achieve the relaxation response, you can employ a variety of techniques—meditation, prayer, progressive relaxation, autogenic training, self-hypnosis, and/or biofeedback. Choose the type of relaxation technique(s) best for you. The important thing is to set aside 5 to 10 minutes each day for a relaxation technique. These sessions remind us to breath in a relaxed, effective manner. When we are confronted with stressors, sometimes simply breathing in this relaxed manner triggers tremendous relaxation and ability to cope.

One of the most popular techniques for producing the relaxation response is progressive relaxation. The technique is based on a very simple procedure of comparing tension and relaxation. Many people are not aware of the sensation of relaxation. In progressive relaxation, you are taught what it feels like to relax by comparing relaxation to muscle tension.

First you are asked to forcefully contract a muscle for 1 to 2 seconds and then give way to a feeling of relaxation. Since the procedure goes progressively through all the muscles of the body, eventually a deep state of relaxation results. The procedure begins by contracting the muscles of your face and neck, holding the contraction 1 to 2 seconds and then relaxing the muscles. Next you contract the upper arms and chest muscles, then relax, followed by the lower arms and hands. Repeat this process progressively down your body—abdomen, buttocks, thighs, calves, and feet. Repeat the entire process two or three times. Many people use this technique in the treatment of anxiety and insomnia.

Progressive relaxation, deep breathing exercises, or some other stress-reduction technique is an important component of a healthy lifestyle. Again, set aside at least 5 to 10 minutes each day just to relax.

47

Aortic Glycosaminoglycans

The aorta is the main artery of the body. It arises directly from the heart and supplies oxygenated blood to all the other arteries. The mucopolysaccharides or glycosaminoglycans (GAGs) of the aorta are the ground substance components responsible for providing structural support. A mixture of highly purified, bovine-derived glycosaminoglycans naturally present in the aorta—including dermatan sulfate, heparan sulfate, hyaluronic acid, chondroitin sulfate, and related hexosaminoglycans—protect and promote normal artery and vein function. Many Americans could benefit from improved health of their arteries and veins, and over 50 clinical studies show an orally administered complex of aortic GAGs is effective in a number of vascular disorders, including cerebral and peripheral arterial insufficiency; venous insufficiency and varicose veins; hemorrhoids; vascular retinopathies, including macular degeneration; and postsurgical edema. Significant improvements in both symptoms and blood flow have been noted.

Atherosclerosis

Atherosclerosis and its complications are the major causes of death in the United States and have reached epidemic proportions throughout all of the Western world. Heart disease alone accounts for 36 percent of all deaths in the United States and ranks as our number one killer. Strokes, another complication of atherosclerosis, are the third most common cause of death. All together, atherosclerosis is responsible for at least 43 percent of all deaths in the United States. Because atherosclerosis is largely a disease of diet and lifestyle, many of these deaths could be significantly delayed through a healthy diet and lifestyle.

Consistent with the theory behind modern glandular therapy (like cures like), the use of extracts rich in aortic glycosaminoglycans may be beneficial in the treatment of atherosclerosis. There is considerable evidence to support the clinical effectiveness of aortic GAGs in improving arterial function and blood flow. In addition, there is evidence indicating aortic GAGs address many of the underlying features that contribute to the development of atherosclerosis. Most clinical studies have utilized a mixture of highly-purified, bovine-derived glycosaminoglycans naturally present in the aorta, including dermatan sulfate, heparan sulfate, hyaluronic acid, chondroitin sulfate, and related hexosaminoglycans.

To fully understand the important role aortic GAGs play in the health of the artery and in the treatment of vascular disease, it is necessary to examine closely the structure of an artery and the process of atherosclerosis.

Arterial Structure

An artery is divided into three major layers:

- **Intima**   Represents the endothelium (internal lining of the artery) and consists of a layer of endothelial cells. GAGs are naturally present on the vessel surface, where they protect the endothelial cells from damage and promote repair. Beneath the surface cells is the internal elastic membrane composed of a layer of GAGs and other ground substance compounds. It provides support to the endothelial cells and separates the endothelium from the smooth muscle layer.

- **Media**   Consists primarily of smooth muscle cells. Interposed among the cells are GAGs and other ground substance structures that provide support and elasticity to the artery.

- **Adventitia**   External elastic membrane, consists primarily of connective tissue (including glycosaminoglycans) and provides structural support and elasticity to the artery (see Figure 47.1).

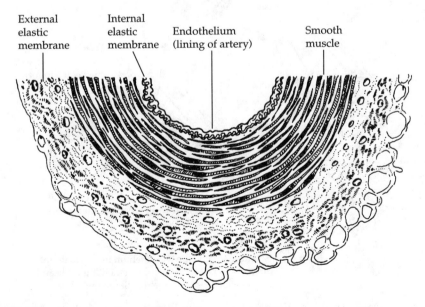

FIGURE 47.1   Structure of an artery.

Development of Atherosclerosis

No single theory of the development of atherosclerosis that has been formulated satisfies all investigators. However, the most widely accepted explanation theorizes that the lesions of atherosclerosis are initiated in response to injury of the cells lining the artery, the arterial endothelium. Figure 47.2 illustrates the progression in detail as follows:

1. The initial step in the development of atherosclerosis is damage to the endothelium by free radicals. Immune, physical, mechanical, viral, chemical, and drug factors all can induce damage that can lead to plaque development.

2. Once the endothelium has been damaged, sites of injury become more permeable to plasma constituents, especially lipoproteins (fat-carrying proteins). The binding of lipoproteins to glycosaminoglycans leads to a breakdown in the integrity of the ground substance matrix and causes an increased affinity for cholesterol. Once significant damage has occurred, monocytes (large white blood cells) and platelets adhere to the damaged area, where they release growth factors that stimulate smooth muscle cells to migrate from the media into the intima and replicate.

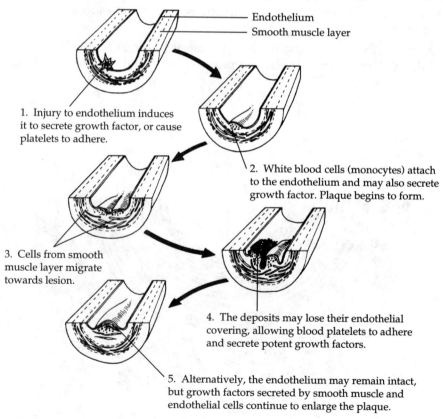

Endothelium
Smooth muscle layer

1. Injury to endothelium induces it to secrete growth factor, or cause platelets to adhere.

2. White blood cells (monocytes) attach to the endothelium and may also secrete growth factor. Plaque begins to form.

3. Cells from smooth muscle layer migrate towards lesion.

4. The deposits may lose their endothelial covering, allowing blood platelets to adhere and secrete potent growth factors.

5. Alternatively, the endothelium may remain intact, but growth factors secreted by smooth muscle and endothelial cells continue to enlarge the plaque.

FIGURE 47.2   Stages in the development of atherosclerosis.

3. The local concentration of lipoproteins, monocytes, and platelets leads to the migration of smooth muscle cells from the media into the intima, where they undergo proliferation. The smooth muscle cells dump cellular debris into the intima, leading to further development of plaque.

4. The formation of a fibrous cap (consisting of collagen, elastin, and glycosaminoglycans) over the intimal surface occurs. Fat and cholesterol deposits accumulate.

5. The plaque continues to grow until eventually it blocks the artery. Blockage is usually around 90 percent before symptoms of atherosclerosis are apparent.

Arterial Disorders

Aortic GAGs are essential for maintaining arterial health. In addition, aortic GAGs have many important effects that interfere with the progression of atherosclerosis, including preventing damage to the surface of the artery, formation of damaging blood clots, migration of smooth muscle cells into the intima, and formation of fat and cholesterol deposits. They also lower total cholesterol levels while raising HDL cholesterol.[1-6]

Studies in animals indicate aortic GAGs are effectively absorbed orally and incorporated into vessels where they dramatically improve the integrity and function of arteries.[7] As for human use, a number of clinical studies demonstrate that supplementing the diet with aortic GAGs has remarkable effect in improving the structure, function, and integrity of arteries and improves blood flow.[8-11] Aortic GAGs can be effective in improving both cerebral (brain) and peripheral (hands and feet) vascular insufficiency. Significant improvements in both symptoms and blood flow have been noted.

Symptoms of cerebral vascular insufficiency can include short-term memory loss, vertigo, headache, ringing in the ears, and depression. These symptoms are often referred to as "symptoms of aging" and represent almost entirely a reduced supply of blood and oxygen to the brain because of atherosclerosis. Symptoms of peripheral vascular disease can include coldness of hands or feet, pain, muscle cramps, and impotence (in males).

Venous Disorders

Veins are fairly frail structures. Defects in a vein's wall lead to dilation of the vein and damage to the valves. When the valves become damaged, the increased pressure results in bulging veins known as varicose veins. Varicose veins affect nearly 50 percent of middle-aged adults. The veins just under the skin of the legs are the veins most commonly affected because of the tremendous strain standing has on these veins. When an individual stands for long periods of time, the pressure exerted against the vein can increase up to ten times. Hence, individuals with occupations that require long periods of standing are at greatest risk for developing varicose veins.

Women are affected about four times as frequently as men; obese individuals have a much greater risk; and the risk increases with age because of loss of tissue tone, loss of muscle mass, and weakening of the venous walls. Pregnancy may also lead to the development of varicose veins because pregnancy increases venous pressure in the legs.

Several theories exist to explain the cause of varicose veins:

- Genetic weakness of the veins or venous valves
- Excessive venous pressure because of a low-fiber-induced increase in straining during defecation
- Long periods of standing and/or heavy lifting
- Damage to the veins or venous valves secondary to thrombophlebitis
- Weakness of the vascular walls because of either abnormalities in the proteoglycans of the connective tissue or excessive release of cellular enzymes that break down the ground substance, resulting in increased capillary permeability and loss of integrity of the venous structure

Glycosaminoglycans provide the skeletal framework of the vein and are therefore essential in maintaining the structure and integrity of veins. Without proper structural support, veins lose their shape and become bulging and unsightly. Aortic GAGs demonstrate impressive clinical results in improving the function and structure of veins.[12–16] Individuals with poor venous function of the legs typically experience such symptoms as a sense of heaviness in the legs, tingling sensations, fluid retention, itching, and painful cramps. These symptoms are improved with aortic GAGs because of its ability to improve the structure and function of the vein, thereby allowing improved blood flow.

On a final note, two double-blind studies compared aortic GAGs (72 milligrams per day) to flavonoid extracts, hydroxy-ethyl-rutosides (1,000 milligrams per day), and bilberry extract (320 milligrams per day), in the treatment of hemorrhoids and varicose veins. The aortic extract produced far better results. In fact, in the study in hemorrhoids the authors suggested that it should be used as the "drug of first choice" in the nonsurgical treatment of acute hemorrhoidal pain and disease.[17]

Principal Uses

Aortic GAGs may be useful in enhancing the function, structure, and integrity of arteries and veins. Aortic GAGs have many important effects that interfere with the progression of atherosclerosis, including prevention of damage to the surface of the artery, formation of damaging blood clots, migration of smooth muscle cells into the intima, and formation of fat and cholesterol deposits. They also lower total cholesterol levels while raising HDL-cholesterol.

Dosage Ranges

The dosage of highly purified, bovine-derived glycosaminoglycans naturally present in the aorta (including dermatan sulfate, heparan sulfate, hyaluronic acid, chondroitin sulfate, and related hexosaminoglycans) is 100 milligrams daily. Results similar (but not nearly as impressive) to those of aorta extracts in the treatment of atherosclerosis have been noted with chondroitin sulfate at a daily dose of 3 grams (1 gram with meals three times daily).[18]

48

Liver Extracts

The liver is truly an intricate, complex, and remarkable organ. Without question, it is the most important organ of metabolism. To a very large extent, the health and vitality of an individual is determined by the health and vitality of the liver.

The liver's basic functions are threefold: vascular, secretory, and metabolic. Its vascular functions include being a major blood reservoir and filtering over 1 quart of blood per minute. The liver effectively removes bacteria, endotoxins, antigen-antibody complexes, and various other particles from the circulation.

The liver's secretory functions involve the synthesis and secretion of bile. Each day the liver manufactures about 1 quart of bile. Bile is necessary for the absorption of fat-soluble substances, including many vitamins. Although the majority of the bile secreted into the intestines is reabsorbed, many toxic substances are effectively eliminated from the body by the bile.

The metabolic functions of the liver are immense because the liver is intricately involved in carbohydrate, fat, and protein metabolism; the storage of vitamins and minerals; the formation of numerous physiologic factors; and the detoxification or excretion into the bile of various chemical compounds (hormones such as thyroxine, cortisol, estrogen, and aldosterone; histamine; drugs; and pesticides).

Beneficial Effects

Liver is the richest natural source of many vitamins and minerals, including iron. Iron is critical to human life. It plays the central role in the hemoglobin molecule of our red blood cells, where it functions in transporting oxygen from the lungs to the body's tissues and carbon dioxide from the tissues to the lungs. Iron also functions in several key enzymes in energy production and metabolism, including DNA synthesis.[1,2] For more information on iron, see Chapter 26.

Iron and Other Nutrients

Iron supplementation is often required, especially during pregnancy and in young menstruating women. Liver extracts provide the best form of iron (heme iron) and are therefore considered by many experts to be the best iron supplements. Liver extracts contain not only iron but also other nutritional and physiological substances that promote healthy red blood cells. Many liver extracts provide the benefit of heme iron without the calories and fat that would be required to achieve similar amounts of heme iron from meats.

Liver is also a rich source of other nutrients critical in building blood, including vitamin B_{12} and folic acid. These nutrients also function in maintaining a healthy nervous system and increasing energy levels.

Endurance Enhancement

Dr. B. H. Ershoff of the University of Southern California performed several experiments that demonstrated raw liver has phenomenal antifatigue effects. In one of Dr. Ershoff's classic experiments, three groups of laboratory rats were fed different diets over a 12-week period. The first group was fed a usual laboratory diet to which 11 different vitamins were added. The second group was fed the same diet plus all known B vitamins. The third group was fed the original diet with 10 percent raw liver in place of the vitamins.

At the end of the 12 weeks, each group of rats was placed in drums of water that they could not climb out of. The first group of rats swam for an average of 13.3 minutes; the second group averaged 13.4 minutes before giving up, indicating they had exhausted all available strength and energy. The third group, however, demonstrated amazing results. Three rats swam for 63, 83, and 87 minutes, while the balance of the group was still swimming vigorously at the end of the 2-hour test period.

The mysterious effects of liver have puzzled researchers and scientists for decades. Some scientists believe liver contains an unidentified physiological substance that promotes stamina, strength, and endurance. These attributes have made liver preparations extremely popular among bodybuilders and athletes.

Principal Uses

Most clinical studies utilized hydrolyzed liver extracts produced by exposing the liver material to enzymes that hydrolyze (add water to) the protein bonds. This process basically "liquefies" the liver fraction and is why hydrolyzed extracts are often referred to as "liquid liver extracts." These aqueous liver extracts are used to improve liver function and since 1896 have been used in the treatment of many chronic liver diseases. Numerous scientific investigations into the therapeutic efficacy of liver extracts demonstrate that these extracts possess an ability to improve fat utilization, promote tissue regeneration, and prevent damage to the liver.[3-6] In short, clinical studies demonstrate that oral administration of liquid liver extracts can be quite effective in improving liver function.

For example, one double-blind study involved 556 patients with chronic hepatitis given either 70 milligrams of liver hydrosylate or a placebo three times daily.[6] At the end of 3 months of treatment, the group receiving the liver extract had far lower liver enzyme levels. Since the level of liver enzymes in the blood reflects damage to the liver, it can be concluded that the liver extract is effective in chronic hepatitis via an ability to improve the function of damaged liver cells and prevent further damage to the liver.

A key benefit of liver extracts occurs because the liver is the most important organ of metabolism—when liver function improves, metabolism improves. An improved metabolism creates high energy levels and greater feelings of health and well-being. Liquid liver extracts are a remarkable tonic for well-being.

Dosage Ranges

Dosage depends entirely on the concentration, method of preparation, and quality of the liver extract. The highest quality liver extracts are aqueous (hydrolyzed) extracts because they have had the fat-soluble components removed and typically contain more than 20 times the nutritional content of raw liver, including 3 to 4 milligrams of heme iron per gram.

Safety Issues

Liver extracts should not be used in patients suffering from an iron-storage disorder such as hemochromatosis.

49

Pancreatic Extracts

The pancreas produces enzymatic secretions required for the digestion and absorption of food. Each day the pancreas secretes about 1.5 quarts of pancreatic juice into the small intestine. Enzymes secreted include lipases that digest fat, proteases that digest proteins, and amylases that digest starch molecules.

There is strong evidence the body seeks to conserve its digestive enzymes by reabsorbing them. Numerous human studies show that when supplemental pancreatic enzymes (trypsin and chymotrypsin) are given orally, they are absorbed intact into the bloodstream.[1-5] Even more dramatic is the finding that pancreatic enzymes are not only absorbed intact from the gut, but they are also transported through the bloodstream, taken up intact by pancreatic secretory cells, and resecreted into the intestines by the pancreas.[6] The existence of this circulation of pancreatic enzymes is quite similar to the recycling of bile salts by the liver.

Of further interest is the possibility that oral supplementation with pancreatic enzymes may have a sparing effect on the body's own digestive enzymes, perhaps reducing the stress on the pancreas and allowing the body to redirect energy to other areas.

There are three categories of pancreatic enzymes:

- **Lipases** Enzymes that, along with bile, function in the digestion of fats. Deficiency of lipase results in malabsorption of fats and fat soluble vitamins.
- **Amylases** Enzymes that break down starch molecules into smaller sugars. The salivary glands also secrete mylase.
- **Proteases** These pancreatic enzymes (trypsin, chymotrypsin, and carboxypeptidase) function in digestion by breaking down protein molecules into single amino acids.

Deficiency Signs and Symptoms

Physicians use both physical symptoms and laboratory tests to assess pancreatic function. Common symptoms of pancreatic insufficiency include abdominal bloating and discomfort, gas, indigestion, and the passing of undigested food in the stool. For laboratory diagnosis, most nutrition-oriented physicians use the comprehensive stool and digestive analysis. This comprehensive analysis usually reveals the level of pancreatic enzymes being dumped into the intestines by determining the level of excess fat in the stool, excess nitrogen in the stool, and the presence of any other partially or completely undigested food elements. In addition, the complete stool and digestive analysis also reveals the health of the bacteria flora that often reflects the degree of pancreatic function.

Available Forms

Pancreatic enzyme products are quite popular nutritional supplements. Most commercial preparations are prepared from fresh hog pancreases. The United States Pharmacopoeia (USP) has set strict definition for level of activity. A 1× pancreatic enzyme (pancreatin) product has in each milligram not less than 25 USP units of amylase activity, not less than 2 USP units of lipase activity, and not less than 25 USP units for protease activity. Pancreatin of higher potency is given a whole number multiple indicating its strength. For example, a full-strength undiluted pancreatic extract that is ten times stronger than the USP standard would be referred to as 10× USP.

Full-strength products are preferred to lower potency pancreatin products because lower potency products are often diluted with salt, lactose, or galactose to achieve desired strength (4× or 1×).

Enzyme products are often enteric-coated—coated to prevent digestion in the stomach so the enzymes will be liberated in the small intestine. However, nonenteric-coated enzyme preparations actually outperform enteric-coated products if they are given prior to a meal (for digestive purposes) or on an empty stomach (for anti-inflammatory effects).

Principal Uses

Pancreatic enzymes are most often employed in the treatment of pancreatic insufficiency. Pancreatic insufficiency is characterized by impaired digestion, malabsorption, nutrient deficiencies, and abdominal discomfort. Physicians prescribe pancreatic enzymes in the treatment of cystic fibrosis; inflammatory and autoimmune diseases like rheumatoid arthritis, scleroderma, athletic injuries, tendonitis; cancer; and infections. Clinical uses of pancreatic enzymes include:

- Digestive disturbances
- Pancreatic insufficiency
- Cystic fibrosis
- Food allergies

- Autoimmune disorders
  - Rheumatoid arthritis
  - Lupus
  - Scleroderma
  - Multiple sclerosis
  - Various cancers
- Sports injuries and trauma
- Viral infections
  - *Herpes zoster* (shingles)
  - AIDS

Digestive Aids

The most obvious clinical use of pancreatic extracts is for impaired digestion because of either pancreatic insufficiency or a disease like cystic fibrosis. While cystic fibrosis is a rare inherited disorder, pancreatic insufficiency is relatively common in the elderly.

Starch and fat digestion can be carried out satisfactorily without the help of pancreatic enzymes; however, the proteases are critical to proper protein digestion. Incomplete digestion of proteins creates a number of problems for the body, including the development of allergies and formation of toxic substances produced during putrefaction. Putrefaction refers to the breakdown of protein material by bacteria.

Proteases serve several other important functions. For example, the proteases (as well as other digestive secretions) are largely responsible for keeping the small intestine free from parasites (including bacteria, yeast, protozoa, and intestinal worms).[7] A lack of proteases or other digestive secretions greatly increases an individual's risk of intestinal infection, including an overgrowth of the yeast *Candida albicans*.

Food Allergies

In order for a food molecule to produce an allergic response, it must be a fairly large molecule. In studies performed in the 1930s and 1940s, pancreatic enzymes were quite effective in preventing food allergies.[9] It appears many practitioners are either not aware of, or have forgotten about, these early studies. Typically, individuals who do not secrete enough proteases suffer from multiple food allergies.

Celiac Disease

A recent double-blind study investigated the validity of pancreatic enzyme substitution therapy in the 2 months following the initial diagnosis of celiac disease (gluten enteropathy). The study sought to clarify the benefit of pancreatic enzyme therapy because previous studies had shown pancreatic insufficiency in 8 to 30 percent of celiac patients. The standard treatment of celiac disease is a gluten-free diet. In the study, patients followed a gluten-free diet and received with each meal either two capsules of pancreatic enzymes—5,000 International Units of lipase, 2,900 International Units of amylase, and 330 International Units of protease per capsule—or two placebo capsules. Complete nutritional and anthropomorphic evaluations were conducted at days 0, 30, and 60. Results indicated that pancreatic enzyme supplementation enhanced the clinical benefit of a gluten-free diet during the first 30 days but did not provide any greater benefit than the placebo after 60 days. These results support the use of pancreatic enzyme preparations in the first 30 days after diagnosis of celiac disease.[9]

Inflammation

The proteases are important in preventing tissue damage during inflammation and the formation of fibrin clots. Proteases cause an increase in the breakdown of fibrin, a process known as fibrinolysis. Fibrin's role in the promotion of inflammation is to form a wall around the area of inflammation that results in the blockage of blood and lymph vessels and that leads to swelling. Fibrin can also cause the development of blood clots that may become dislodged and produce strokes or heart attacks. Protease enzymes are often used in the treatment of thrombophlebitis—a disease in which blood clots develop in veins, the veins become inflamed, and the clots dislodge and cause strokes or heart attacks. Pancreatic enzymes and protease enzyme preparations are useful in the treatment of many acute and chronic inflammatory conditions, including sports injuries, tendonitis, and rheumatoid arthritis.[10,11]

Immune Complex Diseases

The proteases are also essential in preventing the deposit of immune complexes in body tissues. Diseases associated with high levels of circulating immune complexes include rheumatoid arthritis, *lupus erythematosus*, periarteritis nodosa, scleroderma, ulcerative colitis, Crohn's disease, multiple sclerosis, and AIDS.[12–14] The presence of immune complexes most likely contribute greatly to the disease process. Experimental and clinical studies show that protease enzyme preparations are extremely effective in reducing circulating immune complex levels in several of these diseases. Furthermore, clinical improvements correspond with decreases in immune complex levels.

For example, in the treatment of multiple sclerosis, pancreatic enzyme preparations produce good effects in reducing the severity and frequency of symptom flare-ups.[12] Especially good results were noted in cases of visual disturbance, urinary bladder and intestinal malfunction, and sensory disturbances. However, there was little effect on spasticity, dizziness, or tremor.

Most of the clinical studies using pancreatic enzyme preparations in inflammatory or autoimmune diseases have used enzyme preparations that are relatively weak in potency when compared to a number of enzyme preparations available in the United States. Presumably by using a higher-potency products individuals experience more impressive results than those provided by weaker preparations.

Cancer

One of the most controversial uses of pancreatic enzymes is cancer treatment. Enzyme preparations have been promoted by numerous alternative cancer practitioners for many years, but most recently by William Kelley, D.D.S., and Nicholas Gonzalez, M.D. There is little evidence in the scientific literature, however, to support their use, as is the case with many alternative cancer treatments. Several studies have been conducted in Germany and Austria, but further research is required.[15,16]

Weight Loss

Pancreatin supplementation can result in decreased food intake and a significant loss of body weight in animals.[17] Pancreatin appears to either contain or stimulate the manufacture of compounds that suppress appetite.

Although to my knowledge there are no human studies with pancreatin as a weight-loss aid, I have seen pancreatin supplementation promote dramatic weight loss. My friend Jim lost at least 40 pounds and 6 inches around his waist simply by supplementing his diet with pancreatin. He decided to try pancreatin because he was extremely sensitive to ephedrine and could not use thermogenic formulas.

Shingles

Orally administered pancreatic enzyme preparations have been used in Germany in the treatment of *herpes zoster* (shingles) for over 30 years. However, even in Germany the standard treatment is now oral acyclovir. The positive results obtained in earlier studies with proteolytic enzymes led researchers to study the effectiveness of enzyme therapy versus acyclovir.[5]

The study design was a double-blind, controlled, multicenter trial of 90 immunocompetent patients with *herpes zoster*. Patients were randomly assigned to receive either acyclovir (800 milligrams) or an enzyme preparation (120 milligrams trypsin, 40 milligrams chymotrypsin, and 320 milligrams papain) five times per day for a treatment period of 7 days. The parameters of pain and skin lesions were measured over 14 to 21 days. Results indicated no statistically significant difference in either parameter between the two groups, indicating the enzyme preparation is as effective as acyclovir (Zovirax). The proposed mechanisms of action for the enzyme preparation were stimulation of the breakdown of immune complexes and enhancement of immune function.

Dosage Ranges

Full-strength products are preferred to lower potency pancreatin products because lower potency products are often diluted with salt, lactose, or galactose to achieve desired strength (4× or 1×). The dosage recommendation for a 10× USP pancreatic enzyme product is 500 to 1,000 milligrams three times a day immediately before meals when used as a digestive aid and 10 to 20 minutes before meals or on an empty stomach when anti-inflammatory effects are desired.

Safety Issues

Pancreatic extracts are generally well tolerated and are not associated with any significant side effects.

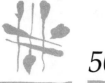

50

Spleen Extracts

The spleen is a fist-sized, spongy, dark purple organ that lies in the upper left abdomen behind the lower ribs. Weighing about 7 ounces, the spleen is the largest mass of lymphatic tissue in the body. At birth, the spleen is deficient in lymphatic components and does not reach its full size or functional capacity until early adulthood. The spleen's functions include producing white blood cells, engulfing and destroying bacteria and cellular debris, and destroying worn-out red blood cells and platelets. The spleen also serves as a blood reservoir. During times of demand (such as hemorrhage), the spleen can release its stored blood and prevent shock.

The spleen accomplishes these functions via extremely unique structure and organization. It is composed of numerous compartments surrounded by a smooth muscle capsule. The compartments are formed by the splenic artery and veins branching out to produce a vascular network with connecting sinusoids, which creates a mechanism to trap cells from circulating blood. The unique structural organization enables the spleen to contract and pump outs stored blood and immune-potentiating compounds under certain physiological conditions.

The spleen has been a source of curiosity since antiquity. Galen, the famous Roman physician, observed the variable size of the spongy, loose organ and could not explain its function. He regarded it as an organ "full of mystery" and believed it was the source of "black bile," or melancholy. In contrast to this view, the Talmud states the spleen induces laughter. The association between the spleen and psyche persists in such expressions as "venting one's spleen."

For centuries physicians believed the spleen had no real value. Although they had been performing splenectomies since 1549 as a therapeutic measure, it was not until 1952 that medicine described the "postsplenectomy syndrome" in children. The modern view of the spleen is it performs vital and essential functions in the reticuloendothelial system (RES), a portion of the immune system responsible for filtering the blood and signaling other arms of the immune system.

Beneficial Effects

As early as the 1930s, researchers knew orally administered bovine spleen extracts possessed some physiological action in increasing white blood cell counts in extreme deficiencies of white blood cells and were of some benefit in patients with malaria and typhoid fever.[1-3] Like thymus extracts, pharmaceutical-grade bovine spleen extracts are now quite popular in Germany for the treatment of infectious conditions and as an immune-enhancing agent in cancer. Spleen tissue extracts may be of benefit in enhancing general immune function because many potent immune system–enhancing compounds secreted by the spleen are peptides of small molecular weight; for example, the potent immunostimulants tuftsin and splenopentin are composed of only four and five amino acids, respectively.

Both tuftsin and splenopentin exert profound immune-enhancing activity. Tuftsin stimulates specialized white blood cells known as macrophages. Macrophages are actually a type of white blood cell (monocyte) that resides in specific tissues like the liver, spleen, and lymph nodes. These large cells engulf and destroy foreign particles, including bacteria, cancer cells, and cellular debris. Macrophages are essential in protecting against invasion by microorganisms and cancer cells. Tuftsin also helps mobilize other white blood cells to fight against infection and cancer. A deficiency of tuftsin is associated with signs and symptoms of frequent infections.[4]

Splenopentin, like tuftsin, also demonstrates significant immune-enhancing effects, primarily directed toward enhancing the immune system's response to regulating compounds known as "colony-stimulating factors."[5] Colony-stimulating factors like interleukin-3 and granulocyte/macrophage colony-stimulating factors stimulate the production of white blood cells. Splenopentin is probably the factor responsible for the results noted in those clinical studies during the 1930s with spleen extracts in the treatment of depressed white blood cell counts.

Splenopentin also can enhance natural killer cell activity.[6] Natural killer cells received their name because of their ability to destroy cells that have become cancerous or infected with viruses. They are the body's first line of defense against cancer development.

In addition to tuftsin and splenopentin, hydrolyzed (predigested) spleen extracts concentrated for peptides demonstrate impressive immune-restorative properties in mice.[7] In one study, the mice were exposed to radiation, a process that leads to significant destruction of the immune system. Mice treated with the spleen extract recovered within 6 to 8 weeks. In contrast, those treated with a placebo recovered after 10 weeks at the earliest.

Principal Uses

The primary uses of spleen extracts occur after removal of the spleen and in conditions associated with low spleen function (hyposplenia). The spleen plays a vital role in immune function largely through the effects of tuftsin and splenopentin. Spleen extracts may also be useful in the treatment of low white blood cell counts, bacterial infections, and as an adjunct in cancer therapy. Individuals who have had their spleen removed, have low tuftsin levels, or have autoimmune conditions linked to low RES activity should use spleen extracts.

After Spleen Removal

Removal of the spleen (splenectomy) is usually performed after the spleen has been seriously injured, causing severe hemorrhage. The spleen must be removed after significant trauma because it is difficult to repair. It is also removed in the medical treatment of certain diseases, such as idiopathic thrombocytic purpurea (ITP), and to determine the extent of Hodgkin's disease.

A splenectomy is associated with an increased risk for infection. In children and adults, this increased risk of infection makes them particularly susceptible to pneumococcal pneumonia. About 2.5 percent of splenectomy patients die from pneumococcal pneumonia within 5 years after splenectomy. Physicians often recommend that children who have undergone a splenectomy receive a pneumococcal vaccine and receive long-term antibiotic treatment. Use of spleen extracts, especially those rich in tuftsin, may be a natural alternative.

Spleen extracts should probably be viewed as a necessary medicine for people who have undergone a splenectomy. If the thyroid, adrenals, or ovaries are removed, most patients would be prescribed the corresponding hormone. It only makes sense that if the spleen is removed, the body should be supplied with necessary spleen substances like tuftsin and splenopentin.

The increased risk of infection occurs primarily because of a deficiency of tuftsin.[8,9] Tuftsin is produced only in the spleen; without the spleen, there simply is no tuftsin in the circulation. Without tuftsin, the body is without one of its key stimulators of the immune system. Individuals without spleens need an outside source of tuftsin like spleen extracts.

Hyposplenia

Hyposplenia refers to low spleen function. Conditions associated with functional hyposplenia include celiac disease, dermatitis herpetiformis, ulcerative colitis, rheumatoid arthritis, glomerulonephritis, systemic *lupus erythematosus*, vasculitis, and thrombocytopenia. In addition, tuftsin levels are quite low in AIDS patients and are linked to the increased risk of bacterial infection in AIDS patients.[10]

All of these diseases, including AIDS, share a common feature—increased levels of circulating immune complexes. Since one of the primary functions of the RES is to eliminate immune complexes from the circulation, we can assume RES function in patients with these diseases is below normal. This assumption has been proven in all of these conditions. Furthermore, research shows that there is an inverse correlation between spleen function and levels of circulating immune complexes in these autoimmune disorders. Clinical remission is almost always associated with normalization of RES (spleen) function. The increased incidence of autoimmune antibodies in splenectomized patients offers further evidence of the spleen's role in autoimmune disorders.[11]

Dosage Ranges

From a practical viewpoint, hydrolyzed (predigested) products concentrated for tuftsin and splenopentin content are preferable to crude preparations. Based on current clinical research, the daily dose should provide 50 milligrams of tuftsin and splenopentin, or roughly 1.5 grams of total spleen peptides.

Safety Issues

No side effects or adverse reactions have been reported with the use of oral spleen preparations.

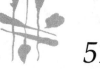

51

Thymus Extracts

The thymus is the major gland of our immune system. It is composed of two soft, pinkish-gray lobes lying in a biblike fashion just below the thyroid gland and above the heart. To a very large extent, the health of the thymus determines the health of the immune system. Individuals who experience frequent infections or suffer from chronic infections typically have impaired thymus activity. Also, people affected with hay fever, allergies, migraine headaches, and rheumatoid arthritis usually have altered thymus function. Before discussing how to support the thymus gland, let's first examine its important roles.

The thymus is responsible for many immune system functions, including the production of T lymphocytes (a type of white blood cell responsible for "cell-mediated immunity"). Cell-mediated immunity refers to immune mechanisms not controlled or mediated by antibodies. It is extremely important in the resistance to infection by moldlike bacteria, yeast (including *Candida albicans*), fungi, parasites, and viruses (including *Herpes simplex*, Epstein-Barr, and viruses that cause hepatitis). If an individual suffers from an infection caused by these organisms, usually their cell-mediated immunity is not functioning up to par. Cell-mediated immunity is also critical for protection against the development of cancer, autoimmune disorders like rheumatoid arthritis, and allergies.

The thymus releases several hormones, such as thymosin, thymopoeitin, and serum thymic factor, that regulate many immune functions. Low blood levels of these hormones are associated with depressed immunity and an increased susceptibility to infection. Typically, thymic hormone levels are very low in the elderly, individuals prone to infection, cancer and AIDS patients, and individuals exposed to undue stress.

If there is evidence that the thymus gland is not functioning at a sufficient level, it steps must be taken to improve thymus function. Promoting optimal thymus gland activity can involve:

- An adequate dietary intake of antioxidant nutrients like carotenes, vitamin C, vitamin E, zinc, and selenium to prevent thymic involution or shrinkage

- Use of nutrients (zinc, vitamin B$_6$, vitamin C) that are required in the manufacture or action of thymic hormones
- Use of products containing concentrates of calf thymus tissue

Principal Uses

A substantial amount of clinical data supports the effectiveness of orally administered thymus extracts. Specifically, numerous clinical trials show oral administration of predigested calf thymus extract rich in thymus-derived polypeptides is effective in:

- Prevention of recurrent respiratory infections in children
- Correction of T-cell defects in human immunodeficiency virus infections (AIDS)
- Treatment of acute hepatitis B infections
- Restoration of the number of peripheral leukocytes in cancer patients with chemotherapy-induced depression of WBC counts
- Treatment of allergies, including asthma, hay fever, and food allergies in children[1,2]

Thymus extract is probably effective in these conditions because it improves thymus gland activity, which in turn enhances the immune system's ability to function. This effect reflects a basic concept of glandular therapy—the oral ingestion of glandular material of a certain animal gland will strengthen the corresponding human gland. The result is a broad general effect indicative of improved glandular function. Amazingly, thymus extract can normalize the ratio of T-helper cells to suppressor cells whether the ratio is low (AIDS, chronic infections, and cancer) or high (allergies, migraine headaches, and autoimmune diseases like rheumatoid arthritis).[1,2]

Chronic Viral Infections

Recurrent or chronic infections, including the so-called "chronic fatigue syndrome" and "chronic postviral syndrome," are characterized by a depressed immune system. What makes it difficult for people to overcome these illnesses is the repetitive cycle—a compromised immune system leads to infection; infection leads to a damaged immune system, further weakening resistance. Thymus extracts may provide the answer to chronic infections by restoring healthy immune function.

Researchers studied the ability of thymus extracts to treat and then reduce the number of recurrent infections in groups of children with a history of recurrent respiratory tract infections. Double-blind studies reveal that orally administered thymus extracts are not only able to effectively eliminate infection, but that treatment over the course of a year significantly reduces the number of respiratory infections and significantly improves numerous immune parameters.[3]

One of the most difficult viral infections for the body to throw off is type B viral hepatitis; however, several double-blind studies indicate thymus extracts can be effective in both acute and chronic cases. In these studies, therapeutic effect was noted by accelerated decreases of liver enzymes (transaminases), elimination of the virus, and antibody changes, signifying clinical remission.[4,5]

The most extreme example of a chronic viral infection is AIDS. Although thymus extracts do not show any real therapeutic benefit in AIDS, studies indicate they can improve several immune parameters, including an ability to raise the T-helper cells, a critical goal in AIDS treatment.[6]

Cancer

The primary application of thymus extracts in cancer is counteraction of the immune suppressing effects of radiation and chemotherapy. The net effect of thymus extract administration is prevention of the tremendous depression of white blood cell levels and activity as a result of chemotherapy or radiation.[2,7]

Allergies

People with allergies often have derangements in the immune system. Levels of the allergic IgE (immunoglobulin gamma E) antibody and allergic white blood cells known as eosinophils are typically elevated. At the same time, levels of suppressor T-cells are typically depressed. These abnormalities are obviously caused by altered immune function.

Double-blind clinical studies indicate the oral administration of thymus extracts can improve the symptoms and course of hay fever, allergic rhinitis, asthma, eczema, and food allergies.[2,8–10] Presumably this clinical improvement is caused by restoration of proper immune function—i.e., reduced levels of IgE and eosinophils and improved ratio of helper to suppressor T-cells. In several double-blind studies, children receiving thymus extracts during food allergy–elimination diets often can tolerate foods previously allergenic and symptom-producing.[9,10]

Autoimmune Disorders

Autoimmune disorders like rheumatoid arthritis are characterized by the body's own antibodies attacking body tissues. Central to this autoimmunity is a high T-helper–to–suppressor–cell ratio. A high T-helper–to–suppressor–cell ratio results in increased antibody formation. The higher the ratio, the higher the number of antibodies being produced that can damage body structures. In one clinical study, rheumatoid arthritis patients with a helper-to-suppressor ratio of 3.30 achieved normal ratios (1.02 to 2.46) after 3 months of therapy with a thymus extract.[4] Although use of a thymus extract may not result in clinical improvement, it can be useful in restoring proper immune function in autoimmune diseases, including rheumatoid arthritis, lupus, and scleroderma.

Dosage Ranges

The dosage of thymus extract varies from one manufacturer to another. There are no quality-control procedures or standards enforced in the glandular industry; it is left up to the individual companies to adopt quality control and good manufacturing procedures.

From a practical view, products concentrated and standardized for polypeptide content are preferable to crude preparations. Based on current clinical research, the daily dose should be equivalent to 120 milligrams pure polypeptides with molecular weights less than 10,000, or roughly 750 milligrams of the crude polypeptide fraction.

Safety Issues

No side effects or adverse reactions have been reported with the use of thymus preparations.

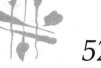

52

Thyroid Extracts

Because thyroid gland hormones regulate metabolism in each body cell, a deficiency of thyroid hormones can affect virtually all body functions. The degree of severity of symptoms in the adult ranges from extremely mild deficiency states that are barely detectable (subclinical hypothyroidism) to severe deficiency states that are life-threatening (myxedema).[1-4]

Deficiency of thyroid hormone may be because of defective hormone synthesis or lack of stimulation by the pituitary gland, which secretes thyroid-stimulating hormone (TSH). When thyroid hormone levels in the blood are low, the pituitary secretes TSH. If thyroid hormone levels are decreased and TSH levels are elevated in the blood, it usually indicates defective thyroid hormone synthesis. This is termed primary hypothyroidism. If TSH levels are low and thyroid hormone levels are also low, this indicates the pituitary gland is responsible for the low thyroid function. This is termed secondary hypothyroidism.

Beneficial Effects

The medical treatment of hypothyroidism in all but its mildest forms involves the use of desiccated thyroid or synthetic thyroid hormone. Although synthetic hormones are popular, many physicians (particularly naturopathic physicians) still prefer the use of desiccated natural thyroid, complete with all thyroid hormones. At this time, it appears that thyroid hormone replacement is necessary in the majority of people with hypothyroidism.

Available Forms

The Food and Drug Administration (FDA) requires the thyroid extracts sold in health-food stores to be thyroxine-free. However, it is nearly impossible to remove all the hormone from the gland. In other words, think of health-food store thyroid preparations as milder forms of desiccated natural thyroid. If you have mild hypothyroidism, these preparations may provide enough support to help you with your thyroid problem.

Since it is important to support the thyroid gland nutritionally by ensuring adequate intake of key nutrients required in the manufacture of thyroid hormone and avoiding goitrogens, most health-food store thyroid products also contain supportive nutrients like iodine, zinc, and tyrosine.

Deficiency Signs and Symptoms

Thyroid supplements may be helpful in the treatment of subclinical hypothyroidism; however, controversy still exists about the diagnosis of hypothyroidism. Before the use of blood measurements, it was common to diagnose hypothyroidism based on basal body temperature (temperature of the body at rest) and Achilles reflex time (reflexes are slowed in hypothyroidism). With the advent of sophisticated laboratory measurement of thyroid hormones in the blood, these "functional" tests fell by the wayside. However, scientists now know the blood tests are not sensitive enough to diagnose milder forms of hypothyroidism. Because mild hypothyroidism is the most common form of hypothyroidism, the majority of people with hypothyroidism are undiagnosed.[3-5]

Undiagnosed hypothyroidism is a serious concern because failure to treat an underlying condition like hypothyroidism reduces the effectiveness of nutritional therapies. For example, in most cases zinc, vitamin A, and essential fatty acids are effective in relieving dry, scaly skin. However, if a person has hypothyroidism, no improvement occurs. It is critical that thyroid function be evaluated because it might be an underlying factor in a large number of diseases.

Basal Body Temperature

The basal body temperature is perhaps the most sensitive functional test of thyroid function.[3,4] Your body temperature reflects your metabolic rate, which is largely determined by hormones secreted by the thyroid gland. The function of the thyroid gland, therefore, can be determined by simply measuring your basal body temperature. All that you need is a thermometer. The simple steps are:

1. At night before going to sleep, shake the thermometer until it registers below 95 degrees and place it by your bed.

2. When you awake, place the thermometer in your armpit for a full 10 minutes. It is important to make as little movement as possible. Lying and resting with your eyes closed is best. Do not get up until the 10-minute test is completed.

3. After 10 minutes, read and record the temperature and date.

4. Record the temperature for at least three mornings (preferably at the same time each day) and give the information to your physician. Menstruating women must

perform the test on the second, third, and fourth days of menstruation. Men and postmenopausal women can perform the test at any time.

Your basal body temperature should be between 97.6 and 98.2 degrees Fahrenheit. Low basal body temperatures are quite common and may reflect hypothyroidism. Common signs and symptoms of hypothyroidism are low basal body temperature, depression, difficulty in losing weight, dry skin, headaches, lethargy or fatigue, menstrual problems, recurrent infections, constipation, and sensitivity to cold.

High basal body temperatures (above 98.6 degrees Fahrenheit) are less common but may be evidence of hyperthyroidism. Common signs and symptoms of hyperthyroidism include bulging eyeballs, fast pulse, hyperactivity, inability to gain weight, insomnia, irritability, menstrual problems, and nervousness.

Occurrence

Most estimates of the occurrence of hypothyroidism are based on measurements of low levels of thyroid hormone in the blood. As stated above, this may mean a large number of people with mild hypothyroidism go undetected. Nonetheless, using blood levels of thyroid hormones as the criteria, it is estimated that between 1 and 4 percent of the adult population has moderate to severe hypothyroidism and another 10 to 12 percent has mild hypothyroidism.[2,6–8] The incidence of hypothyroidism increases steadily with advancing age.

Some popular authors of health texts who use medical history, physical examination, and basal body temperatures along with the blood thyroid levels as the diagnostic criteria estimate the rate of hypothyroidism in the general adult population is approximately 40 percent.[2,3] However, the true rate of hypothyroidism using this criteria is probably somewhere near 25 percent of the population.

Manifestations

Since thyroid hormone affects each body cell, a deficiency usually results in a large number of signs and symptoms. Here is a brief review of the common manifestations of hypothyroid on several body systems.

- **Metabolic** The metabolic manifestations of hypothyroidism reflect a general decrease in the rate of utilization of fat, protein, and carbohydrate. Moderate weight gain combined with cold intolerance is a common finding. Cholesterol and triglyceride levels are increased in even the mildest forms of hypothyroidism.[9] This elevation greatly increases the risk of serious cardiovascular disease. Studies show an increased rate of heart disease because of atherosclerosis in individuals with hypothyroidism.[10,11] It also leads to increased capillary permeability and slow lymphatic drainage. Often this results in swelling of tissue (edema).

- **Endocrine** A variety of hormonal symptoms can exist in hypothyroidism. Perhaps the most common is a loss of libido (sexual drive) in men and menstrual abnormalities in women. Women with mild hypothyroidism have prolonged and heavy menstrual bleeding with a shorter menstrual cycle (time from the start of one period to the next). Infertility may also be a problem. If the hypothyroid woman does become pregnant, miscarriages, premature deliveries, and stillbirths are common. Rarely does a pregnancy terminate in normal labor and delivery in the hypothyroid woman.

- **Skin, Hair and Nails**   Dry, rough skin covered with fine superficial scales is seen in most hypothyroid individuals and the hair is course, dry, and brittle. Hair loss can be quite severe. The nails become thin and brittle and typically show transverse grooves.

- **Psychological**   The brain appears to be quite sensitive to low levels of thyroid hormone. Depression along with weakness and fatigue are usually the first symptoms of hypothyroidism.[5,12] Later, the hypothyroid individual has difficulty concentrating and becomes extremely forgetful.

- **Musculoskeletal**   Muscle weakness and joint stiffness are predominate features of hypothyroidism.[13] Some individuals with hypothyroidism may also experience tenderness and muscle and joint pain.[14]

- **Cardiovascular**   Hypothyroidism probably predisposes one to atherosclerosis because of the increase in cholesterol and triglycerides.[9–11] It can also cause hypertension, reduce the function of the heart, and reduce heart rate.

- **Other Manifestations**   Shortness of breath, constipation, and impaired kidney function are other common features of hypothyroidism.[2]

Dietary Considerations

Thyroid hormone manufacture by the thyroid gland depends on several important nutrients. Deficiency of any of a number of vitamins and minerals (especially iodine) or ingestion of certain foods could result in hypothyroidism. Specifics to consider are:

- **Iodine and Tyrosine**   Thyroid hormones are made from iodine and the amino acid tyrosine. The RDA for iodine in adults is quite small, 150 micrograms.[15] The average intake of iodine in the United States is estimated at over 600 micrograms per day. Too much iodine can actually inhibit thyroid gland synthesis. For this reason, and because the only function of iodine in the body is for thyroid hormone synthesis, it is recommended that dietary levels or supplementation of iodine not exceed 600 micrograms per day for any length of time.

- **Goitrogens**   Some foods contain substances that prevent the utilization of iodine. These foods are termed goitrogens and include such foods as turnips, cabbage, mustard, cassava root, soybean, peanuts, pine nuts, and millet. Cooking usually inactivates goitrogens.[15]

- **Vitamins and Minerals**   Zinc and vitamins E and A function together in many body processes, including the manufacture of thyroid hormone.[16] A deficiency of any of these nutrients results in lower production of active thyroid hormone. Low zinc levels are common in the elderly, as is hypothyroidism.[17] There may be a correlation. Vitamin C and the B vitamins riboflavin (B_2), niacin (B_3), and pyridoxine (B_6) are also necessary for normal thyroid hormone manufacture.[16]

Exercise

Exercise is particularly important in a hypothyroidism treatment program. It stimulates thyroid gland secretion and increases tissue sensitivity to thyroid hormone. Many health benefits of exercise may be a result of improved thyroid function. These benefits are especially important in overweight hypothyroid individuals who are dieting (restricting food intake). A consistent result of dieting is a decrease in the metabolic rate as the body strives to conserve fuel. Exercise can prevent the decline in metabolic rate in response to dieting.[18]

Dosage Ranges

The dosage of commercial thyroid preparations really depends on the potency and level of supportive nutrients. Obviously, these factors vary from one manufacturer to the next. Therefore, it is best to follow the manufacturer's recommendations provided on the product's label. Use your basal body temperature to determine effectiveness of the product.

Safety Issues

Because thyroxine has been removed from health-food store thyroid extracts, the only real concern for safety involves the level of supportive nutrients.

PART SEVEN

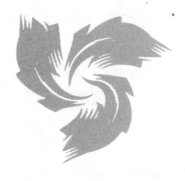

Quick Reference Guide for
Specific Health Conditions

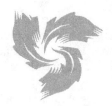

Nutritional supplements are important, but they are only one aspect of health promotion. A positive mental attitude, healthful diet, and exercise are critical to achieving and maintaining good health. The basic outline for each health condition discussed in this section follows this pattern:

- **Description**   A narration and important features.

- **Dietary and Lifestyle Recommendations**   Important dietary and lifestyle considerations. General recommendations for all conditions are
  - Consume a diet that focuses on whole, unprocessed foods (whole grains, legumes, vegetables, fruits, nuts, and seeds).
  - Eliminate alcohol, caffeine, and sugar.
  - Identify and control food allergies.
  - Get regular exercise.
  - Perform a relaxation exercise (deep breathing, meditation, prayer, visualization, etcetera) 10 to 15 minutes each day.
  - Drink at least 48 ounces of water daily.

- **Supplement Protocol**   Unless otherwise specified, the following supplements are recommended:
  - High-potency multiple according to guidelines in Chapter 2
  - Vitamin C, 500 to 1,000 milligrams three times daily
  - Vitamin E, 200 to 400 International Units daily
  - Flaxseed oil, 1 tablespoon daily

These recommendations serve as a strong foundation upon which to build an effective supplementation protocol. It assures a high intake of essential nutrients and antioxidants.

- **Additional Recommendations**   Additional recommendations to consider. Usually they are to be used if there is little or no response to the previous recommendations.

- **Comments**   Interesting facts, contraindications, and general information on the entire program for a particular health condition.

Acne

Acne affects the pores of the skin, canals through which a hair follicle passes. Glands known as sebaceous glands produce sebum, a mixture of oils and waxes, which lubricates the skin and prevents water loss. Sebaceous glands are found in highest concentrations on the face, back, chest, and shoulders. Acne affects the areas of the skin that have sebaceous glands.

Acne occurs in two forms—acne vulgaris, which affects the hair follicles and oil-secreting glands of the skin and manifests as blackheads, whiteheads, inflammation; and acne conglobata, a more severe form, with deep cyst formation and subsequent scaring.

Acne is most common at puberty because of increased levels of the male sex hormone testosterone. Although men have higher levels of testosterone than women, during puberty there is an increase of testosterone in both sexes, which makes girls just as susceptible to acne in this age group. Testosterone causes the sebaceous glands to enlarge and produce more sebum. In addition, the cells that line the skin pore produce more keratin. The combination of increased secretion of sebum and keratin can lead to pore blockage and the formation of a blackhead. With the pore blocked, bacteria can overgrow and release enzymes that break down sebum and promote inflammation. This forms what is known as a whitehead or pimple.

Dietary and Lifestyle Recommendations

- Eliminate all refined and/or concentrated sugars from the diet.
- Do not eat foods containing trans-fatty acids such as milk, milk products, margarine, shortening, and other synthetically hydrogenated vegetable oils; avoid fried foods.
- Avoid milk and foods high in iodized salt.
- Avoid the use of greasy creams or cosmetics.
- Wash the pillowcase regularly in chemical-free (no added colors or fragrances) detergents.

Supplement Protocol

- High-potency multiple according to the guidelines in Chapter 2
- Vitamin C, 500 to 1,000 milligrams three times daily
- Vitamin E, 200 to 400 International Units daily
- Flaxseed oil, 1 tablespoon daily
- Vitamin A, follow guidelines in Chapter 3

- Chromium, 400 to 600 micrograms daily
- Zinc, 45 to 60 milligrams daily

Additional Recommendations

I also recommend washing the face or affected area with a natural soap or cleanser (such as Akne Treatment Cleanser from Enzymatic Therapy) twice daily. For cystic acne and acne rosacea, I recommend a pancrelipase, the fat-digesting enzyme from hog pancreas, at a dosage of 125 milligrams twice daily.

Comments

Do not use high-dosage vitamin A therapy in women of child-bearing age.

Age Spots

Age spots are caused by an accumulation of cellular debris known as lipofuscin within cells. In the skin, the lipofuscin deposits can coalesce or clump together to produce brown spots commonly referred to as "age spots." This process occurs throughout the body; however, we see only the spots on the skin. Typically, the cellular debris in a lipofuscin deposit is composed primarily of molecules partially destroyed by free-radical damage. The number and severity of age spots are a good indication of the level of oxidative damage that has occurred throughout the body.

Dietary and Lifestyle Recommendations

- Avoid excessive sun exposure and use sun-blocking creams when out in the sun.
- Avoid cigarette smoke, fried foods, and other sources of free radicals.
- Consume a diet rich in plant foods, especially high-carotene foods (green leafy vegetables, carrots, yams, sweet potatoes, etcetera).
- Drink at least 48 ounces of water daily.

Supplement Protocol

- High-potency multiple according to guidelines in Chapter 2
- Vitamin C, 500 to 1,000 milligrams three times daily
- Vitamin E, 400 to 800 International Units daily
- Carotene complex, 50,000 to 100,000 International Units daily

Additional Recommendations

- Grape seed extract (95 percent procyanidolic oligomers), 50 milligrams three times daily

Comments

Age spots are indicative of free-radical and oxidative damage internally as well as on the skin. Dr. Julian Whitaker also recommends a product called Imedeen from Scandinavian Naturals. Imedeen is composed of a special protein and glycosaminoglycan concentrate from fish. Several clinical studies show that Imedeen, at an oral dose of 380 to 500 milligrams daily, can significantly improve the health of the skin and help the skin look younger. Also, when a cosmetic effect is desired, Dr. Whitaker recommends the bleaching agent hydroquinone. Reviva Brown Spot Cream is a popular brand.

AIDS and HIV Infection

AIDS (acquired immunodeficiency syndrome) is a severe immune deficiency state due to an infection of the human immunodeficiency virus (HIV). The major methods of transmission of HIV are sexual contact, blood to blood (through blood transfusions or needle sharing in drug addicts), and from woman to fetus.

AIDS is not present in all persons infected with HIV. AIDS represents the end stage of the infection and severe depression of the immune system. The goal is to prevent the progression of the disease by supporting the immune system and inhibiting or slowing down the replication of the virus. The recommendations given below are most suitable for HIV-positive patients not demonstrating AIDS.

Dietary and Lifestyle Recommendations

- Do not have sexual intercourse with persons known to have or suspected of having HIV or who use intravenous drugs.
- Practice safe sex.
- Do not share a toothbrush, razor, or other implement that could become contaminated with blood from someone with an HIV infection.
- Consume a diet that focuses on whole, unprocessed foods (whole grains, legumes, vegetables, fruits, nuts, and seeds).
- Consume adequate protein intake (consider supplementation with a high-quality whey protein at a dosage of 1 gram per 2 pounds body weight).
- Perform a relaxation exercise (deep breathing, meditation, prayer, visualization, etcetera) 10 to 15 minutes each day.
- Get regular exercise (nonstrenuous walking, Tai Chi, stretching, etcetera).
- Eliminate alcohol, caffeine, and sugar.
- Identify and control food allergies.
- Drink at least 48 ounces of water daily.

Supplement Protocol

- High-potency multiple according to guidelines in Chapter 2

- Flaxseed oil, 1 tablespoon daily
- Vitamin C, 3,000 to 12,000 milligrams daily
- Vitamin E, 200 to 400 International Units daily
- Carotene complex, 50,000 to 100,000 International Units daily
- Methylcobalamin (active vitamin B_{12}), 2 milligrams twice daily
- Lipoic acid, 150 milligrams three times daily
- Thymus extract, 750 milligrams of the crude polypeptide fraction daily
- Spleen extract, 1,500 milligrams of spleen polypeptides daily
- Pancreatin (8–10×), 350 to 700 milligrams three times daily between meals

Additional Recommendations

A high-quality whey protein at a dosage of 1 gram per 2 pounds body weight should be used in patients showing signs of muscle wasting or weight loss.

Comments

There is concern over the use of the herb *Echinacea* in patients with HIV and AIDS. Although AIDS is associated with wide-spread depression of the immune system and *Echinacea* can dramatically improve immune function in people with low immune status, there is concern because *Echinacea* can increase levels of tumor-necrosis-factor (TNF). This compound can stimulate replication of the HIV as well. At this time it appears wise for HIV-infected individuals to avoid *Echinacea* until there is more research.

Alcoholism

Alcoholism is defined by the World Health Organization as alcohol consumption by an individual that exceeds the limits accepted by the culture or that injures health or social relationships. Current estimates indicate that alcoholism affects at least 10 million persons in the United States and causes 200,000 deaths each year, making alcoholism one of the most serious health problems today. The total number of people affected, either directly or indirectly, is much greater when one considers disruption of family life, automobile accidents (50 percent of fatal accidents involve a drinking driver), crime, decreased productivity, and mental and physical disease.

Dietary and Lifestyle Recommendations

- Eliminate the consumption of alcohol, refined sugar, and coffee (both caffeinated and decaffeinated).
- Eat less saturated fat and cholesterol by reducing or eliminating the amounts of animal products in the diet.

- Increase the consumption of fiber-rich plant foods (fruits, vegetables, grains, legumes, and raw nuts and seeds).
- Do not smoke.
- Get regular exercise.
- Drink at least 48 ounces of water daily.

Supplement Protocol

- High-potency multiple according to guidelines in Chapter 2
- Vitamin C, 500 to 1,000 milligrams three times daily
- Vitamin E, 200 to 400 International Units daily
- Flaxseed oil, 1 tablespoon daily
- Chromium, 200 to 400 micrograms daily
- Phosphatidylcholine, 500 milligrams three times daily
- L-carnitine, 300 milligrams three times daily

Additional Recommendations

Silymarin, the flavonoid complex from milk thistle (*Silybum marianum*) is also indicated at a dosage of 70 to 210 milligrams of silymarin three times daily. A special silymarin preparation bound to phosphatidylcholine (silymarin phytosome) may offer even better results at a dosage of 100 milligrams two to three times daily.

Comments

Alcohol consumption leads to hypoglycemia. The drop in blood sugar produces a craving for food, particularly foods that quickly elevate blood sugar—sugar and alcohol. Increased sugar consumption aggravates blood sugar control, particularly in the presence of alcohol. Hypoglycemia aggravates the mental and emotional problems of the alcoholic and the withdrawing alcoholic with such symptoms as sweating, tremor, rapid heart beat, anxiety, hunger, dizziness, headache, visual disturbance, decreased mental function, confusion, and depression.

Alzheimer's Disease, Senility, and Dementia

Senility and dementia refer to a general mental deterioration. In the elderly, this mental deterioration is often referred to as "senile dementia." Most often when this term is used, it describes a progressive deterioration of mental function, loss of short-term or recent memory, moodiness and irritability, self-centeredness, and childish behavior. Alzheimer's disease is the best known and most feared type of dementia. Alzheimer's disease can occur at any age, but most commonly after 50. Symptoms occurring before 65 are designated pre–senile dementia of the Alzheimer's type

(PDAT). After 65 it's senile dementia of the Alzheimer's type (SDAT). Current diagnosis of Alzheimer's disease is extremely difficult because the only definitive diagnosis is after-death biopsy of the brain.

Alzheimer's disease is characterized by the general destruction of nerve cells in several key areas of the brain devoted to mental functions. This results in neurofibrillary tangles and plaque formation. The disease's clinical features are probably related to a decrease in acetylcholine, which functions as a transmitting agent in the brain, although there is a general reduction in the concentration of all neurotransmitting substances.

After-death studies demonstrate that about 50 percent of all cases of dementia are the result of Alzheimer's disease. This statistic means approximately 50 percent of dementia patients do not have Alzheimer's. It is not known to what degree patients are erroneously diagnosed as having Alzheimer's, or some other dementia, but it is estimated to be a significant number.

Dietary and Lifestyle Recommendations

- Avoid aluminum (found in many antiperspirants, antacids, and cookware).
- Adopt a general healthful dietary and lifestyle plan.

Supplement Protocol

- High-potency multiple according to guidelines in Chapter 2
- Vitamin C, 500 to 1,000 milligrams three times daily
- Vitamin E, 400 to 800 International Units daily
- Flaxseed oil, 1 tablespoon daily
- Thiamin, 3 to 8 grams daily
- Phosphatidylserine, 100 milligrams three times daily
- Methylcobalamin (active vitamin B_{12}), 1,000 micrograms twice daily

Additional Recommendations

- Get a hair mineral analysis to rule out high lead, aluminum, or other heavy metals.
- *Ginkgo biloba* extract (24 percent ginkgo flavonglycosides) at a dosage of 80 milligrams three times daily can be quite useful in the early stages of Alzheimer's disease.

Comments

Virtually any nutrient deficiency can result in impaired mental function. Nutritional status can be the major factor determining mental function in people over the age of 60. Better nutritional status means better memory and mental function. Correcting an underlying nutritional deficiency can restore normal mental function. A particularly important nutrient in Alzheimer's disease patients is vitamin B_{12}. Vitamin B_{12} works together with folic acid in the manufacture of several nerve transmitters and in nerve cell replication. B_{12} levels are significantly low, and vitamin B_{12} deficiency significantly common, in patients with Alzheimer's disease. Patients with severe mental disorders as a result of a B_{12} deficiency can experience complete recovery upon B_{12} supplementation. Methylcobalamin is the most active form of vitamin B_{12}.

Anemia

Anemia refers to a condition in which the blood is deficient in red blood cells or the hemoglobin (iron-containing) portion of red blood cells. The primary function of the red blood cell (RBC) is to transport oxygen from the lungs to the tissues of the body. There, the RBCs exchange the oxygen for carbon dioxide. Symptoms of anemia, such as extreme fatigue, reflect both a lack of oxygen in the tissues and a buildup of carbon dioxide.

There are several different types of anemia. The major categories are due to excessive blood loss, excessive red blood cell destruction, or deficient red blood cell production. The most common anemias fall into the category of deficient red blood cell production. In most cases, anemia is secondary to blood loss or a nutrient deficiency. Iron deficiency is, by far, the most common nutritional cause of anemia. Deficiencies of folic acid or vitamin B_{12} can also lead to anemia.

Any case of anemia should be properly diagnosed by a physician to identify the cause. Treatment must be directed at the underlying cause.

Supplement Protocol

- Any anemia, hydrolyzed (liquid) liver extract, 500 to 1,500 milligrams before meals
- Iron deficiency anemia, iron (succinate), 15 to 30 milligrams twice daily
- Folic acid deficiency anemia, folic acid, 400 micrograms twice daily
- Vitamin B_{12} deficiency anemia, methylcobalamin (active vitamin B_{12}, 1,000 milligrams twice daily for at least 1 month followed by a daily intake of 1,000 micrograms

Comments

One of the real advantages to hydrolyzed (liquid) liver extracts is they are rich in heme iron as well as folic acid and vitamin B_{12}.

Angina

Angina describes a squeezing or pressurelike pain in the chest. It is caused by an insufficient supply of oxygen to the heart muscle. Since physical exertion and stress cause the heart to need increased oxygen, symptoms of angina are often preceded by these factors. The pain may radiate to the left shoulder blade, left arm, or jaw. The pain typically lasts for only 1 to 20 minutes.

Angina is almost always due to the buildup of cholesterol-containing plaque that progressively narrows and ultimately blocks the blood vessels supplying the heart, the coronary arteries. This blockage results in a decreased blood and oxygen supply to the heart tissue. When the flow of oxygen to the heart muscle is substantially reduced, or when there is an increased need by the heart, it results in angina. The same recommendations for angina also are useful in arrhythmias (altered heart rate or rhythm).

Dietary and Lifestyle Recommendations

- Eat less saturated fat and cholesterol by reducing or eliminating the amounts of animal products in the diet.
- Increase the consumption of fiber-rich plant foods (fruits, vegetables, grains, legumes, and raw nuts and seeds).
- Achieve ideal body weight.
- Participate in regular aerobic exercise under medical supervision.
- Do not smoke.
- Eliminate the consumption of coffee (both caffeinated and decaffeinated).

Supplement Protocol

- High-potency multiple according to guidelines in Chapter 2
- Vitamin C, 500 to 1,000 milligrams three times daily
- Vitamin E, 400 to 800 International Units daily
- Flaxseed oil, 1 tablespoon daily
- Magnesium, 200–400 milligrams three times daily
- Coenzyme Q_{10}, 150 to 300 milligrams daily
- L-carnitine, 500 milligrams three times daily
- Aortic glycosaminoglycans, 50 milligrams twice daily

Comments

Angina is a serious condition that requires strict medical supervision. In the severe case, as well as in the initial stages in the mild to moderate patient, prescription medications may be necessary. Eventually the condition should be manageable with the help of natural measures. If there is significant blockage of the coronary artery, refer to the American College of Advancement in Medicine (ACAM), 23121 Verdugo Drive, Suite 204, Laguna Hills, CA 92653, 1-800 532-3688 (outside California) or 1-800-435-6199 (inside California).

Ankylosing Spondylitis (See Rheumatoid Arthritis)

Anxiety

Anxiety is defined as an unpleasant emotional state ranging from mild unease to intense fear. Anxiety differs from fear. Fear is a rational response to a real danger, while anxiety usually lacks a clear or realistic cause. Though some anxiety is normal and, in fact, healthy, higher levels of anxiety are not only uncomfortable, they can lead to significant problems.

Anxiety is often accompanied by a variety of symptoms. The most common symptoms relate to the chest. These include heart palpitations (awareness of a more forceful or faster heart beat), throbbing or stabbing pains, a feeling of tightness and inability to take in enough air, and a tendency to sigh or hyperventilate. Anxiety can cause tension in the muscles of the back and neck and can lead to headaches, back pains, and muscle spasms. Other symptoms can include excessive sweating, dryness of mouth, dizziness, and symptoms of the irritable bowel syndrome.

Dietary and Lifestyle Recommendations

- Eliminate the intake of caffeine, alcohol, and sugar.
- Identify and control food allergies.
- Perform a relaxation exercise (deep breathing, meditation, prayer, visualization, etcetera) 10 to 15 minutes each day.
- Get regular exercise.

Supplement Protocol

- High-potency multiple according to guidelines in Chapter 2
- Flaxseed oil, 1 tablespoon daily

Additional Recommendations

Kava extract (30 percent kavalactone content) at a dosage of 200 milligrams three times daily can be as effective as drugs like Valium but without the side effects.

Comments

Caffeine must be avoided by patients with anxiety or depression. Caffeine is a stimulant. Even the small amount of caffeine in decaffeinated coffee is enough to affect some people adversely and produce symptoms of anxiety or depression.

Arthritis (See Gout, Osteoarthritis, or Rheumatoid Arthritis)

Arrhythmias (Follow Recommendations for Angina)

Asthma

Asthma is an allergic disorder characterized by spasm of the bronchial tubes and excessive excretion of a viscous mucous in the lungs. This can lead to difficult breathing. Asthma occurs as recurrent attacks that range from mild wheezing to a life-threatening inability to breathe.

The number of Americans suffering from asthma and other allergies has risen dramatically over the last 15 years. Some possible reasons include increased stress on the immune system due to changes in environment (such as greater chemical pollution in the air, water, and food), earlier weaning and earlier introduction of solid foods to infants, food additives, and genetic manipulation of plants resulting in food components with greater allergenic tendencies.

Dietary and Lifestyle Recommendations

- Eliminate food allergies.
- Avoid airborne allergens.
- Follow a vegetarian diet.
- Drink at least 48 ounces of water daily.

Supplement Protocol

- High-potency multiple according to guidelines in Chapter 2
- Vitamin C, 10 to 30 milligrams for every 2 pounds body weight
- Vitamin E, 200 to 400 International Units daily
- Flaxseed oil, 1 tablespoon daily
- Magnesium, 200 to 400 milligrams three times daily
- Adrenal cortex extract, 250 milligrams three times daily

Additional Recommendations

Herbal preparations containing Ma huang (*Ephedra sinensis*) can be quite helpful. The dosage of *Ephedra* depends on the alkaloid content. For asthma, the dosage of ephedrine is 12.5 to 25.0 milligrams two to three times daily.

Comments

Food allergies are a major cause of asthma, especially in children. Milk, corn, wheat, citrus, peanuts, eggs, chocolate, food colorings, and food additives are the major culprits.

In childhood asthma, eliminating food allergies and food additives is often all that is needed.

Airborne allergens such as pollen, dander, and dust mites are often difficult to avoid entirely. Measures can be taken to reduce exposure. Make the bedroom as allergy-proof as possible. Encase the mattress in allergen-proof plastic; wash sheets, blankets, pillowcases, and mattress pads every week; and consider using bedding material made from Ventflex, a special hypoallergenic synthetic material.

Atherosclerosis (See Cholesterol)

Attention Deficit Disorder

Attention deficit disorder is the term currently used to describe a condition that has had multiple labels in the past, including "hyperactivity" and "learning disability." This condition describes three separate disorders: attention deficit disorder without hyperactivity, attention deficit disorder with hyperactivity, and attention deficit disorder residual type. Residual attention deficit disorder (individuals 18 years or older) is viewed primarily as a continuation of the process.

Attention deficit disorder with hyperactivity is the most common. About 3 percent of all school-age children carry this diagnosis. Boys are more likely to be given this diagnosis. In fact, ten boys have it for every one girl. The characteristics of this disorder in order of their frequency are

- Hyperactivity
- Perceptual motor impairment
- Emotional instability
- General coordination deficit
- Disorders of attention
  - Short attention span
  - Distractibility
  - Lack of perseverance
  - Failure to finish things
  - Not listening
  - Poor concentration
- Impulsiveness
  - Action before thought
  - Abrupt shifts in activity
  - Poor organizing
  - Jumping up in class
- Disorders of memory and thinking
- Specific learning disabilities
- Disorders of speech and hearing
- Neurological signs and electroencephalograph (EEG) irregularities

Dietary and Lifestyle Recommendations

Eliminate food allergies and food additives. I refer parents to Dr. William Crook's book *Help for the Hyperactive Child* (Professional Books) or any of the excellent books on attention deficit disorder and hyperactivity written by Dr. Doris Rapp. Also, Meridian Valley Clinical Laboratory (1-206-859-8700) and National Biotech Laboratory (1-800-846-6285) offer a food allergy test that measures both IgE and IgG antibodies, tests for over 100 different foods, comes with detailed dietary instructions, and is reasonably priced at about $120.

Supplement Protocol

Children's high-potency multiple vitamin and mineral preparation.

Additional Recommendations

Numerous studies show that children with attention deficit disorder often have high body stores of heavy metals. I recommend consulting a nutritionally oriented physician to determine whether heavy metals are a factor.

Comments

Nutrient deficiency exists in a significant number of children with attention deficit disorder and learning disabilities. Fortunately, correcting any underlying nutritional deficiency results in an almost immediate improvement in mental function. Even when there is no true nutrient deficiency, taking vitamins and minerals may help improve mental function in children.

Bladder Infections

Over 20 percent of women develop a bladder infection each year. If not treated early and well, the infection may become chronic and spread to the kidneys. The typical symptoms of a bladder infection can include:

- Burning pain on urination
- Increased urinary frequency
- Nighttime urination
- Turbid, foul-smelling or dark urine
- Lower abdominal pain

Most bladder infections are caused by bacteria; however, the diagnosis of bladder infection by culturing the urine for bacteria is imprecise because clinical symptoms and the presence of significant amounts of bacteria in the urine do not always correlate well. Only 60 percent of women with the typical symptoms of urinary tract infection actually have significant levels of bacteria in their urine.

Dietary and Lifestyle Recommendations (Prevention)

- Drink plenty of water (3 quarts or more per day).
- After sexual intercourse, try to urinate as soon as possible.

Supplement Protocol (Acute Infection)

- Calcium bound to Krebs cycle intermediates, 250 milligrams four times daily
- Probiotics, 5 to 10 billion viable *L. acidophilus* or *B. bifidum* cells daily.

Additional Recommendations

Drink unsweetened cranberry juice (16 ounces daily) or take a cranberry extract (follow dosage recommendations on label).

Comments

Although many physicians and women believe acidifying the urine is the best approach, several arguments can be made for alkalinizing the urine. First of all, it is often very difficult to acidify the urine. Many popular methods of attempting to acidify the urine, such as ascorbic acid supplementation and the drinking of cranberry juice, have very little effect on pH at commonly prescribed doses.

The best argument for alkalinizing the urine is that it appears to be more effective, especially in women without evidence of bacteria in their urine. The best method for alkalinizing the urine appears to be a multimineral formula where the minerals are chelated members of the Krebs cycle, such as citrate, malate, fumarate, and succinate.

Blood Clots (See Thrombophlebitis)

Boils

A boil is an inflamed, pus-filled area of skin, usually caused by a hair follicle (the tiny pit from which a hair grows) becoming infected with the bacteria *Staphylococcus auereus*. A boil usually starts as a painful, red lump. As it swells, it fills with pus and becomes rounded, with a yellowish tip (head). Common sites include the back of the neck and moist areas such as the armpits and groin. A more severe and extensive form of a boil is a carbuncle.

Common measures should be taken to prevent the spread of infection, such as cleaning the affected area, taking showers instead of baths, and washing the face and hands several times a day. Towels, linens, and clothing should be kept away from other family members to avoid spreading to others. Do not burst a boil. This may spread infection to deeper tissues. A hot compress applied every 2 hours relieves discomfort and hastens drainage and healing. If the boil is especially large or painful, consult your physician for proper drainage.

Supplement Protocol

- High-potency multiple according to guidelines in Chapter 2
- Vitamin C, 500 to 1,000 milligrams three times daily
- Vitamin E, 200 to 400 International Units daily
- Flaxseed oil, 1 tablespoon daily
- Zinc, 45 to 60 milligrams daily

Additional Recommendations

Apply a hot compress over the area every 2 hours followed by a topical application of pure tea tree oil.

Bronchitis and Pneumonia

Bronchitis refers to an infection or irritation of the bronchial tree, while pneumonia refers to infection or irritation of the lungs. Both are characterized by chills, fever, and chest pain. Pneumonia shows more signs of lung involvement (shallow breathing, cough, abnormal breath sounds, etcetera). X-rays of patients with pneumonia reveal infiltration of fluid and lymph in the lungs. Of the two conditions, pneumonia is by far the more serious.

Dietary and Lifestyle Recommendations

- Avoid cigarette smoke and other respiratory irritants.
- Rest.
- Drink at least 48 ounces of water daily.
- Avoid sugar and dairy products.

Supplement Protocol (Acute Treatment)

- Thymus extract, 750 milligrams of crude polypeptide fraction once or twice daily
- Vitamin C, 500 to 1,000 milligrams every waking hour or to bowel tolerance

Additional Recommendations

Goldenseal root extract (8 to 10 percent berberine content) and bromelain at a dosage of 400 milligrams of each three times daily on an empty stomach.

Comments

One of our main treatment goals in bronchitis and pneumonia is to help the lungs and air passages rid themselves of excessive mucus. I recommend performing the following twice daily: Apply a heating pad, hot water bottle, or a mustard poultice to the chest for up to 20 minutes. A mustard poultice is made by mixing 1 part dry mustard with 3 parts flour and adding enough water to make a paste. Then spread the paste on cotton (an old pillowcase works well) or cheesecloth, fold, and then place on the chest. Check often because the mustard can cause blisters if left on too long. After the hot pack, lie with the top half of the body off the bed, using the forearms as support—this position facilitates drainage of the lungs. Remain in this position for a 5- to 15-minute period and cough and expectorate into a basin or newspaper on the floor.

Bruises

Bruises often result from trauma. If bruises occur without the slightest trauma, it usually reflects thinning of the dermis (the support structure just below the surface of the skin). Regardless of the cause of the bruising, the recommendations below can be of value.

Dietary and Lifestyle Recommendations

- Consume a diet rich in flavonoids by increasing the intake of fresh berries, onions, and citrus fruit.
- Drink at least 48 ounces of water daily.

Supplement Protocol

- High-potency multiple according to guidelines in Chapter 2
- Vitamin C, 500 to 1,000 milligrams three times daily
- Vitamin E, 200 to 400 International Units daily
- Flaxseed oil, 1 tablespoon daily
- PCO extracts or flavonoids according to dosage recommendations in Chapter 37

Additional Recommendations

If additional support is needed, I recommend using the purified triterpenes of gotu cola (*Centella asiatica*) at a dosage of 70 milligrams twice daily.

Bursitis and Tendonitis

Bursitis is inflammation of the bursa, the saclike membrane containing fluid that lubricates the joints. Bursitis may be secondary to trauma, strain, infection, or arthritic conditions. The most common locations are shoulder, elbow, hip, seat, and lower knee. Occasionally the bursa can develop calcified deposits and become a chronic problem.

Tendonitis is an inflammatory condition of a tendon, usually resulting from a strain. Although acute tendonitis usually heals within a few days to 2 weeks, it may become chronic, in which case calcium salts typically deposit along the tendon fibers. The tendons most commonly affected are the Achilles (back of ankle), biceps (front of shoulder), pollicis brevis and longus (thumb), upper patella (knee), posterior tibial (inside of foot), and rotator cuff (shoulder).

The most common cause is sudden excessive tension on a tendon or bursa, although repeated trauma (such as intense sports) can result in similar injury. Some tendonitis may have an anatomical basis because the grooves in which the tendons move may develop bone spurs or other mechanical abnormalities. Proper stretching and warm-up before exercise are important preventive measures.

Supplement Protocol

Manganese, first 2 weeks, 50 to 200 milligrams daily in divided dosages; thereafter, 15 to 30 milligrams daily.

Additional Recommendations

After an injury or sprain, immediate first aid is very important. The acronym RICE summarizes the approach:

- *R*est the injured part immediately to avoid further injury.
- *I*ce the area of pain to decrease swelling and bleeding.
- Compress the area with an elastic bandage, also to limit swelling and bleeding.
- *E*levate the part above heart level to increase fluid drainage out of the injured area.

Proper application of these procedures is important for optimal results. When icing, first cover the injury with a towel, then place an ice pack on it. It is important not to wrap the injured part so tightly that circulation is impaired. The ice and compress should be applied for 30 minutes, followed by 15 minutes without the ice and compress to allow recirculation. Of course, for any serious injury, consult a physician immediately. Indications for a physician include severe pain, injuries to the joints, loss of function, and pain that persists for more than 2 weeks.

Cancer

Cancer refers to an unrestrained growth of cells. Most malignant cancers develop in organs, such as the lungs, breasts, prostate, pancreas, and colon, but they may also develop in other tissues and spread. Standard medical treatment of malignancies can include surgery, chemotherapy, and radiation. Chemotherapy and radiation expose healthy cells and cancer cells to free-radical damage. The result is a great stress to antioxidant mechanisms and depletion of valuable antioxidant enzymes and nutrients. Therefore, nutritional support in the cancer patient must provide additional antioxidants and accessory nutrients that can protect against the damaging effects of chemotherapy and radiation.

Dietary and Lifestyle Recommendations

- Consume a high-fiber, plant-based diet.
- Consume 16 to 24 ounces of fresh vegetable juice daily.
- Get regular exercise.
- Watch comedies, read comics, and try to laugh often.

Supplement Protocol

- High-potency multiple according to guidelines in Chapter 2
- Vitamin C, 3,000 to 12,000 milligrams daily in divided dosages
- Vitamin E, 400 to 800 International Units daily
- Flaxseed oil, 1 to 2 tablespoons daily
- Carotene complex, 50,000 to 100,000 International Units daily
- Thymus extract, 750 milligrams crude polypeptide fraction once or twice daily
- Coenzyme Q_{10}, 150 to 300 milligrams daily during chemotherapy and for 6 months after the last chemotherapy treatment

Additional Recommendations

If the cancer patient has difficulty eating or maintaining his or her body weight, consider supplementing the diet with high-quality whey protein at the dosage recommendation of 1 gram protein per 2 pounds body weight.

Comments

Cancer comes in many different forms. The recommendations provided here are nonspecific, yet apply to most forms. These recommendations are not intended to offer an alternative treatment for cancer. Instead, they are designed to augment other treatments, whether conventional or alternative.

Candidiasis

Candida overgrowth is now recognized as a complex medical syndrome known as the yeast syndrome or chronic candidiasis. This overgrowth can cause a wide variety of symptoms in virtually every system of the body. The gastrointestinal, genitourinary, endocrine, nervous, and immune systems are the most susceptible.

Dietary and Lifestyle Recommendations

- Eliminate the use of antibiotics, steroids, immune-suppressing drugs, and birth control pills (unless there is absolute medical necessity).

- Do not eat foods high in sugar.

- Do not eat foods with a high content of yeast or mold, including alcoholic beverages, cheeses, dried fruits, melons, and peanuts.

- Do not eat milk and milk products because of their high content of lactose (milk sugar) and trace levels of antibiotics.

- Avoid all known or suspected food allergies.

Supplement Protocol

- High-potency multiple according to guidelines in Chapter 2
- Vitamin C, 500 to 1,000 milligrams three times daily
- Vitamin E, 200 to 400 International Units daily
- Flaxseed oil, 1 to 2 tablespoons daily
- Thymus extract, 750 milligrams crude polypeptide fraction once or twice daily
- Probiotics, 1 to 10 billion viable *L. acidophilus* or *B. bifidum* cells daily
- Water-soluble dietary fiber, 3 to 6 grams before bedtime

Comments

Individuals with candidiasis often suffer from lack of hydrochloric acid or pancreatic enzymes. Refer to Indigestion later in this chapter for further recommendations if the above protocol is not completely effective in eliminating gastrointestinal symptoms of candidiasis.

Canker Sores

Canker sores are shallow, painful ulcers found anywhere in the mouth cavity. They can be single or clustered and are anywhere from 1 to 15 millimeters in diameter. The ulcers are surrounded by a reddened border and often are covered by a white membrane.

An occasional canker sore may result from trauma from your toothbrush. Such an ulcer usually resolves in 7 to 21 days. In many people canker sores are recurrent. Canker sores are often confused with cold sores. However, cold sores most often occur on the border of the lips and are linked to the herpes virus.

Dietary and Lifestyle Recommendations

Eliminate wheat and dairy products from the diet; most individuals with recurrent canker sores are sensitive to these foods.

Supplement Protocol

High-potency multiple according to guidelines in Chapter 2

Additional Recommendations

Chewing tablets containing a special licorice extract known as DGL (for deglycyrrhizinated licorice) at a dosage of 380 to 760 milligrams 20 minutes before meals is very effective in healing the ulcers.

Carpal Tunnel Syndrome

Carpal tunnel syndrome is a common painful disorder caused by compression of the median nerve as it passes between the bones and ligaments of the wrist. Compression of the nerve causes weakness; pain when gripping; and burning, tingling, or aching. The sensation may radiate to the forearm and shoulder. Symptoms may be occasional or constant. They occur mostly at night. Carpal tunnel syndrome is found most commonly in people who perform repetitive, strenuous work with their hands, such as grocery store checkers and carpenters.

Supplement Protocol

- High-potency multiple according to guidelines in Chapter 2
- Vitamin C, 500 to 1,000 milligrams three times daily
- Vitamin E, 200 to 400 International Units daily
- Flaxseed oil, 1 to 2 tablespoons daily
- Vitamin B_6, 50 to 100 milligrams daily

Comments

Vitamin B_6 deficiency is a common finding in carpal tunnel syndrome. In double-blind, placebo controlled clinical studies, John Ellis, M.D., Karl Folkers, Ph.D., and their co-workers at the University of Texas have successfully treated hundreds of patients suffering from carpal tunnel syndrome with vitamin B_6. It may take as long as 3 months to produce a benefit, but vitamin B_6 is effective in many cases.

Cataracts

A cataract describes a loss of transparency of the eye lens. The origin of cataract formation is free-radical damage to some of the sulfur-containing proteins in the lens. These delicate protein fibers form white spots when they are damaged—much like sulfur-rich proteins of eggs when they are fried or boiled. The damaged lens cannot transmit light effectively to the retina.

Dietary and Lifestyle Recommendations

- Avoid direct sunlight hitting the lens of the eye by wearing ultraviolet-blocking sunglasses when outdoors.
- Consume a diet rich in fruits and vegetables.
- Drink at least 48 ounces of water daily.

Supplement Protocol

- High-potency multiple according to guidelines in Chapter 2
- Vitamin C, 1,000 milligrams three times daily
- Vitamin E, 400 to 800 International Units daily
- Flaxseed oil, 1 to 2 tablespoons daily
- PCO extracts or flavonoids, according to dosage recommendations in Chapter 37

Additional Recommendations

- Bilberry extract (25 percent anthocyanosides), 40 to 80 milligrams three times daily
- Lipoic acid, 150 milligrams daily

Comments

In the early stages of cataract formation, significant improvement or no further development should be expected.

Cerebrovascular Insufficiency

Cerebrovascular insufficiency refers to a lack of blood flow to the brain. It is extremely common in the elderly as a result of atherosclerosis. The atherosclerotic plaque pinches off the blood flow to the brain. The major symptoms of cerebral vascular insufficiency are impaired mental performance, short-term memory loss, dizziness, headaches, ringing in the ears, and depression. These symptoms are extremely common in the elderly and are often referred to as "symptoms of aging."

Dietary and Lifestyle Recommendations

- Eat less saturated fat and cholesterol by reducing or eliminating the amounts of animal products in the diet.
- Increase the consumption of fiber-rich plant foods (fruits, vegetables, grains, legumes, and raw nuts and seeds).
- Achieve ideal body weight.

- Perform regular aerobic exercise.
- Do not smoke.
- Eliminate the consumption of coffee (both caffeinated and decaffeinated).
- Drink at least 48 ounces of water daily.

Supplement Protocol

- High-potency multiple according to guidelines in Chapter 2
- Vitamin C, 500 to 1,000 milligrams three times daily
- Vitamin E, 400 to 800 International Units daily
- Flaxseed oil, 1 tablespoon daily
- Aorta glycosaminoglycans, 50 milligrams twice daily

Additional Recommendations

- Supplement diet with *Ginkgo biloba* extract (24 percent ginkgo flavonglycosides), 40 to 80 milligrams three times daily.
- If cholesterol levels are elevated, follow recommendations in this chapter for Cholesterol.

Comments

If blockage of blood flow to the brain is severe, consult a qualified EDTA chelation specialist by contacting the American College of Advancement in Medicine (ACAM), 23121 Verdugo Drive, Suite 204, Laguna Hills, CA 92653, 1-800-532-3688 (outside California) or 1-800-435-6199 (inside California).

Chemotherapy (See Cancer)

Cholesterol, Elevated Blood Levels

An elevated cholesterol level is associated with an increased risk of developing atherosclerosis (hardening of the arteries), the major cause of death in the United States. Heart disease and other complications of atherosclerosis have reached epidemic proportions throughout all of the Western world. Heart disease accounts for 36 percent of all deaths in the U.S. and ranks as our number one killer; strokes, another complication of atherosclerosis, are the third most common cause of death. All together, atherosclerosis is responsible for at least 43 percent of all deaths in the U.S. Because atherosclerosis is largely a disease of diet and lifestyle, many of these deaths could be significantly delayed through a healthy diet and lifestyle.

Foremost in the prevention and treatment of heart disease is the reduction of blood cholesterol levels. The evidence overwhelmingly demonstrates that elevated cholesterol levels greatly increase the risk of death due to heart disease. It is currently recommended that the total blood cholesterol level be less than 200 milligrams per deciliter of blood. In addition, LDL cholesterol should be less than 130 milligrams per deciliter, HDL cholesterol greater than 35 milligrams per deciliter, and triglyceride levels less than 150 milligrams per deciliter.

Dietary and Lifestyle Recommendations

- Eat less saturated fat and cholesterol by reducing or eliminating the amount of animal products in the diet.
- Increase the consumption of fiber-rich plant foods (fruits, vegetables, grains, legumes, and raw nuts and seeds).
- Achieve ideal body weight.
- Engage in regular aerobic exercise.
- Do not smoke.
- Eliminate the consumption of coffee (both caffeinated and decaffeinated).
- Drink at least 48 ounces of water daily.

Supplement Protocol

- High-potency multiple according to guidelines in Chapter 2
- Vitamin C, 500 to 1,000 milligrams three times daily
- Vitamin E, 400 to 800 International Units daily
- Flaxseed oil, 1 tablespoon daily
- Inositol hexaniacinate, 500 milligrams three times daily with meals for 2 weeks, then 1,000 milligrams three times daily with meals (diabetics should use pantethine instead)
- Pantethine, 300 milligrams three times daily (for diabetics)
- Phosphatidylcholine, 500 to 900 milligrams three times daily (optional)

Additional Recommendations

Take a commercial garlic preparation at a sufficient dosage to provide the equivalent of 4,000 milligrams of fresh garlic. Look for products that have a guaranteed level of deliverable allicin such as Garlinase 4000, Garlique, and Garlicin.

Comments

Typically, this program produces total cholesterol reduction of 50 to 75 milligrams per deciliter of blood in patients with initial total cholesterol levels above 250 milligrams per deciliter within the first 2 months. In patients with initial cholesterol levels above 300 milligrams per deciliter, it may take 4 to 6 months before cholesterol levels begin to reach recommended levels. Once a patient's cholesterol level is reduced below 200 milligrams per deciliter, then reduce the dosage of niacin, as inositol hexaniacinate, to 500 milligrams three times daily for 2 months. If the cholesterol levels creep up above 200 milligrams per deciliter, then raise the dosage of niacin to 1,000 milligrams three times daily. If the cholesterol level remains below 200 milligrams per deciliter, then withdraw the niacin completely. Recheck the cholesterol levels in 2 months and re-institute niacin therapy if levels have moved up over 200 milligrams per deciliter. Garlic and flaxseed oil supplementation can be continued indefinitely.

Chronic Fatigue Syndrome

Chronic fatigue syndrome (CFS) is a newly established syndrome that describes varying combinations of symptoms, including recurrent sore throats, low-grade fever, lymph node swelling, headache, muscle and joint pain, intestinal discomfort, emotional distress and/or depression, and loss of concentration.

Dietary and Lifestyle Recommendations

- Identify and control food allergies.
- Eliminate consumption of sugar, caffeine, and alcohol.
- Breathe with the diaphragm and hold the body in a posture that is reflective of high energy.
- Drink at least 48 ounces of water daily.
- Follow a regular exercise program.

Supplement Protocol

- High-potency multiple according to guidelines in Chapter 2
- Vitamin C, 500 to 1,000 milligrams three times daily, plus an additional 3,000 to 8,000 milligrams
- Vitamin E, 200 to 400 International Units daily
- Flaxseed oil, 1 tablespoon daily
- Thymus extract, 750 milligrams crude polypeptide fraction once or twice daily
- Magnesium bound to Krebs cycle intermediates, 200 to 300 milligrams three times daily

Additional Recommendations

St.-John's-wort extract (0.3 percent hypericin), 300 milligrams three times daily.

Comments

Chronic fatigue can result from many underlying factors. I refer you to my book, *Chronic Fatigue Syndrome* (Prima), for a complete description of these factors.

Cold Sores

Cold sores are caused by the herpes virus. They are characterized by the appearance of single or multiple clusters of small blisters filled with a clear fluid on a reddened base. Cold sores differ from genital herpes in that the strain of virus is different. Cold sores are usually caused by Herpes simplex virus 1 (HSV1), while genital herpes is usually caused by the type 2 virus (HSV2). Most people, perhaps as high as 90 percent worldwide, are infected by HSV1. After the initial infection, the virus becomes dormant in the nerve cells in most people. In others, however, it can be reactivated. This causes recurring outbreaks, usually following minor infections, trauma, stress, and sun exposure.

Dietary and Lifestyle Recommendations

- Consume a diet that focuses on whole, unprocessed foods (whole grains, legumes, vegetables, and fruits).
- Avoid high arginine-containing foods (chocolate, peanuts, almonds, other nuts, and seeds).
- Eliminate alcohol, caffeine, and sugar.
- Identify and control food allergies.
- Drink at least 48 ounces of water daily.
- Get regular exercise.
- Perform a relaxation exercise (deep breathing, meditation, prayer, visualization, etcetera) 10 to 15 minutes each day.

Supplement Protocol

- High-potency multiple according to guidelines in Chapter 2
- Vitamin C, 500 to 1,000 milligrams three times daily
- Vitamin E, 200 to 400 International Units daily
- Flaxseed oil, 1 tablespoon daily
- PCO extracts or flavonoids, according to dosage recommendations in Chapter 37
- Thymus extract, 750 milligrams of the crude polypeptide fraction daily

Additional Recommendations

Herpilyn is a special cream containing an extract of the herb *Melissa officinalis* that is very effective at healing and preventing cold sores. Apply Herpilyn cream to the lips two to four times a day during an active recurrence. Apply it fairly thickly (1 to 2 millimeters); detailed toxicology studies demonstrate it is extremely safe and suitable for long-term use. In fact, in people with recurrent cold sores, Herpilyn should be used on a daily basis or as soon as the first tingling sensation of a cold sore is noticed.

Herpilyn is available at most health-food stores. You can call 1-800-783-2286 to find a store near you that carries this excellent product.

Common Cold

The common cold is caused by a variety of viruses that infect the oral and nasal passages and the sinuses. The symptoms of a cold are well known: fever, headaches, nasal congestion, sore throat, and/or generalized malaise.

Dietary and Lifestyle Recommendations

- Get plenty of rest.
- Drink plenty of liquids (focus on water, diluted vegetable juices, soups, and herb teas). Try to drink 8 ounces of water every hour.
- Avoid sugar, including natural sugars such as honey, orange juice, and fructose, because simple sugars depress the immune system.

Supplement Protocol (Acute Treatment)

- Vitamin C, 500 to 1,000 milligrams every hour with a glass of water
- Thymus extract, 750 milligrams crude polypeptide fraction once or twice daily

Additional Recommendations

Echinacea is a popular natural remedy for the common cold.

Comments

Colds can be prevented by strengthening the immune system. Getting more than one or two colds a year or having a cold that lasts more than 4 to 5 days is a sign of a weakened immune system. To strengthen the immune system, follow the general Supplement Protocol.

Colitis (See Crohn's Disease and Ulcerative Colitis)

Constipation

Constipation refers to difficulty in defecation. Constipation affects over 4 million people in the United States on a regular basis. The most common cause of constipation is a low-fiber diet.

Dietary and Lifestyle Recommendations

- Increase the consumption of fiber-rich plant foods (fruits, vegetables, grains, legumes, and raw nuts and seeds).
- Drink six to eight glasses of water per day.

Supplement Protocol (Acute Treatment)

Dietary fiber, 1 to 3 grams twice daily.

Additional Recommendations

High doses of Vitamin C are often an effective laxative.

Comments

Listed below are the recommended rules for re-establishing bowel regularity as presented in the *Encyclopedia of Natural Medicine* (Murray, M. T., and Pizzorno, J. E., Prima Publishing). The recommended procedure takes 4 to 6 weeks.

- Find and eliminate known causes of constipation.
- Never repress an urge to defecate.
- Eat a high-fiber diet, particularly fruits and vegetables.
- Drink six to eight glasses of fluid per day.
- Sit on the toilet at the same time every day (even when the urge to defecate is not present), preferably immediately after breakfast or exercise.
- Exercise at least 20 minutes, three times per week.
- Stop using laxatives (except as discussed below to re-establish bowel activity) and enemas.
  - **Week One**   Every night before bed, take a stimulant laxative containing either cascara or senna. Take the lowest amount necessary to reliably ensure a bowel movement every morning.
  - **Weekly**   Each week decrease dosage by one-half. If constipation recurs, go back to the previous week's dosage. Decrease dosage if diarrhea occurs.

Crohn's Disease and Ulcerative Colitis

Crohn's disease and ulcerative colitis are the two major categories of inflammatory bowel disease (IBD). Crohn's disease most often affects the ileum, or terminal portion of the small intestine. Ulcerative colitis affects the lining of the colon. Both diseases are characterized by intestinal pain, diarrhea, and malabsorption of nutrients. Ulcerative colitis is slightly more common than Crohn's disease.

Dietary and Lifestyle Recommendations

Identify and control food allergies.

Supplement Protocol

- High-potency multiple according to guidelines in Chapter 2
- Vitamin C, 3,000 to 8,000 milligrams daily
- Vitamin E, 200 to 400 International Units daily
- Flaxseed oil, 1 tablespoon daily
- Pancreatin (8–10×), 350 to 700 milligrams three times daily between meals

Comments

Diets that eliminate food allergies are extremely effective in the treatment of both Crohn's disease and ulcerative colitis. Meridian Valley Clinical Laboratory (1-206-859-8700) and National Biotech Laboratory (1-800-846-6285) offer a food allergy test that measures both IgE and IgG antibodies, tests for over 100 different foods, and comes with detailed dietary instructions. It is reasonably priced at about $120.

Depression

The official definition of "clinical" depression is based upon the following eight primary criteria:

- Poor appetite with weight loss, or increased appetite with weight gain
- Insomnia or hypersomnia
- Physical hyperactivity or inactivity
- Loss of interest or pleasure in usual activities, or decrease in sexual drive
- Loss of energy and feelings of fatigue
- Feelings of worthlessness, self-reproach, or inappropriate guilt
- Diminished ability to think or concentrate
- Recurrent thoughts of death or suicide

The presence of five of these eight symptoms definitely indicates depression. An individual with four is probably also depressed.

Dietary and Lifestyle Recommendations

- Increase the consumption of fiber-rich plant foods (fruits, vegetables, grains, legumes, and raw nuts and seeds).
- Avoid the intake of caffeine, nicotine, other stimulants, and alcohol.
- Identify and control food allergies.

- Develop a positive, optimistic mental attitude by:
  - Setting goals
  - Using positive self-talk and affirmations
  - Asking yourself empowering questions
  - Seeking the help of a mental health professional

- Exercise regularly.

- Perform a relaxation/stress reduction technique 10 to 15 minutes each day.

- Find ways to interject humor and laughter in your life.

Supplement Protocol

- High-potency multiple according to guidelines in Chapter 2
- Vitamin C, 500 to 1,000 milligrams three times daily
- Vitamin E, 200 to 400 International Units daily
- Flaxseed oil, 1 tablespoon daily
- SAM, 200 milligrams twice daily for the first 2 days, 400 milligrams twice daily days 3 through 9, 400 milligrams three times daily on days 10 through 19, full dosage of 400 milligrams four times daily after 20 days if needed
- Folic acid and vitamin B_{12}, 1,000 micrograms of each daily

Additional Recommendations

- If under the age of 30, St.-John's-wort extract (0.3 percent hypericin), 300 milligrams three times daily
- If over the age of 50, *Ginkgo biloba* extract (24 percent ginkgo flavonglycosides), 80 milligrams three times daily

Comments

St.-John's-wort extract (0.3 percent hypericin content) at a dosage of 300 milligrams three times daily can be as effective as standard antidepressant drugs (including Prozac) without side effects. If you are currently on a prescription antidepressant drug, you absolutely must work with your doctor before discontinuing any drug. Discontinuing an antidepressant drug without medical supervision can be life-threatening. For more detailed information, consult my book *Natural Alternatives to Prozac* (Morrow, 1996).

Diabetes

Diabetes mellitus is a metabolic disease characterized by elevated blood sugar. Diabetics have a greatly increased risk of heart disease, stroke, kidney disease, and loss of nerve function. There are two major types of diabetes. Type 1 is often referred to as insulin dependent or juvenile-onset diabetes. Type 2 is also referred to as noninsulin dependent or adult-onset diabetes.

There are also less frequently encountered forms of diabetes. Secondary diabetes, as the name implies, is secondary to certain conditions and syndromes. These include pancreatic disease, hormone disturbances, drugs, and malnutrition. Gestational diabetes refers to glucose intolerance occurring during pregnancy.

Dietary and Lifestyle Recommendations

- Consume a diet that focuses on whole, unprocessed foods (whole grains, legumes, vegetables, fruits, nuts, and seeds).
- Eliminate alcohol, caffeine, and sugar.
- Get regular exercise.

Supplement Protocol

- High-potency multiple according to guidelines in Chapter 2
- Vitamin C, 500 to 1,000 milligrams three times daily
- Vitamin E, 400 to 800 International Units daily
- Flaxseed oil, 1 tablespoon daily
- GLA source, 240 to 480 milligrams daily
- Magnesium, 250 milligrams two to three times daily
- Methylcobalamin (active vitamin B_{12}), 1,000 micrograms daily
- Lipoic acid, 150 milligrams daily

Additional Recommendations

Take a commercial garlic preparation at a sufficient dosage to provide the equivalent of 4,000 milligrams of fresh garlic. Look for products that have a guaranteed level of deliverable allicin such as Garlinase 4000, Garlique, and Garlicin. If cholesterol or triglyceride levels are elevated, take pantethine, one tablet three times daily.

Comments

The diabetic individual must be monitored carefully, particularly if he or she is on insulin or has relatively uncontrolled diabetes. Careful attention to symptoms, home glucose monitoring, and other blood tests are essential in monitoring the progress of the diabetic individual. It is important to recognize that as the diabetic individual employs some of the suggestions given above, drug dosages need to be altered. The diabetic must establish a good working relationship with his or doctor.

Ear Infections and Chronic Otitis Media

An acute middle ear infection (acute otitis media) is characterized by a sharp, stabbing, dull, and/or throbbing pain in the ear. The pain is due to inflammation, swelling, or infection of the middle ear. Acute ear infections are usually preceded by an upper respiratory infection or allergy. The organisms most commonly cultured from middle ear fluid during acute otitis media include *Streptococcus pneumoniae* (40 percent) and *Haemophilus influenzae* (25 percent).

Chronic otitis media (also known as "glue ear" and serous, secretory, or non-suppurative otitis media with effusion) refers to a constant swelling of the middle ear. Chronic otitis media affect 20 to 40 percent of children under the age of 6. They account for over 50 percent of all visits to pediatricians.

Abnormal eustachian tube function is the underlying cause in virtually all cases of otitis media. The eustachian tube regulates gas pressure in the middle ear. It also protects the middle ear from nose and throat secretions and bacteria and clears fluids from the middle ear. Swallowing causes active opening of the eustachian tube because of action of the surrounding muscles. Since this tube is smaller in diameter and more horizontal in infants and small children, they are particularly susceptible to eustachian tube problems.

Obstruction of the eustachian tube leads first to buildup from fluid in the blood, or serous buildup. If bacteria starts to grow, this leads to bacterial infection. Obstruction results from a variety of causes. The tube can collapse due to weak tissues holding the tube in place and/or an abnormal opening mechanism, or the collapse can occur because of allergic blockage with mucous or infection.

Dietary and Lifestyle Recommendations

- Avoid exposing children to cigarette smoke.
- Identify and eliminate food allergies. The most common allergens are milk, corn, wheat, citrus, eggs, chocolate, and peanut butter.
- Strengthen the immune system by avoiding overconsumption of sugar.

Supplement Protocol (Acute Phase)

- Vitamin C, 10 milligrams for every pound of body weight every 2 hours. Crystalline vitamin C preparations work best. Hyland's offers vitamin C (25 milligrams) in a small chewable tablet for children.
- Probiotics according to guidelines in Chapter 44 (capsules can be emptied into food for infants and young children.
- Children's high-potency multiple vitamin and mineral supplement.

Additional Recommendations

For acute ear infections in children, use a topical herbal-oil combination such as Ear Drops from Eclectic Institute (available at health-food stores). Apply a hot pack to the ear as well. Children can also take *Echinacea* at one-half the adult dosage.

Comments

Acute ear infections require medical supervision.

Eczema

Eczema, also known as atopic dermatitis, is an intensely itchy, inflammatory disease of the skin. It is commonly found on the face, wrists, and insides of the elbows and knees. Although it may occur at any age, it is most common in infants. It completely clears in half the cases by 18 months of age. Eczema affects 2.4 to 7 percent of the population and is often associated with asthma.

Dietary and Lifestyle Recommendations

- Identify and eliminate food allergies (key recommendation).
- Decrease consumption of animal foods, with the exception of cold-water fish (rich source of omega-3 fatty acids).

Supplement Protocol

- High-potency multiple according to guidelines in Chapter 2
- Vitamin C, 500 to 1,000 milligrams three times daily
- Vitamin E, 200 to 400 International Units daily
- Flaxseed oil, 1 tablespoon daily
- Quercetin and bromelain combination, 200 to 400 milligrams of each 5 minutes before meals
- Zinc, 30 to 45 milligrams daily

Additional Recommendations

Natural products containing chamomile and/or licorice extracts such as CamoCare and Simicort can be applied to the affected area two to three times daily.

Comments

The causal role of food allergy in eczema is well established, especially in children. Some researchers have concluded that perhaps 75 percent of the cases of childhood eczema could be resolved merely by shifting some dietary factors. Cow's milk is a major culprit. Other key food allergens in eczema are eggs, tomatoes, and food preservatives and food colorings. Meridian Valley Clinical Laboratory (1-206-859-8700) and National Biotech Laboratory (1-800-846-6285) offer a food allergy test that measures both IgE and IgG antibodies, tests for over 100 different foods, comes with detailed dietary instructions, and is reasonably priced at about $120.

Fibroid (Uterine)

A fibroid is a slow-growing benign tumor of the uterus that consists of smooth muscle bundles and connective tissue. Fibroids may vary in size from the size of a pea to that of a grapefruit. Fibroids occur in about 20 percent of women over the age of 30, making them the most common of tumors. The cause of fibroids is related to an abnormal response to estrogens.

Dietary and Lifestyle Recommendations

- Consume a diet that focuses on whole, unprocessed foods (whole grains, legumes, vegetables, fruits, nuts, and seeds).
- Increase consumption of soy foods.
- Eliminate alcohol, caffeine, and sugar.
- Get regular exercise.
- Perform a relaxation exercise (deep breathing, meditation, prayer, visualization, etc.) 10 to 15 minutes each day.
- Drink at least 48 ounces of water daily.

Supplement Protocol

- High-potency multiple according to guidelines in Chapter 2
- Vitamin C, 500 to 1,000 milligrams three times daily
- Vitamin E, 400 to 800 International Units daily
- Flaxseed oil, 1 to 2 tablespoons daily
- Phosphatidylcholine, 500 milligrams three times daily
- Pancreatin (8–10×), 350 to 700 milligrams three times daily between meals

Additional Recommendations

Remifemin (Cimicifuga extract standardized to contain 1 milligram of 27-deoxyacteine per tablet), two tablets twice daily. Remifemin is available in health food stores.

Fibrocystic Breast Disease

Fibrocystic breast disease (FBD), also known as cystic mastitis, is a mildly uncomfortable to severely painful benign cystic swelling of the breasts. Fibrocystic breast disease is very common. It affects 20 to 40 percent of premenopausal women. It is usually a component of the premenstrual syndrome (PMS) and is considered a minor risk factor for breast cancer. It is not as significant a factor as the classical breast cancer risk factors such as family history, early menarche, and late or no first pregnancy.

The development of fibrocystic breast disease is apparently due to an increased estrogen-to-progesterone ratio. With each menstrual cycle, there is a recurring hormonal stimulation of the breast. As the hormone levels fall after a few days, the breasts normally return to their prestimulation size and function.

Dietary and Lifestyle Recommendations

- Consume a diet that focuses on whole, unprocessed foods (whole grains, legumes, vegetables, fruits, nuts, and seeds).
- Increase consumption of soy foods.
- Eliminate the intake of coffee, tea, cola, chocolate, and caffeinated medications as well as alcohol and sugar.
- Drink at least 48 ounces of water daily.
- Get regular exercise.

Supplement Protocol

- High-potency multiple according to guidelines in Chapter 2
- Vitamin C, 500 to 1,000 milligrams three times daily
- Vitamin E, 400 to 800 International Units daily
- Flaxseed oil, 1 tablespoon daily

Additional Recommendations

Rule out hypothyroidism (See Hypothyroidism).

Food Allergy

Food allergies refer to an allergic reaction caused by food ingestion. It is estimated by some experts that at least 60 percent of Americans suffers from negative reactions to food. Food allergies can be an important cause in a wide range of conditions.

Dietary and Lifestyle Recommendations

An elimination diet can determine if food allergy is playing a major role in a particular health condition. The standard elimination diet consists of lamb, chicken, rice, banana, apple, and a vegetable from the cabbage family. This diet is also called an oligoantigenic diet. The next step is the reintroduction of foods. It is necessary to keep a daily, detailed journal of the dates when new foods are introduced and any adverse responses in the individual's body. Every second day a food can be reintroduced to the diet. If the food is one to which an individual is sensitive, the symptoms of the adverse response reappear (often more strongly than before). The 2-day wait

Symptoms and Diseases Commonly Associated with Food Allergy

System	Symptoms and Diseases
Gastrointestinal	Canker sores, celiac disease, chronic diarrhea, stomach ulcer, gas, gastritis, irritable colon, malabsorption, ulcerative colitis
Genitourinary	Bedwetting, chronic bladder infections, kidney disease
Immune	Chronic infections, frequent ear infections
Brain	Anxiety, depression, hyperactivity, inability to concentrate, insomnia, irritability, mental confusion, personality change, seizures
Musculoskeletal	Bursitis, joint pain, low back pain
Respiratory	Asthma, chronic bronchitis, wheezing
Skin	Acne, eczema, hives, itching, skin rash
Miscellaneous	Irregular heart beats, edema, fainting, fatigue, headache, hypoglycemia, itchy nose or throat, migraines, sinusitis

before reintroducing the next food provides enough time to connect the adverse response to the reintroduced food.

Supplement Protocol

- Flaxseed oil, 1 tablespoon daily
- Pancreatin (8–10×), 350 to 700 milligrams 5 minutes before meals

Additional Recommendations

If a person has multiple food allergies, follow the recommendations given for indigestion.

Comments

Meridian Valley Clinical Laboratory (1-206-859-8700) and National Biotech Laboratory (1-800-846-6285) offer a food allergy test that measures both IgE and IgG antibodies, tests for over 100 different foods, comes with detailed dietary instructions, and is reasonably priced at about $120.

Gallstones

Gallstones are an extremely common occurrence in the U.S. Each year at least 1 million more Americans develop gallstones and another 300,000 gallbladders are removed. The critical factor in gallstone formation is the solubility of the bile within the gallbladder. Bile solubility is based on the relative concentrations of cholesterol, bile acids, phosphatidylcholine (lecithin), and water.

Dietary and Lifestyle Recommendations

- Consume a diet that focuses on whole, unprocessed foods (whole grains, legumes, vegetables, fruits, nuts, and seeds).
- Eliminate the intake of milk.
- Eliminate consumption of food allergies (milk, onions, eggs, and chocolate are the most common in patients with symptoms).
- Drink at least 48 ounces of water daily.
- Avoid use of antacids.
- Get regular exercise.

Supplement Protocol

- High-potency multiple according to guidelines in Chapter 2
- Vitamin C, 500 to 1,000 milligrams three times daily
- Vitamin E, 200 to 400 International Units daily
- Flaxseed oil, 1 tablespoon daily
- Phosphatidylcholine, 500 milligrams three times daily
- Water-soluble fiber, 1 to 3 grams with meals three times daily

Additional Recommendations

Silymarin, the flavonoid complex from milk thistle (*Silybum marianum*) is also indicated, at a dosage of 70 to 210 milligrams three times daily. A special silymarin preparation bound to phosphatidylcholine (silymarin phytosome) may offer even better results at a dosage of 100 milligrams two to three times daily.

Comments

A formula containing menthol and related terpenes (menthone, pinene, borneol, cineol, and camphene) has demonstrated efficacy in several studies in dissolving gallstones. This nonsurgical approach to gallstone removal offers an effective alternative to surgery and is safe even when consumed for prolonged periods of time (up to 4 years). Terpenes, like menthol, help dissolve gallstones by reducing bile cholesterol levels while increasing bile acid and lecithin levels in the gallbladder. Because menthol is the major component of this formula, peppermint oil—especially if enteric-coated—may offer similar benefits.

Glaucoma

Glaucoma refers to the increased pressure within the eye that results from an imbalance between the production and outflow of fluid in the eye. Obstruction of outflow is the main cause of this imbalance in acute glaucoma. A number of physiological abnormalities have been observed in glaucomatous eyes. Sometimes there unusual tissues at the back of the eye through which the optic nerve fibers and blood vessels pass. Other abnormalities occur in the connective tissue network the eye fluid must pass through to leave the eye. Blood vessels might also be problematic. These changes may result in elevated inner eye pressure. Alternatively, they may lead to progressive loss of peripheral vision.

Glaucoma can be acute or chronic, chronic being the most common. In the United States there are approximately 2 million people with glaucoma, 25 percent of which is undetected. Ten percent have the acute, closed-angle type, and 90 percent is the chronic, open-angle type. In chronic glaucoma, usually there are no symptoms until there are significant elevations in pressure readings. Once the pressure of fluids in the eye reaches high enough levels, the person experiences a gradual loss of peripheral vision—in other words, "tunnel vision." Extreme pain, blurred vision, and severely reddened eyes may also be associated with this acute phase of the chronic condition.

An acute case of closed-angle glaucoma is a medical emergency. Usually the individual experiences severe, throbbing eye pain. Vision is markedly blur. Nausea and vomiting are often also associated with its onset. A person who suspects this condition should go immediately to an ophthalmologist or hospital emergency room. Effective therapy must be started within 12 to 48 hours, or permanent loss of vision occurs within 3 to 5 days.

Dietary and Lifestyle Recommendations

- Consume a diet that focuses on whole, unprocessed foods (whole grains, legumes, vegetables, fruits, nuts, and seeds).
- Identify and eliminate consumption of food allergies (milk, onions, eggs, and chocolate are the most common in patients with symptoms).
- Drink at least 48 ounces of water daily.

Supplement Protocol

- High-potency multiple according to guidelines in Chapter 2
- Vitamin C, 500 milligrams for every 2.2 pounds of body weight in divided dosages (work up to this high dosage gradually)
- Vitamin E, 200 to 400 International Units daily
- Flaxseed oil, 1 tablespoon daily
- PCO extracts or flavonoids, according to dosage recommendations in Chapter 37

Comments

High doses of vitamin C can lower pressure levels on the inner eye in many clinical studies. Almost normal tension levels have been achieved in some patients who were unresponsive to standard drug therapies (acetazolamide and pilocarpine).

Gout

Gout is a common type of arthritis caused by an increased concentration of uric acid in biological fluids. Uric acid is the final breakdown product of purine metabolism. The body manufactures purines, and they are also ingested in foods. In gout, uric acid crystals are deposited in joints, tendons, kidneys, and other tissues, where they cause considerable inflammation and damage.

Dietary and Lifestyle Recommendations

- Eliminate alcohol intake.
- Follow a low-purine diet.
- Achieve ideal body weight.
- Eliminate sugar and restrict intake of simple sugars (honey, fructose, fruits, fruit juices, etcetera).
- Consume a diet that focuses on whole, unprocessed foods (whole grains, legumes, vegetables, nuts, and seeds).
- Drink at least 48 ounces of water daily.

Supplement Protocol

- High-potency multiple according to guidelines in Chapter 2
- Vitamin C, 500 to 1,000 milligrams three times daily
- Vitamin E, 200 to 400 International Units daily
- Flaxseed oil, 1 tablespoon daily

Additional Recommendations

- Eating the equivalent of ½ pound of fresh cherries daily is an old nature cure for gout. Health-food stores usually carry cherry extracts in pill or concentrated form.

Comments

Most cases of gout can be treated effectively with diet alone.

Hay Fever

The underlying mechanisms responsible for hay fever are very similar to those that produce asthma. Follow the dosage given for asthma.

Headache (Also See Migraine)

The most common form of headache is referred to as the "tension headache." It is usually caused by a tightening of the muscles of the face, neck or scalp that pinches the nerves. Stress, poor posture, and hypoglycemia can trigger a tension headache, which differs from a migraine in that it is usually associated with a steady, constant pain that starts at the forehead or back of head and can spread pain over the entire head. A migraine, however, tends to be a throbbing pain that pounds sharply in the head of the sufferer.

Dietary and Lifestyle Recommendations

- Consume a diet that focuses on whole, unprocessed foods (whole grains, legumes, vegetables, fruits, nuts, and seeds).
- Eliminate alcohol, caffeine, and sugar.
- Identify and control food allergies.
- Get regular exercise.
- Perform a relaxation exercise (deep breathing, meditation, prayer, visualization, etcetera) 10 to 15 minutes each day.
- Drink at least 48 ounces of water daily.

Supplement Protocol (Acute Treatment)

- Magnesium, 250 to 500 milligrams (up to three times daily).

Additional Recommendations

- Chiropractic adjustments can be quite useful in chronic tension headaches.

Heart Disease (See Cholesterol or Angina)

Hemorrhoids

Hemorrhoids are basically varicose veins of the rectum. They may be near the beginning of the anal canal (internal hemorrhoids) or at the anal opening (external hemorrhoids). Because the venous system supplying the rectal area contains no valves, factors that increase venous congestion in the region can precipitate hemorrhoid formation. This includes increasing intra-abdominal pressure (defecation, pregnancy, coughing, sneezing, vomiting, physical exertion, and portal hypertension due to cirrhosis), a low-fiber diet–induced increase in straining during defecation, and standing or sitting for prolonged periods of time. The symptoms most often associated with hemorrhoids include itching, burning, pain, inflammation, irritation, swelling, bleeding, and seepage.

Dietary and Lifestyle Recommendations

- Consume a diet that focuses on whole, unprocessed foods (whole grains, legumes, vegetables, fruits, nuts, and seeds).
- Get regular exercise.
- Drink at least 48 ounces of water daily.

Supplement Protocol

- Water-soluble fiber, 1 to 2 grams three times daily
- Aortic glycosaminoglycans, 50 milligrams twice daily

Comments

Many over-the-counter products such as suppositories, ointments, and anorectal pads used for hemorrhoids contain primarily natural ingredients, such as witch hazel, vitamin E, shark liver oil, cod liver oil, cocoa butter, Peruvian balsam, zinc oxide, live yeast cell derivative, and allantoin. However, topical therapy provides only temporary relief in most circumstances.

Hepatitis

Hepatitis in most instances is caused by a virus, viral types A, B, and C being the most common. Hepatitis A occurs sporadically or in epidemics and is transmitted primarily through fecal contamination. Hepatitis B is transmitted through infected blood or blood products. It is occasionally transmitted through saliva and sexual secretions. Hepatitis C's (formerly known as hepatitis non-A, non-B) primary route of transmission is through blood transfusion. In fact, about 10 percent of the people who receive blood transfusions develop hepatitis C. Its incubation period is 2 to 20 weeks and although its mortality rate is unclear, it is higher than that of other forms (1 to 12 percent).

Acute viral hepatitis is characterized by loss of appetite, nausea, vomiting, fatigue, and other flulike symptoms; fever; enlarged, tender liver; jaundice (yellowing of skin due to the increased level of bilirubin in the blood); dark urine; and elevated liver enzymes in the blood.

Ten percent of hepatitis B and 10 to 40 percent of hepatitis C cases develop into chronic viral hepatitis forms. The symptomatology varies. The symptoms can be latent and lead to chronic fatigue, serious liver damage, and even death.

Acute Hepatitis Dietary and Lifestyle Recommendations

Consume vegetable broths, soups, and fresh vegetable juices.

Acute Hepatitis Supplement Protocol

- Vitamin C, 500 to 1,000 milligrams every hour or to bowel tolerance
- Thymus extract, 750 milligrams crude polypeptide fraction once or twice daily

Acute Hepatitis Additional Recommendations

Silymarin, the flavonoid complex from milk thistle (*Silybum marianum*) is also indicated at a dosage of 70 to 210 milligrams three times daily. A special silymarin preparation bound to phosphatidylcholine (silymarin phytosome) may offer even better results at a dosage of 100 milligrams two to three times daily.

According to Robert Cathcart, M.D., hepatitis is "one of the easiest diseases for ascorbic acid to cure." Dr. Cathcart demonstrated that vitamin C administered intravenously at very high levels (40 to 100 grams) greatly improved acute viral hepatitis in 2 to 4 days. He showed clearing of jaundice within 6 days. Other studies demonstrate similar benefits. Contact the American College of Advancement in Medicine (ACAM), 23121 Verdugo Drive, Suite 204, Laguna Hills, CA 92653, 1-800-532-3688 (outside California) or 1-800-435-6199 (inside California) for a referral to a physician who can prescribe weekly intravenous vitamin C therapy.

Chronic Hepatitis Dietary and Lifestyle Recommendations

- Consume a diet that focuses on whole, unprocessed foods (whole grains, legumes, vegetables, fruits, nuts, and seeds).
- Eliminate alcohol, caffeine, and sugar.
- Get regular exercise.
- Perform a relaxation exercise (deep breathing, meditation, prayer, visualization, etcetera) 10 to 15 minutes each day.
- Drink at least 48 ounces of water daily.

Chronic Hepatitis Supplement Protocol

- High-potency multiple according to guidelines in Chapter 2
- Vitamin C, 3,000 to 6,000 milligrams per day in divided dosages
- Vitamin E, 200 to 400 International Units daily
- Flaxseed oil, 1 tablespoon daily

- Thymus extract, 750 milligrams crude polypeptide fraction daily

Chronic Hepatitis Additional Recommendations

Silymarin, 70 to 210 milligrams three times daily.

Chronic Hepatitis Comments

Thymus extracts have been effective in several double-blind studies in both acute and chronic cases. In these studies, therapeutic effect was noted by accelerated decreases of liver enzymes (transaminases) and elimination of the virus.

Herpes

The Herpes simplex virus (HSV) can produce a recurrent viral infection on virtually any area of skin or mucous membranes. The most common sites are around the mouth (cold sores) and genitals. Cold sores are usually caused by Herpes simplex virus 1 (HSV1), while genital herpes is usually caused by the type 2 virus (HSV2).

The rash in genital herpes is characterized by the appearance of single or multiple clusters of small blisters filled with a clear fluid on a reddened base. The blisters eventually burst. When they do, they leave small, painful ulcers that heal within 10 to 21 days.

After the initial infection, the virus becomes dormant in the nerve root near the spine. Herpes tends to become reactivated following minor infections, trauma, and stress. The stress can be emotional, dietary, and environmental. While about 40 percent of people never have a second outbreak, others may suffer four or five attacks a year for several years or longer.

Dietary and Lifestyle Recommendations

- Consume a diet that focuses on whole, unprocessed foods (whole grains, legumes, vegetables, and fruits).
- Avoid high arginine-containing foods (chocolate, peanuts, almonds, other nuts, and seeds).
- Eliminate alcohol, caffeine, and sugar.
- Identify and control food allergies.
- Get regular exercise.
- Perform a relaxation exercise (deep breathing, meditation, prayer, visualization, etcetera) 10 to 15 minutes each day.

Supplement Protocol

- High-potency multiple according to guidelines in Chapter 2
- Vitamin C, an additional 3,000 to 8,000 milligrams each day

- Vitamin E, 200 to 400 International Units daily
- Flaxseed oil, 1 tablespoon daily
- PCO extracts or flavonoids, according to dosage recommendations in Chapter 37
- Thymus extract, 750 milligrams crude polypeptide fraction once or twice daily

Additional Recommendations

Apply Herpilyn (see Cold Sores) to affected areas two to four times a day during an active recurrence. Apply it fairly thickly (1 to 2 millimeters); detailed toxicology studies demonstrate it is extremely safe and suitable for long-term use. In fact, people with recurrent cold sores should use Herpilyn on a daily basis or as soon as they notice the first tingling sensation of a cold sore.

High Blood Pressure

A normal blood pressure reading for adults is 120 (systolic)/80 (diastolic). Hypertension or high blood pressure is one of the major risk factors for a heart attack or stroke. Many dietary factors are linked with high blood pressure, including:

- Obesity
- A high sodium-to-potassium ratio
- A high-sugar, low-fiber diet
- A diet high in saturated fats and low in essential fatty acids
- A diet low in calcium and magnesium
- A diet low in vitamin C

Dietary and Lifestyle Recommendations

Consume a diet that focuses on whole, unprocessed foods (whole grains, legumes, vegetables, fruits, nuts, and seeds).

- Avoid salt (sodium chloride).
- Eliminate alcohol, caffeine, and sugar.
- Get regular exercise.
- Perform a relaxation exercise (deep breathing, meditation, prayer, visualization, etcetera) 10 to 15 minutes each day.
- Drink at least 48 ounces of water daily.

Supplement Protocol

- High-potency multiple according to guidelines in Chapter 2
- Vitamin C, 500 to 1,000 milligrams three times daily

- Vitamin E, 400 to 800 International Units daily
- Flaxseed oil, 1 tablespoon daily
- Magnesium, 800 to 1,200 milligrams daily
- Coenzyme Q_{10}, 150 to 300 milligrams daily

Additional Recommendations

Take a commercial garlic preparation at a dosage sufficient to provide the equivalent of 4,000 milligrams of fresh garlic. Look for products that have a guaranteed level of deliverable allicin such as Garlinase 4000, Garlique, and Garlicin.

Comments

Severe hypertension (160+/115+) requires immediate medical attention. A drug may be necessary to achieve initial control. Consider intravenous EDTA chelation therapy (See Angina).

Hives

Hives or urticaria are localized swellings of the skin. Hives usually itch intensely. They are caused by the release of histamine within the skin. About 50 percent of patients with hives develop angioedema. This is a deeper, less-defined swelling that involves tissues beneath the skin.

Hives and angioedema are relatively common conditions. It is estimated that 15 to 20 percent of the general population has had hives at some time. Although persons in any age group may experience acute or chronic hives and/or angioedema, young adults (postadolescence through the third decade of life) are most often affected. Medications are the leading cause of hives in adults. In children, hives are usually due to foods, food additives, or infections.

Dietary and Lifestyle Recommendations

An elimination or low-antigenic diet is of utmost importance in the treatment of most cases of hives, particularly in children. The diet should not only eliminate suspected allergens, but also all food additives. The strictest elimination diets allow only water, lamb, rice, pears, and vegetables. Those foods most commonly associated with inducing urticaria (milk, eggs, chicken, fruits, nuts, and additives) should definitely be avoided.

Supplement Protocol

- High-potency multiple according to guidelines in Chapter 2
- Vitamin C, 500 to 1,000 milligrams three times daily

- Vitamin E, 200 to 400 International Units daily
- Flaxseed oil, 1 tablespoon daily
- Quercetin, 200 to 400 milligrams 5 minutes before meals (capsules can be emptied into food in infants and young children)

Hot Flashes (See Menopause)

Hyperactivity (See Attention Deficit Disorder)

Hypoglycemia

Hypoglycemia refers to a condition of low blood sugar. Because glucose is the primary fuel for the brain, when levels are too low, the brain feels the effects first. Symptoms of hypoglycemia can range from mild to severe. They include such things as headache; depression, anxiety, irritability, and other psychological disturbances; blurred vision; excessive sweating; mental confusion; incoherent speech; bizarre behavior; and convulsions. Some conditions that are linked to hypoglycemia are:

- Depression
- Aggressive and criminal behavior
- Premenstrual syndrome
- Migraine headaches
- Leg cramps
- Angina

Reactive hypoglycemia is the most common form. It is characterized by the development of symptoms of hypoglycemia 2 to 4 hours after a meal.

Dietary and Lifestyle Recommendations

- Consume a diet that focuses on whole, unprocessed foods (whole grains, legumes, vegetables, fruits, nuts, and seeds).
- Eliminate sugar, alcohol, and caffeine.
- Identify and control food allergies.
- Get regular exercise.
- Perform a relaxation exercise (deep breathing, meditation, prayer, visualization, etcetera) 10 to 15 minutes each day.
- Drink at least 48 ounces of water daily.

Supplement Protocol

- High-potency multiple according to guidelines in Chapter 2
- Vitamin C, 500 to 1,000 milligrams three times daily
- Vitamin E, 200 to 400 International Units daily
- Flaxseed oil, 1 tablespoon daily
- Chromium, 400 to 600 micrograms daily

Hypothyroidism (See Chapter 52, Thyroid Extracts)

Impotence

The term "impotence" traditionally has signified the inability of the male to attain and maintain erection of the penis sufficient to permit satisfactory sexual intercourse. Impotence, in most circumstances, is more precisely referred to as erectile dysfunction because this term differentiates itself from loss of libido, premature ejaculation, or inability to achieve orgasm.

An estimated 10 to 20 million men suffer from erectile dysfunction. This number is expected to increase dramatically as the median age of the population increases. Currently, erectile dysfunction probably affects over 25 percent of men over the age of 50.

Although the frequency of erectile dysfunction increases with age, it must be stressed that aging itself is not a cause of impotence. Despite the fact that the amount and force of the ejaculate and the need to ejaculate decrease with age, the capacity for erection is retained. Men are capable of retaining their sexual virility well into their 80s.

Erectile dysfunction may be due to organic or psychogenic factors. In the overwhelming majority of cases, the cause is organic—it is due to some physiological reason. In fact, in men over 50, organic causes are responsible for erectile dysfunction in over 90 percent of cases. Atherosclerosis of the penile artery is the primary cause of impotence in nearly half the men over 50 who have erectile dysfunction.

Dietary and Lifestyle Recommendations

- Consume a diet that focuses on whole, unprocessed foods (whole grains, legumes, vegetables, fruits, nuts, and seeds).
- Eliminate alcohol, caffeine, and sugar.
- Identify and control food allergies.
- Get regular exercise.
- Perform a relaxation exercise (deep breathing, meditation, prayer, visualization, etcetera) 10 to 15 minutes each day.
- Drink at least 48 ounces of water daily.

Supplement Protocol

- High-potency multiple according to guidelines in Chapter 2
- Vitamin C, 500 to 1,000 milligrams three times daily
- Vitamin E, 400 to 800 International Units daily
- Flaxseed oil, 1 tablespoon daily
- Zinc, 30 to 45 milligrams daily

Additional Recommendations

- *Ginkgo biloba* extract (24 percent ginkgo flavonglycosides), 40 to 80 milligrams three times daily.
- If cholesterol levels are elevated, see Cholesterol.
- If diabetes is present, see Diabetes.

Comments

For more information, please consult my book, *Male Sexual Vitality* (Prima, 1995).

Indigestion

The term "indigestion" often describes a feeling of gaseousness or fullness in the abdomen. It can also describe "heartburn." Indigestion can have many causes, including not only increased secretion of acid but also decreased secretion of acid and other digestive juices and enzymes.

Although most people believe that an overacidic stomach is the major cause of indigestion, a very strong case can be made for lack of gastric acid secretion. Deficient production of hydrochloric acid in the stomach is known as hypochlorhydria; achlorhydria refers to a complete absence of gastric acid secretion. Because the ability to secrete gastric acid usually decreases with age, as many as 40 percent of adults may not secrete sufficient levels of hydrochloric acid. Hypochlorhydria has been found in over half of those over age 60. Here are some of the common symptoms, signs, and diseases associated with low hydrochloric acid secretion:

- Symptoms
  - Bloating, belching, burning, and flatulence immediately after meals
  - A sense of "fullness" after eating
  - Indigestion, diarrhea, or constipation
  - Multiple food allergies
  - Nausea after taking supplements

- Signs
  - Itching around the rectum
  - Weak, peeling, and cracked fingernails

- – Dilated blood vessels in the cheeks and nose
  - Acne
- – Iron deficiency
  - Chronic intestinal parasites or abnormal flora
  - Undigested food in stool
  - Chronic *Candida* infections
  - Upper digestive tract gasiness

- Diseases
  - Addison's disease
  - Asthma
  - Celiac disease
  - Dermatitis herpetiformis
  - Diabetes mellitus
  - Eczema
  - Gallbladder disease
  - Graves' disease
  - Chronic autoimmune disorders
  - Hepatitis
  - Chronic hives
  - Lupus erythematosus
  - Myasthenia gravis
  - Osteoporosis
  - Pernicious anemia
  - Psoriasis
  - Rheumatoid arthritis
  - Rosacea
  - Sjogren's syndrome
  - Thyrotoxicosis
  - Hyper- and hypothyroidism
  - Vitiligo

Dietary and Lifestyle Recommendations

Chewing food thoroughly is the first step toward good digestion. Chewing signals other components of the digestive system to get ready to work; it also allows food to mix with saliva. Saliva contains the enzyme salivary amylase, which breaks down starch molecules into smaller sugars.

Supplement Protocol

The best method of diagnosing a lack of hydrochloric acid is a special procedure known as the Heidelberg gastric analysis. This technique uses an electronic capsule attached to a string. The patient swallows the capsule, which measures the stomach's pH and sends a radio message to a receiver that then records the pH level. The response to a bicarbonate challenge is the true test of the functional ability of the stomach to secrete acid. After the test, the capsule is pulled up from the stomach by the attached string.

Since not everyone can have detailed gastric acid analysis to determine the need for gastric acid supplementation, you can use a practical method to determine whether you need hydrochloric acid and how much your body needs for proper digestion. The following is a challenge method modified from the one developed by Dr. Jonathan Wright.

1. Begin by taking one tablet or capsule containing 10 grains (600 milligrams) of hydrochloric acid at your next large meal. If this does not aggravate your symptoms, at each subsequent meal of equal size, take one more tablet or capsule (one at the next meal, two at the meal after that, then three at the next meal).

2. Continue to increase the dose until you reach seven tablets or when you feel a warmth in your stomach, whichever occurs first. A feeling of warmth in the stomach means you have taken too many tablets for that meal and you need to take one less tablet for that meal size. Try the larger dose again at another meal to make sure that it was the hydrochloric acid that caused the warmth and not something else.

3. After you have found the largest dose you can take at your large meals without feeling any warmth, maintain that dose at all meals of similar size—take less at smaller meals.

4. When taking a number of tablets or capsules, take them throughout the meal.

5. As your stomach begins to regain the ability to produce the amount of hydrochloric acid needed for proper digestion, the warm feeling reappears. At that time, cut down the dosage level.

Additional Recommendations

Pancreatin (8–10×), 350 to 700 milligrams 5 minutes before meals.

Infections

An infection refers to a colony of disease-causing organisms establishing a home within the body. Infections can be caused by viruses, bacteria, yeasts, and other microorganisms. The organisms actively reproduce and cause disease directly by damaging cells or indirectly by releasing toxins. It is the function of the immune system to prevent and deal with infections. Different arms of the immune system deal with different microorganisms.

Dietary and Lifestyle Recommendations

- Rest.
- Drink plenty of liquids (focus on water, diluted vegetable juices, soups, and herb teas). Try to drink 8 ounces of water every hour.

- Avoid sugar, including natural sugars such as honey, orange juice, and fructose, because simple sugars depress the immune system.

Acute Viral Infections Supplement Protocol

- Thymus extract, 750 milligrams crude polypeptide fraction once or twice daily
- Vitamin C, 500 to 1,000 milligrams every hour or to bowel tolerance

Acute Bacterial Infections Supplement Protocol

- Spleen extract, 1,500 milligrams spleen peptides daily
- Vitamin C, 500 to 1,000 milligrams every hour or to bowel tolerance

Additional Recommendations

Various herbs are useful in helping fight infection. Most notable for viral infections are *Echinacea* and *Astragalus*. For bacterial infections, goldenseal stands out.

Infertility (Female)

Infertility in females often results from failure to ovulate for no apparent reason or as a result of stress, hormonal imbalance, or a disorder of the ovary, such as a tumor or a cyst. Other, less common causes of infertility are blocked fallopian tubes, endometriosis, or a cervical mucus that is hostile to the partner's sperm.

Dietary and Lifestyle Recommendations

- Consume a diet that focuses on whole, unprocessed foods (whole grains, legumes, vegetables, fruits, nuts, and seeds).
- Eliminate alcohol, caffeine, and sugar.
- Identify and control food allergies.
- Get regular exercise.
- Perform a relaxation exercise (deep breathing, meditation, prayer, visualization, etcetera) 10 to 15 minutes each day.
- Drink at least 48 ounces of water daily.

Absence of Ovulation Supplement Protocol

- High-potency multiple according to guidelines in Chapter 2
- Vitamin C, 500 to 1,000 milligrams three times daily

- Vitamin E, 400 to 800 International Units daily
- Flaxseed oil, 1 tablespoon daily

Additional Recommendations

If the infertility is due to elevated prolactin levels or ovarian insufficiency, an extract of chaste berry (*Vitex agnus-castus*) can be helpful. The usual dosage of chaste berry extract (often standardized to contain 0.5 percent agnuside) is 175 to 225 milligrams daily. It may take chaste berry extract a few months to produce its beneficial effects in restoring female balance. If a woman is ovulating, has no scarring, and still does not conceive, low thyroid function may be a factor.

Infertility (Male)

Most causes of male infertility reflect an abnormal sperm count or quality. In about 90 percent of low sperm count cases, the cause is deficient sperm production. Although it takes only one sperm to fertilize an egg, in an average ejaculate a man ejects nearly 200 million sperm. However, because of the natural barriers in the female reproductive tract, only about 40 or so sperm ever reach the vicinity of an egg. There is a strong correlation between the number of sperm in an ejaculate and fertility.

Sperm formation is closely linked to nutritional and antioxidant status. Since sperm are particularly susceptible to free-radical and oxidative damage, environmental sources of free radicals should be avoided and the diet should be rich in antioxidants.

Dietary and Lifestyle Recommendations

- Consume a diet that focuses on whole, unprocessed foods (whole grains, legumes, vegetables, fruits, nuts, and seeds).
- Eat 1/4 cup of raw sunflower seeds or pumpkin seeds each day.
- Eliminate alcohol, caffeine, and sugar.
- Identify and control food allergies.
- Get regular exercise.
- Perform a relaxation exercise (deep breathing, meditation, prayer, visualization, etcetera) 10 to 15 minutes each day.
- Drink at least 48 ounces of water daily.

Supplement Protocol

- High-potency multiple according to guidelines in Chapter 2
- Vitamin C, 500 to 1,000 milligrams three times daily
- Vitamin E, 400 to 800 International Units daily

- Flaxseed oil, 1 tablespoon daily
- Methylcobalamin (active vitamin B_{12}), 2,000 micrograms daily
- Carnitine, 300 milligrams three times daily

Additional Recommendations

The scrotal sac is supposed to keep the testes at a temperature between 94 and 96 degrees Fahrenheit. If the temperature rises above 96 degrees, sperm production is greatly inhibited or stopped completely. Typically, the mean scrotal temperature of infertile men is significantly higher than fertile men. Reducing scrotal temperature in infertile men is often enough to make them fertile. This temperature reduction is usually achieved by not wearing tight-fitting underwear or tight jeans, avoiding hot tubs, and after exercise allowing the testicles to hang free to allow them to recover from heat buildup.

Comments

For more information, consult my book, *Male Sexual Vitality* (part of the Getting Well Naturally Series from Prima Publishing, 1994).

Insomnia

Insomnia refers to an inability to attain or maintain sleep. Over the course of a year, more than half the U.S. population has difficulty falling asleep. About 33 percent of the population experiences insomnia on a regular basis. Foremost in the natural approach to insomnia is the elimination of those factors known to disrupt normal sleep patterns, such as sources of caffeine, alcohol, and drugs.

Supplement Protocol (Acute Treatment)

- Melatonin, 0.1 to 3 milligrams 30 to 45 minutes before retiring, particularly for the elderly
- Magnesium, 500 milligrams 30 to 45 minutes before retiring

Additional Recommendations

Valerian root extract (0.8 percent valerenic acid), 150 to 300 milligrams 30 to 45 minutes before retiring.

Irritable Bowel Syndrome

The irritable bowel syndrome (IBS) is a very common condition in which the large intestine, or colon, fails to function properly. It is also known as nervous indigestion, spastic colitis, mucous colitis, and intestinal neurosis. IBS has characteristic symptoms that can include a combination of any of the following: abdominal pain and distention, more frequent bowel movements with pain, or relief of pain with bowel movements; constipation; diarrhea; excessive production of mucus in the colon; symptoms of indigestion such as flatulence, nausea, or anorexia; and varying degrees of anxiety or depression. The irritable bowel syndrome (IBS) is an extremely common condition. Estimates suggest that approximately 15 percent of the population has suffered from IBS.

Dietary and Lifestyle Recommendations

- Consume a diet that focuses on whole, unprocessed foods (whole grains, legumes, vegetables, fruits, nuts, and seeds).
- Eliminate alcohol, caffeine, and sugar.
- Identify and control food allergies.
- Get regular exercise.
- Perform a relaxation exercise (deep breathing, meditation, prayer, visualization, etcetera) 10 to 15 minutes each day.
- Drink at least 48 ounces of water daily.

Supplement Protocol

- High-potency multiple according to guidelines in Chapter 2
- Vitamin C, 500 to 1,000 milligrams three times daily
- Vitamin E, 200 to 400 International Units daily
- Flaxseed oil, 1 to 2 tablespoons daily
- Probiotics, 1 to 10 billion viable *L. acidophilus* or *B. bifidum* cells daily (sufficient dosage for most people)
- Water-soluble dietary fiber, 3 to 6 grams at night before bedtime

Additional Recommendations

Enteric-coated peppermint oil, one or two capsules 20 minutes before meals three times daily.

Comments

Avoiding white sugar, consuming a diet rich in complex carbohydrates and dietary fiber, and eliminating food allergies is effective is most cases.

Kidney Stones

In the U.S., most kidney stone are calcium-containing stones composed of calcium oxalate, calcium oxalate mixed with calcium phosphate, or (very rarely) calcium phosphate alone. The high rate of calcium-containing stones in affluent societies is directly associated with the following dietary patterns: low fiber, highly refined carbohydrates, high alcohol consumption, large amounts of animal protein, high fat, high calcium-containing food, high salt, and high vitamin D–enriched food.

Dietary and Lifestyle Recommendations

- Consume a diet that focuses on whole, unprocessed foods (whole grains, legumes, vegetables, fruits, nuts, and seeds).
- Eliminate antacids, alcohol, caffeine, and sugar.
- Drink at least 48 ounces of water daily.

Supplement Protocol

- High-potency multiple according to guidelines in Chapter 2
- Vitamin C, 500 to 1,000 milligrams three times daily
- Vitamin E, 200 to 400 International Units daily
- Flaxseed oil, 1 to 2 tablespoons daily
- Magnesium, 500 to 750 milligrams daily

Lupus

Lupus most often refers to systemic lupus erythematosus, a condition that affects many systems of the body, including the skin, joints, and kidney. Lupus is a classic example of an autoimmune-type disease in which the body's immune system attacks connective tissue. Lupus affects women nine times more often than men. Lupus is life-threatening when the kidneys become involved.

Dietary and Lifestyle Recommendations

- Consume a diet that focuses on whole, unprocessed foods (whole grains, legumes, vegetables, fruits, nuts, and seeds).
- Avoid animal products with the exception of cold-water fish (salmon, mackerel, herring, halibut, etcetera).
- Identify and control food allergies.
- Eliminate alcohol, caffeine, and sugar.
- Get regular exercise.
- Perform a relaxation exercise (deep breathing, meditation, prayer, visualization, etcetera) 10 to 15 minutes each day.
- Drink at least 48 ounces of water daily.

Supplement Protocol

- High-potency multiple according to guidelines in Chapter 2
- Vitamin C, 500 to 1,000 milligrams three times daily
- Vitamin E, 400 to 800 International Units daily
- Flaxseed oil, 1 to 2 tablespoons daily
- Pancreatin (8–10×), 350 to 700 milligrams three times daily between meals
- Adrenal cortex extract, follow recommendations in Chapter 46

Additional Recommendations

The adrenal hormone DHEA (dehydroepiandrosterone) at a dosage of 200 milligrams daily can be of benefit in some cases.

Lyme Disease

Lyme disease is characterized by skin changes, flulike symptoms, and joint inflammation. It was first described in the community of Old Lyme, Connecticut, in 1975. Lyme disease is caused by a bacterium (*Borrelia burgdorferi*) that is transmitted by deer tick bites—deer ticks infest dogs as well as deer. In the acute stage, Lyme disease is best treated with antibiotics to prevent the development of the chronic inflammatory condition. The following dosages are for the chronic form.

Dietary and Lifestyle Recommendations

- Consume a diet that focuses on whole, unprocessed foods (whole grains, legumes, vegetables, fruits, nuts, and seeds).
- Avoid animal products with the exception of cold-water fish (salmon, mackerel, herring, halibut, etcetera).
- Identify and control food allergies.
- Eliminate alcohol, caffeine, and sugar.
- Get regular exercise.
- Perform a relaxation exercise (deep breathing, meditation, prayer, visualization, etcetera) 10 to 15 minutes each day.
- Drink at least 48 ounces of water daily.

Supplement Protocol

- High-potency multiple according to guidelines in Chapter 2
- Vitamin C, 500 to 1,000 milligrams three times daily
- Vitamin E, 400 to 800 International Units daily

- Flaxseed oil, 1 to 2 tablespoons daily
- Pancreatin (8–10×), 350 to 700 milligrams three times daily between meals

Macular Degeneration

The macula is the portion of the eye responsible for fine vision. Degeneration of the macula is the leading cause of severe visual loss in the United States and Europe in persons aged 55 years or older. The risk factors for macular degeneration include aging, atherosclerosis, and high blood pressure. There is no current medical treatment for the most common form of macular degeneration. Laser surgery is used for those individuals who develop a less common type of macular degeneration (exudative macular degeneration).

The origin of macular degeneration is ultimately related to damage caused by free radicals. As with most diseases related to free-radical damage, prevention or treatment at an early stage is more effective than trying to reverse the disease process.

Dietary and Lifestyle Recommendations

- Consume a diet that focuses on whole, unprocessed foods (whole grains, legumes, vegetables, fruits, nuts, and seeds).
- Eliminate alcohol, caffeine, and sugar.
- Get regular exercise.
- Perform a relaxation exercise (deep breathing, meditation, prayer, visualization, etcetera) 10 to 15 minutes each day.
- Drink at least 48 ounces of water daily.

Supplement Protocol

- High-potency multiple according to guidelines in Chapter 2
- Vitamin C, 500 to 1,000 milligrams three times daily
- Vitamin E, 400 to 800 International Units daily
- Flaxseed oil, 1 to 2 tablespoons daily
- PCO extracts or flavonoids, according to dosage recommendations in Chapter 37

Additional Recommendations

Bilberry extract (25 percent anthocyanosides) or *Ginkgo biloba* extract (24 percent ginkgo flavonglycoside), 40 to 80 milligrams three times daily.

Comments

Numerous studies show that individuals consuming more fruits and vegetables are less likely to develop cataracts or macular degeneration than individuals who do not regularly consume fruits and vegetables. Fresh fruits and vegetables are rich in a broad range of antioxidant compounds including vitamin C, carotenes, flavonoids, and glutathione. All these antioxidants are critically involved in important mechanisms that prevent the development of macular degeneration.

Menopause

Menopause denotes the cessation of menstruation in women. It usually occurs when a woman reaches the age of 50. Six to 12 months without a period is the commonly accepted rule for diagnosing menopause. This time period prior to the official designation of menopause is often referred to as perimenopausal, while the time period after menopause is officially designated as postmenopausal.

The current medical view of menopause is that it is a disease rather than a normal physiological process. Current medical treatment of menopause primarily involves the use of hormone replacement therapy featuring the combination of estrogen and progesterone. However, this treatment carries with it significant risk and side effects.

Dietary and Lifestyle Recommendations

- Consume a diet that focuses on whole, unprocessed foods (whole grains, legumes, vegetables, fruits, nuts, and seeds).
- Increase consumption of soy foods.
- Eliminate alcohol, caffeine, and sugar.
- Get regular exercise.
- Perform a relaxation exercise (deep breathing, meditation, prayer, visualization, etcetera) 10 to 15 minutes each day.
- Drink at least 48 ounces of water daily.

Supplement Protocol

- High-potency multiple according to guidelines in Chapter 2
- Vitamin C, 500 to 1,000 milligrams three times daily
- Vitamin E, 400 to 800 International Units daily
- Flaxseed oil, 1 to 2 tablespoons daily

Additional Recommendations

The most widely used and only thoroughly studied natural approach to menopause is Remifemin—a special extract of *Cimicifuga racemosa* (Black cohosh) standardized to contain 1 milligram of triterpenes calculated as 27-deoxyacteine per tablet. Clinical studies show Remifemin relieves not only hot flashes, but also depression and vaginal atrophy. Remifemin is without side effects. The standard dosage in 2 tablets twice daily.

Comments

For those who desire more information, please consult my book on *Menopause* (part of the Getting Well Naturally series from Prima Publishing, 1994).

Menstrual Disorders (See Appropriate Topic, e.g., Infertility, Fibrocystic Breast Disease, or Premenstrual Syndrome)

Migraine Headache

Migraine headaches are vascular headaches characterized by a throbbing pain that pounds sharply in the sufferer's head. In contrast, a tension headache is associated with a steady, constant pain that starts at the forehead or back of the head and can spread pain over the entire head. Sometimes migraines hit without warning. Many who suffer migraines get unusual symptoms called "auras" before the pain hits. The aura may be a tingling or numbness in the body. Alternatively, the individual's vision may become blurred or show bright spots. Thinking may become disturbed. Anxiety or fatigue may suddenly set in. A surprisingly high percentage of Americans suffer from migraines. The percentage is higher for women (25 percent to 30 percent) than for men (14 percent to 20 percent). More than half the sufferers have a family history of the illness.

Dietary and Lifestyle Recommendations

- Consume a diet that focuses on whole, unprocessed foods (whole grains, legumes, vegetables, fruits, nuts, and seeds).
- Avoid animal products with the exception of cold-water fish (salmon, mackerel, herring, halibut, etcetera).
- Identify and control food allergies.
- Eliminate alcohol, caffeine, and sugar.
- Get regular exercise.
- Perform a relaxation exercise (deep breathing, meditation, prayer, visualization, etcetera) 10 to 15 minutes each day.
- Drink at least 48 ounces of water daily.

Supplement Protocol

- High-potency multiple according to guidelines in Chapter 2
- Vitamin C, 500 to 1,000 milligrams three times daily
- Vitamin E, 200 to 400 International Units daily

- Flaxseed oil, 1 tablespoon daily
- Magnesium, 800 to 1,200 milligrams daily

Additional Recommendations

Feverfew is helpful if you select a high-quality product. A recent analysis of the parthenolide content of over 35 different commercial preparations indicates a wide variation in the amount of parthenolide. Use products standardized for parthenolide. The dosage is 600 micrograms of parthenolide daily.

Comments

Rule out hypothyroidism because it can be associated with a tendency toward migraine headaches.

Mononucleosis, Acute Infectious (See Infections)

Multiple Sclerosis

Multiple sclerosis (MS) is a syndrome of progressive nervous system disturbances occurring early in life. The early symptoms of multiple sclerosis may include:

- **Muscular Symptoms** Feeling of heaviness, weakness, leg dragging, stiffness, tendency to drop things, clumsiness
- **Sensory Symptoms** Tingling, "pins and needles" sensation, numbness, dead feeling, bandlike tightness, electrical sensations
- **Visual Symptoms** Blurring, fogginess, haziness, eyeball pain, blindness, double vision
- **Vestibular Symptoms** Light-headedness, feeling of spinning, sensation of drunkenness, nausea, vomiting
- **Genitourinary Symptoms** Incontinence, loss of bladder sensation, loss of sexual function

Despite considerable research, there are still many questions about MS. Mainstream medicine is almost obsessed with finding a viral cause for this disease, although most current work suggests immune disturbances. In MS, the myelin sheath that surrounds nerves is destroyed. For this reason, MS is classified as a "demyelinating" disease. Zones of demyelination (plaques) vary in size and location within the spinal cord. Symptoms correspond in a general way to the distribution of the plaques.

In about two-thirds of the cases, onset is between ages 20 and 40 (rarely is the onset after 50), and women are affected slightly more often than males (60 percent female, 40 percent male). The cause of MS remains to be definitively determined. Many causative factors have been proposed including viruses, autoimmune factors, and diet.

Dietary and Lifestyle Recommendations

- Consume a diet that focuses on whole, unprocessed foods (whole grains, legumes, vegetables, fruits, nuts, and seeds).
- Avoid animal products with the exception of cold-water fish (salmon, mackerel, herring, halibut, etcetera).
- Identify and control food allergies.
- Eliminate alcohol, caffeine, and sugar.
- Get regular exercise.
- Perform a relaxation exercise (deep breathing, meditation, prayer, visualization, etcetera) 10 to 15 minutes each day.
- Drink at least 48 ounces of water daily.

Supplement Protocol

- High-potency multiple according to guidelines in Chapter 2
- Vitamin C, 500 to 1,000 milligrams three times daily
- Vitamin E, 400 to 800 International Units daily
- Flaxseed oil, 1 or 2 tablespoons daily
- Methylcobalamin (active vitamin B_{12}), 1,000 micrograms twice daily
- Pancreatin (8–10×), 350 to 700 milligrams three times daily between meals

Additional Recommendations

Ginkgo biloba extract (24 percent ginkgo flavonglycoside), 40 to 80 milligrams three times daily.

Comments

Dr. Roy Swank, Professor of Neurology, University of Oregon Medical School, has provided convincing evidence that a diet low in saturated fats, maintained over a long period of time (one study lasted over 34 years), tends to halt the disease process. Swank began successfully treating patients with his lowfat diet in 1948. Swank's diet recommends:

- Saturated fat intake of no more than 10 grams per day
- Daily intake of 40 to 50 grams of polyunsaturated oils (margarine, shortening, and hydrogenated oils are not allowed)
- At least 1 teaspoon of cod liver oil daily
- Normal allowance of protein
- Consumption of fish three or more times a week

Osteoarthritis

Osteoarthritis (degenerative joint disease) is the most common form of arthritis. It is seen primarily, but not exclusively, in the elderly. Surveys indicate that over 40 million Americans have osteoarthritis, including 80 percent of persons over 50. Under 45, osteoarthritis is much more common in men; after 45, it is ten times more common in women than men.

The weight-bearing joints and joints of the hands are the joints most often affected by the degenerative changes associated with osteoarthritis. Specifically, there is much cartilage destruction followed by hardening and the formation of large bone spurs in the joint margins. Pain, deformity, and limitation of motion in the joint results. Inflammation is usually minimal.

The onset of osteoarthritis can be very subtle; morning joint stiffness is often the first symptom. As the disease progresses, there is pain on motion of the involved joint that is made worse by prolonged activity and relieved by rest. There are usually no signs of inflammation.

Dietary and Lifestyle Recommendations

- Consume a diet that focuses on whole, unprocessed foods (whole grains, legumes, vegetables, fruits, nuts, and seeds).
- Avoid animal products with the exception of cold-water fish (salmon, mackerel, herring, halibut, etcetera).
- Identify and control food allergies.
- Eliminate alcohol, caffeine, and sugar.
- Get regular exercise. If weight-bearing joints are severely affected, try activities such as swimming, water aerobics, and bike riding.
- Perform a relaxation exercise (deep breathing, meditation, prayer, visualization, etcetera) 10 to 15 minutes each day.
- Drink at least 48 ounces of water daily.

Supplement Protocol

- High-potency multiple according to guidelines in Chapter 2.
- Vitamin C, 500 to 1,000 milligrams three times daily.
- Vitamin E, 400 to 800 International Units daily.
- Flaxseed oil, 1 or 2 tablespoons daily.
- Glucosamine sulfate, 500 milligrams three times daily.
- SAM, 200 milligrams twice daily for the first day, increase to 400 milligrams twice daily on day 3, then 400 milligrams three times daily on day 10. After 21 days at a dosage of 1,200 milligrams daily, reduce dosage to the maintenance dosage of 200 milligrams twice daily.

- Boron (as sodium tetrahydraborate), 6 to 9 milligrams daily.

Osteoporosis

Osteoporosis literally means porous bone. Osteoporosis affects more than 20 million people in the United States. Normally there is a decline in bone mass after 40 in both sexes. This bone loss is accelerated in patients with osteoporosis. Many factors can result in excessive bone loss, and different variants of osteoporosis exist. Post-menopausal osteoporosis in women is the most common form of osteoporosis.

Major risk factors for osteoporosis in women are:

- Postmenopausal
- White or Asian
- Premature menopause
- Positive family history
- Short stature and small bones
- Leanness
- Low calcium intake
- Inactivity
- Nulliparity (never pregnant)
- Gastric or small-bowel resection
- Long-term glucocorticosteroid therapy
- Long-term use of anticonvulsants
- Hyperparathyroidism
- Hyperthyroidism
- Smoking
- Heavy alcohol use

Dietary and Lifestyle Recommendations

- Consume a diet that focuses on whole, unprocessed foods (whole grains, legumes, vegetables, fruits, nuts, and seeds).
- Eliminate alcohol, caffeine, and sugar.
- Do not drink soft drinks.
- Get regular exercise.
- Walk!
- Perform a relaxation exercise (deep breathing, meditation, prayer, visualization, etcetera) 10 to 15 minutes each day.
- Drink at least 48 ounces of water daily.

Supplement Protocol

- High-potency multiple according to guidelines in Chapter 2
- Vitamin C, 500 to 1,000 milligrams three times daily
- Vitamin E, 200 to 400 International Units daily
- Flaxseed oil, 1 or 2 tablespoons daily
- OsteoPrime, two tablets twice daily. (OsteoPrime is a bone-building formula developed by Alan Gaby, M.D., and Jonathan Wright, M.D. It contains a full range of important nutrients for bone health.)
- Boron (as sodium tetrahydraborate), 6 to 9 milligrams daily

Comments

If more information on osteoporosis is desired, I strongly encourage you to read *Preventing and Reversing Osteoporosis* by Alan R Gaby, M.D. (Prima Publishing, 1994).

Parkinson's Disease

Parkinson's disease is a brain disorder that causes muscle tremor, weakness, and stiffness. The characteristic signs are trembling, a rigid posture, slow movements, and a shuffling, unbalanced walk. Parkinson's disease is caused by degeneration of nerve cells due largely to free-radical damage. In all but the initial phases of the diseases, drug therapy is necessary.

Dietary and Lifestyle Recommendations

- Consume a diet that focuses on whole, unprocessed foods (whole grains, legumes, vegetables, fruits, nuts, and seeds).
- Eliminate alcohol, caffeine, and sugar.
- Get regular exercise.
- Perform a relaxation exercise (deep breathing, meditation, prayer, visualization, etcetera) 10 to 15 minutes each day.
- Drink at least 48 ounces of water daily.

Supplement Protocol

- High-potency multiple according to guidelines in Chapter 2
- Vitamin C, 500 to 1,000 milligrams three times daily
- Vitamin E, 400 to 800 International Units daily
- Flaxseed oil, 1 or 2 tablespoons daily

- *Ginkgo biloba* extract (24 percent ginkgo flavonglycoside), 40 to 80 milligrams three times daily
- Phosphatidylserine, 100 milligrams three times daily

Additional Recommendations

Rule out heavy metal toxicity by performing a hair mineral analysis.

Comments

About one-third of the individuals with Parkinson's disease go on to develop dementia. *Ginkgo biloba* extract can be effective in halting this progression.

Pleurisy (See Bronchitis and Pneumonia)

Premenstrual Syndrome

Premenstrual syndrome (PMS), also called premenstrual tension, is a recurrent condition of women characterized by troublesome, yet often ill-defined, symptoms 7 to 14 days before menstruation. Typical symptoms include decreased energy, tension, irritability, depression, headache, altered sex drive, breast pain, backache, abdominal bloating, and swelling of the fingers and ankles. The syndrome affects about one-third of women between 30 and 40, about 10 percent of whom may have a significantly debilitating form.

Although there is a wide spectrum of symptoms, there are common hormonal patterns in PMS patients when compared to symptom-free control groups. Perhaps the most common pattern is an elevation of plasma estrogen and a decrease in plasma progesterone levels 5 to 10 days before the menses.

Dietary and Lifestyle Recommendations

Diet appears to play a major role in the development of PMS. Compared to symptom-free women, PMS patients consume 62 percent more refined carbohydrates, 275 percent more refined sugar, 79 percent more dairy products, 78 percent more sodium, 53 percent less iron, 77 percent less manganese, and 52 percent less zinc. The first step in addressing PMS is limiting the consumption of refined sugar and decreasing or eliminating milk and dairy products.

An additional key dietary dosage for the PMS sufferer includes decreasing salt intake, alcohol and tobacco use, and the intake of caffeine-containing foods and beverages such as coffee, tea, and chocolate. Caffeine intake can produce a dose-dependent effect on the severity of symptoms—the more caffeine consumed, the greater the severity of the symptoms.

Supplement Protocol

- High-potency multiple according to guidelines in Chapter 2
- Vitamin C, 500 to 1,000 milligrams three times daily
- Vitamin E, 400 to 800 International Units daily
- Flaxseed oil, 1 to 2 tablespoons daily

Additional Recommendations

- Chaste berry (*Vitex agnus-castus*) extract (standardized to contain 0.5 percent agnuside), 175 to 225 milligrams daily.
- *Ginkgo biloba* extract (24 percent ginkgo flavonglycoside), 40 to 80 milligrams three times daily for congestive symptoms (water retention, breast tenderness, capillary fragility, etcetera).

Prostate Enlargement (BPH)

Nearly 60 percent of men between 40 and 59 have an enlarged prostate gland, a condition that is known in the medical community as benign prostatic hyperplasia (BPH). Symptoms of BPH typically reflect obstruction of the bladder outlet—progressive urinary frequency, urgency and nighttime awakening to empty the bladder, and hesitancy and intermittence with reduced force and caliber of urine. The condition, if left untreated, eventually obstructs the bladder outlet and results in retention of urine in the blood.

Diet appears to play a critical role in the development of BPH. Paramount to an effective BPH prevention and treatment plan is adequate zinc intake and absorption. Zinc can reduce the size of the prostate (as determined by rectal examination, x-ray, and endoscopy) and reduce symptoms in the majority of patients. The clinical efficacy of zinc is probably because of its critical involvement in many aspects of hormonal metabolism.

Dietary and Lifestyle Recommendations

- Consume a diet that focuses on whole, unprocessed foods (whole grains, legumes, vegetables, fruits, nuts, and seeds).
- Eat $1/4$ cup of raw sunflower seeds or pumpkin seeds each day.
- Eliminate alcohol, caffeine, and sugar.
- Identify and control food allergies.
- Get regular exercise.
- Perform a relaxation exercise (deep breathing, meditation, prayer, visualization, etcetera) 10 to 15 minutes each day.
- Drink at least 48 ounces of water daily, but drink no fluids after 7:00 P.M.

Supplement Protocol

- High-potency multiple according to guidelines in Chapter 2
- Vitamin C, 500 to 1,000 milligrams three times daily
- Vitamin E, 200 to 400 International Units daily
- Flaxseed oil, 1 tablespoon daily
- Zinc, 45 to 60 milligrams daily for 3 months, then 30 milligrams daily

Additional Recommendations

Saw palmetto extract (85 to 95 percent fatty acids and sterols) at a dosage of 160 milligrams twice daily can be effective in roughly 90 percent of cases, making it by far the most effective agent for BPH.

Prostatitis

Prostatitis refers to an infection or inflammation of the prostate. Prostatitis is associated with pain during urination, fever, and a discharge from the penis. The standard medical treatment is antibiotics. With antibiotics alone, the condition is typically of a chronic nature and difficult to clear. Frequent or chronic prostate infections may be a sign of low zinc levels because the prostatic fluid contains a powerful zinc-containing, anti-infective substance.

Dietary and Lifestyle Recommendations

- Consume a diet that focuses on whole, unprocessed foods (whole grains, legumes, vegetables, fruits, nuts, and seeds).
- Eat $^1/_4$ cup of raw sunflower seeds or pumpkin seeds each day.
- Eliminate alcohol, caffeine, and sugar.
- Identify and control food allergies.
- Get regular exercise.
- Perform a relaxation exercise (deep breathing, meditation, prayer, visualization, etcetera) 10 to 15 minutes each day.
- Drink at least 48 ounces of water daily.

Supplement Protocol

- High-potency multiple (according to guidelines in Chapter 2)
- Vitamin C, 500 to 1,000 milligrams three times daily
- Vitamin E, 200 to 400 International Units daily
- Flaxseed oil, 1 tablespoon daily
- Zinc, 45 to 60 milligrams daily for 3 months, then 30 milligrams daily

Additional Recommendations

Cernilton, a flower pollen extract, has been used for decades with great success in prostatitis in Europe. Call 1-800-831-9505 for more information. If antibiotics have been used, probiotic supplementation is indicated.

Psoriasis

Psoriasis is a condition caused by a pileup of skin cells that have replicated too rapidly. Psoriasis is an extremely common skin disorder. Its rate of occurrence in the U.S. is between 2 and 4 percent of the population. A number of dietary factors appear to be responsible for psoriasis, including incomplete protein digestion, alcohol consumption, and excessive consumption of animal fats.

Dietary and Lifestyle Recommendations

- Consume a diet that focuses on whole, unprocessed foods (whole grains, legumes, vegetables, fruits, nuts, and seeds).
- Avoid animal products with the exception of cold-water fish (salmon, mackerel, herring, halibut, etcetera).
- Identify and control food allergies.
- Eliminate alcohol, caffeine, and sugar.
- Get regular exercise.
- Perform a relaxation exercise (deep breathing, meditation, prayer, visualization, etcetera) 10 to 15 minutes each day.
- Drink at least 48 ounces of water daily.

Supplement Protocol

- High-potency multiple according to guidelines in Chapter 2
- Vitamin C, 500 to 1,000 milligrams three times daily
- Vitamin E, 200 to 400 International Units daily
- Flaxseed oil, 1 or 2 tablespoons daily
- Pancreatin (8–10×), 350 to 700 milligrams three times daily between meals
- Zinc, 45 to 60 milligrams daily for 3 months, then 30 milligrams daily

Additional Recommendations

I have had good results using Simicort, a natural alternative to corticosteroid creams. Apply Simicort to the affected area two to three times daily. The components of Simicort have demonstrated an effect equal or superior to cortisone when applied topically. Unlike cortisone creams, Simicort is without side effects.

Rheumatoid Arthritis

Rheumatoid arthritis (RA) is a chronic inflammatory condition that affects the entire body, but especially the synovial membranes of the joints. It is a classic example of an "autoimmune disease," a condition in which the body's immune system attacks the body's own tissue.

In RA, the joints typically involved are the hands and feet, wrists, ankles, and knees. Somewhere between 1 and 3 percent of the population is affected, female patients outnumber males almost three to one, and the usual age of onset is 20 to 40 (although it may begin at any age).

The onset of rheumatoid arthritis is usually gradual, but occasionally it is quite abrupt. Fatigue, low-grade fever, weakness, joint stiffness, and vague joint pain may proceed the appearance of painful, swollen joints by several weeks. Several joints are usually involved in the onset, typically in a symmetrical fashion—both hands, wrists, or ankles. In about one-third of persons with RA, initial involvement is confined to one or a few joints.

Involved joints characteristically are quite warm, tender, and swollen. The skin over the joint takes on a ruddy, purplish hue. As the disease progresses, joint deformities result in the hands and feet. Terms used to describe these deformities include swan neck, boutenniere, and cockup toes.

There is abundant evidence that rheumatoid arthritis is an autoimmune reaction, where antibodies develop against components of joint tissues. Yet what triggers this autoimmune reaction remains largely unknown. Speculation and investigation has centered around genetic susceptibility, abnormal bowel permeability, lifestyle and nutritional factors, food allergies, and microorganisms. Rheumatoid arthritis is a classic example of a multifactorial disease where there is an interesting assortment of genetic and environmental factors that contribute to the disease process. For a full discussion of all these factors, read my book on *Arthritis* (part of the Getting Well Naturally series, Prima Publishing, 1994).

Dietary and Lifestyle Recommendations

- Consume a diet that focuses on whole, unprocessed foods (whole grains, legumes, vegetables, fruits, nuts, and seeds).
- Avoid animal products with the exception of cold-water fish (salmon, mackerel, herring, halibut, etcetera).
- Identify and control food allergies.
- Eliminate alcohol, caffeine, and sugar.
- Get regular exercise.
- Perform a relaxation exercise (deep breathing, meditation, prayer, visualization, etcetera) 10 to 15 minutes each day.
- Drink at least 48 ounces of water daily.

Supplement Protocol

- High-potency multiple according to guidelines in Chapter 2
- Vitamin C, 500 to 1,000 milligrams three times daily
- Vitamin E, 400 to 800 International Units daily
- Flaxseed oil, 1 to 2 tablespoons daily
- Pancreatin (8–10×), 350 to 700 milligrams three times daily between meals
- Adrenal cortex extract, dosage recommendations in Chapter 46

Additional Recommendations

- If corticosteroids have been used at either high dosages or long-term, I recommend whole adrenal extracts as discussed in Chapter 46.
- DHEA supplementation may be useful (See Lupus).
- Try topical preparations containing a pungent principal called capsaicin, which is isolated from cayenne pepper (*Capsicum frutescens*). When applied to the skin, capsaicin stimulates and then blocks the transmission of the pain impulse. It does this by depleting the nerves of a messenger substance called substance P (the *P* stands for pain). In addition to playing a key role in the pain impulse, substance P activates inflammatory mediators into joint tissues in rheumatoid arthritis.

Rosacea

Rosacea is a chronic acnelike eruption on the face of middle-aged and older adults associated with facial flushing. The primary involvement occurs over the flush areas of the cheeks and nose. It is more common in women (a ratio of three to one), but more severe in men. Many factors are suspect as a cause of acne rosacea: alcoholism, menopausal flushing, local infection, B-vitamin deficiencies, and decreased secretion of digestive factors. Most cases are associated with moderate to severe seborrhea (excess flow of sebum).

Dietary and Lifestyle Recommendations

- Eliminate all refined and/or concentrated sugars from the diet.
- Do not eat fried foods or foods containing trans fatty acids such as milk, milk products, margarine, shortening, and other synthetically hydrogenated vegetable oils.
- Avoid milk and foods high in iodized salt.
- Avoid the use of greasy creams or cosmetics.
- Wash the pillowcase regularly in chemical-free (no added colors or fragrances) detergents.

Supplement Protocol

See Acne.

Scleroderma

Scleroderma refers to an autoimmune disorder that can affect many body tissues, particularly the skin, arteries, kidneys, heart, lungs, gastrointestinal tract, and joints. Symptoms are the result of abnormal collagen formation. The number and severity of the symptoms can vary drastically. The most common symptom is Raynaud's phenomena, a painful response of the hands or feet to cold exposure.

Dietary and Lifestyle Recommendations

- Consume a diet that focuses on whole, unprocessed foods (whole grains, legumes, vegetables, fruits, nuts, and seeds).
- Avoid animal products with the exception of cold-water fish (salmon, mackerel, herring, halibut, etcetera).
- Identify and control food allergies.
- Eliminate alcohol, caffeine, and sugar.
- Get regular exercise.
- Perform a relaxation exercise (deep breathing, meditation, prayer, visualization, etcetera) 10 to 15 minutes each day.
- Drink at least 48 ounces of water daily.

Supplement Protocol

- High-potency multiple according to guidelines in Chapter 2
- Vitamin C, 500 to 1,000 milligrams three times daily
- Vitamin E, 400 to 800 International Units daily
- Flaxseed oil, 1 to 2 tablespoons daily
- Pancreatin (8–10×), 350 to 700 milligrams three times daily between meals

Additional Recommendations

If corticosteroids have been used at either high dosages or for long-term, I recommend whole adrenal extracts according to the guidelines in Chapter 46.

DHEA supplementation may be useful (See Lupus).

The purified triterpenes of gotu kola (*Centella asiatica*) has been tested in several trials in the treatment of scleroderma (including systemic sclerosis). In addition to decreasing skin hardening, patients have noticed a lessening of joint pain and improved finger motility. Presumably the positive therapeutic response is a result of *Centella*'s balancing effect on connective tissue that prevents the excessive collagen synthesis observed in scleroderma. Dosage for the purified triterpenes is 70 milligrams twice daily.

Sinus Infection

An acute sinus infection is characterized by nasal congestion and discharge; fever; chills; frontal headache; and pain, tenderness, redness, and swelling over the involved sinus. A chronic infection may produce no symptoms other than mild postnasal discharge, a musty odor, or a nonproductive cough.

The most common predisposing factor in acute bacterial sinusitis is viral upper respiratory tract infection (the common cold). Allergies and other factors that interfere with normal protective mechanisms may precede the viral infection and, therefore, are also likely predisposing factors. Any factor that induces swelling and fluid retention of the mucous membranes of the sinuses may cause drainage blockage. In this scenario, bacterial overgrowth occurs. In chronic sinus infections (sinusitis), an allergic background is commonly present, and in 25 percent of chronic maxillary sinusitis there is an underlying dental infection.

Dietary and Lifestyle Recommendations

- Avoid cigarette smoke and other respiratory irritants.
- Rest.
- Drink at least 48 ounces of water daily.
- Avoid sugar and dairy products.

Supplement Protocol (Acute Treatment)

- Thymus extract, 750 milligrams crude polypeptide fraction once or twice daily
- Vitamin C, 500 to 1,000 milligrams every waking hour or to bowel tolerance

Additional Recommendations

I recommend the following be performed twice daily: Apply a heating pad, hot water bottle, or a mustard poultice to the chest for up to 20 minutes. A mustard poultice is made by mixing 1 part dry mustard with 3 parts flour and adding enough water to make a paste. Then spread the paste on cotton (an old pillowcase works well) or cheesecloth, fold, and then place on the chest. Check often because the mustard can cause blisters if left on too long. After the hot pack, lie with the top half of the body off the bed, using the forearms as support—this position facilitates drainage of the lungs. Remain in this position for a 5- to 15-minute period and cough and expectorate into a basin or newspaper on the floor.

Sports Injuries (See Bursitis and Tendonitis)

Strokes (See Cerebrovascular Insufficiency)

Sore Throat and Tonsillitis (See Infection)

Surgery Preparation and Recovery

Any surgical procedure requires special nutritional attention. Major surgeries, especially abdominal surgery, can benefit by natural measures designed to reduce inflammation and swelling while promoting proper wound healing. These measures not only improve recovery but also help prevent adhesion and excessive scar formation.

Supplement Protocol

- High-potency multiple according to guidelines in Chapter 2
- Vitamin C, 500 to 1,000 milligrams three times daily
- Flaxseed oil, 1 tablespoon daily
- PCO extracts or flavonoids, according to dosage recommendations in Chapter 37

In preparation for surgery, begin the above supplement protocol at least 2 weeks prior to surgery. After surgery, continue supplements and add bromelain (the protein-digesting enzyme from pineapple), 250 to 750 milligrams twice daily between meals. Continue for at least 1 month after surgery.

Ulcer

An ulcer usually refers to a peptic ulcer, a term that refers to a group of ulcerative disorders of the upper gastrointestinal tract. The major forms of peptic ulcer are chronic duodenal and gastric (stomach) ulcer. Although duodenal and gastric ulcerations occur at different locations, they appear to be the result of similar mechanisms. Specifically, the development of a duodenal or gastric ulcer is generally thought to be the result of pepsin and stomach acids damaging the lining of the duodenum or stomach. Normally there are enough protective factors to prevent the ulcer formation; however, when there is a decrease in the integrity of these protective factors, ulceration occurs.

Although symptoms of a peptic ulcer may be absent or quite vague, most often peptic ulcers are associated with abdominal discomfort noted 45 to 60 minutes after meals or during the night. In the typical case, the pain is described as gnawing, burning, cramplike, aching, or as "heartburn." Eating or using antacids usually results in great relief.

Individuals with any symptoms of a peptic ulcer need competent medical care. Peptic ulcer complications such as hemorrhage, perforation, and obstruction represent medical emergencies that require immediate hospitalization. Patients with peptic ulcers should be monitored by a physician even when following the natural approaches discussed here.

The natural approach to peptic ulcers is to first identify and then eliminate or reduce all factors that can contribute to the development of peptic ulcers: food allergy, low-fiber diet, cigarette smoking, stress, and drugs such as aspirin and other nonsteroidal analgesics. Once the causative factors have been controlled or eliminated, the focus is directed at healing the ulcers and promoting tissue resistance.

Dietary and Lifestyle Recommendations

- Consume a diet that focuses on whole, unprocessed foods (whole grains, legumes, vegetables, fruits, nuts, and seeds).
- Eliminate milk and other dairy products.
- Get regular exercise.
- Drink at least 48 ounces of water daily.

Supplement Protocol

- High-potency multiple according to guidelines in Chapter 2
- Vitamin C, 500 to 1,000 milligrams three times daily
- Vitamin E, 200 to 400 International Units daily
- Flaxseed oil, 1 tablespoon daily

Additional Recommendations

Chewing tablets containing a special licorice extract known as DGL (for deglycyrrhizinated licorice) at a dosage of 380 to 760 milligrams 20 minutes before meals in very effective in healing ulcers. In fact, clinical studies show DGL is more effective than standard anti-ulcer drugs.

Varicose Veins

Varicose veins affect nearly 50 percent of all middle-aged adults. The veins just under the skin of the legs are the veins most commonly affected because of the tremendous strain that standing produces on these veins. When an individual stands for long periods of time, the pressure exerted against the vein can increase up to ten times. Hence, individuals with occupations that require long periods of standing are at greatest risk for developing varicose veins.

Women are affected about four times as frequently as men; obese individuals have a much greater risk; and the risk increases with age due to loss of tissue tone, loss of muscle mass, and weakening of the walls of the veins. Pregnancy may also lead to the development of varicose veins because pregnancy increases venous pressure in the legs.

Dietary and Lifestyle Recommendations

- Consume a diet that focuses on whole, unprocessed foods (whole grains, legumes, vegetables, fruits, nuts, and seeds).
- Get regular exercise.
- Drink at least 48 ounces of water daily.

Supplement Protocol

- High-potency multiple according to guidelines in Chapter 2
- Vitamin C, 500 to 1,000 milligrams three times daily
- Vitamin E, 200 to 400 International Units daily
- Flaxseed oil, 1 tablespoon daily
- PCO extracts or flavonoids, according to dosage recommendations in Chapter 37
- Aorta glycosaminoglycans, 50 milligrams twice daily

Comments

In general, varicose veins pose little harm if the involved vein is small and near the surface. These types of varicose veins are, however, cosmetically unappealing. Although significant symptoms are not common, the legs may feel heavy, tight, and tired. Larger varicose veins and varicose veins that involve obstruction and valve defects of the leg's deeper veins need medical attention.

References

1   The Emerging Role of Nutritional Supplementation in Medicine

1. Block G, *et al.*, Vitamin supplement use, by demographic characteristics. *Am J Epidemiol* **127**, 297–309, 1988.
2. National Research Council, *Diet and Health: Implications for Reducing Chronic Disease Risk.* National Academy Press, Washington, DC, 1989.
3. National Research Council, *Recommended Dietary Allowances, 10th Edition*, National Academy Press, Washington, DC, 1989.

3   Vitamin A and Carotenes

1. Olson R, ed., *Nutrition Reviews' Present Knowledge in Nutrition, 6th Edition*. Nutrition Foundation, Washington, DC, 1989, pp. 96–107.
2. Underwood B, Vitamin A in animal and human nutrition. *The Retinoids, Vol 1*, Sporn M, Roberts A, and Goodman S (eds.). Academic Press, Orlando, FL, 1984, Chapter 6, pp. 282–392.
3. Brown ED, *et al.*, Plasma carotenoids in normal men after a single ingestion of vegetables or purified beta-carotene. *Am J Clin Nutr* **49**, 1258–1265, 1989.
4. Simpson KL and Chichester CO, Metabolism and significance of carotenoids. *Ann Rev Nutr* **1**, 351–374, 1981.
5. Krause MV and Mahan LK, *Food, Nutrition and Diet Therapy, 5th Edition*. WB Saunders, Philadelphia, PA, 1984, pp. 103–107, 224.
6. Brubacher GB and Weiser H, The vitamin A activity of beta-carotene. *Int J Vit Nutr Res* **55**, 5–15, 1984.
7. Ganguly J and Sastry PS, Mechanism of conversion of beta-carotene into Vitamin A—Central cleavage versus random cleavage. *Wld Rev Nutr Diet* **45**, 198–220, 1985.
8. Olson JA, Serum levels of vitamin A and carotenoids as reflectors of nutritional status. *JNCI* **73**, 1439–1444, 1984.
9. Cullum ME and Zile MH, Acute polybrominated biphenyl toxicosis alters vitamin A homeostasis and enhances degradation of vitamin A. *Toxicol Appl Pharmacol* **81**, 177–181, 1985.
10. Thunberg T, Ahlborg UG, and Wahlstrom B, Comparison of the effects of 2,3,7,8-tetrachlorodibenzo-p-dioxin and six other compounds on vitamin A storage, the UDP-gluconosyltransferase and aryl hydrocarbon hydroxylase activity in the rat liver. *Arch Toxicol* **55**, 16–19, 1984.

11. Folman Y, et al., The effect of dietary and climatic factors on fertility, and on plasma progesterone and oestradiol-17B levels in dairy cows. *J Steroid Biochem* **19**, 863–868, 1983.

12. Editor, Metabolism of beta-carotene by the bovine corpus luteum. *Nutr Rev* **41**, 357, 358, 1983.

13. Lotthammer KH, Importance of beta-carotene for the fertility of dairy cattle. *Feedstuffs* **51**, 16–19, 1979.

14. O'Fallon JV and Chew BP, The subcellular distribution of β-Carotene in bovine corpus luteum. *Proc Soc Exp Biol Med* **177**, 406–411, 1984.

15. Sherman BM and Korenman SG, Inadequate corpus luteum function: A pathophysiological interpretation of human breast cancer epidemiology. *Cancer* **33**, 1306–1312, 1974.

16. Cew BP, Hollen LL, Hillers JK, et al., Relationship between vitamin A and β-carotene in blood plasma and milk and mastitis in Holsteins. *J Dairy Science* **65**, 2111–2118, 1982.

17. Semba RD, Vitamin A, immunity, and infection. *Clin Inf Dis* **19**, 489–499, 1994.

18. Bendich A, Beta-carotene and the immune response. *Proc Nutr Soc* **50**, 263–274, 1991.

19. Krinsky NI, Antioxidant function of carotenoids. *Free Rad Biol Med* **7**, 627–635, 1989.

20. Cutler RG, Carotenoids and retinol: Their possible importance in determining longevity of primate species. *Proc Natl Acad Sci* **81**, 7627–7631, 1984.

21. Murakoshi M, et al., Potent preventive action of alpha-carotene against carcinogenesis. *Cancer Res* **52**, 6583–6587, 1992.

22. Di Mascio P, Kaiser S, and Sies H, Lycopene as the most efficient biological carotenoid singlet oxygen quencher. *Arch Biochem Biophysics* **274**, 532–538, 1989.

23. Franceschi S, et al., Tomatoes and risk of digestive-tract cancers. *Int J Cancer* **59**, 181–184, 1994.

24. Mangels AR, et al., Carotenoid content of fruits and vegetables: An evaluation of analytic data. *J Am Diet Assoc* **93**, 284–286, 1993.

25. Ben-Amotz, et al., Bioavailability of a natural isomer mixture as compared with synthetic all-trans beta-carotene in rats and chicks. *J Nutr* **119**, 1013–1019, 1989.

26. Mokady S, Avron M, and Ben-Amotz A, Accumulation in chick livers of 9-cis versus all-trans beta-carotene. *J Nutr* **120**, 889–892, 1990.

27. Carughi A and Hooper FG, Plasma carotenoid concentrations before and after supplementation with a carotenoid mixture. *Am J Clin Nutr* **59**, 896–899, 1994.

28. Morinobu T, et al., Changes in beta-carotene levels by long-term administration of natural beta-carotene derived from *Dunaliella bardawil* in humans. *J Nutr Sci Vitaminol* **40**, 421–430, 1994.

29. Fawzi WW, et al., Vitamin A supplementation and child mortality. *JAMA* **269**, 898–903, 1993.

30. Arrieta AC, et al., Vitamin A levels in children with measles in Long Beach, California. *J Pediatr* **121**, 75–78, 1992.

31. Neuzil KM, et al., Safety and pharmacokinetics of vitamin A therapy for infants with respiratory syncytial infections. *Antimicrob Agents Chemother* **39**, 1191–1193, 1995.

32. Semba RD, et al., Increased mortality associated with vitamin A deficiency during human immunodeficiency virus type 1 infection. *Arch Intern Med* **153**, 2149–2154, 1993.

33. Ullrich R, et al., Serum carotene deficiency in HIV-infected patients. *AIDS* **8**, 661–665, 1994.

34. Vahlquist A, Clinical use of vitamin A and its derivatives—physiological and pharmacological aspects. *Clin Exp Derm* **10**, 133–143, 1985.

35. Kligman AM, et al., Oral vitamin A in Acne vulgaris. *Int J Derm* **20**, 278–285, 1981.

36. Thomas JR, Cooke J, and Winkelmann RK, High-dose vitamin A in Darier's disease. *Arch Dermatol* **118**, 891–894, 1982.

37. Randle HW, Diaz-Perez J, and Winkelmann RK, Toxic doses of vitamin A for pityriasis rubra pilaris. *Arch Dermatol* **116**, 888–892, 1980.

38. Winkelmann RK, Thomas JR, and Randle HW, Further experience with toxic vitamin A therapy in pityriasis rubra pilaris. *Cutis* **31**, 621–629, 1983.

39. Rengstorff RH, Topical treatment of external eye disorders with preparations containing vitamin A. *Practical Optometry* **4**, 163–165, 1993.

40. Westerhout D, Treatment of dry eyes with aqueous antioxidant eye drops. *Contact Lens J* **19**, 165–173, 1989.

41. Ziegler RG, A review of the epidemiologic evidence that carotenoids reduce the risk of cancer. *J Nutr* **119**, 116–122, 1989.

42. National Research Council, *Diet and Health. Implications for Reducing Chronic Disease Risk.* National Academy Press, Washington, DC, 1989, pp. 313, 314.

43. Gerster H, Anticarcinogenic effect of common carotenoids. *Internat J Vit Nutr Res* **63**, 93–121, 1993.

44. The Alpha-tocopherol, Beta-carotene Cancer Prevention Study Group, The effect of vitamin E and beta-carotene on incidence of lung cancer and other cancers in male smokers. *N Engl J Med* **330**, 1029–1035, 1994.

45. Leo MA, *et al.*, Interaction of ethanol with beta-carotene: Delayed blood clearance and enhanced hepatotoxicity. *Hepatology* **15**, 883–891, 1992.

46. Krinsky NI, The biological properties of carotenoids. *Pure Appl Chem* **66**, 1003–1010, 1994.

47. Krinsky NI, Antioxidant functions of carotenoids. *Free Rad Biol Med* **7**617–7635, 1989.

48. Omenn GS, *et al.*, The beta-carotene and retinol efficacy trial (CARET) for chemoprevention of lung cancer in high risk populations: Smokers and asbestos-exposed workers. *Cancer Res* **54** (Suppl.), 2038S–2043S, 1994.

49. Rowe PM, Beta-carotene takes a collective beating. *Lancet* **347**, 249, 1996.

50. Garewal H and Shamdas GJ, Intervention trials with beta-carotene in precancerous conditions of the upper aerodigestive tract. In: *Micronutrients in Health and Disease Prevention*, Bendich A and Butterworth CE (eds.). Marcel Dekker, New York, 1991, pp. 127–140.

51. Toma S, *et al.*, Treatment of oral leukoplakia with beta-carotene. *Oncology* **49**, 77–81, 1992.

52. Blot WJ, *et al.*, The Linxian trials: Mortality rates by vitamin-mineral intervention group. *Am J Clin Nutr* **62** (Suppl. 6), 1424S–1426S, 1995.

53. Blot WJ, *et al.*, Nutrition intervention trials in Linxian, China: Supplementation with specific vitamin/mineral combinations, cancer incidence, and disease-specific mortality in the general population. *J Nat Canc Inst* **85**, 1483–1491, 1993.

54. Street DA, *et al.*, Serum antioxidants and myocardial infarction. *Circulation* **90**, 1154–1161, 1994.

55. Hennekens CH and Gaziano JM, Antioxidants and heart disease: Epidemiology and clinical evidence. *Clin Cardio* **16** (Suppl. 1), 10–15, 1993.

56. Reaven PD, *et al.*, Effect of dietary antioxidant combinations in humans. Protection of LDL by vitamin E but not by beta-carotene. *Arterioscl Thrombosis* **13**, 590–600, 1993.

57. Clausen SW, Carotenemia and resistance to infection. *Trans Am Pediatr Soc* **43**, 27–30, 1931.

58. Alexander M, Newmark H, and Miller RG, Oral beta-carotene can increase the number of OKT4+ cells in human blood. *Immunol Letters* **9**, 221–224, 1985.

59. Brevard PB, Beta-carotene affects white blood cells in human peripheral blood. *Nutr Rep Internat* **40**, 139–150, 1989.

60. Mikhail MS, *et al.*, Decreased beta-carotene levels in exfoliated vaginal epithelial cells in women with vaginal candidiasis. *Am J Reproductive Immunol* **32**, 221–225, 1994.

61. Mathews-Roth MM, *et al.*, Beta-carotene as an oral photoprotective agent in erythropoietic protoporphyria. *JAMA* **228**, 1004–1008, 1974.

62. Mathews-Roth MM, *et al.*, Beta-carotene therapy for erythropoietic protoporphyria and other photosensitivity diseases. *Arch Dermatol* **113**, 1229–1232, 1977.

63. Mathews-Roth MM, Photosensitization by porphyrins and prevention of photosensitization by carotenoids. *JNCI* **69**, 279–285, 1982.

64. Mathews-Roth MM, Treatment of erythropoietic protoporphyria with beta-carotene. *Photodermatol* **1**, 318–321, 1984.

65. Wennersten G, Carotenoid treatment for light sensitivity: A reappraisal and six years experience. *Acta Dermatovener* **60**, 251–255, 1980.

66. Swanback G and Wennersten G, Treatment of polymorphous light eruptions with beta-carotene. *Acta Dermatovener* **52**, 462–466, 1972.

67. Newbold PC, Beta-carotene in the treatment of *discoid lupus erythematosus*. *Br J Dermatol* **100**, 187, 188, 1976.
68. Fusaro RM and Johnson JA, Hereditary polymorphic light eruption in American Indians—Photoprotection and prevention of streptococcal pyoderma and glomerulonephritis. *JAMA* **244**, 156–159, 1980.
69. Mathews-Roth MM, *et al.*, A clinical trial of the effects of oral beta-carotene on the responses of human skin to solar radiation. *J Invest Dermatol* **59**, 349–353, 1972.
70. Rothman KJ, *et al.*, Teratogenecity of high vitamin A intake. *N Engl J Med* **333**, 1369–1373, 1995.
71. Hatoff DE, Gertler SL, Miyai K, *et al.*, Hypervitaminosis A unmasked by acute viral hepatitis. *Gastroenterol* **82**, 124–128, 1982.
72. Harris WA and Erdman JW, Protracted hypervitaminosis A following long-term, low level intake. *JAMA* **247**, 1317, 1318, 1982.
73. Shoenfeld Y, *et al.*, Neutropenia induced by hypercarotenemia. *Lancet* **1**, 1245, 1982.
74. Kemmann E, Pasquale SA, Skaf R, Amenorrhea associated with carotenemia. *JAMA* **249**, 926–929, 1983.
75. Mathews-Roth MM, Neutropenia and beta-carotene. *Lancet* **ii**, 222, 1982.
76. Stampfer MJ, Willett W, and Hennekens CH, Carotene, carrots, and neutropenia. *Lancet* **ii**, 615, 1982.
77. Mathews-Roth MM, Abraham AA, and Gabuzda TG, Beta-carotene content of certain organs from two patients receiving high doses of beta-carotene. *Clin Chem* **22**, 922–924, 1976.
78. Mathews-Roth MM, Amenorrhea associated with carotenemia. *JAMA* **250**, 731, 1983.
79. Poh-Fitzpatrick MB and Barbera LG, Absence of crystalline retinopathy after long-term therapy with B-carotene. *J Am Acad Dermatol* **11**, 111–113, 1984.
80. Heywood R, Palmer AK, Gregson RL, *et al.*, The toxicity of beta-carotene. *Toxicology* **36**, 91–100, 1985.

4 Vitamin D

1. Gloth FM and Tobin HD, Vitamin D deficiency in older people. *J Am Geriatr Soc* **43**, 822–828, 1995.
2. Lore F, Nuti R, Vattimo A, and Caniggia, Vitamin D metabolites in postmenopausal osteoporosis. *Horm Metabol Res* **16**, 58, 1984.
3. DeLuca HF, The vitamin D story: A collaborative effort of basic science and clinical medicine. *FASEB J* **2**, 224–236, 1988.
4. Pols HAP, *et al.*, Vitamin D: A modulator of cell proliferation and differentiation. *J Steroid Biochem Mol Biol* **37**, 873–876, 1990.
5. Reichel H, Koeffler HP, and Norman AW, The role of vitamin-D endocrine system in health and disease. *New Engl J Med* **320**, 980, 981, 1989.
6. Garland CF and Garland FC, Do sunlight and vitamin D reduce the likelihood of colon cancer? *Int J Epidemiol* **9**, 227–231, 1980.
7. Seelig MS, Magnesium deficiency with phosphate and vitamin D excess: Role in pediatric cardiovascular nutrition. *Cardio Med* **3**, 637–650, 1978.

5 Vitamin E

1. Horwitt MK, Vitamin E: A re-examination. *Am J Clin Nutr* **29**, 569–578, 1976.
2. Ingold KU, *et al.*, Biokinetics of and discrimination between dietary RRR- and SRRR-alpha-tocopherols in the male rat. *Lipids* **22**, 163–172, 1987.
3. Burton GW and Traber MG, Vitamin E: Antioxidant activity, biokinetics, and bioavailability. *Annu Rev Nutr* **10**, 357–382, 1992.
4. Komiyama K, *et al.*, Studies on the biological activity of tocotrienols. *Chem Pharm Bull* **37**, 1369–1381, 1989.

5. Ohrvall M, Sundlof G, and Vessby B, Gamma, but not alpha, tocopherol levels in serum are reduced in coronary heart disease patients. *J Int Med* **239**, 111–117, 1996.
6. Nasr SZ, *et al.*, Correction of vitamin E deficiency with fat-soluble versus water-miscible preparations of vitamin E in patients with cystic fibrosis. *J Pediatr* **122**, 810–812, 1993.
7. Gey KF, *et al.*, Inverse correlation between plasma vitamin E and mortality from ischemic heart disease in cross-cultural epidemiology. *Am J Clin Nutr* **53**, 326S–334S, 1991.
8. Stampfer MJ, *et al.*, Vitamin E consumption and the risk of coronary heart disease in women. *New Engl J Med* **328**, 1444–1449, 1993.
9. Rimm EB, *et al.*, Vitamin E consumption and the risk of coronary heart disease in men. *New Engl J Med* **328**, 1450–1456, 1993.
10. Bellizzi MC, *et al.*, Vitamin E and coronary heart disease: The European paradox. *Eur J Clin Nutr* **48**, 822–831, 1994.
11. Princen HMG, *et al.*, Supplementation with low doses of vitamin E protects LDL from lipid peroxidation in men and women. *Arterioscler Thromb Vasc Biol* **15**, 325–333, 1995.
12. Abbey M, Nestel PJ, and Baghurst P, Antioxidant vitamins and low density lipoprotein oxidation. *Am J Clin Nutr* **58**, 525–332, 1993.
13. Princen HMG, *et al.*, Supplementation with vitamin E, but not beta-carotene, *in vivo* effects low density lipoprotein from lipid peroxidation *in vitro*. Effect of cigarette smoking. *Arterioscler Thromb* **12**, 554–562, 1992.
14. Stampfer MJ, *et al.*, Vitamin E consumption and the risk of coronary disease in women. *New Engl J Med* **328**, 1444–1448, 1993.
15. Rimm EB, Vitamin E consumption and the risk of coronary heart disease in men. *New Engl J Med* **328**, 1450–1455, 1993.
16. Hodis HN, *et al.*, Serial coronary angiographic evidence that antioxidant vitamin intake reduces progression of coronary artery atherosclerosis. *JAMA* **273**, 1849–1854, 1995.
17. Gaby SK and Machlin LJ, Vitamin E. In: *Vitamin Intake and Health: A Scientific Review*, Gaby SK, *et al.* (eds.). Marcel Dekker, New York, 1991, pp. 72–89.
18. Knecht P, *et al.*, Vitamin E in cancer prevention. *Am J Clin Nutr* **53** (Suppl. 1), 283S–286S, 1991.
19. Paolisso G, *et al.*, Chronic intake of pharmacological doses of vitamin E might be useful in the therapy of elderly patients with coronary heart disease. *Am J Clin Nutr* **61**, 848–852, 1995.
20. Paolisso G, *et al.*, Pharmacologic doses of vitamin E improve insulin action in healthy subjects and non-insulin-dependent diabetic patients. *Am J Clin Nutr* **57**, 650–656, 1993.
21. London RS, *et al.*, Endocrine parameters and alpha-tocopherol therapy of patients with mammary dysplasia. *Cancer Res* **41**, 3811–3813, 1981.
22. London RS, *et al.*, The effect of alpha-tocopherol on premenstrual symptomatology: A double-blind study, II, Endocrine correlates. *J Am Col Nutr* **3**, 351–356, 1984.
23. Christy CJ, Vitamin E in menopause. *Am J Ob Gyn* **50**, 84–87, 1945.
24. McLaren HC, Vitamin E in the menopause. *Br Med J* ii, 1378–1381, 1949.
25. Finkler RS, The effect of vitamin E in the menopause. *J Clin Endocrinol Metab* **9**, 89–94, 1949.
26. Schroeder DJ, Hart LL, and Miyagi SL, Vitamin E in tardive dyskinesia. *Annals Pharmacol* **27**, 311, 312, 1993.
27. Egan MF, *et al.*, Treatment of tardive dyskinesia with vitamin E. *Am J Psychiatry* **149**, 773–777, 1992.
28. Adler LA, *et al.*, Vitamin E treatment of tardive dyskinesia. *Am J Psychiatry* 150, 1405–1407, 1993.
29. Meydani SN, *et al.*, Assessment of the safety of high-dose, short-term supplementation with vitamin E in healthy older adults. *Am J Clin Nutr* **60**, 704–709, 1994.

6 Vitamin K

1. Suttie JW, Vitamin K and human nutrition. *J Am Diet Assoc* **92**, 585–590, 1992.
2. Rafsky HA and Krieger CI, The treatment of intestinal diseases with solutions of water-soluble chlorophyll. *Rev Gastroenterol* **15**, 549–553, 1945.

3. Smith L and Livingston A, Chlorophyll: An experimental study of its water soluble derivatives in wound healing. *Am J Surg* **62**, 358–369, 1943.

4. Nahata MC, Sleccsak CA, and Kamp J, Effect of chlorophyllin on urinary odor in incontinent geriatric patients. *Drug Intel Clin Pharm* **17**, 732–734, 1983.

5. Young RW and Beregi JS, Use of chlorophyllin in the care of geriatric patients. *J Am Ger Soc* **28**, 46, 47, 1980.

6. Patek A, Chlorophyll and regeneration of the blood. *Arch Int Med* **57** 73–76, 1936.

7. Gubner R and Ungerleider HE, Vitamin K therapy in menorrhagia. *South Med J* **37**, 556–558, 1944.

8. Ong T, Whong WZ, Stewart J, and Brockman HE, Chlorophyllin: A potent antimutagen against environmental and dietary complex mixtures. *Mutation Research* **173**, 111–115, 1986.

9. Bitensky L, Hart JP, Catterall A, *et al.*, Circulating vitamin K levels in patients with fractures. *J Bone Joint Surg* **70-B**, 663, 664, 1988.

10. Price PA, Role of vitamin-K-dependent proteins in bone metabolism. *Ann Rev Nutr* **8**, 565–583, 1988.

11. Gubner R and Ungerleider HE, Vitamin K therapy in menorrhagia. *South Med J* **37**, 556–558, 1944.

12. von Kries RV and Gobel U, Vitamin K prophylaxis: Oral or parenteral? *Am J Dis Child* **142**, 13–25, 1988.

7 Vitamin C

1. Cheraskin E, *Vitamin C—Who Needs It?* Arlington Press, Birminham, AL, 1993.

2. Levine M, New concepts in the biology and biochemistry of ascorbic acid. *New Engl J Med* **314**, 892–902, 1986.

3. Bendich A, Vitamin C and immune responses. *Food Technol* **41**, 112–114, 1987.

4. Ginter E, Optimum intake of vitamin C for the human organism. *Nutr Health* **1**, 66–77, 1982.

5. Frei B, England L, and Ames BN, Ascorbate is an outstanding antioxidant in human blood plasma. *Proc Natl Acad Sci* **86**, 6377–6381, 1989.

6. Jain A, *et al.*, Effect of ascorbate or N-acetylcysteine treatment in a patient with hereditary glutathione synthetase deficiency. *J Pediatr* **124**, 229–233, 1994.

7. Kleinveld HA, Demacker PNM, and Stalenhoef AFH, Failure of N-acetylcystein to reduce low-density lipoprotein oxidizability in healthy subjects. *Eur J Clin Pharmacol* **43**, 639–642, 1992.

8. Witschi A, *et al.*, The systemic availability of oral glutathione. *Eur J Clin Pharmacol* **43**, 667–669, 1992.

9. Johnston CJ, Meyer CG, and Srilakshmi JC, Vitamin C elevates red blood cell glutathione in healthy adults. *Am J Clin Nutr* **58**, 103–105, 1993.

10. Whitehead, *et al.*, Effect of red wine ingestion on the antioxidant capacity of serum. *Clin Chem* **41**, 32–35, 1995.

11. Johnston CS and Luo B, Comparison of the absorption and excretion of three commercially available sources of vitamin C. *J Am Diet Assoc* **94**, 779–781, 1994.

12. Vinson JA and Bose P, Comparative bioavailability to humans of ascorbic acid alone or in a citrus extract. *Am J Clin Nutr* **48**, 601–604, 1988.

13. Hatch GE, Asthma, inhaled oxidants, and dietary antioxidants. *Am J Clin Nutr* **61** (Suppl.), 625S–630S, 1995.

14. Bielory L and Gandhi R, Asthma and vitamin C. *Annals Allergy* **73**, 89–96, 1994.

15. Johnston CS, Martin LJ, and Cai X, Antihistamine effect of supplemental ascorbic acid and neutrophil chemotaxis. *J Am Coll Nutr* **11**, 172–176, 1992.

16. National Research Council, Diet and Health. *Implications for Reducing Chronic Disease Risk.* National Academy Press, Washington, DC, 1989, pp. 331–334.

17. Simon JA, Vitamin C and cardiovascular disease: A review. *J Am Coll Nutr* **11**, 107–125, 1992.

18. Engstrom JE, Kanim LE, and Klein MA, Vitamin C intake and mortality among a sample of the United States population. *Epidemiol* **3**, 194–202, 1992.

19. Harats D, *et al.*, Effect of vitamin C and E supplementation on susceptibility of plasma lipoproteins to peroxidation induced by acute smoking. *Atherosclerosis* **85**, 47–54, 1990.

20. Howard PA and Meyers DG, Effect of vitamin C on plasma lipids. *Pharmacother* **29**, 1129–1136, 1995.

21. Jacques PF, *et al.*, Ascorbic acid and plasma lipids. *Epidemiol* **5**, 19–26, 1994.

22. Hallfrisch J, *et al.*, High plasma vitamin C associated with high plasma HDL and HDL2 cholesterol. *Am J Clin Nutr* **60**, 100–105, 1994.

23. Jacques PF, *et al.*, Effect of vitamin C supplementation on lipoprotein cholesterol, apolipoprotein, and triglyceride concentrations. *Ann Epidemiol* **5**, 52–59, 1995.

24. Pierkle JL, Schwartz J, Landis JR, and Harlan WR, The relationship between blood lead levels and blood pressure and its cardiovascular risk implications. *Am J Epid* **121**, 246–258, 1985.

25. Ballmer PE, *et al.*, Depletion of plasma vitamin C but not vitamin E in response to cardiac operations. *J Thorac Cardiovasc Surg* **108**, 308–311, 1994.

26. Block G, Vitamin C and cancer prevention: The epidemiologic evidence. *Am J Clin Nutr* **53**, 270S–282S, 1991.

27. Block G, Vitamin C, cancer and aging. *Age Ageing* **16**, 55–58, 1993.

28. Howe GR, *et al.*, Dietary factors and risk of breast cancer: Combined analysis of 12-case control studies. *J Natl Cancer Inst* **82**, 561–569, 1990.

29. Wassertheil-Smoller S, *et al.*, Dietary vitamin C and uterine cervical dysplasia. *Am J Epid* **114**, 714–724, 1981.

30. Romney S, *et al.*, Plasma vitamin C and uterine cervical dysplasia. *Am J Ob Gyn* **151**, 978–980, 1985.

31. Schiffman MH, Diet and faecal genotoxicity. *Cancer Surv* **6**, 653–672, 1987.

32. Cameron E and Pauling L, Supplemental ascorbate in the supportive treatment of cancer: Prolongation of survival times in terminal human cancer. *Proc Natl Acad Sci* **73**, 3685, 1976.

33. Cameron E and Campbell A, Innovation vs. quality control. An "unpublishable" clinical trial of supplemental ascorbate in incurable cancer. *Med Hypothesis* **36**, 185–189, 1991.

34. Moertel CG, *et al.*, High-dose vitamin C versus placebo in the treatment of patients with advanced cancer who have had no prior chemotherapy. *New Engl J Med* **312**, 137–141, 1985.

35. Taylor A, Cataract: Relationships between nutrition and oxidation. *J Am Coll Nutr* **12**, 138–146, 1993.

36. Bouton S, Vitamin C and the aging eye. *Arch Int Med* **63**, 930–945, 1939.

37. Ringvold A, Johnsen H, and Blika S, Senile cataract and ascorbic acid loading. *Acta Opthalmol* **63**, 277–280, 1985.

38. Pauling L, *Vitamin C and the Common Cold*. Freeman. San Francisco, CA, 1970.

39. Hemila H, Vitamin C and the common cold. *Br J Nutr* **67**, 3–16, 1992.

40. Hemila H and Herman, Vitamin C and the common cold: A retrospective analysis of Chalmers' review. *J Am Coll Nutr* **14**, 116–123, 1995.

41. Hunt C, *et al.*, The clinical effects of vitamin C supplementation in elderly hospitalized patients with acute respiratory infections. *Internat J Vit Nutr Res* **64**, 212–219, 1994.

42. Cathcart RF, The third face of vitamin C. *J Orthomol Med* **7**, 197–200, 1992.

43. Cathcart RF, The method of determining proper doses of vitamin C for the treatment of disease by titrating to bowel tolerance. *J Orthomol Psychiat* **10**, 125–132, 1981.

44. Klenner FR, Observations on the dose of administration of ascorbic acid when employed beyond the range of a vitamin in human pathology. *J Applied Nutr* **23**, 61–88, 1971.

45. Baetgen D, Results of the treatment of epidemic hepatitis in children with high doses of ascorbic acid for the years 1957–1958. *Medizinische Monatchrift* **15**, 30–36, 1961.

46. Baur H and Staub H, Treatment of hepatitis with infusions of ascorbic acid: Comparison with other therapies. *JAMA* **156**, 565, 1954.

47. Sinclair AJ, *et al.*, Low plasma ascorbate levels in patients with type 2 diabetes mellitus consuming adequate dietary vitamin C. *Diabet Med* **11**, 893–898, 1994.

48. Eriksson J and Kohvakka A, Magnesium and ascorbic acid supplementation in diabetes mellitus. *Ann Nutr Metab* **39**, 217–223, 1995.

49. Seghieri G, *et al.*, Renal excretion of ascorbic acid in insulin dependent diabetes mellitus. *Int J Vitam Nutr Res* **64**, 119–124, 1994.
50. Sinclair AJ, *et al.*, Modulators of free radical activity in diabetes mellitus: Role of ascorbic acid. *EXS* **62**, 342–352, 1992.
51. Cunningham JJ, *et al.*, Vitamin C: An aldose reductase inhibitor that normalizes erythrocyte sorbitol in insulin-dependent diabetes mellitus. *J Am Coll Nutr* 13, 344–350, 1994.
52. Wang H, *et al.*, Experimental and clinical studies on the reduction of erythrocyte sorbitol-glucose ratios by ascorbic acid in diabetes mellitus. *Diabetes Res Clin Pract* **28**, 1–8, 1995.
53. Paolisso G, *et al.*, Metabolic benefits deriving from chronic vitamin C supplementation in aged non-insulin dependent diabetics. *J Am Coll Nutr* **14**, 387–392, 1995.
54. Davie SJ, Gould BJ, and Yudkin JS, Effect of vitamin C on glycosylation of proteins. *Diabetes* **41**, 167–173, 1992.
55. Fraga C, *et al.*, Ascorbic acid protects against endogenous oxidative DNA damage in human sperm. *Proc Natl Acad Sci* 88, 11003–11006, 1991.
56. National Research Council, *Recommended Dietary Allowances, 10th Edition.* National Academy Press, Washington, DC, 1989.
57. Dawson E, Harris W, and Powell L, Effect of vitamin C supplementation on sperm quality of heavy smokers. *FASEB J* **5**, A915, 1991.
58. Dawson EB, *et al.*, Effect of ascorbic acid on male fertility. *Ann NY Acad Sci* **498**, 312–323, 1987.
59. Fahn S, A pilot trial of high-dose alpha-tocopherol and ascorbate in early Parkinson's disease. *Annals of Neurology* 32, S128–S132, 1992.
60. Goode HF, Burns E, and Walker BE, Vitamin C depletion and pressure sores in elderly patients with femoral neck fracture. *BMJ* **305**, 925–927, 1992.
61. Taylor TV, *et al.*, Ascorbic acid supplementation in the treatment of pressure sores. *Lancet* **ii**, 544–546, 1974.
62. Mikhail MS, *et al.*, Preeclampsia and antioxidant nutrients: Decreased plasma levels of reduced ascorbic acid, alpha-tocopheral, and beta-carotene in women with preeclampsia. *Am J Obstet Gynecol* **171**, 150–157, 1994.
63. Barrett BM, *et al.*, Potential role of ascorbic acid and beta-carotene in the prevention of preterm rupture of fetal membranes. *Int J Vit Ntr Res* **64**, 192–197, 1994.
64. Rivers JM, Safety of high level vitamin C ingestion. *Int J Vit Ntr Res* **30** (Suppl.), 95–102, 1989.
65. Wanzilak TR, *et al.*, Effect of high dose vitamin C on urinary oxalate levels. *J Urol* **151**, 834–837, 1994.
66. Shklar G, *et al.*, The effectiveness of a mixture of beta-carotene, alpha-tocopherol, glutathione, and ascorbic acid for cancer prevention. *Nutr Cancer* **20**, 145–151, 1993.

8 Thiamin (Vitamin B$_1$)

1. Butterworth RF, Effects of thiamine deficiency on brain metabolism: Implications for the pathogenesis of Wernicke-Korsakoff syndrome. *Alcohol Alcoholism* **24**, 271–279, 1989.
2. Carner MWP, Vitamin deficiency and mental symptoms. *Br J Psychiatr* **156**, 878–882, 1990.
3. Meador KJ, *et al.*, Evidence for a central cholinergic effect of high dose thiamine. *Ann Neurol* **34**, 724–726, 1993.
4. Meador K, Preliminary findings of high-dose thiamine in dementia of Alzheimer's type. *J Geriatr Psychiatry Neurol* **6**, 222–229, 1993.
5. Benton D, Fordy J, and Haller J, The impact of long-term vitamin supplementation on cognitive functioning. *Psychopharmacol* **117**, 298–305, 1995.
6. Botez MI, *et al.*, Thiamine and folate treatment of chronic epileptic patients: A controlled study with the Wechsler IQ scale. *Epilepsy Res* **16**, 157–163, 1993.

9 Riboflavin (Vitamin B$_2$)

1. Munoz N, *et al.*, Effect of riboflavin, retinol, and zinc on the micronuclei of buccal mucosa and of esophagus: A randomized double-blind intervention study in China. *J Nat Cancer Inst* **79**, 687–691, 1987.

2. Schoenen J, Lenaerts M, and Bastings E, High-dose riboflavin as a prophylactic treatment of migraine: Results of an open pilot study. *Cephalalgia* **14**, 328, 329, 1994.
3. Skalka H and Prchal J, Cataracts and riboflavin deficiency. *Am J Clin Nutr* **34**, 861–863, 1981.
4. Prchal J, Conrad M, and Skalka H, Association of pre-senile cataracts with heterozygousity for galactosemic states and riboflavin deficiency. *Lancet* **1**, 12, 13, 1978.
5. Ajayi OA, George BO, and Ipadeola T, Clinical trial of riboflavin in sickle cell disease. *East Afr Med J* **70**, 418–421, 1993.

10   Niacin (Vitamin B₃)

1. DiPalma JR and Thayer WS, Use of niacin as a drug. *Annu Rev Nutr* **11**, 169–187, 1991.
2. The Coronary Drug Project Group, Clofibrate and niacin in coronary heart disease. *JAMA* **231**, 360–381, 1975.
3. Canner PL, *et al.*, Fifteen year mortality in Coronary Drug Project patients: Long-term benefit with niacin. *J Am Coll Cardiol* **8**, 1245–1255, 1986.
4. Committee of Principal Investigators, World Health Organization Clofibrate Trial: A cooperative trial in the primary prevention of ischemic heart disease using clofibrate. *Br Heart J* **40**, 1069–1118, 1978.
5. Lovastatin Study Groups I through IV, Lovastatin 5-year safety and efficacy study. *Arch Intern Med* **153**, 1079–1087, 1993.
6. Illingworth DR, *et al.*, Comparative effects of lovastatin and niacin in primary hypercholesterolemia. *Arch Intern Med* **154**, 1586–1595, 1994.
7. Scanu AM and Fless GM, Lipoprotein(a): A genetic risk factor for premature coronary heart disease. *JAMA* **267**, 3326–3329, 1992.
8. Schaefer EJ, *et al.*, Lipoprotein(a) levels and risk of coronary heart disease in men. The Lipid Research Clinics Coronary Primary Prevention Trial. *JAMA* **271**, 999–1003, 1994.
9. Carlson LA, Hamsten A, and Asplund A, Pronounced lowering of serum levels of lipoprotein Lp(a) in hyperlipidaemic subjects treated with nicotinic acid. *J Intern Med* **226**, 271–276, 1989.
10. Lal SM, *et al.*, Effects of nicotinic acid and lovastatin in renal transplant patients: A prospective, randomized, open-labeled crossover trial. *Am J Kidney Dis* **25**, 616–622, 1995.
11. Vega GL and Grundy SM, Lipoprotein responses to treatment with lovastatin, gemfibrozil, and nicotinic acid in normolipidemic patients with hypoalphalipoproteinemia. *Arch Intern Med* **154**, 73–82, 1994.
12. Welsh AL and Ede M, Inositol hexanicotinate for improved nicotinic acid therapy. *Int Record Med* **174**, 9–15, 1961.
13. El-Enein AMA, *et al.*, The role of nicotinic acid and inositol hexaniacinate as anticholesterolemic and antilipemic agents. *Nutr Rep Intl* **28**, 899–911, 1983.
14. Sunderland GT, Belch JJF, Sturrock RD, *et al.*, A double blind randomized placebo controlled trial of hexopal in primary Raynaud's disease. *Clin Rheumatol* **7**, 46–49, 1988.
15. O'Hara J, Jolly PN, and Nicol CG, The therapeutic effect of inositol nicotinate (Hexopal) in intermittent claudication: A controlled trial. *Br J Clin Practice* **42**, 377–383, 1988.
16. Gerstein HC, Cow's milk exposure and type I diabetes mellitus. A critical review of the clinical literature. *Diabetes Care* **17**, 13–19, 1994.
17. Leslie DG and Elliott RB, Early environmental events as a cause of IDDM. *Diabetes* **43**, 843–850, 1994.
18. Goday A, *et al.*, Effects of a short prednisone regime at clinical onset of type 1 diabetes. *Diabetes Res Clin Pract* **20**, 39–46, 1993.
19. Secchi A, *et al.*, Prednisone administration in recent onset type I diabetes. *J Autoimmun* **3**, 593–600, 1990.
20. Mistura L, *et al.*, Prednisone treatment in newly diagnosed type I diabetic children: 1-yr follow-up. *Diabetes Care* **10**, 39–43, 1987.
21. Silverstein J, *et al.*, Immunosuppression with azathioprine and prednisone in recent-onset insulin-dependent diabetes mellitus. *N Engl J Med* **319**, 599–604, 1988.

22. Lazarow A, Liambies L, and Tausch AJ, Protection against diabetes with nicotinamide. *J Lab Clin Med* **36**, 249–258, 1950.
23. Pozzilli P and Andreani D, The potential role of nicotinamide in the secondary prevention of IDDM. *Diabetes Metabol Rev* **9**, 219–230, 1993.
24. Andersen HU, *et al.*, Nicotinamide prevents interleukin-1 effects on accumulated insulin release and nitric oxide production in rat islets of langerhans. *Diabetes* **43**, 770–777, 1994.
25. Bingley PJ, *et al.*, Nicotinamide and insulin secretion in normal subjects. *Diabetologia* **36**, 675–677, 1993.
26. Vague PH, *et al.*, Nicotinamide may extend remission phase in insulin dependent diabetes. *Lancet* **I**, 619, 1987.
27. Pozzili P, *et al.*, Nicotinamide increases C-peptide secretion in patients with recent onset type 1 diabetes. *Diabetic Med* **6**, 568, 1989.
28. Mendola G, Casamitjana R, and Gomis R, Effect of nicotinamide therapy upon beta-cell function in newly diagnosed type 1 (insulin-dependent) diabetic patients. *Diabetologia* **32**, A160, 1989.
29. Chase HP, *et al.*, A trial of nicotinamide in newly diagnosed patients with type 1 (insulin dependent) diabetes mellitus. *Diabetologia* **33**, 444–446, 1990.
30. Pozzili P, *et al.*, The IMDIAB I multicenter study in newly diagnosed insulin dependent diabetic patients: Final results. *Diabetologia* **34** (Suppl. 2):A29, 1991.
31. Lewis CM, *et al.*, Double-blind randomized trial of nicotinamide on early onset diabetes. *Diabetes Care* **15**, 121–123, 1992.
32. Herskowitz RD, *et al.*, Pilot trial to prevent type 1 diabetes: Progression to overt IDDM despite oral nicotinamide. *J Autoimmun* **2**, 733–737, 1989.
33. Elliot RB and Chase HP, Prevention or delay of type 1 (insulin-dependent) diabetes mellitus in children using nicotinamide. *Diabetologia* **34**, 362–365, 1991.
34. Manna R, *et al.*, Nicotinamide treatment in subjects at high risk of developing IDDM improves insulin secretion. *Br J Clin Practice* **46**, 177–179, 1992.
35. Elliot RB and Pilcher CC, Prevention of diabetes in normal school children. *Diabetes Res Clin Pract* **14**, S85, 1991.
36. Mandrup Paulsen T, *et al.*, Nicotinamide in the prevention of insulin dependent diabetes mellitus. *Diabetes Metabol Rev* **9**, 295–309, 1993.
37. Rubin RJ, *et al.*, Health care expenditures for people with diabetes mellitus, 1992. *J Clin Endocrinol Metab* **78**, 809A–809F, 1994.
38. Vialettes B, *et al.*, A preliminary multicentre study of the treatment of recently diagnosed type 1 diabetes by combination nicotinamide-cyclosporin therapy. *Diabet Med* **7**, 731–735, 1990.
39. Pozzili P, *et al.*, Combination of nicotinamide and steroid versus nicotinamide in recent-onset IDDM. *Diabetes Care* **17**, 897–900, 1994.
40. Kaufman, W, *The Common Form of Joint Dysfunction: Its Incidence and Treatment*. E. L. Hildreth Company, Brattleboro, VT, 1949.
41. Hoffer, A, Treatment of arthritis by nicotinic acid and nicotinamide. *Canadian Medical Association Journal* **81**; 235–239, 1959.
42. McKenney JM, *et al.*, A comparison of the efficacy and toxic effects of sustained- vs. immediate-release niacin in hypercholesterolemic patients. *JAMA* **271**, 672–677, 1994.

11   Pyridoxine (Vitamin B$_6$)

1. Driskell JA, Vitamin B$_6$ requirements of humans. *Nutr Res* **14**, 293–324, 1994.
2. Middleton HM, Intestinal absorption of pyridoxal-5-phosphate, Disappearance from perfused segments of rat jejunum *in vivo. J Nutr* **109**, 975–981, 1979.
3. Labadarios D, *et al.*, Vitamin B$_6$ deficiency in chronic liver disease—evidence for increased degradation of pyridoxal-5-phosphate. *Gut* 18, 23–27, 1977.
4. Collip PJ, Goldzier III S, Weiss N, *et al.*, Pyridoxine treatment of childhood asthma. *Ann Allergy* **35**, 93–97, 1975.

5. Reynolds RD and Natta CL, Depressed plasma pyridoxal-5-phosphate concentrations in adult asthmatics. *Am J Clin Nutr* **41**, 684–688, 1985.

6. Shimizu T, *et al.*, Theophylline attenuates circulating vitamin B$_6$ levels in children with asthma. *Pharmacol* **49**, 392–397, 1994.

7. Bartel PR, *et al.*, Vitamin B$_6$ supplementation and theophylline-related effects in humans. *Am J Clin Nutr* **60**, 93–99, 1994.

8. Rimland B, Callaway E, and Dreyfuss P, The effects of high doses of vitamin B$_6$ on autistic children: A double-blind crossover study. *Am J Psychiatry* **135**, 472–475, 1979.

9. Lipton M, Mailman R, and Numeroff C, Vitamins, megavitamin therapy, and the nervous system. In: *Nutrition and the Brain, Vol 3*, Wurtman R and Wurtman J (eds.). Raven Press, New York, NY, 1979, pp. 183–264.

10. Lelord G, Callaway E, and Muh J, Clinical and biological effects of high doses of vitamin B$_6$ and magnesium on autistic children. *Acta Vitaminol Enzymol* **4**, 27–44, 1982.

11. Barthelemy C, *et al.*, Behavioral and biochemical effects of oral magnesium, vitamin B$_6$ and magnesium. Vitamin B$_6$ administration in autistic children. *Magnesium Bulletin* **3**, 23, 24, 1981.

12. Martineau J, *et al.*, Vitamin B$_6$, magnesium, and combined B$_6$-magnesium: Therapeutic effects in childhood autism. *Biol Psychiatry* **20**, 467, 468, 1985.

13. Kok FJ, *et al.*, Low vitamin B$_6$ status in patients with acute myocardial infarction. *Am J Cardiol* **63**, 513–6, 1989; Robinson K, *et al.*, Hyperhomocysteinemia and low pyridoxal phosphate. *Circulation* **92**, 2825–2830, 1995.

14. Levene CI and Murray JC, The aetiological role of maternal B$_6$ deficiency in the development of atherosclerosis. *Lancet* **i**, 628, 629, 1977.

15. Lam SCT, Harfenist EJ, Packham MA, *et al.*, Investigation of possible mechanisms of pyridoxal 5′-phosphate inhibition of platelet reactions. *Thrombosis Res* **20**, 633–645, 1980.

16. Sermet A, *et al.*, Effect of oral pyridoxine hydrochloride supplementation on *in vitro* platelet sensitivity to different agonists. *Arzneim Forsch* **45**, 19–21, 1995.

17. Ayback M, *et al.*; Effect of oral pyridoxine hydrochloride supplementation on arterial blood pressure in patients with essential hypertension. *Arzneim Forsch* **45**, 1271–1273, 1995.

18. Ellis JM, *et al.*, Response of vitamin B$_6$ deficiency and the carpal tunnel syndrome to pyridoxine. *Proc Natl Acad Sci USA* **79**, 7494–7498, 1982.

19. Folkers K, Ellis J, Successful therapy with vitamin B$_6$ and Vitamin B$_2$ of the carpal tunnel syndrome and need for determination of the RDA's for vitamin B$_6$ and B$_2$ disease states. *Annals NY Acad Sci* **585**, 295–301, 1990.

20. Ellis JM, Folkers K, Clinical aspects of treatment of carpal tunnel syndrome with B$_6$. *Annals NY Acad Sci* **585**, 302–320, 1990.

21. Phalen, GS, The birth of a syndrome, or carpal tunnel syndrome revisited. *J Hand Surg* **6**, 109, 110, 1981.

22. Folkers K, *et al.*, Biochemical evidence for a deficiency of vitamin B$_6$ in subjects reacting to monosodium glutamate by the Chinese restaurant syndrome. *Biochem Biophys Res Common* **100**, 972–977, 1981.

23. Russ C, Hendricks T, Chrisley B, Kalin N, and Driskell J, Vitamin B$_6$ status of depressed and obsessive-compulsive patients. *Nutr Rep Intl* **27**, 867–873, 1983.

24. Carney M, Williams D, and Sheffield B, Thiamin and pyridoxine lack in newly admitted psychiatric patients. *Br J Psychiatr* **135**, 249–254, 1979.

25. Nobbs B, Pyridoxal phosphate status in clinical depression. *Lancet* **i**, 405, 1974.

26. Wynn V, *et al.*, Tryptophan, depression and steroidal contraception. *J Steroid Biochem* **6**, 965–970, 1975.

27. Bermond P, Therapy of side effects of oral contraceptive agents with vitamin B$_6$. Acta Vitaminol-Enzymol **4**, 45–54, 1982.

28. Jones CL and Gonzalez V, Pyridoxine deficiency: A new factor in diabetic neuropathy. *J Am Pod Assoc* **68**, 646–653, 1978.

29. Solomon LR and Cohen K, Erythrocyte $_2$ transport and metabolism and effects of vitamin B$_6$ therapy in type II diabetes mellitus. *Diabetes* **38**, 881–886, 1989.

30. Coelingh-Bennick HJT and Schreurs WHP, Improvement of oral glucose tolerance in gestational diabetes. *Br Med J* **3**, 13–15, 1975.

31. Crowell GF and Roach ES, Pyridoxine-dependent seizures. *Amer Fam Physic* **27**, 183–187, 1983.

32. Goutieres F and Aicardi J, Atypical presentations of pyridoxine-dependent seizures: A treatable cause of intractable epilepsy in infants. *Ann Neurol* **17**, 117–120, 1985.

33. Bankier A, Turner M, and Hopkins IJ, Pyridoxine dependent seizures: A wider clinical spectrum. *Arch Dis Child* **58**, 415–418, 1983.

34. Nakazawa M, Tadataka M, Takeda H, *et al.*, High-dose vitamin B_6 therapy for infantile spasms—The effect and adverse reactions. *Brain Development* **5**, 193–197, 1983.

35. Hansson O and Sillanpaa M, Pyridoxine and serum concentrations of phenytoin and phenobarbitone. *Lancet* **i**, 256, 1976.

36. Beisel W, Edelman R, Nauss K, and Suskind R, Single-nutrient effects of immunologic functions. *JAMA* **245**, 53–58, 1981.

37. Bum MK, *et al.*, Association of vitamin B_6 status with parameters of immune function in early HIV-1 infection. *J AIDS* **4**, 122–132, 1991.

38. Prien E and Gershoff S, Magnesium oxide-pyridoxine therapy for recurrent calcium oxalate calculi. *J Urol* **112**, 509–512, 1974.

39. Gershoff S and Prien E, Effect of daily MgO and Vitamin B_6 administration to patients with recurring calcium oxalate stones. *Am J Clin Nutr* **20**, 393–399, 1967.

40. Will E and Bijvoet L, Primary oxalosis: Clinical and biochemical response to high-dose pyridoxine therapy. *Metab* **28**, 542–548, 1979.

41. Lyon E, *et al.*, Calcium oxalate lithiasis produced by pyridoxine deficiency and inhibition with high magnesium diets. *Invest Urol* **4**, 133–142, 1966.

42. Murthy M, *et al.*, Effect of pyridoxine supplementation on recurrent stone formers. *Int J Clin Pharm Ther Tox* **20**, 434–437, 1982.

43. Azowry L, *et al.*, May enzyme activity in urine play a role in kidney stone formation? *Urol Res* **10**, 185–189, 1982.

44. Sarig S, Azoury R, and Garti N, Biological control to diminish dangers of urolithiasis. *Urol Int* **40**, 274–276, 1985.

45. Vutyananich T, Wongtra-ngan S, and Rung-aroon R, Pyridoxine for nausea and vomiting of pregnancy: A randomized, double-blind, placebo-controlled trial. *Am J Obstet Gynecol* **173**, 881–884, 1995.

46. Fischer-Rasmussen W, *et al.*, Ginger treatment of hyperemesis gravidarum. *Eur J Obstet Gynecol Reprod Biol* **38**, 19–24, 1990.

47. Benke PH, *et al.*, Osteoporotic bone disease in the pyridoxine-deficient rat. *Biochem Med* **6**, 526–535, 1972.

48. Berman MK, *et al.*, Vitamin B_6 in premenstrual syndrome. *J Am Diet Assoc* **90,** 859–861, 1990.

49. Kliejnen J, Ter Riet G, and Knipschild P, Vitamin B_6 in the treatment of premenstrual syndrome—a review. *Br J Obstet Gynaecol* **97**, 847–852, 1990.

50. Barr W, Pyridoxine supplements in the premenstrual syndrome. *Practitioner* **228**, 425–427, 1984.

51. Snider B and Dieteman D, Pyridoxine therapy for premenstrual acne flare. *Arch Dermatol* **110**, 103–111, 1974.

52. Zempleni J, Pharmacokinetics of vitamin B_6 supplements in humans. *J Am Coll Nutr* **14**, 579–586, 1995.

53. Cohen M and Bendich A, Safety of pyridoxine—A review of human and animal studies. *Toxicol Letters* **34**, 129–139, 1986.

54. Parry GJ and Bredesen DE, Sensory neuropathy with low-dose pyridoxine. *Neurology* **35**, 1466–1468, 1985.

55. Waterston JA and Gilligan BS, Pyridoxine neuropathy. *Med J Aust* **146**, 640–642, 1987.

56. Dalton K and Dalton MJT, Characteristics of pyridoxine overdose neuropathy syndrome. *Acta Neurol Scand* **76**, 8, 1987.

12 Biotin

1. Hochman LG, *et al.*, Brittle nails: Response to daily biotin supplementation. *Cutis* **51**, 303–307, 1993.
2. Nisenson A, Seborrheic dermatitis of infants and Leiner's disease: A biotin deficiency. *J Ped* **51**, 537–549, 1957.
3. Nisenson A, Treatment of seborrheic dermatitis with biotin and vitamin B complex. *J Ped* **81**, 630, 631, 1972.
4. Reddi A, DeAngelis B, Frank O, *et al.*, Biotin supplementation improves glucose and insulin tolerances in genetically diabetic KK mice. *Life Sciences* **42**, 1323–1230, 1988.
5. Coggeshall JC, Heggers JP, Robson MC, and Baker H, Biotin status and plasma glucose in diabetics. *Annals NY Acad Sci* **447**, 389–392, 1985.
6. Maebashi M, Makino Y, Furukawa Y, *et al.*, Therapeutic evaluation of the effect of biotin on hyperglycemia in patients with non-insulin dependent diabetes mellitus. *J Clin Biochem Nutr* **14**, 211–218, 1993.
7. Koutsikos D, Agroyannis B, and Tzanatos-Exarchou H, Biotin for diabetic peripheral neuropathy. *Biomed Pharmacother* **44**, 511–514, 1990.
8. Noda H, Akasak N, and Ohsugi M, Biotin production by bifidobacteria. *J Nutr Sci Vitaminol* **40**, 181–188, 1994.

13 Pantothenic Acid (Vitamin B$_5$) and Pantethine

1. Fry PC, *et al.*, Metabolic response to a pantothenic acid deficient diet in humans. *J Nutr Sci Vitaminol* **22**, 339–346, 1976.
2. Barton-Wright EC and Elliott WA, The pantothenic acid metabolism of rheumatoid arthritis. *Lancet* **ii**, 862, 863, 1963.
3. General Practitioner Research Group, Calcium pantothenate in arthritic conditions. *Practitioner* **224**, 208–211, 1980.
4. Arsenio L, Bodria P, Magnati G, *et al.*, Effectiveness of long-term treatment with pantethine in patients with dyslipidemias. *Clin Ther* **8**, 537–545, 1986.
5. Gaddi A, Descovich G, Noseda, *et al.*, Controlled evaluation of pantethine, a natural hypolipidemic compound, in patients with different forms of hyperlipoproteinemia. *Atherosclerosis* **50**, 73–83, 1984.
6. Arsenio L, *et al.*, Effectiveness of long-term treatment with pantethine in patients with dyslipidemia. *Clin Ther* **8(5)**, 537–545, 1986.
7. Donati C, *et al.*, Pantethine improves the lipid abnormalities of chronic hemodialysis patients: Results of a multicenter clinical trial. *Clin Nephrol* **25(2)**, 70–74, 1986.
8. Gaddi A, *et al.*, Controlled evaluation of pantethine, a natural hypolipidemic compound, in patients with different forms of hyperlipoproteinemia. *Atherosclerosis* **50(1)**, 73–83, 1984.
9. Bertolini S, *et al.*, Lipoprotein changes induced by pantethine in hyperlipoproteinemic patients: Adults and children. *Int J Clin Pharmacol Ther Toxicol* **24(11)**, 630–637, 1986.
10. Binaghi P, *et al.*, Evaluation of the cholesterol-lowering effectiveness of pantethine in women in perimenopausal age. *Min Med* **81(6)**, 475–479, 1990.
11. Cattin L, *et al.*, Treatment of hypercholesterolemia with pantethine and fenofibrate: An open randomized study on 43 subjects. *Curr Ther Res* **38**, 386–395, 1985.
12. Cighetti G, *et al.*, Effects of pantethine on cholesterol synthesis from mevalonate in isolated rat hepatocytes. *Atherosclerosis* **60(1)**, 67–77, 1986.
13. Cighetti G, *et al.*, Pantethine inhibits cholesterol and fatty acid syntheses and stimulates carbon dioxide formation in isolated rat hepatocytes. *J Lipid Res* **28(2)**, 152–161, 1987.
14. Coronel F, *et al.*, Treatment of hyperlipemia in diabetic patients on dialysis with a physiological substance. *Am J Nephrol* **11(1)**, 32–36, 1991.
15. Donati C, Bertieri RS, and Barbi G, Pantethine, diabetes mellitus and atherosclerosis. Clinical study of 1045 patients. *Clin Ther* **128(6)**, 411–422, 1989.

16. Arsenio L, *et al.*, Hyperlipidemia, diabetes and atherosclerosis: Efficacy of treatment with pantethine. *Acta Biomed Ateneo Parmense* **55**, 25–42, 1984.
17. Coronel F, *et al.*, Treatment of hyperlipemia in diabetic patients on dialysis with a physiological substance. *Am J Nephrol* **11(1)**, 32–36, 1991.
18. Hiramatsu K, Nozaki H, and Arimori S, Influence of pantethine on platelet volume, microviscosity, lipid composition and functions in diabetes mellitus with hyperlipidemia. *Tokai J Exp Clin Med* **6(1)**, 49–57, 1981.
19. Prisco D, *et al.*, Effect of oral treatment with pantethine on platelet and plasma phospholipids in IIa hyperlipoproteinemia. *Angiology* **38(3)**, 241–247, 1987.
20. Gensini GF, *et al.*, Changes in fatty acid composition of the single platelet phospholipids induced by pantethine treatment. *Int J Clin Pharmacol Res* **5(5)**, 309–318, 1985.

14   Folic Acid

1. Bailey LB, *Folate in Health and Disease*, Marcel Dekker, New York, NY, 1995.
2. Nilsson K, *et al.*, Plasma homocysteine in relationship to serum cobalamin and blood folate in a psychogeriatric population. *Eur J Clin Invest* **24**, 600–606, 1994.
3. Werler MM, Shapiro S, and Mitchell AA, Periconceptional folic acid exposure and risk of occurrent neural tube defects. *JAMA* **269**, 1257–1261, 1993.
4. Milunsky A, *et al.*, Multivitamin/folic acid supplementation in early pregnancy reduces the prevalence of neural tube defects. *JAMA* **262**, 2847–2852, 1989.
5. Hibbard ED and Smithells RW, Folic acid metabolism and human embryopathy. *Lancet* **i**, 1254, 1965.
6. Smithells RW, Sheppard S, and Schorah CJ, Vitamin deficiencies and neural tube defects. *Arch Dis Child* **51**, 944–950, 1976.
7. Laurence KM, *et al.*, Double-blind randomized controlled trial of folate treatment before conception to prevent recurrence of neural tube defects. *Br Med J* **282**, 1509–1511, 1981.
8. Smithells RW, *et al.*, Further experience of vitamin supplementation for the prevention of neural tube defects. *Lancet* **I**, 1027–1033, 1983.
9. Glueck CJ, *et al.*, Evidence that homocysteine is an independent risk factor for atherosclerosis in hyperlipidemic patients. *Am J Cardiol* **75**, 132–136, 1995.
10. Clarke R, *et al.*, Hyperhomocysteinemia: An independent risk factor for vascular disease. *New Engl J Med* **324**, 1149–1155, 1991.
11. Landgren F, *et al.*, Plasma homocysteine in acute myocardial infarction: Homocysteine-lowering effect of folic acid. *J Int Med* **237**, 381–388, 1995.
12. Ubbink JB, *et al.*, Vitamin B_{12}, vitamin B_6, and folate nutritional status in men with hyperhomocysteinemia. *Am J Clin Nutr* **57**, 47–53, 1993.
13. Ubbink JB, van der Merwe WJ, and Delport R, Hyperhomocysteinemia and the response to vitamin supplementation. *Clin Invest* **71**, 993–998, 1993.
14. Gaby AR, *Preventing and Reversing Osteoporosis*. Prima Publishing, Rocklin, CA, 1994.
15. Brattstrom LE, Hultberg BL, and Hardebo JE, Folic acid responsive postmenopausal homocysteinemia. *Metabolism* **34**, 1073–1077, 1985.
16. Van Niekerk W, Cervical cytological abnormalities caused by folic acid deficiency. *Acta Cytol* **10**, 67–73, 1966.
17. Kitay D and Wentz B, Cervical cytology in folic acid deficiency of pregnancy. *Am J Ob Gyn* **104**, 931–938, 1969.
18. Streiff R, Folate deficiency and oral contraceptives. *JAMA* **214**, 105–108, 1970.
19. Whitehead N, Reyner F and Lindenbaum J, Megaloblastic changes in the cervical epithelium association with oral contraceptive therapy and reversal with folic acid. *JAMA* **226**, 1421–1424, 1973.
20. Butterworth C, Hatch K, Gore H, *et al.*, Improvement in cervical dysplasia associated with folic acid therapy in users of oral contraceptives. *Am J Clin Nutr* **35**, 73–82, 1982.
21. Crellin R, Bottiglieri T, and Reynolds EH, Folates and psychiatric disorders. Clinical potential. *Drugs* **45**, 623–636, 1993.

22. Carney MWP, *et al.*, Red cell folate concentrations in psychiatric patients. *J Affective Disorders* **19**, 207–213, 1990.
23. Reynolds E, *et al.*, Folate deficiency in depressive illness. *Br J Psychiat* **117**, 287–292, 1970.
24. Godfrey PSA, *et al.*, Enhancement of recovery from psychiatric illness by methyl folate. Lancet **336**, 392–395, 1990.
25. Thornton WE and Thornton BP, Geriatric mental function and folic acid, a review and survey. *Southern Med J* **70**, 919–922, 1977.
26. Wesson VA, *et al.*, Change in folate status with antidepressant treatment. *Psychiatry Res* **53**, 313–322, 1994.
27. Zucker D, *et al.*, B$_{12}$ deficiency and psychiatric disorders: A case report and literature review. *Biol Psychiatry* **16**, 197–205, 1981.
28. Kivela SL, Pahkala K, and Eronen A, Depression in the aged: Relation to folate and vitamins C and B$_{12}$. *Biol Psychiatry* **26**, 209–213, 1989.
29. Curtius H, Muldner H, and Niederwieser A, Tetrahydrobiopterin: Efficacy in endogenous depression and Parkinson's disease. *J Neural Trans* **55**, 301–308, 1982.
30. Curtius H, *et al.*, Successful treatment of depression with tetrahydrobiopterin. *Lancet* **i**, 657, 658, 1983.
31. Leeming R, *et al.*, Tetrahydrofolate and hydroxycobalamin in the management of Dihydropteridine reductase deficiency. *J Ment Def Res* **26**, 21–25, 1982.
32. Botez M, *et al.*, Effect of folic acid and vitamin B$_{12}$ deficiencies on 5-hydroxyindoleacetic acid in human cerebrospinal fluid. *Ann Neurol* **12**, 479–84, 1982.
33. Reynolds E and Stramentinoli G, Folic acid, S-adenosylmethionine and affective disorder. *Psychol Med* **13**, 705–710, 1983.
34. Reynolds E, Carney M, and Toone B, Methylation and mood. *Lancet* **ii**, 196–199, 1983.
35. Russell RM, *et al.*, Impairment of folic acid absorption by oral pancreatic extracts. *Dig Dis Sci* **25**, 369–373, 1980.

15   Cobalamin (Vitamin B$_{12}$)

1. Van Goor, *et al.* Review, Cobalamin deficiency and mental impairment in elderly people. *Age Ageing* **24**, 536–542, 1995.
2. Shevell MI and Rosenblatt DS, The neurology of cobalamin. *Can J Neurol Sci* **19**, 472–486, 1992.
3. Yao Y, *et al.*, Decline of serum cobalamin levels with increasing age among geriatric outpatients. *Arch Fam Med* **3**, 918–922, 1994.
4. Savage DG, *et al.*, Sensitivity of serum methylmalonic acid and total homocysteine determinations for diagnosing cobalamin deficiency. *Am J Med* **96**, 239–246, 1994.
5. Norman EJ and Morrison JA, Screening elderly populations for cobalamin (vitamin B$_6$) deficiency using the urinary methylmalonic acid assay by gas chromatography mass spectrophotometry. *Am J Med* **94**, 589–594, 1993.
6. Glueck CJ, *et al.*, Evidence that homocysteine is an independent risk factor for atherosclerosis in hyperlipidemic patients. *Am J Cardiol* **75**, 132–136, 1995.
7. Clarke R, *et al.*, Hyperhomocysteinemia: An independent risk factor for vascular disease. *New Engl J Med* **324**, 1149–1155, 1991.
8. Ubbink JB, *et al.*, Vitamin B$_{12}$, vitamin B$_6$, and folate nutritional status in men with hyperhomocysteinemia. *Am J Clin Nutr* **57**, 47–53, 1993; Ubbink JB, van der Merwe WJ, and Delport R, Hyperhomocysteinemia and the response to vitamin supplementation. *Clin Invest* **71**, 993–998, 1993.
9. Nilsson K, *et al.*, Plasma homocysteine in relationship to serum cobalamin and blood folate in a psychogeriatric population. *Eur J Clin Invest* **24**, 600–606, 1994.
10. Tsao CS and Myashita K, Influence of cobalamin on the survival of mice bearing ascites tumor. *Pathobiology* **61**, 104–108, 1993.
11. Lederly FA, Oral cobalamin for pernicious anemia: Medicine's best kept secret. *JAMA* **265**, 94, 95, 1991.

12. Lowenstein L, *et al.*, An immunological basis for acquired resistance to oral administration of hog intrinsic factor and vitamin B_{12} in pernicious anemia. *J Clin Invest* **40**, 1656–1662, 1961.

13. Doscherholmen A, *et al.*, A dual mechanism of vitamin B_{12} plasma absorption. *J Clin Invest* 36, 1551–1557, 1957.

14. Reisner EH, *et al.*, Oral treatment of pernicious anemia with vitamin B_{12} without intrinsic factor. *N Eng J Med* 253, 502–506, 1955.

15. McIntyre PA, *et al.*, Treatment of pernicious anemia with orally administered cyanocobalamin (vitamin B_{12}). *Arch Intern Med* **106**, 280–292, 1960.

16. Waife SO, *et al.*, Oral vitamin B_{12} without intrinsic factor in the treatment of pernicious anemia. *Ann Intern Med* **58**, 810–817, 1963.

17. Berlin H, Berlin R, and Brante G, Oral treatment of pernicious anemia with high doses of vitamin B_{12} without intrinsic factor. *Acta Med Scand* **184**, 247, 248, 1968.

18. Berlin R, *et al.*, Vitamin B_{12} body stores during oral and parenteral treatment of pernicious anemia. *Acta Med Scand* **204**, 81–84, 1978.

19. Bethell FH, *et al.*, Present status of treatment of pernicious anemia, Ninth announcement of USP Ani-Anemia Preparations Advisory Board. *JAMA* **171**, 2092–2094, 1959.

20. Robertson KR, *et al.*, Vitamin B_{12} deficiency and nervous system disease in HIV infection. *Arch Neurol* **50**, 807–811, 1993.

21. Palteil O, *et al.*, Clinical correlates of subnormal vitamin B_{12} levels in patients infected with the human immunodeficiency virus. *Am J Hematol* **49**, 318–322, 1995.

22. Rule SAJ, Serum vitamin B_{12} and transcobalamin levels in early HIV disease. *Am J Hematol* **47**, 167–171, 1994.

23. Weinberg JB, *et al.*, Inhibition of productive human immunodeficiency virus-1 infection by cobalamins. *Blood* **86**, 1281–1287, 1995.

24. Nilsson K, *et al.*, Plasma homocysteine in relationship to serum cobalamin and blood folate in a psychogeriatric population. *Eur J Clin Invest* **24**, 600–606, 1994.

25. Healton EB, *et al.*, Neurologic aspects of cobalamin deficiency. *Medicine* **70**, 229–245, 1991.

26. Martin DC, *et al.*, Time dependency of cognitive recovery with cobalamin replacement: A report of a pilot study. *J Am Geriatric Soc* **40**, 168–172, 1992.

27. Levitt AJ and Karlinsky H, Folate, vitamin B_{12} and cognitive impairment in patients with Alzheimer's disease. *Acta Psychiatr Scand* **86**, 301–305, 1992.

28. Abalan F and Delile JM, B_{12} deficiency in presenile dementia. *Biol Psychiatry* **20**, 1247–1251, 1985.

29. Cole MG and Parchal JF, Low serum vitamin B_{12} in Alzheimer-type dementia. *Age Ageing* **13**, 101–105, 1984.

30. Personal communication with Jonathan Wright, M.D., Kent, Washington.

31. Simon SW, Vitamin B_{12} therapy in allergy and chronic dermatoses. *J Allergy* **2**, 183–185, 1951.

32. Garrison R and Somer E, Vitamin Research: Selected Topics. *The Nutrition Desk Reference, Chapter 5,* Keats Publ., New Canann, CN, 1985, pp. 93, 94.

33. Abalan F, *et al.*, Frequency of deficiencies of vitamin B_{12} and folic acid in patients admitted to a geriatric-psychiatry unit. *Encephale* **10**, 9–12, 1984.

34. Zucker D, *et al.*, B_6 deficiency and psychiatric disorders: A case report and literature review. *Biol Psychiatry* **16**, 197–205, 1981.

35. Kivela SL, Pahkala K, and Eronen A, Depression in the aged: Relation to folate and vitamins C and B_6. *Biol Psychiatry* **26**, 209–213, 1989.

36. Curtius H, Muldner H, and Niederwieser A, Tetrahydrobiopterin: Efficacy in endogenous depression and Parkinson's disease. *J Neural Trans* **55**, 301–308, 1982.

37. Curtius H, *et al.*, Successful treatment of depression with tetrahydrobiopterin. *Lancet* **i**, 657, 658, 1983.

38. Leeming R, *et al.*, Tetrahydrofolate and hydroxycobalamin in the management of Dihydropteridine reductase deficiency. *J Ment Def Res* **26**, 21–25, 1982.

39. Davidson S, The use of vitamin B_{12} in the treatment of diabetic neuropathy. *J Flor Med Assoc* **15**, 717–720, 1954.

40. Sancetta SM, Ayres PR, and Scott RW, The use of vitamin B$_{12}$ in the management of the neurological manifestations of diabetes mellitus, with notes on the administration of massive doses. *Ann Intern Med* **35**, 1028–1048, 1951.

41. Yoshioka K and Tanaka K, Effect of methylcobalamin on diabetic neuropathy as assessed by power spectral analysis of heart rate variations. *Horm Metab Res* **27**, 43, 44, 1995.

42. Yaqub BA, Siddique A, and Sulimani R, Effects of methylcobalamin on diabetic neuropathy. *Clin Neurol Neurosurg* **94**, 105–111, 1992.

43. Yamane K, *et al.*, Clinical efficacy of intravenous plus oral mecobalamin in patients with peripheral neuropathy using vibration perception thresholds as an indicator of improvement. *Curr Ther Res* **56**, 656–670, 1995.

44. Bhatt HR, Linnell JC, and Matt DM, Can faulty vitamin B$_{12}$ (cobalamin) metabolism produce diabetic retinopathy? *Lancet* **2**, 572, 1983.

45. Sandler B and Faragher B, Treatment of oligospermia with vitamin B$_{12}$. *Infertility* **7**, 133–138, 1984.

46. Kumamoto Y, *et al.*, Clinical efficacy of mecobalamin in treatment of oligospermia. Results of a double-blind comparative clinical study. *Acta Urol Japan* **34**, 1109–1132, 1988.

47. Sandyk R and Awerbuch G, Vitamin B$_{12}$ and its relationship to age of onset of multiple sclerosis. *Int J Neurosci* **71**, 93–99, 1993.

48. Reynolds E, Multiple sclerosis and vitamin B$_{12}$ metabolism. *J Neuroimmunol* **40**, 225–230, 1992.

49. Reynolds EH, *et al.*, Vitamin B$_{12}$ metabolism in multiple sclerosis. *Arch Neurol* **49**, 649–652, 1992.

50. Kira J, Tobimatsu S, and Goto I, Vitamin B$_{12}$ metabolism and massive-dose methyl vitamin B$_{12}$ therapy in Japanese patients with multiple sclerosis. *Int Med* **33**, 82–86, 1994.

51. Simpson CA, Newell DJ, and Miller H, The treatment of multiple sclerosis with massive doses of hydroxocobalamin. *Neurology* **15**, 599–602, 1965.

52. Shemish A, *et al.*, Vitamin B$_{12}$ deficiency in patients with chronic-tinnitus and noise-induced hearing loss. *Am J Otolarygol* **14**, 94–99, 1994.

53. Honma K, *et al.*, Effects of vitamin B$_{12}$ on plasma melatonin rhythm in humans: Increased light sensitivity phase-advances the circadian clock? *Experentia* **48**, 716–720, 1992.

54. Okawa M, *et al.*, Vitamin B$_{12}$ treatment for sleep-wake rhythm disorders. *Sleep* **13**, 1–23, 1990.

16 Choline

1. Canty DJ and Zeisel SH, Lecithin and choline in human health and disease. *Nutr Reviews* **52**, 327–339, 1994.

2. Zeisel SH, *et al.*, Choline, an essential nutrient for humans. *FASEB J* **5**, 2093–2098, 1991.

3. Essentiale, *Essentiale forte'*. Natterman International GMBH, P.O. Box 350120, Cologne 5000, Germany, 1989.

4. Lieber CS and Rubin E, Alcoholic fatty liver. *N Engl J Med* **280**, 705–708, 1969.

5. Brook JG, Linn S, and Aviram M, Dietary soya lecithin decreases plasma triglyceride levels and inhibits collagen- and ADP-induced platelet aggregation. *Biochem Med Metabol Biol* **35**, 31–39, 1986.

6. Lipostabil. Natterman International GMBH, P.O. Box 350120, Cologne 5000, Germany, 1990.

7. Wojcicki J, *et al.*, Clinical evaluation of lecithin as a lipid-lowering agent. *Phytotherapy Res* **9**, 597–599, 1995.

8. Rosenberg G and Davis KL, The use of cholinergic precursors in neuropsychiatric diseases. *Am J Clin Nutr* **36**, 709–720, 1982.

9. Levy R, Little A, Chuaqui P, and Reith M, Early results from double blind, placebo controlled trial of high dose phosphatydylcholine in Alzheimer's Disease. *Lancet* **1**, 474–476, 1982.

10. Sitaram N, Weingartner B, Gaine ED, and Cillin JC, Choline: Selective enhancement of serial learning and encoding of low imagery words in man. *Life Sci* **22**, 1555–1560, 1978.

11. Wurtman R, Barbeau A, and Growdon J, Choline and lecithin in brain disorders. *Nutrition and the Brain, Vol. 5.* Raven Press, New York, NY, 1979.
12. Cohen B, Miller A, Lipinski J, and Pope H, Lecithin in mania : A preliminary report. *Am J Psychiat* **137**, 242, 243, 1980.
13. Cohen B, Lipinski J, and Altesman R, Lecithin in the treatment of mania: Double-blind, placebo controlled trials. *Am J Psychiat* **139**, 1162–1164, 1982.
14. Jope R, Tolbert L, Wright S, and Walter-Ryan W, Biochemical RBC abnormalities in drug-free and lithium-treated manic patients. *Am J Psychiat* **142**, 356–358, 1985.
15. Daily JW and Sachan DS, Choline supplementation alters carnitine homeostasis in humans and guinea pigs. *J Nutr* **125**, 1938–1944, 1995.
16. Varela-Mreiras G, *et al.*, Effect of chronic choline deficiency on liver folate content and distribution. *J Nutr Biochem* **3**, 519–522, 1992.

17 Inositol

1. Shasuddin AM, Inositol phosphates have novel anticancer function. *J Nutr* **125**, 725–732, 1995.
2. Benjamin J, *et al.*, Inositol treatment in psychiatry. *Psychopharmacol Bull* **31**, 167–175, 1995.
3. Levine J, *et al.*, Double-blind, controlled trial of inositol treatment of depression. *Am J Psychiatry* **152**, 792–794, 1995.
4. Benjamin J, *et al.*, Double-blind, placebo-controlled, crossover trial of inositol treatment for panic disorder. *Am J Psychiatry* **152**, 1084–1086, 1995.
5. Gegersen G, Harb H, Helles A, and Christensen J, Oral supplementation of myoinositol: Effects on peripheral nerve function in human diabetics and on the concentration in plasma, erythrocytes, urine and muscle tissue in human diabetics and normals. *Acta Neurol Scand* **67**, 164–171, 1983.

18 Calcium

1. Heaney RP and Weaver CM, Calcium absorption from kale. *Am J Clin Nutr* **51**, 656, 657, 1990.
2. Bourgoin BP, Evans DR, Cornett JR, *et al.*, Lead content in 70 brands of dietary calcium supplements. *Am J Public Health* **83**, 1155–1160, 1993.
3. Grossman M, Kirsner J, and Gillespie I, Basal and histalog-stimulated gastric secretion in control subjects and in patients with peptic ulcer or gastric cancer. *Gastroenterology* **45**, 15–26, 1963.
4. Recker R, Calcium absorption and achlorhydria. *N Engl J Med* **313**, 70–73, 1985.
5. Nicar MJ and Pak CYC, Calcium bioavailability from calcium carbonate and calcium citrate. *J Clin Endocrinol Metabol* **61**, 391–393, 1985.
6. Harvey JA, *et al.*, Superior calcium absorption from calcium citrate that calcium carbonate using external forearm counting. *J Am Coll Nutr* **9**, 583–587, 1990.
7. Pak CYC, *et al.*, Long-term treatment of calcium nephrolithiasis with potassium citrate. *J Urol* **134**, 11–19, 1985.
8. Pak CYC and Fuller C, Idiopathic hypocitraturic calcium-oxalate nephrolithiasis successfully treated with potassium citrate. *Ann Intern Med* **104**, 33–37, 1986.
9. Lore F, Nuti R, Vattimo A, and Caniggia, Vitamin D metabolites in postmenopausal osteoporosis. *Horm Metabol Res* 16:58, 1984.
10. Gallagher J, Riggs L, Eisman J, *et al.*, Intestinal calcium absorption and serum vitamin D metabolites in normal subjects and osteoporotic patients: Effect of age and dietary calcium. *J Clin Invest* 64, 729–736, 1979.
11. Brautbar N, Osteoporosis: Is 1,25-$(OH)_2D_3$ of value in treatment? *Nephron* **44**, 161–166, 1986.
12. Ellis F, Holesh S, and Ellis J, Incidence of osteoporosis in vegetarians and omnivores. *Am J Clin Nutr* **25**, 55–58, 1972.

13. Marsh A, *et al.*, Bone mineral mass in adult lactoovovegetarian and omnivorous adults. *Am J Clin Nutr* **37**, 453–456, 1983.

14. Licata A, *et al.*, Acute effects of dietary protein on calcium metabolism in patients with osteoporosis. *J Gerontol* **36**, 14–19, 1981.

15. Thom J, Morris J, Bishop A, and Blacklock, The influence of refined carbohydrate on urinary calcium excretion. *Br J Urol* **50**, 459–464, 1978.

16. Lee CJ, Lawler GS, and Johnson GH, Effects of supplementation of the diets with calcium and calcium-rich foods on bone density of elderly females with osteoporosis. *Am J Clin Nutr* **34**, 819–823, 1981.

17. Gaby AR, *Preventing and Reversing Osteoporosis*. Prima Publishing, Rocklin, CA, 1994.

18. Aloia JF, *et al.*, Calcium supplementation with and without hormone replacement therapy to prevent postmenopausal bone loss. *Annals Intern Med* **120**, 97–103, 1994.

19. Liberman UA, *et al.*, Effect of oral endronate on bone mineral density and the incidence of fractures in postmenopausal osteoporosis. *New Engl J Med* **333**, 1437–1443, 1995.

20. Reid IR, *et al.*, Long-term effects of calcium supplementation on bone loss and fractures in postmenopausal women: A randomized controlled trial. *Am J Med* **98**, 331–335, 1995.

21. Cappuccio FP, *et al.*, Epidemiologic association between dietary calcium intake and blood pressure: A meta-analysis of published data. *Am J Epidemiol* **142**, 935–945, 1995.

22. Zhou C; *et al.*, Clinical observation of treatment of hypertension with calcium. *Am J Hypertens* **7**, 363–367, 1994.

23. Galloe AM, Effect of oral calcium supplementation on blood pressure in patients with previously untreated hypertension: A randomized, double-blind, placebo-controlled, crossover study. *J Hum Hypertens* **7**, 43–45, 1993.

24. Cappuccio FP, *et al.*, Oral calcium supplementation and blood pressure: An overview of randomized controlled trials. *J Hypertens* **7**, 941–946, 1989.

25. Grobbee DE and Hofman A, Effect of calcium supplementation on diastolic blood pressure in young people with mild hypertension. *Lancet* **ii**, 703–707, 1986.

26. Zoccali C, *et al.*, Double-blind randomized, crossover trial of calcium supplementation in essential hypertension. *J Hypertens* **6**, 451–455, 1988.

27. Cappuccio FP, *et al.*, Does oral calcium supplementation lower high blood pressure? A double blind study. *J Hypertens* **5**, 67–71, 1987.

28. Strazzullo P, *et al.*, Controlled trial of long-term oral calcium supplementation in essential hypertension. *Hypertension* **8**, 1084–1088, 1986.

29. McCarron DA and Morris CD, Blood pressure response to oral calcium in persons with mild to moderate hypertension. A randomized, double-blind, placebo-controlled, crossover trial. *Ann Intern Med* **103**, 825–833, 1985.

30. Meese RB, *et al.*, The inconsistent effects of calcium supplements upon blood pressure in primary hypertension. *Am J Med Sci* **294** 219–224, 1987.

31. Sowers JR, *et al.*, Calcium and hypertension. *J Lab Clin Med* **114**, 338–348.

32. Takagi Y, *et al.*, Calcium treatment of essential hypertension in elderly patients evaluated by 24 H monitoring. *Am J Hypertens* **4**, 836–839, 1991.

33. van den Elzen HJ, *et al.*, Calcium metabolism, calcium supplementation and hypertensive disorders of pregnancy. *Eur J Obstet Gynecol Reprod Biol* **59**, 5–16, 1995.

34. Editorial, Calcium supplementation prevents hypertensive disorders of pregnancy. *Nutr Rev* **50**, 233–236, 1992.

35. Belizan JM, *et al.*, Calcium supplementation to prevent hypertensive disorders of pregnancy. *N Engl J Med* **325**, 1399–1405, 1991.

36. Knight KB and Keith RE, Calcium supplementation on normotensive and hypertensive pregnant women. *Am J Clin Nutr* **55**, 891–895, 1992.

19 Magnesium

1. Lindberg JS, *et al.*, Magnesium bioavailability from magnesium citrate and magnesium oxide. *J Am Coll Nutr* **9**, 48–55, 1990.

2. Bohmer T, *et al.*, Bioavailability of oral magnesium supplementation in female students evaluated from elimination of magnesium in 24-hour urine. *Magnes Trace Elem* **9**, 272–278, 1990.

3. Gullestad L, *et al.*, Oral versus intravenous magnesium supplementation in patients with magnesium deficiency. *Magnes Trace Elem* **10**, 11–16, 1991.

4. Skobeloff EM, *et al.*, Intravenous magnesium sulfate for the treatment of acute asthma in the emergency department. *JAMA* **262**, 1210–1213, 1989.

5. Okayama H, *et al.*, Bronchodilating effect of intravenous magnesium sulfate in bronchial asthma. *JAMA* **257**, 1076–1078, 1987.

6. Noppen M, *et al.*, Bronchodilating effect of intravenous magnesium sulfate in acute severe bronchial asthma. *Chest* **97**, 373–376, 1990.

7. Skorodin MS, *et al.*, Magnesium sulfate in exacerbations of chronic obstructive pulmonary disease. *Arch Intern Med* **155**, 496–500, 1995.

8. McLean RM, Magnesium and its therapeutic uses: A review. *Am J Med* **96**, 63–76, 1994.

9. Altura BM, Basic biochemistry and physiology of magnesium: A brief review. *Magnes Trace Elem* **10**, 167–171, 1991.

10. Purvis JR and Movahed A, Magnesium disorders and cardiovascular disease. *Clin Cardiol* **15**, 556–568, 1992.

11. Altura BM, Ischemic heart disease and magnesium. *Magnesium* **7**, 57–67, 1988.

12. Hampton EM, Whang DD, and Whang R, Intravenous magnesium therapy in acute myocardial infarction. *Ann Pharmacother* **28**, 212–219, 1994.

13. Teo KK and Yusuf S, Role of magnesium in reducing mortality in acute myocardial infarction. A review of the evidence. *Drugs* **46**, 347–359, 1993.

14. Schecter M, Kaplinsky E, and Rabinowitz B, The rationale of magnesium supplementation in acute myocardial infarction. A review of the literature. *Arch Intern Med* **152**, 2189–2196, 1992.

15. Turlapaty PDMV and Altura BM, Magnesium deficiency produces spasms of coronary arteries: Relationship to etiology of sudden death ischemic heart disease. *Science* **208**, 199, 200, 1980.

16. Goto K, *et al.*, Magnesium deficiency detected by intravenous loading test in variant angina pectoris. *Am J Cardiol* **65**, 709–712, 1990.

17. Brodsky MA, *et al.*, Magnesium therapy in new-onset atrial fibrillation. *Am J Cardiol* **73**, 1227–1229, 1994.

18. Perticone F, *et al.*, Antiarrhythmic short-term protective magnesium treatment in ischemic dilated cardiomyopathy. *J Am Coll Nutr* **9**, 492–499, 1990.

19. Gottlieb SS, *et al.*, Prognostic importance of serum magnesium concentration in patients with congestive heart failure. *J Am Coll Cardiol* **16**, 827–831, 1990.

20. Gottlieb SS, Importance of magnesium in congestive heart failure. *Am J Cardiol* **63**, 39G–42G, 1989.

21. Whelton PK and Klag, Magnesium and blood pressure: Review of the epidemiologic and clinical trial experience. *Am J Cardiol* **63**, 26G–30G, 1989.

22. Joffres MR, Reed DM, and Yano K, Relationship of magnesium intake and other dietary factors to blood pressure: The Honolulu Heart Study. *Am J Clin Nutr* **45**, 469–475, 1987.

23. Witteman JCM, *et al.*, Reduction of blood pressure with oral magnesium supplementation in women with mild to moderate hypertension. *Am J Clin Nutr* **60**, 129–135, 1994.

24. Motoyama T, Sano H, and Fukuzaki H, Oral magnesium supplementation in patients with essential hypertension. *Hypertension* **13**, 227–232, 1989.

25. Howard JMH, Magnesium deficiency in peripheral vascular disease. *J Nutr Med* **1**, 39–49, 1990.

26. Davis WH, *et al.*, Monotherapy with magnesium increases abnormally low high density lipoprotein cholesterol: A clinical essay. *Clin Ther Res* **36**, 341–346, 1984.

27. Galland LD, Baker SM, and McLellan RK, Magnesium deficiency in the pathogenesis of mitral valve prolapse. *Magnesium* **5**, 165–174, 1986.

28. Fernandes JS, *et al.*, Therapeutic effect of a magnesium salt in patients suffering from mitral valvular prolapse and latent tetany. *Magnesium* **4**, 283–289, 1985.

29. Altura BT and Altura BM, The role of magnesium in etiology of strokes and cerebrovasospasm. *Magnesium* **1**, 277–291, 1982.

30. Paolisso G, Sgambato S, Gambardella A, *et al.*, Daily magnesium supplements improve glucose handling in elderly subjects. *Am J Clin Nutr* **55**, 1161–1167, 1992.

31. White JR and Campbell RK, Magnesium and diabetes: A review. *Ann Pharmacother* **27**, 775–780, 1993.

32. Djurhuus MS, *et al.*, Insulin increases renal magnesium excretion: A possible cause of magnesium depletion in hyperinsulinaemic states. *Diabetic Med* **12**, 664–669, 1995.

33. Consensus Statement, Magnesium supplementation in the treatment of diabetes. *Diabetes Care* **19** (Suppl. 1), S93–S95, 1996.

34. Clauw DJ, *et al.*, Magnesium deficiency in the eosinophilia-myalgia syndrome. *Arth Rheum* **9**, 1331–1334, 1994.

35. Cox IM, Campbell MJ and Dowson D, Red blood cell magnesium and chronic fatigue syndrome. *Lancet* **337**, 757–760, 1991.

36. Ahlborg H, Ekelund LG, and Nilsson CG, Effect of potassium-magnesium aspartate on the capacity for prolonged exercise in man. *Acta Physiologica Scand* **74**, 238–245, 1968.

37. Hicks JT, Treatment of fatigue in general practice: A double blind study. *Clin Med Jan*, 85–90, 1964.

38. Friedlander HS, Fatigue as a presenting symptom: Management in general practice. *Curr Ther Res* **4**, 441–449, 1962.

39. Shaw DL, Management of fatigue: A physiologic approach. *Am J Med Sci* **243**, 758–769, 1962.

40. Abraham G, Management of fibromyalgia: Rationale for the use of magnesium and malic acid. *J Nutr Med* **3**, 49–59, 1992.

41. Gaspar AZ, Gasser P, and Flammer J, The influence of magnesium on visual field and peripheral vasospasm in glaucoma. *Ophthalmologica* **209**, 11–13, 1995.

42. Attias J, *et al.*, Oral magnesium intake reduces permanent hearing loss induced by noise exposure. *Am J Otolaryngol* **15**, 26–32, 1994.

43. Johansson G, Backman U, Danielson B, *et al.*, Biochemical and clinical effects of the prophylactic treatment of renal calcium stones with magnesium hydroxide. *J Urol* **124**, 770–774, 1980.

44. Wunderlich W, Aspects of the influence of magnesium ions on the formation of calcium oxalate. *Urol Res* **9**, 157–160, 1981.

45. Hallson P, Rose G, and Sulaiman, Magnesium reduces calcium oxalate crystal formation in human whole urine. *Clin Sci* **62**, 17–19, 1982.

46. Johansson G, Backman U, Danielson B, *et al.*, Magnesium metabolism in renal stone formers. Effects of therapy with magnesium hydroxide. *Scand J Urol Nephrol* **53**, 125–130, 1980.

47. Prien E and Gershoff S, Magnesium oxide-pyridoxine therapy for recurrent calcium oxalate calculi. *J Urol* **112**, 509–512, 1974.

48. Gershoff S and Prien E, Effect of daily MgO and Vitamin B_6 administration to patients with recurring calcium oxalate stones. *Am J Clin Nutr* **20**, 393–399, 1967.

49. Pak CYC and Fuller C, Idiopathic hypocitraturic calcium-oxalate nephrolithiasis successfully treated with potassium citrate. *Annals Int Med* **104**, 33–37, 1986.

50. Pak CYC, *et al.*, Long-term treatment of calcium nephrolithiasis with potassium citrate. *J Urol* **134**, 11–19, 1985.

51. Swanson DR, Migraine and magnesium: Eleven neglected connections. *Perspect Biol Med* **31**, 526–557, 1988.

52. Ramadan NM, et al., Low brain magnesium in migraine. Headache 29, 590–593, 1989.

53. Gallai V, et al., Magnesium content of mononuclear blood cells in migraine patients. Headache 34, 160–165, 1994.

54. Cohen L and Kitzes R, Infrared spectroscopy and magnesium content of bone mineral in osteoporotic women. *Isr J Med Sci* **17**, 1123–1125, 1981.

55. Rude RK, Adams JS, Ryzen E, *et al.*, Low serum concentration of 1,25-dihydroxyvitamin D in human magnesium deficiency. *J Clin Endo Metabol* **61**, 933–940, 1985.

56. Altura BM, *et al.*, Magnesium deficiency-induced spasm of umbilical vessels: Relation to preeclampsia, hypertension, growth retardation. *Science* **221**, 376–378, 1983.

57. Conradt A, Weidinger H, and Algayer H, ON: The role of magnesium in fetal hypertrophy, pregnancy-induced hypertension, and preeclampsia. *Mag Bull* **6**, 68–76, 1984.
58. Kiss V, *et al.*, Effect of maternal magnesium supply on spontaneous abortion and premature birth and on intrauterine fetal development: Experimental epidemiological study. *Mag Bull* **3**, 73–79, 1981.
59. Spatling L and Spatling G, Magnesium supplementation in pregnancy. A double-blind study. *Br J Obstet Gynaecol* **95**, 120–125, 1988.
60. Rudnicki M, *et al.*, The effect of magnesium on maternal blood pressure in pregnancy-induced hypertension. A randomized double-blind placebo-controlled trial. *Acta Obstet Gynecol Scand* **70**, 445–450, 1991.
61. Martin RW and Morrison JC, Oral magnesium for tocolysis. *Contemp Ob/Gyn* **30**, 111–118, 1987.
62. Sibai BM, *et al.*, Magnesium supplementation during pregnancy: A double-blind randomized controlled clinical trial. *Am J Obstet Gynecol* **161**, 115–119, 1989.
63. Abraham GE, Nutritional factors in the etiology of the premenstrual tension syndromes. *J Repro Med* **28**, 446–464, 1983.
64. Piesse JW, Nutritional factors in the premenstrual syndrome. *Int Clin Nutr Rev* **4**, 54–81, 1984.
65. Rosenstein DL, *et al.*, Magnesium measures across the menstrual cycle in premenstrual syndrome. *Biol Psychiatr* **35**, 557–561, 1994.
66. Facchinetti F, *et al.*, Oral magnesium successfully relieves premenstrual mood changes. *Obstet Gynecol* **78**, 177–181, 1991.
67. Goei GS and Abraham GE, Effect of nutritional supplement, Optivite, on symptoms of premenstrual tension. *J Repro Med* **28**, 527–531, 1983.
68. Majumdar P and Boylan M, Alteration of tissue magnesium levels in rats by dietary vitamin B_6 supplementation. *Int J Vit Ntr Res* **59**, 300–303, 1989.
69. Seelig MS, Magnesium deficiency with phosphate and vitamin D excess: Role in pediatric cardiovascular nutrition. *Cardio Med* **3**, 637–650, 1978.

20 Potassium

1. Jansson B, Dietary, total body, and intracellular potassium-to-sodium ratios and their influence on cancer. *Cancer Detect Prevent* **14**, 563–565, 1991.
2. Khaw KT and Barrett-Connor E, Dietary potassium and stroke-associated mortality. *N Engl J Med* **316**, 235–240, 1987.
3. National Research Council, Diet and Health. *Implications for Reducing Chronic Disease Risk*. National Academy Press, Washington, DC, 1989, pp. 421–423.
4. Skrabal F, Aubock J, and Hortnagl H, Low sodium/high potassium diet for prevention of hypertension: Probable mechanisms of action. *Lancet* **ii**, 895–900, 1981.
5. Iimura O, *et al.*, Studies on the hypotensive effect of high potassium intake in patients with essential hypertension. *Clin Sci* **61** (Suppl. 7), S77–S80, 1981.
6. Sangiorgi GB, *et al.*, Serum potassium levels, red-blood-cell potassium and alterations of the repolarization phase of electrocardiography in old subjects. *Age Ageing* **13**, 309–312, 1984.
7. Langford HG, Dietary potassium and hypertension, Epidemiological data. *Ann Intern Med* **98**, 770–772, 1990.
8. MacGregor SA, *et al.*, Moderate potassium supplementation in essential hypertension. *Lancet* **ii**, 567–570, 1982.
9. Kaplan NM, Potassium supplementation in hypertensive patients with diuretic-induced hypokalemia. *New Engl J Med* **312**, 746–749, 1985.
10. Matlou SM, *et al.*, Potassium supplementation in blacks with mild to moderate essential hypertension. *J Hypertens* **4**, 61–64, 1986.
11. Oble AO, Placebo controlled trial of potassium supplements in black patients with mild essential hypertension. *J Cardiovasc Pharmacol* **14**, 294–296, 1989.

12. Patki PS, *et al.*, Efficiacy of potassium and magnesium in essential hypertension: A double-blind, placebo-controlled, crossover study. *Br J Med* **301**, 521–523, 1990.
13. Fotherby MD and Potter JF, Potassium supplementation reduces clinic and ambulatory blood pressure in elderly hypertensive patients. *J Hypertens* **10**, 1403–1408, 1992.
14. Thijs L, *et al.*, Age-related effects of placebo and active treatment in patients beyond the age of 60 years: The need for a proper control group. *J Hypertens* **8**, 997–1002, 1990.

21   Zinc

1. Prasad A, Clinical, biochemical and nutritional spectrum of zinc deficiency in human subjects: An update. *Nutrition Reviews* **41**, 197–208, 1983.
2. Sandstead H, Zinc nutrition in the United States. *Am J Clin Nutr* **26**, 1251–1260, 1973.
3. Nordstrom J, Trace mineral nutrition in the elderly. *Am J Clin Nutr* **36**, 788–795, 1982.
4. Loeffel E and Koya D, Cutaneous manifestations of gastrointestinal disease. *Cutis* **21**, 852–861, 1978.
5. Tuormaa TE, Adverse effect of zinc deficiency: A review from the literature. *J Orthomol Med* **10**, 149–162, 1995.
6. Pfeiffer C, Mental and Elemental Nutrients. Keats Pub, New Canaan, CT, 1975.
7. Davies S, Assessment of zinc status. *Int Clin Nutr Rev* **4**, 122–129, 1984.
8. Goldenber RL, *et al.*, The effect of zinc supplementation on pregnancy outcome. *JAMA* **274**, 463–468, 1995.
9. Dardenne M, *et al.*, Contribution of zinc and other metals to the biological activity of the serum thymic factor. *Proc Natl Acad Sci* **79**, 5370–5373, 1982.
10. Bogden JD, *et al.*, Zinc and immunocompetence in the elderly: Baseline data on zinc nutriture and immunity in unsupplemented subjects. *Am J Clin Nutr* **46**, 101–109, 1987.
11. Boukaiba N, *et al.*, A physiological amount of zinc supplementation: Effects on nutritional, lipid, and thymic status in an elderly population. *Am J Clin Nutr* **57**, 566–572, 1993.
12. Eby GA, Davis DR, and Halcomb WW, Reduction in duration of common colds by zinc gluconate lozenges in a double-blind study. *Antimicrob Agents Chemother* **25**, 20–24, 1984.
13. Prasad AS, Zinc in growth and development and spectrum of human zinc deficiency. *J Am Coll Nutr* **7**, 377–384, 1988.
14. Tikkiwal M, *et al.*, Effect of zinc administration on seminal zinc and fertility of oligospermic males. *Ind J Physiol Pharmacol* **31**, 30–34, 1987.
15. Takihara H, *et al.*, Zinc sulfate therapy for infertile males with or without varicocelectomy. *Urology* **29**, 638–641, 1987.
16. Netter A, *et al.*, Effect of zinc administration on plasma testosterone, dihydrotestosterone and sperm count. *Arch Androl* **7**, 69–73, 1981.
17. Pandley SP, Bhattacharya SK, and Sundar S, Zinc in rheumatoid arthritis. *Indian Journal of Medical Research* **81**, 618–620, 1985.
18. Simkin PA, Treatment of rheumatoid arthritis with oral zinc sulfate. *Agents and Actions* (Suppl.) **8**, 587–595, 1981.
19. Mattingly PC and Mowat AG, Zinc sulphate in rheumatoid arthritis. *Annals of the Rheumatic Diseases* **41**, 456–457, 1982.
20. Michaelsson G, Vahlquist A, and Juhlin L, Serum zinc and retinol-binding protein in acne. *Br J Dermatol* **96**, 283–286, 1977.
21. Michaelson G, Juhlin L, and Ljunghall K, A double blind study of the effect of zinc and oxytetracycline in acne vulgaris. *Br J Dermatol* **97**, 561–565, 1977.
22. Cunliffe WJ, *et al.*, A double-blind trial of a zinc sulphate/citrate complex and tetracycline in the treatment of acne. *Br J Dermatol* **101**, 321–325, 1979.
23. Dreno B, Amblard P, Agache P, *et al.*, Low doses of zinc gluconate for inflammatory acne. *Acta Derm Venereol* **69**, 541–543, 1989.
24. Weimar V, Puhl S, Smith W, and Broeke J, Zinc sulphate in acne vulgaris. *Arch Dermatol* **114**, 1776–1778, 1978.
25. Newsome DA, *et al.*, Oral zinc in macular degeneration. *Arch Ophthalmol* **106**, 192–198, 1988.

26. Constantinidis J, The hypothesis of zinc deficiency in the pathogenesis of neurofibrillary tangles. *Med Hypoth* **35**, 319–323, 1991.
27. Constantinidis J, Treatment of Alzheimer's disease by zinc compounds. *Drug Develop Res* **27**, 1–14, 1992.
28. Brewer GJ, Practical recommendations and new therapies for Wilson's disease. *Drugs* **50**, 240–249, 1995.

22 Boron

1. Ellis F, Holesh S, and Ellis J, Incidence of osteoporosis in vegetarians and omnivores. *Am J Clin Nutr* **25**, 55–58, 1972.
2. Marsh A, Sanchez T, Chaffe F, *et al.*, Bone mineral mass in adult lactoovovegetarian and omnivorous adults. *Am J Clin Nutr* **37**, 453–456, 1983.
3. Block G, Dietary guidelines and the results of food consumption surveys. *Am J Clin Nutr* **53**, 356S–357S, 1991.
4. Lore F, Nuti R, Vattimo A, and Caniggia, Vitamin D metabolites in postmenopausal osteoporosis. *Horm Metabol Res* **16**, 58, 1984.
5. Gallagher J, Riggs L, Eisman J, *et al.*, Intestinal calcium absorption and serum vitamin D metabolites in normal subjects and osteoporotic patients: Effect of age and dietary calcium. *J Clin Invest* **64**, 729–736, 1979.
6. Neilsen FH, Hunt CD, Mullen LM, and Hunt JR, Effect of dietary boron on mineral, estrogen, and testosterone metabolism in postmenopausal women. *FASEB J* **1**, 394–397, 1987.
7. Nielsen FH, Gallagher SK, Johnson LK, and Nielsen EJ, Boron enhances and mimics some of the effects of estrogen therapy in postmenopausal women. *J Trace Elem Exp Med* **5**, 237–246, 1992.
8. Meacham SL, *et al.*, Effect of boron supplementation on blood and urinary calcium, magnesium, and phosphorus, urinary boron in athletic and sedentary women. *Am J Clin Nutr* **61**, 341–345, 1995.
9. Travers RL, Rennie GC, and Newnham RE, Boron and arthritis: The results of a double-blind pilot study. *J Nutr Med* **1**, 127–132, 1990.
10. Newnham RE, Arthritis or skeletal fluorosis and boron. *Int Clin Nutr Rev* **11**, 68–70, 1991.

23 Chromium

1. Mertz W, Chromium in human nutrition: A review. *J Nutr* **123**, 626–633, 1993.
2. Evans GW, Chromium picolinate is an efficacious and safe supplement. *Int J Sport Nutr* **3**, 117–122, 1993.
3. Abraham AS, Brooks BA, and Eylath U, The effects of chromium supplementation on serum glucose and lipids in patients with and without non-insulin dependent diabetes. *Metabolism* **41**, 768–771, 1992.
4. Mossop RT, Effects of chromium (III) on fasting blood glucose, cholesterol, and cholesterol HDL levels in diabetics. *Centr Afr J Med* **29**, 80–82, 1983.
5. Rabinowitz MB, *et al.*, Effect of chromium and yeast supplements on carbohydrate metabolism in diabetic men. *Diabetes Care* **6**, 319–327, 1983.
6. Anderson RA, Chromium, glucose tolerance, and diabetes. *Biological Trace Element Research* **32**, 19–24, 1992.
7. Anderson RA, *et al.*, Effects of supplemental chromium on patients with symptoms of reactive hypoglycemia. *Metabolism* **36**, 351–355, 1987.
8. Lee NA and Reasner CA, Beneficial effect of chromium supplementation on serum triglyceride levels in NIDDM. *Diabetes Care* **17**, 1449–1452, 1994.
9. Offenbach E and Pistunyer F, Beneficial effect of chromium-rich yeast on glucose tolerance and blood lipids in elderly patients. *Diabetes* **29**, 919–925, 1980.
10. Press RI, Geller J, and Evans GW, The effect of chromium picolinate on serum cholesterol and apolipoprotein fractions in human subjects. *Western J Med* **152,** 41–45, 1993.

11. Wang MM, *et al.*, Serum cholesterol of adults supplemented with brewer's yeast or chromium chloride. *Nutr Res* **9**, 989–998, 1989.
12. Roeback JR, *et al.*, Effects of chromium supplementation on serum high-density lipoprotein cholesterol levels in men taking beta-blockers. *Annals Int Med* **115**, 917–924, 1991.
13. Lefavi RG, *et al.*, Lipid-lowering effect of a dietary chromium (III) nicotinic acid complex in male athletes. *Nutr Res* **13**, 239–249, 1993.
14. McCarthy MF, Hypothesis: Sensitization of insulin-dependent hypothalamic glucoreceptors may account for the fat-reducing effects of chromium picolinate. *J Optimal Nutr* **21**, 36–53, 1993.
15. Evans GW and Pouchnik DJ, Composition and biological activity of chromium-pyridine carbosylate complexes. *J Inorgranic Biochemistry* **49**, 177–187, 1993.
16. Katts GR, Ficher JA, and Blum K, The effects of chromium picolinate supplementation on body composition in different age groups. *Age* **14**, 138(Abstract #40), 1991.
17. Abdel KM, *et al.*, Glucose tolerance in blood and skin of patients with acne vulgaris. *Ind J Derm* **22**, 139–149, 1977.
18. Cohen J and Cohen A, Pustular acne staphyloderma and its treatment with tolbutamide. *Can Med Assoc J* **80**, 629–632, 1959.
19. McCarthy M, High chromium yeast for acne? *Med Hypoth* **14**, 307–310, 1984.
20. Schrauzer GN, Shrestha KP, and Flores MP, Somatopsychological effects of chromium supplementation. *J Nutr Med* **3**, 43–48, 1992.
21. Seaborn C and Stoecker B, Effects of antacid or ascorbic acid on tissue accumulation and urinary excretion of chromium. *Nutr Res* **10**, 1401–1407, 1990.

24   Copper

1. Solomons NW, Biochemical, metabolic, and clinical role of copper in human nutrition. *J Am Coll Nutr* **4**, 83–105, 1985.
2. Klevay LM, Dietary copper: A powerful determinant of cholesterolemia. *Medical Hypothesis* **24**, 111–119, 1987.
3. Reiser S, *et al.*, Effect of copper intake on blood cholesterol and its lipoprotein distribution in men. *Nutr Rep Intl* **36**, 641–649, 1987.
4. Kivirikko K and Peltonen L, Abnormalities in copper metabolism and disturbances in the synthesis of collagen and elastin. *Med Biol* **60**, 45–48, 1982.
5. Walker WR and Keats DM, An investigation of the therapeutic value of the "copper bracelet"—dermal assimilation of copper in arthritic/rheumatoid conditions. *Agents and Actions* **6**, 454–458, 1976.
6. Finley EB and Cerklewski FL, Influence of ascorbic acid supplementation on copper status in young adult men. *Am J Clin Nutr* **47**, 96–101, 1988.

25   Iodine

1. Boyages SC, Iodine deficiency disorders. *J Clin Endocrinol Metabol* **77**, 587–591, 1993.
2. Ghent WR, *et al.*, Iodine replacement in fibrocystic disease of the breast. *Can J Surg* **36**, 453–460, 1993.
3. Paul T, *et al.*, The effect of small increases in dietary iodine on thyroid function in euthyroid subjects. *Metabolism* **37**, 121–124, 1988.
4. Chow CC, *et al.*, Effect of low dose iodide supplementation on thyroid function in potentially susceptible subjects. Are dietary iodide levels in Britain acceptable? *Clin Endocrinol* **34**, 413–416, 1991.
5. Hitch JM, Acneform eruptions induced by drugs and chemicals. *JAMA* **200**, 879, 880, 1967.

26   Iron

1. Krause MV and Mahan KL, *Food, Nutrition and Diet Therapy, 7th Edition*. WB Saunders, Philadelphia, PA, 1984, pp. 128–131, 157–164, 585–599.

2. Fairbanks VF and Beutler E, Iron. In: *Modern Nutrition in Health and Disease, 7th Edition.* Shils ME and Young VR (eds.). Lea and Febiger, Philadelphia, PA, 1988, pp. 193–226.
3. Morley JE, Nutritional status of the elderly. *Am J Med* **81**, 679–695, 1986.
4. Jacobs AM and Owen GM, The effect of age on iron absorption. *J Gerontol* **24**, 95, 96, 1969.
5. Bezwoda W, *et al.*, The importance of gastric hydrochloric acid in the absorption of non-heme iron. *J Lab Clin Med* **92**, 108–116, 1978.
6. Arvidsson B, *et al.*, Iron prophylaxis in menorrhagia. *Acta Ob Gyn Scand* **60**, 157–160, 1981.
7. Taymor ML, Sturgis SH, and Yahia C, The etiological role of chronic iron deficiency in production of menorrhagia. *JAMA* **187**, 323–327, 1964.
8. Cook JD and Lynch SR, The liabilities of iron deficiency. *Blood* **68**, 803–809, 1986.
9. Viteri FE and Torun B, Anaemia and physical work capacity. *Clin Haematol* **3**, 609–626, 1974.
10. Basta SS, *et al.*, Iron deficiency anemia and the productivity of adult males in Indonesia. *Am J Clin Nutr* **32**, 6–25, 1979.
11. Gardner GW, *et al.*, Physical work capacity and metabolic stress in subjects with iron deficiency anemia. *Am J Clin Nutr* **30**, 910–917, 1977.
12. O'Keeffe ST, Gaavin K, and Lavan JN, Iron status and restless legs syndrome in the elderly. *Age Ageing* **23**, 200–203, 1994.
13. Salonen JT, *et al.*, High stored iron levels are associated with excess risk of myocardial infarction in Eastern Finnish men. *Circulation* **86**, 803–811, 1992.
14. Gordeuk V, *et al.*, Iron overload: Causes and consequences. *Annual Rev Nutr* **7**, 485–508, 1987.

27   Manganese

1. Keen CL and Zidenberg-Cherr S, Manganese. In: *Present Knowledge in Nutrition, 6th Edition.* Brown ML (ed.). International Life Sciences Institute, Washington, DC, 1990, pp. 279–286.
2. Rosa GD, *et al.*, Regulation of superoxide dismutase activity by dietary manganese. *J Nutr* **110**, 795–804, 1980.
3. Menander-Huber KB, Orgotein in the treatment of rheumatoid arthritis. *Eur J Rheumatol Inflam* **4**, 201–211, 1981.
4. Zidenberg-Cherr S, *et al.*, Dietary superoxide dismutase does not affect tissue levels. *Am J Clin Nutr* **37**, 5–7, 1983.
5. Pasquier C, *et al.*, Manganese-containing superoxide-dismutase deficiency in polymorphonuclear leukocytes of adults with rheumatoid arthritis. *Inflammation* **8**, 27–32, 1984.
6. Hurley LS, Wooley DE, Rosenthal F, *et al.*, Influence of manganese on susceptibility of rats to convulsions. *Am J Physiol* **204**, 493–496, 1963.
7. Carl EG, Keen BB, Gallagher BB, *et al.*, Association of low blood manganese concentrations with epilepsy. *Neurology* **336**, 1584–1587, 1986.
8. Dupont CL and Tanaka Y, Blood manganese levels in children with convulsive disorder. *Biochem Med* **33**, 246–255, 1985.
9. Sampson P, Low manganese level may trigger epilepsy. *JAMA* **238**, 1805, 1977.
10. Papavasiliou P, *et al.*, Seizure disorders and trace metals: Manganese in epileptics. *Neurology* **29**, 1466–1473, 1979.
11. Sohler A and Pfeiffer CC, A direct method for the determination of manganese in whole blood: Patients with seizure activity have low blood levels. *J Orthomol Psych* **8**, 275–280, 1979.
12. Wimhurst JM and Manchester KL, Comparison of ability of Mg and Mn to activate the key enzymes of glycolysis. *FEBS Letters* **27**, 321–326, 1972.
13. Editor, Manganese and glucose tolerance. *Nutr Rev* **26**, 207–210, 1968.
14. Mooradian AD and Morley JE, Micronutrient status in diabetes mellitus. *Am J Clin Nutr* **45**, 877–895, 1987.

15. Rubinstein AH, Levin NW, and Elliott GA, Manganese-induced hypoglycemia. *Lancet* **2**, 1348–1351, 1962.
16. Freeland-Graves JH and Lin PH, Plasma uptake of manganese as affected by oral loads of manganese, calcium, milk, phosphorus, copper, and zinc. *J Am Coll Nutr* **10**, 38–43, 1991.

28 Molybdenum

1. Sardesai VM, Molybdenum: An essential trace element. *Nutr Clin Pract* **8**, 277–281, 1993.
2. Turnlund JR, Keyes WR, and Peiffer GL, Molybdenum absorption, excretion, and retention studied with stable isotopes in young men at five intakes of dietary molybdenum. *Am J Clin Nutr* **62**, 790–796, 1995.
3. Simon RA, Sulfite sensitivity. *Annals Allergy* **56**, 281–288, 1986.
4. Yang CS, Research on esophageal cancer in China: A review. *Cancer Res* **40**, 2633–2644, 1980.
5. Berg JW, Jaenzel W, and Devesa SS, Epidemiology of gastrointestinal cancer. *Proc Natl Cancer Congr* **7**, 459–463, 1973.
6. Luo XM, Wei HJ, and Yang SP, Inhibitory effects of molybdenum on esophageal and forestomach carcinogenesis in rats. *J Natl Cancer Inst* **71**, 75–80, 1983.
7. Komada K, *et al.*, Effect of dietary molybdenum on esophageal carcinogenesis in rats induced by N-methyl-N-benzylnitrosamine. *Cancer Res* **50**, 2418–2422, 1990.
8. Losee FL and Adkins BL, A study of the mineral environment of caries-resistant navy recruits. *Caries Res* **3**, 23–31, 1969.
9. Jenkins GN, Molybdenum. In: *Trace Elements and Dental Disease*. Curzon MEJ and Cutress TW (eds.). John Wright, Boston, MA, 1983, pp. 149–166.
10. Brewer GJ, Practical recommendations and new therapies for Wilson's disease. *Drugs* **50**, 240–249, 1995.
11. Brewer GJ, *et al.*, Treatment of Wilson's disease with ammonium tetrathiomolybdate; I, Initial therapy in 17 neurologically affected patients. *Arch Neurol* **51**, 545–554, 1994.

29 Selenium

1. Fan AM and Kizer KW, Selenium: Nutritional, toxicological, and clinical aspects. *West J Med* **153**, 160–167, 1990.
2. Burk RF, Recent developments in trace element metabolism and function: Newer roles of selenium in nutrition. *J Nutr* **119**, 1051–1054, 1989.
3. Contempre B, *et al.*, Effect of selenium supplementation on thyroid hormone metabolism in an iodine and selenium deficient population. *Clin Endocrinol* **36**, 579–583, 1992.
4. Andersen O and Nielsen JB, Effects of simultaneous low-level dietary supplementation with inorganic and organic selenium on whole-body, blood, and organ levels of toxic metals in mice. *Environ Health Perspect* **102** (Suppl. 3), 321–324, 1994.
5. Thomson CD, *et al.*, Effect of prolonged supplementation with daily supplements of selenomethionine and sodium selenite on glutathione peroxidase activity in blood of New Zealand residents. *Am J Clin Nutr* **36**, 24–31, 1982.
6. Lavender OA, *et al.*, Bioavailability of selenium to Finnish men as assessed by platelet glutathione peroxidase activity and other blood parameters. *Am J Clin Med* **37**, 887–897, 1983.
7. Mutanen M, Bioavailability of selenium. *Annals Clin Res* **18**, 48–54, 1986.
8. National Research Council, Diet and Health. *Implications for Reducing Chronic Disease Risk.* National Academy Press, Washington, DC, 1989, pp. 376–379.
9. Hocman G, Chemoprevention of cancer: Selenium. *Int J Biochem* **20**, 123–132, 1988.
10. Wasowicz W, Selenium concentration and glutathione peroxidase activity in blood of children with cancer. *J Trace Elem Electrolytes Health Dis* **8**, 53–57, 1994.

11. Fex G, Petterson B, and Akesson B, Low plasma selenium as a risk factor for cancer death in middle-age men. *Nutr Cancer* **10**, 221–229, 1987.

12. Kok FJ, *et al.*, Is serum selenium a risk factor for cancer in men only? *Am J epidemiol* **125**, 12–16, 1987.

13. Kiremidjian-Schumacher L and Stotsky G, Selenium and immune responses. *Environmental Res* **42**, 277–303, 1987.

14. Kiremidjian-Schumacher L, *et al.*, Supplementation with selenium and human immune cell functions; II, Effect on cytotoxic lymphocytes and natural killer cells. *Biol Trace Elem Res* **41**, 115–127, 1994.

15. Roy M, Supplementation with selenium and human immune cell functions; I, Effect on lymphocyte proliferation and interleukin 2 receptor expression. *Biol Trace Elem Res* **41**, 103–114, 1994.

16. Kok FJ, *et al.*, Decreased selenium levels in acute myocardial infarction. *JAMA* **261**, 1161–1164, 1989.

17. Salonen JT, Association between cardiovascular death and myocardial infarction and serum selenium in a matched-pair longitudinal study. *Lancet* **2**, 175–179, 1982.

18. Beaglehole R, *et al.*, Decreased blood selenium and risk of myocardial infarction. *Int J Epid* **19**, 918–922, 1990.

19. Luoma PV, *et al.*, Serum selenium, glutathione peroxidase activity and high-density lipoprotein cholesterol—effect of selenium supplementation. *Res Commun Chem Pathol Pharmacol* **46**, 469–472, 1984.

20. Stead NW, *et al.*, Selenium (Se) balance in the dependent elderly. *Am J Clin Nutr* **39**, 677, 1984.

21. Korpela H, *et al.*, Effect of selenium supplementation after acute myocardial infarction. *Res Commun Chem Pathol Pharmacol* **65**, 249–252, 1989.

22. Tarp U, *et al.*, Low selenium level in severe rheumatoid arthritis. *Scand J Rheumatol* **14**, 97–101, 1985.

23. Hinks LJ, *et al.*, Trace element status in eczema and psoriasis. *Clin Exp Derm* **12**, 93–97, 1987.

24. Tarp U, *et al.*, Selenium treatment in rheumatoid arthritis. *Scand J Rheumatol* **14**, 364–368, 1985.

25. Munthe E and Aseth J, Treatment of rheumatoid arthritis with selenium and vitamin E. *Scand J Rheumatol* **53** (Suppl.), 103, 1984.

26. Swanson A and Truesdale A, Elemental analysis in normal and cataractous human lens tissue. *Biochem Biophys Res Comm* **45**, 1488–1496, 1971.

27. Karakucuk S, *et al.*, Selenium concentrations in serum, lens, and aqueous humour of patients with senile cataract. *Arch Opthalmol Scand* **73**, 329–332, 1995.

28. Karunanithy R, Roy AC, and Ratnam SS, Selenium status in pregnancy: Studies in amniotic fluid from normal pregnant women. *Gynecol Obstet Invest* **27**, 148–150, 1989.

29. Lockitch G, *et al.*, Selenium deficiency in low birth weight neonates: An unrecognized problem. *J Pediatr* **114**, 865–870, 1989.

30. McGlashan ND, Low selenium status and cot deaths. *Med Hypothesis* **35**, 311–314, 1991.

31. Kariks J, Cardiac lesions in sudden infant death syndrome. *Forensic Sci Int* **39**, 211–215, 1988.

32. Money DFL, Vitamin E and selenium deficiencies and their possible aetological role in the sudden infant death syndrome. *NZ Med J* **71**, 32–34, 1970.

33. Lemke R, Schafer A, and Makropoulos W, Postmortem serum selenium concentrations and their possible etiological role in sudden infant death (SID). *Forensic Sci Int* **60**, 179–182, 1993.

34. Centers for Disease Control, Selenium intoxication. *MMWR* **33**, 157, 1984.

30 Silicon

1. Brown ML (ed.), *Present Knowledge in Nutrition, 6th Edition*. International Life Sciences Institute, Nutrition Foundation. Washington, DC, 1990, pp. 301–302.

2. Nielsen FH, Ultratrace elements in nutrition. *Annu Rev Nutr* **4**, 21–41, 1984.

3. Fessenden RJ and Fessenden JS, The biological properties of silicon compounds. *Adv Drug Res* **4**, 95, 1987.

4. Lassus A, Colloidal silicic acid for oral and topical treatment of aged skin, fragile hair and brittle nails in females. *J Int Med Res* **21**, 209–215, 1993.

5. Hershey CO, Hershey LA, Varnes A, *et al.*, Cerebrospinal fluid trace element content in dementia: Clinical, radiologic, and pathologic correlations. *Neurology* **33**, 1350–1353, 1983.

6. Candy JM, Klinowski J, Perry RH, *et al.*, Aluminosilicates and senile plaque formation in Alzheimer's disease. *Lancet* **i**, 354–357, 1986.

31 Vanadium

1. Harland BF and Harden-Williams BA, Is vanadium of human nutritional importance yet? *J Am Diet Assoc* **94**, 891–894, 1994.

2. Brichard SM and Henquin JC, The role of vanadium in the management of diabetes. *Trends Pharmacol Sci* **16**, 265–270, 1995.

3. Cohen N, *et al.*, Oral vanadyl sulfate improves hepatic and peripheral insulin sensitivity in patients with non-insulin-dependent diabetes mellitus. *J Clin Invest* **95**, 2501–2509, 1995.

32 Understanding Fats and Oils

1. Willett WC, *et al.*, Intake of trans fatty acids and risk of coronary heart disease among women. *Lancet* **341**, 581–585, 1993.

2. Longnecker MP, Do trans fatty acids in margarine and other foods increase the risk of coronary heart disease? *Epidemiology* **4**, 492–495, 1993.

3. Booyens J and Van Der Merwe CF, Margarines and coronary artery disease. *Med Hypothesis* **37**, 241–244, 1992.

4. Mensink RP and Katan MB, Effect of dietary trans fatty acids on high-density and low-density lipoprotein cholesterol levels in healthy subjects. *New Engl J Med* **323**, 439–445, 1990.

5. Robbins SL, Cotran RS, and Kumar V, *Pathologic Basis of Disease, 3rd Edition*. WB Saunders, Philadelphia, PA, 1984, p. 9.

6. Pelikanova T, *et al.*, Fatty acid composition of serum lipids and erythrocyte membranes in type 2 (non-insulin-dependent) diabetic men. *Metab Clin Exp* **40**, 175–180, 1991.

7. National Research Council, Diet and Health. *Implications for Reducing Chronic Disease Risk*. National Academy Press, Washington, DC, 1989.

8. Borkman M, *et al.*, The relationship between insulin sensitivity and the fatty acid composition of skeletal-muscle phospholipids. *N Engl J Med* **328**, 238–244, 1993.

9. Pelikanova T, *et al.*, Insulin secretion and insulin action are related to the serum phospholipid fatty acid pattern in healthy men. *Metab Clin Exp* **38**, 188–192, 1989.

10. Feskens EJM, Bowles CH, and Kromhout D, Inverse association between fish intake and risk of glucose intolerance in normoglycemic elderly men and women. *Diabetes Care* **14**, 935–941, 1991.

11. Storlien LH, *et al.*, Influence of dietary fat composition on the development of insulin resistance in rats, relation to muscle triglyceride and omega-3 fatty acids in muscle phospholipid. *Diabetes* **40**, 280–289, 1991.

12. Vessby B, *et al.*, The risk to develop NIDDM is related to the fatty acid composition of the serum cholesterol esters. *Diabetes* **43**, 1353–1357, 1994.

13. Hennekens CH and Gaziano JM, Antioxidants and heart disease: Epidemiology and clinical evidence. *Clin Cardiol* **16** (Suppl. 1), 10–15, 1993.

14. Stahelin HB, *et al.*, Plasma antioxidant vitamins and subsequent cancer mortality in the 12-year follow-up of the prospective Basel Study. *Am J epidemiol* **133**, 766–775, 1991.

15. Diplock AT, Antioxidant nutrients and disease prevention: An overview. *Am J Clin Nutr* **53**, 189S–193S, 1991.

33 Essential Fatty Acid Supplementation

1. Nettleton JA, Omega-3 fatty acids: Comparison of plant and seafood sources in human nutrition. *J Am Diet Assoc* **91**, 331–337, 1991.

2. Cunnane SC, *et al.*, Alpha-linolenic acid in humans: Direct functional role or dietary precursor. *Nutrition* **7**, 437–439, 1991.
3. Mantzioris E, *et al.*, Dietary substitution with alpha-linolenic acid-rich vegetable oil increases eicosapentaenoic acid concentrations in tissues. *Am J Clin Nutr* **59**, 1304–1309, 1994.
4. Janti J, Evening primrose oil in rheumatoid arthritis: Changes in serum lipids and fatty acids. *Annals Rheum Dis* **48**, 124–127, 1989.
5. The Gamma-Linolenic Acid Multicenter Trial Group, Treatment of diabetic neuropathy with gamma-linolenic acid. *Diabetes Care* **16**, 8–15, 1993.
6. Schlomo Y and Carasso RL, Modulation of learning, pain thresholds, and thermoregulation in the rat by preparations of free purified alpha-linolenic and linoleic acids: Determination of the optimal w3-to-w6 ratio. *Proc Natl Acad Sci* **90**, 10345–10347 ,1993.
7. Von Schacky C, Prophylaxis of atherosclerosis with marine omega-3 fatty acids. A comprehensive strategy. *Annals Int Med* **107**, 890–899, 1987.
8. Simopoulos AP, Omega-3 fatty acids in health and disease and in growth and development. *Am J Clin Nutr* **54**, 438–463, 1991.
9. Bjerve KS, *et al.*, Clinical studies with alpha-linolenic acid and long chain n-3 fatty acids. *Nutrition* **8**, 130–132, 1992.
10. Bierenbaum ML, *et al.*, Reducing atherogenic risk in hyperlipemic humans with flax seed supplementation: A preliminary report. *J Am Coll Nutr* **12**, 501–504, 1993.
11. Schmidt EB and Dyerberg J, Omega-3 fatty acids: Current status in cardiovascular medicine. *Drugs* **47**, 405–424, 1994.
12. Cobias L, *et al.*, Lipid, lipoprotein, and hemostatic effects of fish vs fish oil w-3 fatty acids in mildly hyperlipidemic males. *Am J Clin Nutr* **53**, 1210–1216, 1991.
13. Shukla VKS and Perkins EG, The presence of oxidative polymeric materials in encapsulated fish oils. *Lipids* **26**, 23–26, 1991.
14. Fritshe KL and Johnston PV, Rapid autoxidation of fish oil in diets without added antioxidants. *J Nutr* **118**, 425–426, 1988.
15. Harats D, *et al.*, Fish oil ingestion in smokers and nonsmokers enhances peroxidation of plasma lipoproteins. *Atherosclerosis* **90**, 127–139, 1991.
16. Kromann N and Green A. Epidemiological studies in the Upernavik district, Greenland. *Acta Med Scand* **208**, 401–406, 1980.
17. Kromhout D, Bosscheiter EB, and De Lezenne-Coulander C, Inverse relation between fish oil consumption and 20 year mortality from coronary heart disease. *N Engl J Med* **312**, 1205–1209, 1985.
18. Seidelin KN, Myrup B, and Fischer-Hansen B, N-3 fatty acids in adipose tissue and coronary artery disease are inversely correlated. *Am J Clin Nutr* **55**, 1117–1119, 1992.
19. Ornish D, *et al.*, Can lifestyle changes reverse coronary heart disease. *Lancet* **336** 129–133, 1990.
20. Burr ML, *et al.*, Effects of changes in fat, fish, and fiber intakes on death and myocardial reinfarction: Diet and reinfarction trial (DART). *Lancet* **334**, 757–761, 1989.
21. de Lorgeril M, *et al.*, Mediterranean alpha-linolenic acid-rich diet in secondary prevention of coronary heart disease. *Lancet* **343** 1454–1459, 1994.
22. Sandker GN, *et al.*, Serum cholesterol ester fatty acids and their relation with serum lipids in elderly men in Crete and the Netherlands. *Eur J Clin Nutr* **47**, 201–208, 1993.
23. Kagawa Y, *et al.*, Eicosapolyenoic acids of serum lipids of Japanese Islanders with low incidence of cardiovascular diseases. *J Nutr Sci Vitaminol* **28**, 441–453, 1982.
24. Ernst E, Fibrinogen: An important risk factor for atherothrombotic diseases. *Annals Med* **26**, 15–22, 1994.
25. Radack K, Deck C, and Huster G, The comparative effects of n-3 and n-6 polyunsaturated fatty acids on plasma fibrinogen levels: A controlled clinical trial in hypertriglyeridemic subjects. *J Am Coll Nutr* **9**, 352–357, 1990.
26. Schmidt EB and Dyerberg J, Omega-3 fatty acids. Current status in cardiovascular medicine. *Drugs* **47**, 405–424, 1994.
27. Appel LJ, *et al.*, Does supplementation of diet with "fish oil" reduce blood pressure? A meta-analysis of controlled clinical trials. *Arch Intern Med* **153**, 1429–1438, 1993.

28. Singer P, Alpha-linolenic acid vs. long-chain fatty acids in hypertension and hyperlipidemia. *Nutrition* **8**, 133–135, 1992.
29. Chan JK, Bruce VM, and McDonald BE, Dietary-alpha-linolenic acid is as effective as oleic acid and linoleic acid in lowering blood cholesterol in normolipidemic men. *Am J Clin Nutr* **53**, 1230–1234, 1991.
30. Berry EM and Hirsch J, Does dietary linolenic acid influence blood pressure. *Am J Clin Nutr* **44**, 336–340, 1986.
31. Jantti J, *et al.*, Evening primrose oil in rheumatoid arthritis: Changes in serum lipids and fatty acids. *Annals Rheum Dis* **48**, 124–127, 1989.
32. Brzeski M, Madhok R, and Capell HA, Evening primrose oil in patients with rheumatoid arthritis and side effects of non-steroidal anti-inflammatory drugs. *Br J Rheumatol* **30**, 371–372, 1991.
33. Belch JF, *et al.*, Effects of altering dietary essential fatty acids on requirements for non-steroidal anti-inflammatory drugs in patients with rheumatoid arthritis: A double blind placebo controlled study. *Annals Rheum Dis* **47**, 96–104, 1988.
34. Levanthal LJ, *et al.*, Treatment of rheumatoid arthritis with gammalinoleic acid. *Annals Int Med* **119**, 867–873, 1993.
35. Kremer J, *et al.*, Effects of manipulation of dietary fatty acids on clinical manifestation of rheumatoid arthritis. *Lancet* **i**, 184–187, 1985.
36. Kremer J, *et al.*, Fish-oil supplementation in active rheumatoid arthritis: A double-blinded, controlled cross-over study. *Ann Intern Med* **106**, 497–502, 1987.
37. Sperling R, *et al.*, Effects of dietary supplementation with marine fish oil on leukocyte lipid mediator generation and function in rheumatoid arthritis. *Arth Rheum* **30**, 988–997, 1987.
38. Cleland LG, *et al.*, Clinical and biochemical effects of dietary fish oil supplements in rheumatoid arthritis. *J Rheumatol* **15**, 1471–1475, 1988.
39. Magaro M, *et al.*, Influence of diet with different lipid composition on neutrophil composition on neutrophil chemiluminescence and disease activity in patients with rheumatoid arthritis. *Annals Rheum Dis* **47**, 793–796, 1988.
40. van der Temple H, *et al.*, Effects of fish oil supplementation in rheumatoid arthritis. *Annals Rheum Dis* **49**, 76–80, 1990.
41. Kremer JM, *et al.*, Dietary fish oil and olive oil supplementation in patients with rheumatoid arthritis. *Arth Rheum* **33**, 810–820, 1990.
42. Lau CS, *et al.*, Maxepa on nonsteroidal anti-inflammatory drug usage in patients with mild rheumatoid arthritis. *Br J Rheumatol* **30**, 137, 1991.
43. Nielsen GL, *et al.*, The effects of dietary supplementation with n-3 polyunsaturated fatty acids in patients with rheumatoid arthritis: A randomized, double-blind trial. *Eur J Clin Invest* **22**, 687–791, 1992.
44. Nordstrom DCE, *et al.*, Alpha-linolenic acid in the treatment of rheumatoid arthritis. A double-blind placebo-controlled and randomized study: flaxseed vs. safflower oil. *Rheumatol Int* **14**, 231–234, 1995.
45. Kelley DS, Alpha-linolenic acid and immune response. *Nutrition* **8**, 215–217, 1992.
46. Simopoulos AP, Omega-3 fatty acids in health and disease and in growth and development. *Am J Clin Nutr* **54**, 438–463, 1991.
47. Cunane SC (ed.), Symposium Proceedings: Third Toronto Essential Fatty Acid Workshop on Alpha-Linolenic Acid in Human Nutrition and Disease. May 17–18, 1991, University of Toronto, Toronto, Ontario, Canada. *Nutrition* **7**, 435, 446, 1991.
48. Swank RL, Multiple sclerosis: Fat-oil relationship. *Nutrition* **7**, 368–376, 1991.
49. Swank RL and Pullen MH, *The Multiple Sclerosis Diet Book*. Doubleday, Garden City, NY, 1977.
50. Millar ZHD, Zilkha KJ, Langman MJS, *et al.*, Double-blind trial of linolate supplementation of the diet in multiple sclerosis. *Br Med J* **i**, 765–768, 1973.
51. Bates D, Fawcett PRW, Shaw DA, and Weightman D, Polyunsaturated fatty acids in treatment of acute remitting multiple sclerosis. *Br Med J* **ii**, 1390, 1391, 1978.
52. Paty DW, Cousin HK, Read S, and Adlakkha K, Linoleic acid in multiple sclerosis: Failure to show any therapeutic benefit. *Acta Neurol Scand* **58**, 53–58, 1978.

53. Swank RL, *et al.*, Multiple sclerosis in rural Norway: Its geographic distribution and occupational incidence in relation to nutrition. *NEJM* **246**, 721–728, 1952.
54. Esparza ML, Sasaki S, and Kesteloot H, Nutrition, latitude, and multiple sclerosis: An ecological study. *Am J epidemiol* **142**, 733–737, 1995.
55. Horrobin DF, Multiple sclerosis: The rational basis for treatment with colchicine and evening primrose oil. *Med Hypothesis* **5**, 365–378, 1979.
56. Bates D, *et al.*, Polyunsaturated fatty acids in treatment of acute remitting multiple sclerosis. *Br Med J* **ii**, 1390, 1391, 1978.
57. Thompson LU, *et al.*, Mammalian lignan production from various foods. *Nutr Cancer* **16**, 43–52, 1991.
58. Setchell KDR and Adlercreutz H, Mammalian lignans and phytoestrogens: Recent studies on their formation, metabolism, and biological role in health and disease. *Role of Gut Flora in Toxicology and Cancer*, Rowland IR (ed.). Academic Press, London, UK, 1988, pp. 315–343.
59. Lampe JW, *et al.*, Urinary lignan and isoflavonoid excretion in premenopausal women consuming flaxseed powder. *Am J Clin Nutr* **60**, 122–128, 1994.
60. Serraino M and Thompson LU, The effect of flaxseed on early risk markers for mammary carcinogenesis. *Cancer Letters* **60**, 135–142, 1991.
61. Serraino M and Thompson LU, Flaxseed supplementation and early markers of colon carcinogenesis. *Cancer Letters* **63**, 159–165, 1992.
62. Serraino M and Thompson LU, The effect of flaxseed supplementation on the initiation and promotional stages of mammary tumorigenesis. *Nutr Cancer* **17**, 153–159, 1992.
63. Adlercreutz H, *et al.*, Determination of urinary lignans and phytoestrogen metabolites, potential antiestrogens and anticarcinogens, in urine of women in various habitual diets. *J Steroid Biochem* **25**, 791–797, 1986.
64. Bougnoix P, *et al.*, Alpha-linolenic acid content of adipose breast tissue: A host determinant of the risk of early metastasis in breast cancer. *Br J Cancer* **70**, 330–334, 1994.
65. Rose DP and Hatala MA, Dietary fatty acids and breast cancer invasion and metastasis. *Nutr Cancer* **21**, 103–111, 1994.
66. Kelley DS, Alpha-linolenic acid and immune response. *Nutrition* **8**, 215–217, 1992.
67. Benquet C, *et al.*, Modulation of exercise-induced immunosuppression by dietary polyunsaturated fatty acids in mice. *J Toxicol Env Health* **43**, 225–237, 1994.
68. Enig MG, Trans tatty acids: An update. *Nutrition Quarterly* **17**, 79–95, 1993.
69. King J, Geary B, and List GR, A solution thermodynamic study of soybean oil/solvent systems by inverse gas chromatography. *JAOCS* **67**, 424–230, 1990.
70. Fabio F, Mazzanti M, and King J, Super critical carbon dioxide extraction of evening primrose oil. *JAOCS* **68**, 422–427, 1991.
71. List GR, Friedrich JP, and King J, Oxidative stability of seed oils extracted with supercritical carbon dioxide. *JAOCS* **66**, 98–100, 1989.
72. List GR, Friedrich JP and King J, Supercritical CO_2 extraction and processing of oilseeds. *Oil Mill Gazette* **Dec**, 28–34, 1989.
73. Stitt P, Efficacy of feeding flax to humans and other animals. *Proceedings Flax Institute* **52**, 37–40, 1988.
74. Carter JF, Potential of flaxseed and flaxseed oil in baked goods and other products in human nutrition. *Cereal Foods World* **38**, 753–759, 1993.

34 Carnitine

1. Bremer J, Carnitine—metabolism and function. *Physiol Rev* **63**, 1420–1480, 1983.
2. Bamji MS, Nutritional and health implications of lysine carnitine relationship. *Wld Rev Nutr Diet* **44**, 185–211, 1984.
3. Borum PR, Carnitine. *Ann Rev Nutr* **3**, 233–259, 1983.
4. Carter HE, *et al.*, Chemical studies on vitamin BT isolation and characterization as carnitine. *Arch Biochem Biophys* **38**, 405–416, 1952.

5. Scholte HR, Stinis JT, and Jennekens FGI, Low carnitine levels in serum of pregnant women. *NEJM* **299**, 1079, 1080, 1979.

6. Cederblad G, Fahraeus L, and Lindgren K, Plasma carnitine and renal-carnitine clearance during pregnancy. *Am J Clin Nutr* **44**, 379–383, 1986.

7. Warshaw JB and Curry E, Comparison of serum carnitine and ketone body concentrations in breast and in formula-fed infants. *J Pediatr* **97**, 122–125, 1980.

8. Ardissone P, et al., The effects of treatment with L-carnitine of hypoglycemia in pre-term AGA infants. *Curr Ther Res* **38**, 256–264, 1985.

9. Engel AG and Angelini C, Carnitine deficiency of human skeletal muscle with associated lipid storage myopathy: A new syndrome. *Science* **179**, 899–902, 1973.

10. Borum PR and Bennett SG, Carnitine as an essential nutrient. *J Am Coll Nutr* **5**, 177–182, 1986.

11. Gilbert EF, Carnitine deficiency. *Pathology* **17**, 161–169, 1985.

12. Winter SC, et al., Plasma carnitine deficiency, clinical observations in 51 pediatric patients. *AJDC* **141**, 660–665, 1987.

13. Glasgow AM, Eng G, and Engel AG, Systemic carnitine deficiency simulating recurrent Reye syndrome. *J Pediatr* **96**, 889–891, 1980.

14. Chapoy PR, et al., Systemic carnitine deficiency: A treatable inherited lipid storage disease presenting as Reye's syndrome. *NEJM* **303**, 1389–1394, 1980.

15. Rebouche CJ and Engel AG, Carnitine metabolism and deficiency syndromes. *Mayo Clin Proc* **58**, 533–540, 1983.

16. Siliprandi N, et al., Transport and function of L-carnitine and L-propionylcarnitine: Relevance to some cardiac myopathies and cardiac ischemia. *Z Cardiol* **76** (Suppl. 5), 34–40, 1987.

17. Paulson DJ, et al., Protection of the ischaemic myocardium by L-propionylcarnitine: Effects on the recovery of cardiac output after ischaemia and repurfusion, carnitine transport, and fatty acid oxidation. *Cardiovasc Res* **20**, 356–341, 1986.

18. Opie LH, Role of carnitine in fatty acid metabolism of normal and ischemic myocardium. *Am Heart J* **97**, 373–378, 1979.

19. Goa KL and Brogden RN, L-carnitine—A preliminary review of its pharmacokinetics, and its therapeutic use in ischemic cardiac disease and primary and secondary carnitine deficiencies in relationship to its role in fatty acid metabolism. *Drugs* **34**, 1–24, 1987.

20. Pola P, et al., Statistical evaluation of long-term L-carnitine therapy in hyperlipoproteinemias. *Drugs Exp Clin Res* **9**, 925–934, 1983.

21. Pola P, et al., Carnitine in the therapy of dyslipidemic patients. *Curr Ther Res* **27**, 208–215, 1980.

22. Silverman NA, Schmitt G, Vishwanath M, et al., Effect of carnitine on myocardial function and metabolism following global ischemia. *Ann Thor Surg* **40**, 20–25, 1985.

23. Cherchi A, et al., Effects of L-carnitine on exercise tolerance in chronic stable angina: A multicenter, double-blind, randomized, placebo controlled crossover study. *Int J Clin Pharm Ther Tox* **23**, 569–572, 1985.

24. Orlando G and Rusconi C, Oral L-carnitine in the treatment of chronic cardiac ischemia in elderly patients. *Clin Trials J* **23**, 338–344, 1986.

25. Kamikawa T, et al., Effects of L-carnitine on exercise tolerance in patients with stable angina pectoris. *Jap Heart J* **25**, 587–597, 1984.

26. Kosolcharoen P, et al., Improved exercise tolerance after administration of carnitine. *Curr Ther Res* **30**, 753–764, 1981.

27. Pola P, et al., Use of physiological substance, acetyl-carnitine, in the treatment of angiospastic syndromes. *Drugs Exp Clin Res* **X**, 213–217, 1984.

28. Lagioia R, et al., Propionyl-L-carnitine: A new compound in the metabolic approach to the treatment of effort angina. *Int J Cardiol* **34**, 167–172, 1992.

29. Bartels GL, et al., Effects of L-propionylcarnitine on ischemia-induced myocardial dysfunction in men with angina pectoris. *Am J Cardiol* **74**, 125–130, 1994.

30. Cacciatore L, et al., The therapeutic effect of L-carnitine in patients with exercise-induced stable angina: A controlled study. *Drugs Exp Clin Res* **17**, 225–335, 1991.

31. Davini P, et al., Controlled study on L-carnitine therapeutic efficacy in post-infarction. *Drugs Exp Clin Res* **18**, 355–365, 1992.

32. Iliceto S, et al., Effects of L-carnitine administration on left ventricular remodeling after acute anterior myocardial infarction: The L-Carnitine Ecocardiografia Digitalizzata Infarto Miocardico (CEDIM) Trial. *J Am Coll Cardiol* **26**, 380–387, 1995.

33. Mancini M, et al., Controlled study on the therapeutic efficacy of propionyl-L-carnitine in patients with congestive heart failure. *Arzneim Forsch* **42**, 1101–1104, 1992.

34. Pucciarelli G, et al., The clinical and hemodynamic effects of propionyl-L-carnitine in the treatment of congestive heart failure. *Clin Ther* **141**, 379–384, 1992.

35. Brevetti G, et al., Superiority of L-propionylcarnitine vs L-carnitine in improving walking capacity in patients with peripheral vascular disease: An acute, intravenous, double-blind, cross-over study. *Eur Heart J* **13**, 251–255, 1992.

36. Sabba C, et al., Comparison between the effect of L-propionylcarnitine, L-acetylcarnitine and nitroglycerin in chronic peripheral arterial disease: A haemodynamic double blind echo-Doppler study. *Eur Heart J* **15**, 1348–1352, 1994.

37. Brevetti G, et al., Increases in walking distance in patients with peripheral vascular disease treated with L-carnitine: A double-blind, cross-over study. *Circulation* **77**, 767–773, 1988.

38. Dragan AM, et al., Studies concerning some acute biological changes after exogenous administration of 1 g L-carnitine in elite athletes. *Physiologie* **24**, 231–234, 1987.

39. Dragan GI, et al., Studies concerning acute and chronic effects of L-carnitine on some biological parameters. *Physiologie* **24**, 23–28, 1987.

40. Dragan GI, Wagner W, and Ploesteanu E, Studies concerning the ergogenic value of protein supply and L-carnitine in elite junior cyclists. *Physiologie* **25**, 129–132, 1988.

41. Soop M, et al., Influence of carnitine supplementation on muscle substrate and carnitine metabolism during exercise. *J Appl Physiol* **64**, 2394–2399, 1988.

42. Greig C, et al., The effect of oral supplementation with L-carnitine on maximum and submaximum exercise capacity. *Eur J Appl Physiol* **54**, 131–135, 1985.

43. Marconi C, et al., Effects of L-carnitine loading on the aerobic and anaerobic performance of endurance athletes. *Eur J Appl Physiol* **54**, 131–135, 1985.

44. Huertas R, et al., Respiratory chain enzymes in muscle of endurance athletes: Effect of L-carnitine. *Biochem Biophys Res Comm* **188**, 102–107, 1992.

45. Dal Negro R, et al., Changes in physical performance of untrained volunteers: effects of L-carnitine. *Clin Trials J* **23**, 242–248, 1986.

46. Bowman B, Acetyl-carnitine and Alzheimer's disease. *Nutrition Reviews* **50**, 142–144, 1992.

47. Carta A, et al., Acetyl-L-carnitine and Alzheimer's disease. Pharmacological considerations beyond the cholinergic sphere. *Ann NY Acad Sci* **695**, 324–326, 1993.

48. Calvani M, et al., Action of acetyl-L-carnitine in neurodegneration and Alzheimer's disease. *Ann NY Acad Sci* **663**, 483–486, 1993.

49. Pettegrew JW, et al., Clinical and neurochemical effects of acetyl-L-carnitine in Alzheimer's disease. *Neurobiol Aging* 16, 1–4, 1995.

50. Sano M, et al., Double-blind parallel design pilot study of acetyl levocarnitine in patients with Alzheimer's disease. *Arch Neurol* **49**, 1137–1141, 1992.

51. Spagnoli A, et al., Long-term acetyl-L-carnitine treatment in Alzheimer's disease. *Neurology* **41**, 1726–1732, 1991.

52. Vecchi GP, et al., Acetyl-L-carnitine treatment of mental impairment in the elderly: Evidence from a multicenter study. *Arch Gerontol Geriatr* **2** (Suppl.), 159–168, 1991.

53. Salvioli G and Neri M, L-acetylcarnitine treatment of mental decline in the elderly. *Drugs Exp Clin Res* **20**, 169–176, 1994.

54. Cipolli C and Chiari G, Effects of L-acetylcarnitine on mental deterioration in the aged: Initial results. *Clin Ther* **132**, 479–510, 1990.

55. Garyza G, et al., Evaluation of the effects of L-acetylcarnitine on senile patients suffering from depression. *Drugs Exp Clin Res* **101**–106, 1990.

56. Tempesta E, et al., L-acetylcarnitine in depressed elderly subjects. A cross-over study vs. placebo. *Drugs Exp Clin Res* **8**, 417–423, 1987.

57. De Falco FA, *et al.*, Effect of the chronic treatment with L-acetylcarnitine in Down's syndrome. *Clin Ther* **144**, 123–127, 1994.

58. Gjuarnieri GF, *et al.*, Lipid-lowering effect of carnitine in chronically uremic patients treated with maintenance hemodialysis. *Am J Clin Nutr* **33**, 1489–1492, 1980.

59. Lacour B, *et al.*, Carnitine improves lipid abnormalities in haemodialysis patients. *Lancet* ii:763–765, 1980.

60. Bertoli M, *et al.*, Carnitine deficiency induced during hemodialysis and hyperlipidemia: Effect of replacement therapy. *Am J Clin Nutr* **34**, 1496–1500, 1981.

61. Vacha GM, *et al.*, Favorable effects of L-carnitine treatment on hypertriglyceridemia in hemodialysis patients: Decisive role of low levels of high-density lipo-protein cholesterol. *Am J Clin Nutr* **38**, 532–540, 1983.

62. Bellinghieri G, *et al.*, Correlation between increased serum and tissue L-carnitine levels and improved muscle symptoms in hemodialyzed patients. *Am J Clin Nutr* **38**, 523–531, 1983.

63. Donatelli M, *et al.*, Effects of L-carnitine on chronic anemia and erythrocyte adenosine triphosphate concentration in hemodialyzed patients. *Curr Ther Res* **41**, 620–624, 1987.

64. Golper TA, *et al.*, Multicenter trial of L-carnitine in maintenance hemodialysis. *Kidney International* **38**, 904–918, 1990.

65. Labonia D, L-carnitine effects on anemia in hemodialyzed patients treated with erythropoietin. *Am J Kidney Dis* **26**, 757–764, 1995.

66. Cederblad G, Hermansson G, and Ludvigsson J, Plasma and urine carnitine in children with diabetes mellitus. *Clin Chim Acta* **125**, 207–217, 1982.

67. Greco AV, *et al.*, Effect of propionyl-L-carnitine in the treatment of diabetic angiopathy: Controlled double blind trial versus placebo. *Drugs Exp Clin Res* **18**, 69–80, 1992.

68. Sachan DS, Rhew TH, and Ruark RA, Ameliorating effects of carnitine and its precursors on alcohol-induced fatty liver. *Am J Clin Nutr* **39**, 738–744, 1984.

69. Sachan DA and Rhew TH, Lipotropic effect of carnitine on alcohol-induced hepatic stenosis. *Nutr Rep Int* **27**, 1221–1226, 1983.

70. Noto R, *et al.*, Free fatty acids and carnitine in patients with liver disease. *Curr Ther Res* **40**, 35–39, 1986.

71. Borum PR, Broquist HP, and Roelofs RI, Muscle carnitine levels in neuromuscular disease. *J Neurol Sci* **34**, 279–286, 1977.

72. Carrier HN and Berthiller G, Carnitine levels in normal children and adults and in patients with diseased muscle. *Muscle Nerve* **3**, 326–334, 1980.

73. Bresolin N, *et al.*, Carnitine and acyltransferase in experimental neurogenic atrophies: Changes with treatment. *J Neurol* **231**, 170–175, 1984.

74. Bornman MS, *et al.*, Seminal carnitine, epididymal function and spermatozoal motility. *S Afr Med J* **75**, 20, 21, 1989.

75. Menchini Fabris GF, *et al.*, Free L-carnitine in human semen: Its variability in different andologic pathologies. *Fertil Steril* **42**, 263–267, 1984.

76. Costa M, *et al.*, L-carnitine in idiopathic asthenozoospermia: A multicenter study. *Andrologia* **26**, 155–159, 1994.

77. Dal Negro R, *et al.*, L-carnitine and physiokinesiotherapy in chronic respiratory insufficiency. *Clinical Trials J* **22**, 353–360, 1985.

78. De Simone C, *et al.*, Carnitine depletion in peripheral blood mononuclear cells from patients with AIDS: Effect of oral L-carnitine. *AIDS* **8**, 655–660, 1994.

79. Semino-Mora MC, *et al.*, Effect of L-carnitine on the zidovidine-induced destruction of human myotubes. *Lab Invest* **71**, 102–112, 1994.

80. De Simone C, *et al.*, High dose L-carnitine improves immunologic and metabolic parameters in AIDS patients. *Immunopharmacol Immunotoxicol* **15**, 1–12, 1993.

81. Seccombe DW, James L, and Booth F, L-carnitine treatment in glutaric aciduria type I. *Neurology* **36**, 264–267, 1986.

82. Sousa CD, *et al.*, The response to L-carnitine and glycine therapy in isovaleric acidemia. *Eur J Pediatr* **144**, 451–456, 1986.

83. Roe CR and Bohon TP, L-carnitine therapy in propionicacidemia. *Lancet* **i**, 1411–1412, 1982.

84. Roe CR, *et al.*, Metabolic response to carnitine in methylmalonic aciduria. *Arch Dis Child* **58**, 916–920, 1983.

85. Furitano G, *et al.*, Polygraphic evaluation of effects of carnitine in patients on Adriamycin treatment. *Drugs Exp Clin Res* **10**, 107–111, 1984.

86. O'Conner JE, *et al.*, Influence of the route of administration on the protective effect of L-carnitine on acute hyperammonemia. *Biochem Pharmacol* **18**, 3173–3176, 1986.

87. Matsuda I, Ohtani Y, and Ninomiya N, Renal handling of carnitine in children with carnitine deficiency and hyperammonemia associated with valproate therapy. *J Pediatr* **109**, 131–134, 1986.

88. Freeman JM, Does carnitine administration improve the symptoms attributed to anticonvulsant medications? A double-blinded, crossover study. *Pediatrics* **93**, 893–895, 1994.

89. Weschler A, *et al.*, High dose of L-carnitine increases platelet aggregation and plasma triglyceride levels in uremic patients on hemodialysis. *Nephron* **38**, 120–124, 1984.

90. Bazzato G, *et al.*, Myasthenia-like syndrome associated with carnitine in patients on long-term dialysis. *Lancet* i, 1041–1042, 1979.

91. Paulson DJ and Shug AL, Tissue specific depletion of L-carnitine in rat heart and skeletal muscle by D-carnitine. *Life Sci* **28**, 2931–2938, 1981.

92. Watanable S, *et al.*, Effects of L- and DL-carnitine on patients with impaired exercise tolerance. *Jap Heart J* **36**, 319–331, 1995.

93. Bertelli A, *et al.*, L-carnitine and coenzyme Q_{10} protective action against ischaemia and reperfusion of working rat heart. *Drugs Exp Clin Res* **18**, 431–436, 1992.

94. Gleeson JM, *et al.*, Effect of carnitine and pantethine on the metabolic abnormalities of acquired total lipodystrophy. *Curr Ther Res* **41**, 83–88, 1987.

95. Daily JW III; Sachan DS, Choline supplementation alters carnitine homeostasis in humans and guinea pigs. *J Nutr* **125**, 1938–1944, 1995.

35 Coenzyme Q_{10}

1. Frei B, Kim MC, and Ames BN, Ubiquinol-10 is an effective lipid-soluble antioxidant at physiological concentrations. *Proc Natl Acad Sci* **87**, 4879–4883, 1990.

2. Weber C, *et al.*, Effect of dietary coenzyme Q_{10} as an antioxidant in human plasma. *Mol Aspects Med* **15** (Suppl.), S97–S102, 1994.

3. Weber C, *et al.*, Antioxidative effect of dietary coenzyme Q_{10} in human blood plasma. *Int J Vitam Nutr Res* **64**, 311–315, 1994.

4. Littarru GP, *et al.*, Metabolic implications of coenzyme Q_{10} in red blood cells and plasma lipoproteins. *Mol Aspects Med* **15** (Suppl.), S67–S72, 1994.

5. Alleva R, *et al.*, The roles of coenzyme Q_{10} and vitamin E on the peroxidation of human low density lipoprotein subfractions. *Proc Natl Acad Sci USA* **92**, 9388–9891, 1995.

6. Weis M, Bioavailability of four oral coenzyme Q_{10} formulations in healthy volunteers. *Mol Aspects Med* **15** (Suppl.), S273–S280, 1994.

7. Kitamura N, *et al.*, Myocardial tissue level of coenzyme Q_{10} in patients with cardiac failure. In: *Biomedical and Clinical Aspects of Coenzyme Q, Vol 4*. Folkers K and Yamamura Y (eds.). Elsevier Science Publ, Amsterdam, 1984, pp. 243–252.

8. Littarru GP, Ho L and Folkers K, Deficiency of coenzyme Q_{10} in human heart disease, Part II. *Int J Vit Nutr Res* **42**, 413, 1972.

9. Folkers K, *et al.*, Evidence for a deficiency of coenzyme Q_{10} in human heart disease. *Int J Vit Res* **40**, 380, 1970.

10. Folkers K, Vadhanavikit S, and Mortensen SA, Biochemical rationale and myocardial tissue data on the effective therapy of cardiomyopathy with coenzyme Q_{10}. *Proc Natl Acad Sci* **82**, 901, 1985.

11. Langsjoen H, *et al.*, Usefulness of coenzyme Q_{10} in clinical cardiology: A long-term study. *Mol Aspects Med* **15** (Suppl.), S165–S175, 1994.

12. Ishiyama T, *et al.*, A clinical study of the effect of coenzyme Q on congestive heart failure. *Jap Heart J* **17**, 32, 1976.

13. Tsuyusaki T, Noro C, and Kikawada R, Mechanocardiography of ischemic or hypertensive heart failure. In: *Biomedical and Clinical Aspects of Coenzyme Q, Vol 2*. Yamamura Y, Folkers K, and Ito Y, (eds.). Elsevier/North-Holland Biomedical Press, Amsterdam, 1980, pp. 273–288.

14. Judy WV, *et al.*, Myocardial effects of Co-enzyme Q_{10} in primary heart failure. In: *Biomedical and Clinical Aspects of Coenzyme Q, Vol 4*. Folkers K and Yamamura Y (eds.). Elsevier Science Publ, Amsterdam, 1984, pp. 353–367.

15. Vanfraechem JHP, Picalausa C, and Folkers K, Coenzyme Q_{10} and physical performance in myocardial failure. In: *Biomedical and Clinical Aspects of Coenzyme Q, Vol 4*. Folkers K and Yamamura Y (eds.). Elsevier Science Publ, Amsterdam, 1984, pp. 281–290.

16. Hofman-Bang C, Rehnquist N, and Swedberg K, Coenzyme Q_{10} as an adjunctive treatment of congestive heart failure. *J Am Coll Cardiol* **19**, 216A, 1992.

17. Morisco C, Trimarco B, and Condorelli M, Effect of coenzyme Q_{10} therapy in patients with congestive heart failure: A long-term multicenter randomized study. *Clin Invest* **71** (Suppl. 8), S134–S136, 1993.

18. Baggio E, *et al.*, Italian multicenter study on the safety and efficacy of coenzyme Q_{10} as adjunctive therapy in heart failure. CoQ_{10} Drug Surveillance Investigators. *Mol Aspects Med* **15** (Suppl.), S287–S294, 1994.

19. Digiesi V, *et al.*, Mechanism of action of coenzyme Q_{10} in essential hypertension. *Curr Ther Res* **51**, 668–672, 1992.

20. Langsjoen P, *et al.*, Treatment of essential hypertension with coenzyme Q_{10}. *Mol Aspects Med* **15** (Suppl.), S265–S272, 1994.

21. Digiesi V, *et al.*, Coenzyme Q_{10} in essential hypertension. *Mol Aspects Med* **15** (Suppl.), S257–S263, 1994.

22. Langsjoen PH, Vadhanavikit S, and Folkers K, Response of patients in classes III and IV of cardiomyopathy to therapy in a blind and crossover trial with coenzyme Q_{10}. *Proc Natl Acad Sci* **82**, 4240, 1985.

23. Oda T and Hamamoto K, Effect of coenzyme Q_{10} on the stress-induced decrease of cardiac performance in pediatric patients with mitral valve prolapse. *Jap Circ J* **48**, 1387, 1984.

24. Chello M, *et al.*, Protection of coenzyme Q_{10} from myocardial reperfusion injury during coronary artery bypass grafting. *Ann Thorac Surg* **58**, 1427–1432, 1994.

25. Kamikawa T, *et al.*, Effects of coenzyme Q_{10} on exercise tolerance in chronic stable angina pectoris. *Am J Cardiol* **56**, 247, 1985.

26. Kishi T, *et al.*, Bioenergetics in clinical medicine, XI, Studies on coenzyme Q and diabetes mellitus. *J Med* **7**, 307, 1976.

27. Shigeta Y, Izumi K, and Abe H, Effect of coenzyme Q_7 treatment on blood sugar and ketone bodies of diabetics. *J Vitaminol* **12**, 293, 1966.

28. Nakamura R, *et al.*, Study of Co Q_{10}-enzymes in gingiva from patients with periodontal disease and evidence for a deficiency of coenzyme Q_{10}. *Proc Natl Acad Sci* **71**, 1456, 1974.

29. Hansen IL, *et al.*, Bioenergetics in clinical medicine, IX, Gingival and leukocytic deficiencies of coenzyme Q_{10} in patients with periodontal disease. *Res Commun Chem Pathol Pharmacol* **14**, 729, 1976.

30. Littarru GP, Nakamura R, and Ho L, *et al.*, Deficiency of coenzyme Q_{10} in gingival tissue from patients with periodontal disease. *Proc Natl Acad Sci* **68**, 2332, 1971.

31. Nakamura R, Littarru GP, Folkers K, and Wilkinson EG, Deficiency of coenzyme Q in gingiva of patients with periodontal disease. *Int J Vit Nutr Res* **43**, 84, 1973.

32. Wilkinson EG, Arnold RM, and Folkers K, Treatment of periodontal and other soft tissue diseases of the oral cavity with coenzyme Q. In: *Biomedical and Clinical Aspects of Coenzyme Q, Vol 1*. Folkers K and Yamamura Y (eds.). Elsevier/North-Holland Biomedical Press, Amsterdam, 1977, pp. 251–265.

33. Wilkinson EG, *et al.*, Bioenergetics in clinical medicine, II, Adjunctive treatment with coenzyme Q in periodontal therapy. *Res Commun Chem Pathol Pharmacol* **12**, 111, 1975.

34. Shizukuishi S, *et al.*, Therapy by coenzyme Q_{10} of experimental periodontitis in a dog-model supports results of human periodontitis therapy. In: *Biomedical and Clinical Aspects*

of Coenzyme Q, Vol 4. Folkers K and Yamamura Y (eds.). Elsevier Science Publ, Amsterdam, 1984, pp. 153–162.

35. Tsunemitsu A and Matsumura T, Effect of coenzyme Q administration on hypercitricemia of patients with periodontal disease. *J Dent Res* **46**, 1382, 1967.

36. Hanioka T, *et al.*, Effect of topical application of coenzyme Q_{10} on adult periodontitis. *Mol Aspects Med* **15** (Suppl.), S241–S248, 1994.

37. Mayer P, Hamberger H, and Drews J, Differential effects of ubiquinone Q_7 and ubiquinone analogs on macrophage activation and experimental infections in granulocytopenic mice. *Infection* **8**, 256, 1980.

38. Saiki I, Tokushima Y, Nishimura K, and Azuma I, Macrophage activation with ubiquinones and their related compounds in mice. *Int J Vit Nutr Res* **53**, 312, 1983.

39. Bliznakov E, Casey A, and Premuzic E, Coenzymes Q: Stimulants of the phagocytic activity in rats and immune response in mice. *Experientia* **26**, 953, 1970.

40. Block LH, Georgopoulos A, Mayer P, and Drews J, Nonspecific resistance to bacterial infections, Enhancement by ubiquinone-8. *J Exp Med* **148**, 1228, 1978.

41. Bliznakov E, Casey A, Kishi T, *et al.*, Coenzyme Q deficiency in mice following infection with Friend leukemia virus. *Int J Vit Nutr Res* **45**, 388, 1975.

42. Bliznakov EG, Effect of stimulation of the host defense system by coenzyme Q_{10} on dibenzpyrene-induced tumors and infection with Friend leukemia virus in mice. *Proc Natl Acad Sci* **70**, 390, 1973.

43. Bliznakov EG, *et al.*, Coenzyme Q deficiency in aged mice. *J Med* **9**, 337, 1978.

44. Bliznakov EG, Immunological senescence in mice and its reversal by coenzyme Q_{10}. *Mech Aging Dev* **7**, 189, 1978.

45. Folkers K, *et al.*, Increase in levels of IgG in serum of patients treated with coenzyme Q_{10}. *Res Commun Chem Pathol Pharmacol* **38**, 335, 1982.

46. Lockwood K, Moesgaard S, and Folkers K, Partial and complete regression of breast cancer in patients in relation to dosage of coenzyme Q_{10}. *Biochem Biophys Res Comm* **199**, 1504–1508, 1994.

47. Combs AB, *et al.*, Reduction by coenzyme Q_{10} of the acute toxicity of adriamycin in mice. *Res Commun Chem Pathol Pharmacol* **18**, 565, 1977.

48. Judy WV, *et al.*, Coenzyme Q_{10} reduction of adriamycin cardiotoxicity. In: *Biomedical and Clinical Aspects of Coenzyme Q, Vol 4.* Folkers K and Yamamura Y (eds.). Elsevier Science Publ, Amsterdam, 1984, pp. 231–241.

49. Iarussi D, *et al.*, Protective effect of coenzyme Q_{10} on anthracyclines cardiotoxicity: Control study in children with acute lymphoblastic leukemia and non-Hodgkin lymphoma. *Mol Aspects Med* **15** (Suppl.), S207–S212, 1994.

50. van Gaal L, de Leeuw ID, Vadhanavikit S, and Folkers K, Exploratory study of coenzyme Q_{10} in obesity. In: *Biomedical and Clinical Aspects of Coenzyme Q, Vol 4.* Folkers K and Yamamura Y (eds.). Elsevier Science Publ, Amsterdam, 1984, pp. 369–373.

51. Folkers K, Wolaniuk J, Simonsen R, *et al.*, Biochemical rationale and the cardiac response of patients with muscle disease to therapy with coenzyme Q_{10}. *Proc Natl Acad Sci* **82**, 4513, 1985.

52. Folkers K and Simonsen R, Two successful double-blind trials with coenzyme Q_{10} (vitamin Q_{10}) on muscular dystrophies and neurogenic atrophies. *Biochem Biophys Acta* **1271**, 281–286, 1995.

53. Vanfraechem JHP and Folkers K, Coenzyme Q_{10} and physical performance. In: *Biomedical and Clinical Aspects of Coenzyme Q, Vol 3.* Folkers K and Yamamura Y (eds.) Elsevier/North-Holland Biomedical Press, Amsterdam, 1981, pp. 235–241.

54. Bargossi AM, *et al.*, Exogenous CoQ_{10} supplementation prevents plasma ubiquinone reduction induced by HMG-CoA reductase inhibitors. *Mol Aspects Med* **15** (Suppl.), S187–S193, 1994.

55. Kishi T, Kishi H, and Folkers K, Inhibition of cardiac CoQ_{10}-enzymes by clinically used drugs and possible prevention. In: *Biomedical and Clinical Aspects of Coenzyme Q, Vol 1.* Folkers K and Yamamura Y (eds.). Elsevier/North-Holland Biomedical Press, Amsterdam, 1977, pp. 47–62.

56. Hamada M, Kazatani Y, Ochi T, *et al.*, Correlation between serum CoQ$_{10}$ level and myocardial contractility in hypertensive patients. In: *Biomedical and Clinical Aspects of Coenzyme Q, Vol 4*. Folkers K and Yamamura Y (eds.). Elsevier Science Publ, Amsterdam, 1984, pp. 263–270.

57. Kishi T, Makino K, Okamoto T, *et al.*, Inhibition of myocardial respiration by psychotherapeutic drugs and prevention by coenzyme Q. In: *Biomedical and Clinical Aspects of Coenzyme Q, Vol 2*. Yamamura Y, Folkers K, and Ito Y (eds.). Elsevier/North-Holland Biomedical Press, Amsterdam, 1980, pp. 139–154.

36 Fiber Supplements

1. Spiller GA, *Dietary Fiber in Health and Nutrition*. CRC Press, Boca Raton, FL, 1994.

2. Trowell H and Burkitt D, *Western Diseases: Their Emergence and Prevention*. Harvard University Press, Boston, MA, 1981.

3. Trowell H, Burkitt D, and Heaton K, *Dietary Fibre, Fibre-depleted Foods and Disease*. Academic Press, New York, NY, 1985.

4. US Dept of Health and Human Services, *The Surgeon General's Report on Nutrition and Health*. Prima, Rocklin, CA, 1988.

5. National Research Council, Diet and Health. *Implications for Reducing Chronic Disease Risk*. National Academy Press, Washington, DC, 1989.

6. Price W, *Nutrition and Physical Degeneration*. Price-Pottinger Foundation, 1970.

7. Glore SR, *et al.*, Soluble fiber and serum lipids: A literature review. *J Am Diet Assoc* **94**, 425–436, 1994.

8. Ripsin CM, Keenan JM, and Jacobs DR, *et al.*, Oat products and lipid lowering, a meta-analysis. *JAMA* **267**, 3317–3325, 1992.

9. Krotkiewski M, Effect of guar on body weight, hunger ratings and metabolism in obese subjects. *Clinical Science* **66**, 329–336, 1984.

10. Krotkiewski M and Smith U, Dietary fibre in obesity. In: *Dietary Fiber Perspectives, Reviews and Bibliography*. Leeds AR and Avenell A (eds.). John Libbey, London, 1985, pp. 61.

11. Krotkiewski M, Effect of guar gum on body-weight, hunger ratings and metabolism in obese subjects. *Br J Nutr* **52**, 97–105, 1984.

12. Anonymous, Better than oat bran. *Science News* **145**, 28, 1994.

13. Walsh DE, Yaghoubian V, and Behforooz A, Effect of glucomannan on obese patients: A clinical study. *Int J Obesity* **8**, 289–293, 1984.

14. Biancardi G, Palmiero L, and Ghirardi PE, Glucomannan in the treatment of overweight patients with osteoarthrosis. *Curr Ther Res* **46**, 908–912, 1989.

15. El-Shebini SM, *et al.*, The role of pectin as a slimming agent. *J Clin Biochem Nutr* **4**, 255–262, 1988.

16. Solum TT, *et al.*, The influence of a high-fibre diet on body weight, serum lipids and blood pressure in slightly overweight persons: A randomized, double-blind, placebo-controlled investigation with diet and fibre tablets (DumoVital). *Int J Obesity* **11** (Suppl. 1), 67–71, 1987.

17. Ryttig KR, Larsen S, and Haegh L, Treatment of slightly to moderately overweight persons: A double-blind placebo-controlled investigation with diet and fibre tablets (DumoVital). *Tidsskr Nor Laegeforen* **104**, 989–991, 1984.

18. Rossner S, *et al.*, Weight reduction with dietary fibre supplements: Results of two double-blind studies. *Acta Med Scand* **222**, 83–88, 1987.

19. Ryttig KR, *et al.*, A dietary fibre supplement and weight maintenance after weight reduction: A randomized, double-blind, placebo-controlled long-term trial. *Int J Obesity* **14**, 763–769, 1989.

20. Rigaud D, *et al.*, Mild overweight treated with energy restriction and a dietary fiber supplement: A 6-month randomized, double-blind, placebo-controlled trial. *Int J Obesity* **14**, 763–769, 1990.

21. Halama WH and Maudlin JL, Distal esophageal obstruction due to a guar gum preparation. *South Med J* **85**, 642–646, 1992.

22. Henry CA, *et al.*, Glucomannan and risk of oesophageal obstruction. *Br Med J* **292**, 591–592, 1986.

37 Flavonoids

1. Hertog MG, *et al.*, Dietary antioxidant flavonoids and risk of coronary heart disease: The Zutphen Elderly Study. *Lancet* **342**, 1007–1011, 1993.
2. Havsteen B, Flavonoids, a class of natural products of high pharmacological potency. *Biochem Pharmacol* **32**, 1141–1148, 1983.
3. Middleton E, The flavonoids. *Trends Pharmaceut Sci* **5**, 335–338, 1984.
4. Schwitters B and Masquelier J, *OPC in Practice: Biflavanols and Their Application.* Alfa Omega, Rome, Italy, 1993.
5. Masquelier J, Procyanidolic oligomers. *J Parfums Cosm Arom* **95**, 89–97, 1990.
6. Masquelier J, Dumon MC, and Dumas J, Stabilization of collagen by procyanidolic oligomers. *Acta Therap* **7**, 101–105, 1981.
7. Tixier JM, *et al.*, Evidence by *in vivo* and *in vitro* studies that binding of pycnogenols to elastin affects its rate of degradation by elastases. *Biochem Pharmacol* **33**, 3933–3939, 1984.
8. Meunier MT, Duroux E, and Bastide P, Free-radical scavenger activity of procyanidolic oligomers and anthocyanosides with respect to superoxide anion and lipid peroxidation. *Plant Med Phytother* **4**, 267–274, 1989.
9. Facino RM, *et al.*, Free radicals scavenging action and anti-enzyme activities of procyanidines from Vitis vinifera: A mechanism for their capillary protective action. *Arzneim Forsch* **44**, 592–601, 1994.
10. Ferrandiz ML and Alcaraz MJ, Anti-inflammatory activity and inhibition of arachidonic acid metabolism by flavonoids. *Agents Action* **32**, 283–287, 1991.
11. Middleton E and Drzewieki G, Flavonoid inhibition of human basophil histamine release stimulated by various agents. *Biochem Pharmacol* **33**, 3333–3338, 1984.
12. Middleton E and Drzewieki G, Naturally occurring flavonoids and human basophil histamine release. *Int Arch Allergy Appl Immunol* **77**, 155–157, 1985.
13. Amella M, Bronner C, Briancon F, *et al.*, Inhibition of mast cell histamine release by flavonoids and bioflavonoids. *Planta Medica* **51**, 16–20, 1985.
14. Pearce F, Befus AD, and Bienenstock J, Mucosal mast cells, III, Effect of quercetin and other flavonoids on antigen-induced histamine secretion from rat intestinal mast cells. *J Allergy Clin Immunol* **73**, 819–123, 1984.
15. Busse WW, Kopp DE, and Middleton E, Flavonoid modulation of human neutrophil function. *J Allergy Clin Immunol* **73**, 801–809, 1984.
16. Yoshimoto T, *et al.*, Flavonoids: Potent inhibitors of arachidonate 5-lipoxygenase. *Biochem Biophys Res Common* **116**, 612–618, 1983.
17. Chaundry PS, *et al.*, Inhibition of human lens aldose reductase by flavonoids, sulindac and indomethacin. *Biochem Pharmacol* **32**, 1995–1998, 1983.
18. Varma SD, Mizuno A, and Kinoshita JH, Diabetic cataracts and flavonoids. *Science* **195**, 87–89, 1977.
19. Mucsi I and Pragai BM, Inhibition of virus multiplication and alteration of cyclic AMP level in cell cultures by flavonoids. *Experentia* **41**, 930–931, 1985.
20. Kaul T, Middleton E, and Ogra P, Antiviral effects of flavonoids on human viruses. *J Med Virol* **15**, 71–79, 1985.
21. Beladi I, *et al.*, *In vitro* and *in vivo* antiviral effects of flavonoids. In: *Flavonoids and Bioflavonoids.* Farkas L, Gabor M, Kallay F, and Wagner H (eds.). Elsevier, New York, NY, 1982, pp. 443–450.
22. Guttner J, Veckenstedt A, Heinecke H, and Pusztai R, Effect of quercetin on the course of mengo virus infection in immunodeficient and normal mice: A histological study. *Arch Virol* **26**, 148–155, 1982.
23. Elangovan V, *et al.*, Studies on the chemopreventive potential of some naturally-occurring bioflavonoids in 7,12-dimethylbenz(a)anthracene-induced carcinogens in mouse skin. *J Clin Biochem Nutr* **17**, 153–160, 1994.

24. Verma K, *et al.*, Inhibition of 7,12-dimethylbenz(a)anthracene and N-nitrosomethyl urea in-duced rat mammary cancer by dietary flavonol quercetin. *Cancer Res* **48**, 5754–5758, 1988.

25. Stavric B, Quercetin in our diet: from potent mutagen to probable anticarcinogen. *Clin Biochem* **27**, 245–248, 1994.

26. Larocca LM, *et al.*, Growth-inhibitory effect of quercetin and presence of type II estrogen binding sites in primary human transitional cell carcinomas. *J Urol* **152**, 1029–1033, 1994.

27. Ho C, *et al.*, Antioxidative effect of polyphenol extract prepared from various Chinese teas. *Prev Med* **21**, 520–525, 1992.

28. Khan SG, *et al.*, Enhancement of antioxidant and phase II enzymes by oral feeding of green tea polyphenols in drinking water to SKH-1 hairless mice: Possible role in cancer chemoprevention. *Cancer Res* **52**, 4050–4052, 1992.

29. Katiyar SK, Agarwal R, and Mukhtar H, Green tea in chemoprevention of cancer. *Compr Ther* **18**, 3–8, 1992.

30. Mukhtar H, *et al.*, Tea components: Antimutagenic and anticarcinogenic effects. *Prev Med* **21**, 351–360, 1992.

31. Wang ZY, *et al.*, Protection against polycyclic aromatic hydrocarbon-induced skin tumor initiation in mice by green tea polyphenols. *Carcinogenesis* **10**, 411–415, 1989.

32. Komori A, *et al.*, Anticarcinogenic activity of green tea polyphenols. *Jap J Clin Oncol* 23(3), 186–190, 1993.

33. Yang CS and Wang ZY, Tea and cancer. *J Natl Cancer Inst* **85(13)**, 1038–1049, 1993.

34. Stich HF, Teas and tea components as inhibitors of carcinogen formation in model sys-tems and man. *Prev Med* **21**, 377–384, 1992.

35. Xu GP, Song PJ, and Reed PI. Effects of fruit juices, processed vegetable juice, orange peel and green tea on endogenous formation of N-nitrosoproline in subjects from a high-risk area for gastric cancer in Moping County, China. *Eur J Cancer Prev* **2(4)**, 327–335, 1993.

36. Henriet JP, Veno-lymphatic insufficiency: 4,729 patients undergoing hormonal and pro-cyanidol oligomer therapy. *Phlebologie* **46**, 313–325, 1993.

37. Baruch J, Effect of Endotelon in postoperative edema: Results of a double-blind study versus placebo in 32 female patients. *Ann Chir Plast Esthet* **29**, 393–395, 1984.

38. Lagrue G, Oliver-Martin F, and Grillot A, A study of the effects of procyanidol oligomers on capillary resistance in hypertension and in certain nephropathies. *Sem Hosp Paris* **57**, 1399–1401, 1981.

39. Gomez Trillo JT, Varicose veins of the lower extremities: Symptomatic treatment with a new vasculotrophic agent. *Prensa Med Mex* **38**, 293–296, 1973.

40. Soyeux A, *et al.*, Endotelon: Diabetic retinopathy and hemorrheology (preliminary study). *Bull Soc Ophtalmol Fr* **87**, 1441–1444, 1987.

41. Proto F, *et al.*, Electrophysical study of *Vitis vinifera* procyanoside oligomers effects on reti-nal function in myopic subjects. *Ann Ott Clin Ocul* **114**, 85–93, 1988.

42. Corbe C, Boisin JP, and Siou A, Light vision and chorioretinal circulation: Study of the ef-fect of procyanidolic oligomers (Endotelon). *J Fr Ophtalmol* **11**, 453–460, 1988.

43. Boissin JP, Corbe C, and Siou A, Chorioretinal circulation and dazzling: use of pro-cyanidol oligomers. *Bull Soc Ophtalmol Fr* **88**, 173–174, 177–179, 1988.

44. Wegrowski J, Robert AM, and Moczar M, The effect of procyanidolic oligomers on the composition of normal and hypercholesterolemic rabbit aortas. *Biochem Pharmacol* **33**, 3491–3497, 1984.

45. Chang WC and Hsu FL, Inhibition of platelet aggregation and arachidonate metabolism in platelets by procyanidins. *Prostagland Leukotri Essential Fatty Acids* **38**, 181–188, 1989.

46. Meunier MT, *et al.*, Inhibition of angiotensin I converting enzyme by flavanolic com-pounds, *In vitro* and *in vivo* studies. *Planta Medica* **54**, 12–15, 1987.

47. Petrakis PL, Kallianos AG, Wender SH, *et al.*, Metabolic studies of quercetin labeled with C_{14}. *Arch Biochem Biophys* **85**, 264–271, 1959.

48. Gugler R, Leshik M, and Dengler HJ, Disposition of quercetin in man after single oral and intravenous doses. *Eur J Clin Pharmacol* **9**, 229–234, 1975.

49. Hollman PCH, *et al.*, Absorption of dietary quercetin glycosides and quercetin in health ileostomy volunteers. *Am J Clin Nutr* **62**, 1276–1282, 1995.

50. Lagrue E, Behar A, and Maurel P, Edematous syndromes caused by capillary hyper-permeability. *J Mal Vasc* **14**, 231–235, 1989.

51. Horoschak A, Nocturnal leg cramps, easy bruisability and epistaxis in menopausal patients: Treated with hesperidin and ascorbic acid. *Del State Med J* **Jan**, 19–22, 1959.

52. Cragin RB, The use of bioflavonoids in the prevention and treatment of athletic injuries. *Med Times* **90**, 529–530, 1962.

53. Beretz A and Cazenave J, The effect of flavonoids on blood vessel wall interactions. In: *Plant Flavonoids in Biology and Medicine II: Biochemical, Cellular, and Medicinal Properties.* Cody V, Middleton E, Harborne JB, and Beretz A (eds.). Alan R Liss, New York, NY, 1988, pp. 187–200.

54. Wadworth AN and Faulds D, Hydroxyethylrutosides: A review of its pharmacology, and therapeutic efficacy in venous insufficiency and related disorders. *Drugs* **44**, 1013–1032, 1992.

55. Poynard T and Valterio C, Meta-analysis of hydroxyethylrutosides in the treatment of chronic venous insufficiency. *Vasa* **23**, 244–250, 1994.

56. Boisseau MR, *et al.*, Fibrinolysis and hemorrheology in chronic venous insufficiency: A double blind study of troxerutin efficiency. *J Cardiovasc Surg* **36**, 369–374, 1995.

57. Neumann HA and van den Broek MJ, A comparative clinical trial of graduated compression stockings and O-(beta-hydroxyethyl)-rutosides (HR) in the treatment of patients with chronic venous insufficiency. *Z Lymphol* **19**, 8–11, 1995.

58. Renton S, *et al.*, The effect of hydroxyethylrutosides on capillary filtration in moderate venous hypertension: A double blind study. *Int Angiol* **13**, 259–262, 1994.

59. MacLennan WJ, *et al.*, Hydroxyethylrutosides in elderly patients with chronic venous insufficiency: Its efficacy and tolerability. *Gerontology* **40**, 45–52, 1994.

60. Bergstein NAM, Clinical study on the efficacy of O-(beta-hydroxyethyl)-rutoside (HR) in varicosis of pregnancy. *J Int Med Res* **3**, 189–193, 1975.

61. Wijayanegara H, *et al.*, A clinical trial of hydroxyethylrutosides in the treatment of haemorrhoids of pregnancy. *J Int Med Res* **20**, 54–60, 1992.

62. Annoni F, *et al.*, Treatment of acute symptoms of haemorrhoidal disease with high dose O-(beta-hydroxyethyl)-rutoside. *Min Med* **77**, 1663–1668, 1986.

63. Belcaro G and Candiani C, Chronic effects of O-(beta-hydroxyethyl)-rutosides on microcirculation and capillary filtration in diabetic microangiopathy. *Curr Ther Res* **49**, 131–139, 1991.

64. Agolini G and Cavallini GM, Treatment of long-term retinal vasculopathies with high oral dosage of O-(beta-hydroxyethyl)-rutosides. *Clin Ther* **120**, 101–110, 1987.

65. La Vecchia C, *et al.*, Tea consumption and cancer risk. *Nutr Cancer* **17**, 27–31, 1992.

66. Heilbrun LK, Nomura A, and Stemmermann GN, Black tea consumption and cancer risk: A prospective study. *Br J Cancer* **54**, 677–683, 1986.

67. Masquelier J, *Historical Note on OPC.* Martillac, France, October 1991.

68. Tarayre JP and Lauressergues H, Advantages of a combination of proteolytic enzymes, flavonoids and ascorbic acid in comparison with non-steroid anti-inflammatory agents. *Arzneim Forsch* **27**, 1144–1149, 1977.

69. Stoewsand GS, *et al.*, Quercetin: A mutagen, not a carcinogen, in Fischer rats. *J Toxicol Env Health* **14**, 105–114, 1984.

70. Hirono I, Ueno H, Hosaka S, *et al.*, Carcinogenicity examination of quercetin and rutin in ACI rats. *Cancer Letters* **13**, 15–21, 1981.

71. Kato K, *et al.*, Lack of promotive effect of quercetin on methlazoxy acetate carcinogenesis in rats. *J Toxicol Sci* **9**, 319–325, 1984.

72. Kato K, *et al.*, Absence of initiating activity by quercetin in the rat liver. *Ecotoxicol Environ Safety* **10**, 63–69, 1985.

73. Hosaka S and Hirono I, Carcinogenicity test of quercetin by pulmonary-adenoma bioassay in Starin A mice. *Gann* **72**, 327–328, 1981.

74. Hirose M, *et al.*, Effect of quercetin on two-stage carcinogenesis of the rat urinary bladder. *Cancer Letters* **21**, 23–27, 1983.

75. Willhite CC, Teratogenic potential of quercetin in the rat. *Food Chem Toxicol* **20**, 75–79, 1982.

76. Fuhr U and Kummert AL, The fate of naringin in humans: A key to grapefruit juice-drug interactions? *Clin Pharmacol Ther* **58**, 365–373, 1995.

38   Gamma-oryzanol

1. Pussayanawin V and Wetzel DL, High-performance liquid chromatographic determination of ferulic acid in wheat milling fractions as a measure of bran contamination. *J Chromatography* **391**, 243–255, 1987.

2. Graf E, Antioxidant potential of ferulic acid. *Free Rad Biol Med* **13**, 435–448, 1992.

3. Scott BC, *et al.*, Evaluation of the antioxidant actions of ferulic acid and catechins. *Free Rad Res Comms* **19**, 241–253, 1993.

4. Yagi K and Ohishi N, Action of ferulic acid and its derivatives as antioxidant. *J Nutr Sci Vitaminol* **25**, 127–130, 1979.

5. Tanaka T, *et al.*, Inhibition of 4-nitroquinoline-1-oxide-induced rat tongue carcinogenesis by the naturally occurring plant phenolics caffeic, ellagic, chlorogenic and ferulic acids. *Carcinogenesis* **14**, 1321–1325, 1993.

6. Asanoma M, *et al.*, Inhibitory effect of topical application of polymerized ferulic acid, a synthetic lignin, on tumor promotion in mouse skin two stage tumorigenesis. *Carcinogenesis* **15**, 2069–2071, 1994.

7. Ieiri T, *et al.*, The effects of gamma-oryzanol on the hypothalamo-pituitary axis in the rat. *Folia Endocrinol* **58**, 1350–1356, 1982.

8. Shimomura Y, *et al.*, Effect of gamma-oryzanol on serum TSH concentrations in primary hypothyroidism. *Endocrinol Jap* **27**, 83–86, 1980.

9. Takayanagi H and Honda Y, Effect of gamma-oryzanol on prolactin secretion. *Horumon To Rinsho* **29**, 91–93, 1981.

10. Yamauchi J, *et al.*, Inhibition of LH secretion by gamma-oryzanol in rat. *Horm Metabol Res* **13**, 185, 1981.

11. Chawla AS, *et al.*, Anti-inflammatory action of ferulic acid and its esters in carrageenan-induced rat paw edema model. *Ind J Exp Biol* **25**, 187–189, 1987.

12. Hiraga Y, *et al.*, Effect of the rice bran-derived phytosterol cycloartenol ferulic acid ester on the central nervous system. *Arzneim Forsch* **43**, 715–721, 1993.

13. Fujiwara S, *et al.*, Mass fragmentographic determination of ferulic acid in plasma after oral administration of gamma-oryzanol. *Chem Pharm Bull* **30**, 973–979, 1982.

14. Murase Y and Iishima H, Clinical studies of oral administration of gamm-oryzanol on climacteric complaints and its syndrome. *Obtet Gynecol Prac* **12**, 147–149, 1963.

15. Ishihara M, Effect of gamma-oryzanol on serum lipid peroxide levels and climacteric disturbances. *Asia Oceania J Obstet Gynecol* **10**, 317, 1984.

16. Yoshino G, Kazumi T, Amano M, *et al.*, Effects of gamma-oryzanol on hyperlipidemic subjects. *Curr Ther Res* **45**, 543–552, 1989.

17. Yoshino G, *et al.*, Effects of gamma-oryzanol and probucol on hyperlipidemia. *Curr Ther Res* **45**, 975–982, 1989.

18. Sasaki J, *et al.*, Effects of gamma-oryzanol on serum lipids and apolipoproteins in dyslipidemic schizophrenics receiving major tranquilizers. *Clin Ther* **12**, 263–268, 1990.

19. Seetharamaiah GS and Chandrasekhara N, Effect of oryzanol on cholesterol absorption & biliary & fecal bile acids in rats. *Ind J Med Res* **92**, 471–475, 1990.

20. Sakamoto K, *et al.*, Effects of gamma-oryzanol and cycloartenol ferulic acid ester on cholesterol diet induced hyperlipidemia in rats. *Jap J Pharmacol* **45**, 559–565, 1987.

21. Oguni C, *et al.*, Clinical effects of gamma-oryzanol on vegetative neurosis. *Clin Gynecol Obstet* **16**, 57–63, 1962.

22. Minakuchi C, *et al.*, Clinical effectiveness of gamma-oryzanol on gastric system complaints. *Shiyaku To Rinsho* **25**, 29–33, 1976.

23. Oota K, *et al.*, Clinical studies of Hi-Z pills on indefinite complaints of gastrointestinal neurosis. *Yakuri Chiryo* **3**, 133–137, 1976.
24. Sasagawa T, *et al.*, Clinical tests of gamma-oryzanol (Hi-Z pills) on gastrointestinal neurosis. *Yakuri Chiryo* **4**, 118–122, 1976.
25. Takemoto T, *et al.*, Clinical trial of Hi-Z pills on gastrointestinal symptoms at 375 hospitals. *Shiyaku To Rinsho* **26**, 25–27, 1977.
26. Sasagawa T, *et al.*, Clinical studies on gamma-oryzanol in the treatment of gastro-entero neurosis. *Basic Pharmacol Ther* **4**, 588–591, 1980.
27. Arai T, Effect of gamma-oryzanol on indefinite complaints in the gastrointestinal symptoms in patients with chronic gastritis: Studies on the endocrinological environment. *Horumon To Rinsho* 30, 271–279, 1982.
28. Bucci LR, *Nutrients as Ergogenic Aids for Sport and Exercise*. CRC Press, Boca Raton, FL, 1993, pp. 90, 91.
29. Bucci LR, *et al.*, Effect of ferulate on strength and body composition of weightlifters. *J Appl Sport Sci Res* **4**, 104–109, 1990.
30. Bonner B, Warren B, and Bucci L, Influence of ferulate supplementation on post-exercise stress hormone levels after repeated exercise stress. *J Appl Sport Sci Res* **4**, 110–114, 1990.
31. Tamagawa M, *et al.*, Carcinogenicity study of gamma-oryzanol in B6C3F1 mice. *Food Chem Toxicol* **30**, 49–56, 1992.
32. Tamagawa M, *et al.*, Carcinogenicity study of gamma-oryzanol in F344 rats. *Food Chem Toxicol* **30**, 41–48, 1992.

39 Glucosamine

1. Setnikar I, *et al.*, Pharmacokinetics of glucosamine in man. *Arzneim Forsch* **43(10)**, 1109–1113, 1993.
2. Setnikar I, *et al.*, Pharmacokinetics of glucosamine in the dog and man. *Arzneim Forsch* **36(4)**, 729–735, 1986.
3. Setnikar I, Antireactive properties of "chondroprotective" drugs. *Int J Tissue React* **14(5)**, 253–261, 1992.
4. Karzel K and Domenjoz R, Effect of hexosamine derivatives and uronic acid derivatives on glycosaminoglycan metabolism of fibroblast cultures. *Pharmacol* **5**, 337–345, 1971.
5. Vidal Y and Plana RR, *et al.*, Articular cartilage pharmacology, I, *In vitro* studies on glucosamine and non steroidal anti-inflammatory drugs. *Pharmacol Res Comm* **10**, 557–569, 1978.
6. Capps JC, *et al.*, Hexosamine metabolism, II, Effect of insulin and phlorizin on the absorption and metabolism, *in vivo*, of D-glucosamine and N-acetyl-glucosamine in the rat. *Biochem Biophys Acta* **127**, 205–212, 1966.
7. Capps JC, *et al.*, Hexosamine metabolism, I, The absorption and metabolism, *in vivo* of orally administered D-glucosamine and N-acetyl-D-glucosamine in the rat. *Biochem Biophys Acta* **127**, 194–204, 1966.
8. Shetlar MR, *et al.*, Incorporation of radioactive glucosamine into the serum proteins of intact rats and rabbits. *Biochem Biophys Acta* **83**, 93–101, 1964.
9. Richmond JE, Studies on the metabolism of plasma glycoproteins. *Biochemistry* **2(4)**, 676–683, 1963.
10. Capps JC and Shetlar MR, *In vivo* incorporation of D-glucosamine-1-C_6 into acid mucopolysachharides of rabbit liver. *Proc Soc Exptl Biol Med* **114,** 118–120, 1963.
11. Shetlar MR, *et al.*, Fate of radioactive glucosamine administered parenterally to the rat. *Proc Soc Exptl Biol Med* **109**, 335–337, 1962.
12. Kohn P, *et al.*, Metabolism of D-glucosamine and N-acetyl-D-glucosamine in the intact rat. *J Biol Chem* **237(2)**, 304–308, 1962.
13. McGarrahan JF and Maley F, Hexosamine metabolism. *J Biol Chem* **237(8)**, 2458–2465, 1962.
14. Shetlar MR, *et al.*, Incorporation of [1-$_{14}$C]glucosamine into serum proteins. *Biochem Biophys Acta* **53**, 615, 616, 1961.

15. Tesoriere G, *et al.*, Intestinal absorption of glucosamine and N-acetylglucosamine. *Experientia* **28**, 770, 771, 1972.

16. Setnikar I, *et al.*, Antiarthritic effects of glucosamine sulfate studied in animal models. *Arzneim Forsch* **41**, 542–545, 1991.

17. Setnikar I, *et al.*, Antireactive properties of glucosamine sulfate. *Arzneim Forsch* **41(2)**, 157–161, 1991.

18. Burton AF and Anderson FH, Decreased incorporation of 14C-glucosamine relative to 3H-N-acetylglucosamine in the intestinal mucosa of patients with inflammatory bowel disease. *Am J Gastroenterol* **78**, 19–22, 1983.

19. McDermott RP, *et al.*, Glycoprotein synthesis and secretion by mucosal biopsies of rabbit colon and human rectum. *J Clin Invest* **54**, 545–554, 1974.

20. Sullivan MX and Hess WC, Cystine content of finger nails in arthritis. *J Bone Joint Surg* **16**, 185–188, 1935.

21. Senturia BD, Results of treatment of chronic arthritis and rheumatoid conditions with colloidal sulfur. *J Bone Joint Surg* **16**, 119–125, 1934.

22. Brandt KD, Effects of nonsteroidal anti-inflammatory drugs on chondrocyte metabolism *in vitro* and *in vivo*. *Am J Med* **83** (Suppl. 5A), 29–34, 1987.

23. Shield MJ, Anti-inflammatory drugs and their effects on cartilage synthesis and renal function. *Eur J Rheumatol Inflam* **13**, 7–16, 1993.

24. Brooks PM, Potter SR, and Buchanan WW, NSAID and osteoarthritis—help or hindrance. *J Rheumatol* **9**, 3–5, 1982.

25. Newman NM and Ling RSM, Acetabular bone destruction related to non-steroidal anti-inflammatory drugs. *Lancet* **ii**; 11–13, 1985.

26. Solomon L, Drug induced arthropathy and necrosis of the femoral head. *J Bone Joint Surg* **55B**, 246–251, 1973.

27. Ronningen H and Langeland N, Indomethacin treatment in osteoarthritis of the hip joint. *Acta Orthop Scand* **50**, 169–174, 1979.

28. Crolle G and D'este E, Glucosamine sulfate for the management of arthrosis: A controlled clinical investigation. *Curr Med Res Opin* **7**, 104–109, 1980.

29. Pujalte JM, *et al.*, Double-blind clinical evaluation of oral glucosamine sulphate in the basic treatment of osteoarthrosis. *Curr Med Res Opin* **7**, 110–114, 1980.

30. Drovanti A, *et al.*, Therapeutic activity of oral glucosamine sulfate in osteoarthrosis: A placebo-controlled double-blind investigation. *Clin Ther* **3**, 260–272, 1980.

31. Vajaradul Y, Double-blind clinical evaluation of intra-articular glucosamine in outpatients with gonarthosis. *Clin Ther* **3**, 336–343, 1981.

32. Vaz AL, Double-blind clinical evaluation of the relative efficacy of ibuprofen and glucosamine sulfate in the management of osteoarthrosis of the knee in out-patients. *Curr Med Res Opin* **8**, 145–149, 1982.

33. D'Ambrosia ED *et al.*, Glucosamine sulphate: A controlled clinical investigation in arthrosis. *Pharmatherapeutica* **2**, 504–508, 1982.

34. Reichelt A, *et al.*, Efficacy and safety of intramuscular glucosamine sulfate in osteoarthritis of the knee. A randomized, placebo-controlled, double-blind study. *Arzneim Forsch* **44**, 75–80, 1994.

35. Tapadinhas MJ, *et al.*, Oral glucosamine sulfate in the management of arthrosis: Report on a multi-centre open investigation in Portugal. *Pharmatherapeutica* **3**, 157–168, 1982.

36. Morrison M, Therapeutic applications of chondroitin-4-sulfate, appraisal of biologic properties. *Folia Angiol* **25**, 225–232, 1977.

40   Lipoic Acid

1. Kagan VE, *et al.*, Dihydrolipoic acid—A universal antioxidant both in the membrane and in the aqueous phase. Biochem Pharmacol 44, 1637–1649, 1992.

2. Packer L, Witt EH, and Tritschler HJ, Alpha-Lipoic acid as a biological antioxidant. *Free Rad Biol Med* **19**, 227–250, 1995.

3. Ou P, Tritschler HJ, and Wolff SP, Thioctic (lipoic) acid: A therapeutic metal-chelating antioxidant? *Biochem Pharmacol* **50**, 123–126, 1995.

4. Matsugo S, *et al.*, Elucidation of antioxidant activity of alpha-lipoic acid toward hydroxyl radical. *Biochem Biophys Res Comm* **208**, 161–167, 1995.

5. Scott BC, *et al.*, Lipoic and dihydrolipoic acids as antioxidants: A critical evaluation. *Free Rad Res* **20**, 119–133, 1994.

6. Podda M, *et al.*, Alpha-lipoic acid supplementation prevents symptoms of vitamin E deficiency. *Biochem Biophys Res Comm* **204**, 98–104, 1994.

7. Packer L, Antioxidant properties of lipoic acid and its therapeutic effects in prevention of diabetes complications and cataracts. *Annals NY Acad Sci* **738**, 257–264, 1994.

8. Kahler W, *et al.*, Diabetes mellitus—a free radical-associated disease: Results of adjuvant antioxidant supplementation. *Gesamte Inn Med* **48**, 223–232, 1993.

9. Nagamatsu M, *et al.*, Lipoic acid improves nerve blood flow, reduces oxidative stress, and improves distal nerve conduction in experimental diabetic neuropathy. *Diabetes Care* **18**, 1160–1167, 1995.

10. Jacob S, *et al.*, Enhancement of glucose disposal in patients with type 2 diabetes by alpha-lipoic acid. *Arzneim Forsch* **45**, 872–874, 1995.

11. Kawabata T and Packer L, Alpha-lipoate can protect against glycation of serum albumin, but not low density lipoprotein. *Biochem Biophys Res Comm* **203**, 99–104, 1994.

12. Suzuki YJ, Tsuchiya M, and Packer L, Lipoate prevents glucose-induced protein modifications. *Free Rad Res Comms* **17**, 211–217, 1992.

13. Fuchs J, *et al.*, Studies on lipoate effects on blood redox state in human immunodeficiency virus infected patients. *Arzneim Forsch* **43**, 1359–1362, 1993.

14. Baur A, *et al.*, Alpha-lipoic acid is an effective inhibitor of human immuno-deficiency virus (HIV-1) replication. *Klin Wochenschr* **69**, 722–724, 1991.

15. Suzuki YJ, Aggarwal BB, and Packer L, Alpha-lipoic acid is a potent inhibitor of NF-kB activation in human T cells. *Biochem Biophys Res Comm* **189**, 1709–1715, 1992.

41   Medium-Chain Triglycerides

1. Bach AC and Babayan VK, Medium-chain triglycerides: An update. *Am J Clin Nutr* **36**, 950–962, 1982.

2. Baba N, Bracco EF, and Hashim SA, Enhanced thermogenesis and diminished deposition of fat in response to overfeeding with diet containing medium chain triglyceride. *Am J Clin Nutr* **35**, 678–682, 1982.

3. Hill JO, *et al.*, Thermogenesis in humans during overfeeding with medium-chain triglycerides in man. *Amer J Clin Nutr* **44**, 630–634, 1986.

4. Hill JO, *et al.*, Thermogenesis in man during overfeeding with medium chain triglycerides. *Metabolism* **38**, 641–648, 1989.

5. Seaton TB, *et al.*, Thermic effect of medium-chain and long-chain triglycerides in man. *Am J Clin Nutr* **44**, 630–634, 1986.

6. Barborha CJ, Ketogenic diet treatment of epilepsy in adults. *JAMA* **91**, 73–78, 1928.

7. Barborha CJ, Epilepsy in adults, results of treatment by ketogenic diet in one hundred cases. *Arch Neurol Psych* **23**, 904–914, 1930.

8. Signore, Ketogenic diet with medium chain triglycerides. *J Am Diet Assoc* **62**, 285–290, 1973.

42   Melatonin

1. Yu HS and Reiter RJ (eds.), *Melatonin Biosynthesis, Physiological Effects and Clinical Applications*. CRC Press, Boca Raton, FL, 1993.

2. Waldhauser F, Ehrhart B, and Forster E, Clinical aspects of the melatonin action. *Experentia* **49**, 671–681, 1993.

3. Reiter RJ, *et al.*, A review of the evidence supporting melatonin's role as an antioxidant. *J Pineal Res* **18(1)**, 1–11, 1995.

4. Arendt J, *et al.*, Some effects of jet-lag and their alleviation by melatonin. *Ergonomics* **30**, 1379–1393, 1987.

5. Claustrat B, *et al.*, Melatonin and jet lag: Confirmatory result using a simplified protocol. *Biol Psychiatry* **32**, 705–711, 1992.

6. Petrie K, *et al.*, Effect of melatonin on jet lag after long haul flights. *Br Med J* **298**, 705–707, 1989.

7. Lino A, *et al.*, Melatonin and jet lag: Treatment schedule. *Biol Psychiatry* **34**, 587, 1993.

8. Petrie K, *et al.*, A double-blind trial of melatonin as a treatment for jet lag in international cabin crew. *Biol Psychiatry* **33**, 526–530, 1993.

9. Waldhauser F, Saletu B, and Trinchard-Lugan I, Sleep laboratory investigations on hypnotic properties of melatonin. *Psychopharmacol* **100**, 222–226, 1990.

10. Zhdanova IV, *et al.*, Sleep-inducing effects of low doses of melatonin ingested in the evening. *Clin Pharmacol Ther* **57**, 552–558, 1995.

11. Dahlitz M, *et al.*, Delayed sleep phase syndrome response to melatonin. *Lancet* **337**, 1121–1124, 1991.

12. MacFarlane JG, *et al.*, The effects of exogenous melatonin on the total sleep time and daytime alertness of chronic insomniacs: A preliminary study. *Biol Psychiatry* **30**, 371–376, 1991.

13. James SP, *et al.*, Melatonin administration in insomnia. *Neuropsychopharmacology* **3**, 19–23, 1990.

14. Nave R, Peled R, and Lavie P, Melatonin improves evening napping. *Eur J Pharmacol* **275**, 213–216, 1995.

15. Haimov I, *et al.*, Sleep disorders and melatonin rhythms elderly people. *BMJ* **309**, 167, 1994.

16. Molis TM, *et al.*, Melatonin modulation of estrogen-regulated proteins, growth factors, and proto-oncogenes in human breast cancer. *J Pineal Res* **18(2)**, 93–103, 1995.

17. Reiter RJ, Melatonin suppression by static and extremely low frequency electromagnetic fields: Relationship to the reported increased incidence of cancer. *Rev Environ Health* **10**, 3, 4, 171–186, 1994.

18. Lissoni P, *et al.*, A randomized study with subcutaneous low-dose interleukin 2 alone vs interleukin 2 plus the pineal neurohormone melatonin in advanced solid neoplasms other than renal cancer and melanoma. *Br J Cancer* **69**, 196–199, 1994.

19. Lissoni P, *et al.*, A randomized study of neuroimmunotherapy with low-dose subcutaneous interleukin-2 plus melatonin compared to supportive care alone in patients with untreatable metastatic solid tumor. *Support Care Cancer* **3(3)**, 194–197, 1995.

20. Neri B, *et al.*, Modulation of human lymphoblastoid interferon activity by melatonin in metastatic renal cell carcinoma: A phase II study. *Cancer* **73(12)**, 3015–3019, 1994.

21. Brackowski R, *et al.*, Preliminary study on modulation of the biological effects of tumor necrosis factor-alpha in advanced cancer patients by the pineal hormone melatonin. *J Biol Regul Homeost Agents* **8(3)**, 77–80, 1994.

22. Lissoni P, *et al.*, Modulation of cancer endocrine therapy by melatonin: A phase II study of tamoxifen plus melatonin in metastatic breast cancer patients progressing under tamoxifen alone. *Br J Cancer* **71(4)**, 854–856, 1995.

23. Lissoni P, *et al.*, Randomized study with the pineal hormone melatonin versus supportive care alone in advanced non-small cell lung cancer resistant to a first-line chemotherapy containing cisplatin. *Oncology* **49**, 336–339, 1992.

24. Lissoni P, *et al.*, Clinical results with the pineal hormone melatonin in advanced cancer resistant to standard antitumor therapies. *Oncology* **48**, 448–450, 1991.

25. Lissoni P, *et al.*, A randomized study with the pineal hormone melatonin versus supportive care alone in patients with brain metastases due to solid neoplasms. *Cancer* **73**, 699–701, 1994.

26. Maurizi C, Disorder of the pineal gland associated with depression, peptic ulcers, and sexual dysfunction. *Southern Med J* **77**, 1516–1518, 1984.

27. Wetterberg L, The relationship between the pineal gland and the pituitary-adrenal axis in health, endocrine and psychiatric conditions. *Psychoneuroendocrinology* **8**, 75–80, 1983.
28. Beck F, *et al.*, Serum melatonin in relation to clinical variables in patients with major depressive mood and a hypothesis of low melatonin syndrome. *Acta Psychiatr Scand* **71**, 319–330, 1985.
29. Rubin RL, *et al.*, Neuroendocrine aspects of primary endogenous depression, XI, Serum melatonin measures in patients and matched control subjects. *Arch Gen Psychiat* **49**, 558–567, 1992.
30. Thompsom C, *et al.*, A comparison of melatonin secretion in depressed patients and normal subjects. *Br J Psychiatry* **152**, 260–265, 1988.
31. Waterman GS, *et al.*, Nocturnal urinary excretion of 6-hydroxymelatonin sulfate in prepubertal major depressive disorder. *Biol Psychiatry* **31**, 582–590, 1992.
32. Mallo C, *et al.*, Effects of a four-day nocturnal melatonin treatment on the 24 h plasma melatonin, cortisol and prolactin profiles in humans. *Acta Endocrinologia* **119**, 474–480, 1988.
33. Carman JS, *et al.*, Negative effects of melatonin on depression. *Am J Psychiatry* **133**, 1181–1186, 1976.
34. Dollins AB, *et al.*, Effect of pharmacological daytime doses of melatonin on human mood and performance. *Psychopharmacol* **112**, 490–496, 1993.
35. Dollins AB, *et al.*, Effect of inducing nocturnal serum melatonin concentrations in daytime on sleep, mood, body temperature, and performance. *Proc Natl Acad Sci USA* **91**, 1824–1828, 1994.
36. Fellenberg AJ, Phillipou G, and Seamark RF, Measurement of urinary production rates of melatonin as an index of human pineal function. *Endocr Res Comm* **7**, 167–175, 1980.
37. Honma K, *et al.*, Effects of vitamin B_{12} on plasma melatonin rhythm in humans: Increased light sensitivity phase-advances the circadian clock? *Experentia* **48**, 716–720, 1992.
38. Okawa M, *et al.*, Vitamin B_{12} treatment for sleep-wake rhythm disorders. *Sleep* **13**, 1–23, 1990.

43 Phosphatidylserine

1. Vannucchi MG, Casamenti F, and Pepeu G, Decrease of acetylcholine release from cortical slices in aged rats: Investigations into its reversal by phosphatidylserine. *J Neurochem* **55**, 819–825, 1990.
2. Valzelli L, *et al.*, Activity of phosphatidylserine on memory retrieval and on exploration in mice. *Meth Find Exptl Clin Pharmacol* **9**, 657–660, 1987.
3. Nunzi MG, *et al.*, Effects of phosphatidylserine administration on age-related structural changes in the rat hippocampus and septal complex. *Pharmacopsychiat* **22**, 125–128, 1989.
4. Cenacchi T, *et al.*, Cognitive decline in the elderly: A double-blind, placebo-controlled multicenter study on efficacy of phosphatidylserine administration. *Aging* **5**, 123–133, 1993.
5. Engel RR, *et al.*, Double-blind cross-over study of phosphatidylserine vs. placebo in patients with early dementia of the Alzheimer type. *Eur Neuropsychopharmacol* **2**, 149–155, 1992.
6. Crook T, *et al.*, Effects of phosphatidylserine in Alzheimer's disease. *Psychopharmacol Bull* **28**, 61–66, 1992.
7. Crook TH, *et al.*, Effects of phosphatidylserine in age-associated memory impairment. *Neurology* **41**, 644–649, 1991.
8. Funfgeld EW, *et al.*, Double-blind study with phosphatidylserine (PS) in parkinsonian patients with senile dementia of Alzheimer's type (SDAT). *Prog Clin Biol Res* **317**, 1235–1246, 1989.
9. Maggioni M, *et al.*, Effects of phosphatidylserine therapy in geriatric patients with depressive disorders. *Acta Psychiatr Scand* **81**, 265–270, 1990.
10. Monteleone P, *et al.*, Effects of phosphatidylserine on the neuroendocrine response to physical stress in humans. *Neuroendocrinology* **52**, 243–248, 1990.

11. Monteleone P, *et al.*, Blunting chronic phosphatidylserine administration of the stress-induced activation of the hypothalamo-pituitary-adrenal axis in healthy men. *Eur J Clin Pharamacol* **41**, 385–388, 1992.
12. Nerozzi D, *et al.*, Early cortisol escape phenomenon reversed by phosphatidylserine in elderly normal subjects. *Clinical Trials J* **26**, 33–38, 1989.
13. Hofferberth B, The efficacy of Egb761 in patients with senile dementia of the Alzheimer type: A double-blind, placebo-controlled study on different levels of investigation. *Human Psychopharmacol* **9**, 215–222, 1994.

44 Probiotics

1. Metchnikoff E, *The Prolongation of Life*. Arna Press, New York, NY, 1908 (1977 reprint).
2. Hentges DJ (ed.), Human Intestinal Microflora. In: *Health and Disease*. Academic Press, New York, NY, 1983.
3. Shahani KM and Ayebo AD, Role of dietary *lactobacilli* in gastrointestinal microecology. *Am J Clin Nutr* **33**, 2448–2457, 1980.
4. Shahani KM and Friend BA, Nutritional and therapeutic aspects of *lactobacilli*. *J Appl Nutr* **36**, 125–152, 1984.
5. Hughes VL and Hillier SL, Microbiologic characteristics of *Lactobacillus* products used for colonization of the vagina. *Obstet Gynecol* **75**, 244–248, 1990.
6. Mitsuoka T, Intestinal flora and host. *Asian Med J* **31**, 400–409, 1988.
7. Barefoot SF, and Klaenhammer TR, Detection and activity of lacticin B, a bacteriocin produced by *Lactobacillus acidophilus*. *Appl Environ Microbiol* **45**, 1808–1815, 1983.
8. Klaenhammer TR, Microbiological considerations in the selection of preparations of *lactobacillus* strains for use in dietary adjuncts. *J Dairy Sci* **65**, 1339–1349, 1982.
9. Klaenhammer TR, Bacteriocins of lactic acid bacteria. *Biochemie* **70**, 337–349, 1988.
10. Upreti GC and Hinsdill RD, Isolation and characterization of a bacteriocin from a homofermentative *Lactobacillus*. *Antimicrob Agents Chemother* **4**, 487–494, 1973.
11. Upreti GC and Hinsdill RD, Production and mode of action of lactocin 27, Bacteriocin from a homofermentative *Lactobacillus*. *Antimicrob Agents Chemother* **7**, 139–145, 1975.
12. DeKlerk HC, Bacteriocinogency in *Lactobacillus fermenti*. *Nature* **214**, 609, 1967.
13. DeKlerk HC and Smit JA, Properties of a *Lactobacillus fermenti* bacteriocin. *J Gen Microbiol* **48**, 309–316, 1967.
14. Friend BA and Shahani KM, Nutritional and therapeutic aspects of *lactobacilli*. *J Appl Nutr* **36**, 125–152, 1984.
15. Shahani KM, Vakil JR, and Kilara A, Natural antibiotic activity of *Lactobacillus acidophilus* and *bulgaricus*, II, Isolation of acidophilin from *L. acidophilus*. *Cult Dairy Prod J* **12**, 8, 1977.
16. Shahani KM, Vakil JR, and Kilara A, Natural antibiotic activity of *Lactobacillus acidophilus* and *Lactobacillus bulgaricus*. *Cult Dairy Prod J* **11**, 14–17, 1976.
17. Dahiya RS and Speck ML, Hydrogen peroxide formation by *lactobacilli* and its effect on *Staphylococcus aureus*. *J Dairy Sci* **51**, 1568, 1968.
18. Price RJ and Lee JS, Inhibition of *pseudomonas* species by hydrogen peroxide producing *lactobacilli*. *J Milk Food Technol* **33**, 13, 1970.
19. Vesely R, Negri R, Bianchi-Salvadori B, *et al.*, Influence of a diet addition with yogurt on the mouse immune system. *EOS J Immunol Immunopharmacol* **5**, 30–35, 1985.
20. Vincent JG, Veonett RC, and Riley RG, Antibacterial activities associated with *Lactobacillus acidophilus*. *J Bacterioll* **78**, 477, 1959.
21. Perdigon G, N de Macias ME, Alvarez S, *et al.*, Enhancement of immune response in mice fed with *Streptococcus thermophilus* and *Lactobacillus acidophilus*. *J Diary Sci* **70**, 919–926, 1987.
22. Weir D and Blackwell C, Interaction of bacteria with the immune system. *J Clin Lab Immunol* **10**, 1–12, 1983.
23. Perdigon G, de Macias N, Alvarez S, *et al.*, Systemic augmentation of the immune response in mice by feeding fermented milks with *Lactobacillus casei* and *Lactobacillus acidophilus*. *Immunol* **63**, 17–23, 1988.

24. Perdigon G, *et al.*, Symposium: Probiotic bacteria for humans: Clinical systems for evaluation of effectiveness: Immune system stimulation by probiotics. *J Dairy Sci* **78**, 1597–1606, 1995.

25. Clements ML, Levine MM, Black RE, *et al.*, *Lactobacillus prophylaxis* for diarrhea due to enterotoxinogenic *Escherichia coli*. *Antimicrob Agents Chemother* **20**, 104–108, 1981.

26. Dios Pozo-Olano JD, Warram JH, Gomez RG and Cavazos MG, Effect of a *lactobacilli* preparation on traveler's diarrhea: A randomized, double blind clinical trial. *Gastroenterol* **74**, 829–830, 1978.

27. Thompson GE, Control of intestinal flora in animals and humans: Implications for toxicology and health. *J Environ Path Toxicol* **1**, 113–123, 1977.

28. Clements ML, Levine MM, and Ristaino PA, Exogenous *lactobacilli* fed to man: Their fate and ability to prevent diarrheal disease. *Prog Food Nutr Sci* **7**, 29–37, 1983.

29. Tomomatsu H, Health effects of oligosaccharides. *Food Technol* October, 61–65, 1994.

30. Gibson GR, *et al.*, Selective stimulation of *bifidobacteria* in the human colon by oligofructose and inulin. *Gastroenterology* **108**, 975–982, 1995.

31. Zoppi G, Deganello A, Benoni G, and Saccomani F, Oral bacteriotherapy in clinical practice, I, The use of different preparations in infants treated with antibiotics. *Eur J Ped* **139**, 18–21, 1982.

32. Gotz VP, Romankiewics JA, Moss J, and Murray HW, Prophylaxis against ampicillin-induced diarrhea with a *lactobacillus* preparation. *Am J Hosp Pharm* **36**, 754–757, 1979.

33. Zoppi G, Balsamo V, Deganello A, *et al.*, Oral bacteriotherapy in clinical practice, I, The use of different preparations in the treatment of acute diarrhea. *Eur J Ped* **139**, 22–24, 1982.

34. Collins EB and Hardt P, Inhibition of *Candida albicans* by *Lactobacillus acidophilus*. *J Dairy Sci* **63**, 830–832, 1980.

35. Neri A, Sabah G, and Samra Z, Bacterial vaginosis in pregnancy treated with yoghurt. *Acta Obstet Gynecol* **72**, 17–19, 1993.

36. Butler C and Beakley JW, Bacterial flora in the vagina. *Am J Obstet Gynecol* **79**, 432, 1960.

37. Lock FR, Yow MD, Griffith MI, and Stout M, Bacteriology of the vagina in 75 normal young adults. *Surg Gyn Obs* **87**, 410, 1948.

38. Rogosa M and Sharp ME, Species differentiation of human vaginal lactobacilli. *J Gen Microbiol* **23**, 197, 1960.

39. Wylie JG and Henderson A, Identity of glycogen-fermenting ability of *lactobacilli* isolated from the vagina of pregnant women. *J Med Microbiol* **2**, 363, 1969.

40. Huppert M, Cazin J, and Smith H, Pathogenesis of *C. albicans* infections following antibiotic therapy. *J Bacteriol* **70**, 440–447, 1955.

41. Reid G, Bruce AW, and Taylor M, Influence of three-day antimicrobial therapy and *lactobacillus* vaginal suppositories on recurrence of urinary tract infections. *Clin Ther* **14**, 11–16, 1992.

42. IARC Intestinal Microecology Group, Dietary fibre, transit time, fecal bacteria, steroids, and colon cancer in two Scandinavian populations. *Lancet* **ii**, 207–210, 1977.

43. Bogdanov IG, Velichkov VT, Daley PG, *et al.*, Antitumor action of glycopeptides from cell wall of *Lactobacillus bulgaricus*. *Bull Exp Biol* **84**, 1750, 1977.

44. Bailey PJ and Shahani KM, Inhibitory effect of *acidophilus* cultured colostrum and milk upon the proliferation of ascites tumor. *Proc 71st Ann Meet Am Dairy Sci Assoc*, 41, 1979.

45. Ayebo AD, Angelo IA, Shahani KM, and Kies C, Effect of feeding Lactobacillus acidophilus milk upon fecal flora and enzyme activity in humans. *J Dairy Sci* **62** (Suppl. 1), 44, 1979.

46. Aso Y, *et al.*, Preventive effect of *Lactobacillus casei* preparation on the recurrence of superficial bladder cancer in a double-blind trial. *Eur Urol* **27**, 104–109, 1995.

47. Salminen E, *et al.*, Preservation of intestinal integrity during radiotherapy using live *Lactobacillus acidophilus* cultures. *Clin Radiology* **39**, 435–437, 1988.

48. Daikos GK, Kontomichalou P, Bilalis D, and Pimenidou L, Intestinal flora ecology after oral use of antibiotics. *Chemotherapy* **13**, 146–160, 1968.

49. Pradhan A and Majumdar MK, Metabolism of some drugs by intestinal *lactobacilli* and their toxicological considerations. *Acta Pharmacol Toxicol* **58**, 11–15, 1986.

45 S-Adenosylmethionine (SAM)

1. Strementinoli G, Pharmacological aspects of S-adenosylmethionine: Pharmacokinetics and pharamcodynamics. *Am J Med* **83** (Suppl. 5A), 35–42, 1987.
2. Bombardieri G, *et al.*, Intestinal absorption of S-adenosyl-L-methionine in humans. *Int J Clin Pharmacol Ther Toxicol* **21**, 186–188, 1983.
3. Baldessarini RJ, Neuropharmacology of S-adenosyl-L-methionine. *Am J Med* **83** (Suppl. 5A), 95–103, 1987.
4. Reynolds E, Carney M, and Toone B, Methylation and mood. *Lancet* **ii**, 196–199, 1983.
5. Bottiglieri T, Laundry M, Martin R, *et al.*, S-adenosylmethionine influences monoamine metabolism. *Lancet* **ii**, 224, 1984.
6. Janicak PG, *et al.*, Parenteral S-adenosylmethionine in depression: A literature review and preliminary report. *Psychopharmacology Bulletin* **25**, 238–241, 1989.
7. Friedel HA, Goa KL, and Benfield P, S-adenosylmethionine. *Drugs* **38**, 3889–3417, 1989.
8. Carney MWP, Toone BK, and Reynolds EH, S-adenosylmethionine and affective disorder. *Am J Med* **83** (Suppl. 5A), 104–106, 1987.
9. Vahora SA and Malek-Ahmadi P, S-adenosylmethionine in depression. *Neurosci Biobehav Rev*, **12**, 139–141, 1988.
10. Kagan BL, *et al.*, Oral S-adenosylmethionine in depression: A randomized, double-blind placebo-controlled trial. *Am J Psychiatry* **147**, 591–595, 1990.
11. Rosenbaum JF, *et al.*, An open-label pilot study of oral S-adenosylmethionine in major depression. *Psychopharmacol Bull* **24**, 189–194, 1988.
12. De Vanna M and Rigamonti R, Oral S-adenosyl-L-methionine in depression. *Curr Ther Res* **52**, 478–485, 1992.
13. Salmaggi P, *et al.*, Double-blind, placebo-controlled study of S-adenosyl-L-methionine in depressed postmenopausal women. *Psychother Psychosom* **59**, 34–40, 1993.
14. Bell KM, *et al.*, S-adenosylmethionine blood levels in major depression: Changes with drug treatment. *Acta Neurol Scand* **154** (Suppl.), 15–18, 1994.
15. Cerutti R, *et al.*, Psychological distress during peurperium: A novel therapeutic approach using S-adenosylmethionine. *Curr Ther Res* **53**, 707–717, 1993.
16. Lo Russo A, *et al.*, Efficacy of S-adenosyl-L-methionine in relieving psychological distress associated with detoxification in opiate abusers. *Curr Ther Res* **55**, 905–913, 1994.
17. Brandt KD, Effects of nonsteroidal anti-inflammatory drugs on chondrocyte metabolism *in vitro* and *in vivo*. *Am J Med* **83** (Suppl. 5A), 29–34, 1987.
18. Shield MJ, Anti-inflammatory drugs and their effects on cartilage synthesis and renal function. *Eur J Rheumatol Inflam* **13**, 7–16, 1993.
19. Brooks PM, Potter SR, and Buchanan W, NSAID and osteoarthritis—help or hindrance. *J Rheumatol* **9**, 3–5, 1982.
20. Newman NM and Ling RSM, Acetabular bone destruction related to non-steroidal anti-inflammatory drugs. *Lancet* **ii**; 11–13, 1985.
21. Solomon L, Drug induced arthropathy and necrosis of the femoral head. *J Bone Joint Surg* **55B**, 246–251, 1973.
22. Harmand MF, *et al.*, Effects of S-adenosylmethionine on human articular chondrocyte differentiation: An *in vitro* study. *Am J Med* **83** (Suppl. 5A), 48–54, 1987.
23. Konig H, *et al.*, Magnetic resonance tomography of finger polyarthritis: Morphology and cartilage signals after ademetionine therapy. *Aktuelle Radiol* **5**, 36–40, 1995.
24. Muller-Fassbender H, Double-blind clinical trial of S-adenosylmethionine versus ibuprofen in the treatment of osteoarthritis. *Am J Med* **83** (Suppl. 5A), 81–83, 1987.
25. Glorioso S, *et al.*, Double-blind multicentre study of the activity of S-adenosylmethionine in hip and knee osteoarthritis. *Int J Clin Pharmacol Res* **5**, 39–49, 1985.

26. Marcolongo R, *et al.*, Double-blind multicentre study of the activity of S-adenosyl-methionine in hip and knee osteoarthritis. *Curr Ther Res* **37**, 82–94, 1985.

27. Domljan Z, *et al.*, A double-blind trial of ademetionine vs naproxen in activated go-narthrosis. *Int J Clin Pharmacol Ther Toxicol* **27**, 329–333, 1989.

28. Caruso I and Pietrogrande V, Italian double-blind multicenter study comparing S-adenosylmethionine, naproxen, and placebo in the treatment of degenerative joint disease. *Am J Med* **83** (Suppl. 5A), 66–71, 1987.

29. Vetter G, Double-blind comparative clinical trial with S-adenosylmethionine and indomethacin in the treatment of osteoarthritis. *Am J Med* **83** (Suppl. 5A), 78–80, 1987.

30. Maccagno A, Double-blind controlled clinical trial of oral S-adenosylmethionine versus piroxicam in knee osteoarthritis. *Am J Med* **83** (Suppl. 5A), 72–77, 1987.

31. Konig B, A long-term (two years) clinical trial with S-adenosylmethionine for the treatment of osteoarthritis. *Am J Med* **83** (Suppl. 5A), 89–94, 1987.

32. Berger R and Nowak H, A new medical approach to the treatment of osteoarthritis: Report of an open phase IV study with ademetionine (Gumbaral). *Am J Med* **83** (Suppl. 5A), 84–88, 1987.

33. Tavoni A, *et al.*, Evaluation of S-adenosylmethionine in primary fibromyalgia: A double-blind crossover study. *Am J Med* **83** (Suppl. 5A), 107–110, 1987.

34. Jacobsen S, *et al.*, Oral S-adenosylmethionine in primary fibromyalgia: Double-blind clinical evaluation. *Scand J Rheumatol* **20**, 294–302, 1991.

35. Di Benedetto P, Iona LG, and Zidarich V, Clinical evaluation of S-adenosyl-L-methionine versus transcutaneous nerve stimulation in primary fibromyalgia. *Curr Ther Res* **53**, 222–229, 1993.

36. Mazzanti R, *et al.*, On the antisteatosic effects of S-adenosyl-L-methionine in various chronic liver diseases: A multicenter study. *Curr Ther Res* **25**, 25–32, 1979.

37. Frezza M, *et al.*, Oral S-adenosylmethionine in the symptomatic treatment of intrahepatic cholestasis: A double-blind, placebo-controlled study. *Gastroenterology* **99**, 211–215, 1990.

38. Adachi Y, *et al.*, The effects of S-adenosyl-methionine on intrahepatic cholestasis. *Jap Arch Int Med* **33**, 185–192, 1986.

39. Padova C, Tritapepe R, Padova F, *et al.*, S-adenosyl-L-methionine antagonizes oral contraceptive-induced bile cholesterol supersaturation in healthy women: Preliminary report of a controlled randomized trial. *Am J Gastroenterol* **79**, 941–944, 1984.

40. Frezza M, Pozzato G, Chiesa L, *et al.*, Reversal of intrahepatic cholestasis of pregnancy in women after high dose S-adenosyl-L-methionine (SAMe) administration. *Hepatology* **4**, 274–278, 1984.

41. Frezza M, *et al.*, S-adenosylmethionine counteracts oral contraceptive hepatotoxicity in women. *Am J Med Sci* **293**, 234–238, 1987.

42. Bombardieri G, Milani A, Bernardi L, and Rossi L, Effects of S-adenosyl-L-methionine (SAMe) in the treatment of Gilbert's syndrome. *Curr Ther Res* **37**, 580–585, 1985.

43. Angelico M, *et al.*, Oral S-adenosyl-L-methionine (SAMe) administration enhances bile salt conjugation with taurine in patients with liver cirrhosis. *Scand J Clin Lab Invest* **54**, 459–464, 1994.

44. Kakimoto H, *et al.*, Changes in lipid composition of erythrocyte membranes with administration of S-adenosyl-L-methionine in chronic liver disease. *Gastroenterolia Japonica* **27**, 508–513, 1992.

45. Loguercio C, *et al.*, Effect of S-adenosyl-L-methionine administration on red blood cell cysteine and glutathione levels in alcoholic patients with and without liver disease. *Alcohol Alcoholism* **29**, 597–604, 1994.

46. Pascale RM, *et al.*, Chemoprevention of rat liver carcinogenesis by S-adenosyl-L-methionine: A long-term study. *Cancer Res* **52**, 4979–4986, 1992.

47. Gatto G, *et al.*, Analgesizing effect of a methyl donor (S-adenosylmethionine) in migraine: An open clinical trial. *Int J Clin Pharmacol Res* **6**, 15–17, 1986.

48. Reicks M and Hathcock JN, Effects of methionine and other sulfur compounds on drug conjugations. *Pharmac Ther* **37**, 67–79, 1988.

Part Six Introduction—Glandular Product Profiles

1. Gardener MLG, Gastrointestinal absorption of intact proteins. *Ann Rev Nutr* **8**, 329–350, 1988.
2. Gardner MLG, Intestinal assimilation of intact peptides and proteins from the diet—a neglected field? *Biol Rev* **59**, 289–331, 1984.
3. Udall JN and Walker WA, The physiologic and pathologic basis for the transport of macromolecules across the intestinal tract. *J Pediatr Gastroenterol Nutr* **1**, 295–301, 1982.
4. Kleine MW, Stauder GM, and Beese EW, The intestinal absorption of orally administered hydrolytic enzymes and their effects in the treatment of acute herpes zoster as compared with those of oral acyclovir therapy. *Phytomedicine* **2**, 7–15, 1995.
5. Hemmings WA and Williams EW, Transport of large breakdown products of dietary protein through the gut wall. *Gut* **27**, 715–723, 1986.
6. Ambrus JL, *et al.*, Absorption of exogenous and endogenous proteolytic enzymes. *Clin Pharmacol Ther* **8**, 362–368, 1967.
7. Kabacoff BB, *et al.*, Absorption of chymotrypsin from the intestinal tract. *Nature* **199**, 815–817, 1963.
8. Ormiston BJ, Clinical effects of TRH and TSH after i.v. and oral administration in normal volunteers and patients with thyroid disease. In: *Thytropin Releasing Hormone (Frontiers of Hormone Research, Vol. I)*, R Hal *et al.* (eds.). Karger, Basel, Switzerland, 1972, pp. 45–52.
9. Amoss M, *et al.*, Release of gonadotrophins by oral administration of synthetic LRF or tripeptide fragment of LRF. *J Clin Endocrinol Metab* **35**, 175–177, 1977.
10. Seifert J, *et al.*, Mucosal permeation of macromolecules and particles. *Angiology* **17**, 505–513, 1966.
11. Laskowski M, *et al.*, Effect of trypsin inhibitor on passage of insulin across the intestinal barrier. *Science* **127**, 1115, 1116, 1958.

46 Adrenal Extracts

1. Seyle H, *Stress in Health and Disease*. Buttersworth, London, UK, 1976.
2. Britton SW and Silvette H, Further experiments on cortico-adrenal extract: Its efficacy by mouth. *Science* **74**, 440, 441, 1931.

47 Aortic Glycosaminoglycans

1. Stevens RL, *et al.*, The glycosaminoglycans of the human artery and their changes in atherosclerosis. *J Clin Invest* **58**, 470–481, 1976.
2. Tammi M, *et al.*, Connective tissue components in normal and atherosclerotic human coronary arteries. *Atherosclerosis* **29**, 191–194, 1978.
3. Day CE, Powell JR, and Levy RS, Sulfated polysaccharide inhibition of aortic uptake of low density lipoproteins. *Artery* **1**, 126–137, 1975.
4. Pernigotti LM, *et al.*, Effect of mesoglycan on clotting, fibrinolysis and platelet aggregation in normal subjects and hyperaggregating arteriosclerosis. In: *Current Aspects of Atherosclerosis. Lipids, Lipoproteins, Platelets, Prostaglandins, and Experimental Findings*. Widhalm K and Sinzinger H (eds.). Verlag Wilhelm, Madrich, 1983, pp. 164–175.
5. Postiglione A, *et al.*, Effect of oral mesoglycan-sulphate on plasma lipoprotein concentration and on lipoprotein concentration in primary hyperlipidemia. *Pharmacol Res Comm* **16**, 1–8, 1984.
6. Saba P, *et al.*, Hypolipidemic effect of mesoglycan in hyperlipidemic patients. *Curr Ther Res* **40**, 761–768, 1986.
7. Zanolo G, *et al.*, Pharmacokinetic aspect of tritium-labeled glycosaminoglycans (mesoglycan), their absorption in rat and monkey and tissue distribution in rat. *Boll Chim Farm* **123**, 223–235, 1984.
8. Abate G, *et al.*, Controlled multicenter study on the therapeutic effectiveness of mesoglycan in patients with cerebrovascular disease. *Min Med* **82(3)**, 101–105, 1991.

9. Mansi D, *et al.*, Open trial of mesoglycan in the treatment of cerebrovascular ischemic disease. *Acta Neurol* **10**, 108–112, 1988.
10. Laurora G, *et al.*, Delayed arteriosclerosis progression in high risk subjects treated with mesoglycan: Evaluation of intima-media thickness. *J Cardiovasc Surg* **34(4)**, 313–318, 1993.
11. Vecchio F, *et al.*, Mesoglycan in treatment of patients with cerebral ischemia: Effects on hemorrheologic and hematochemical parameters. *Acta Neurol* **15(6)**, 449–456, 1993.
12. De Donato G and Sangiuolo P, Instrumental evaluation of the mesoglycan effects in phlebopathic patients: Prospective randomized double-blind study. *Min Med* **77**, 1927–1931, 1986.
13. Oddone G, Fiscella GF, and De Franceschi T, Assessment of the effects of oral mesoglycan sulphate in patients with chronic venous pathology of the lower extremities. *Gazzetta Medica Italiana* **146**, 111–114, 1987.
14. Prandoni P, Cattelan AM, and Carta M, Long-term sequelae of deep venous thrombosis of the legs: Experience with mesoglycan. *Ann Ital Med Int* **4(4)**, 378–385, 1989.
15. Sangrigoli V, Mesoglycan in acute and chronic venous insufficiency of the legs. *Clin Ther* **129(3)**, 207–209, 1989.
16. Petruzezellis V and Velon A, Therapeutic action of oral doses of mesoglycan in the pharmacological treatment of varicose syndrome and its complications. *Min Med* **76**, 543–548, 1985.
17. Saggloro A, *et al.*, Treatment of hemorrhoidal syndrome with mesoglycan. *Min Diet Gastr* **31**, 311–315, 1985.
18. Nakazawa K and Murata K, The therapeutic effect of chondroitin polysulphate in elderly atherosclerotic patients. *J Int Med Res* **6**, 217–225, 1978.

48   Liver Extracts

1. Krause MV and Mahan KL, *Food, Nutrition and Diet Therapy, 7th Edition*. WB Saunders, Philadelphia, PA, 1984, pp. 128–131, 157–164, 585–599.
2. Fairbanks VF and Beutler E, Iron. In: *Modern Nutrition in Health and Disease, 7th Edition*. Shils ME and Young VR (eds.). Lea and Febiger, Philadelphia, PA, 1988, pp. 193–226.
3. Nagai K, A study of the excretory mechanism of the liver—effect of liver hydrolysate on BSP excretion. *Jap J Gastroenterol* **67**, 633–638, 1970.
4. Ohbayashi A, Akioka T, and Tasaki H, A study of effects of liver hydrolysate on hepatic circulation. *J Therapy* **54**, 1582–1585, 1972.
5. Sanbe K, *et al.*, Treatment of liver disease—with particular reference to liver hydrolysates. *Jap J Clin Exp Med* **50**, 2665–2676, 1973.
6. Fujisawa K, *et al.*, Therapeutic effects of liver hydrolysate preparation on chronic hepatitis—A double blind, controlled study. *Asian Med J* **26**, 497–526, 1984.

49   Pancreatic Extracts

1. Ambrus JL, *et al.*, Absorption of exogenous and endogenous proteolytic enzymes. *Clin Pharmacol Ther* **8**, 362–368, 1967.
2. Kabacoff BB, *et al.*, Absorption of chymotrypsin from the intestinal tract. *Nature* **199**, 815–817, 1963.
3. Martin GJ, *et al.*, Further *in vivo* observations with radioactive trypsin. *Am J Pharm* **129**, 386–392, 1964.
4. Avakian S, Further studies on the absorption of chymotrypsin. *Clin Pharmacol Ther* **5**, 712–715, 1964.
5. Kleine MW, Stauder GM, and Beese EW, The intestinal absorption of orally administered hydrolytic enzymes and their effects in the treatment of acute *herpes zoster* as compared with those of oral acyclovir therapy. *Phytomedicine* **2**, 7–15, 1995.
6. Liebow C and Rothman SS, Enteropancreatic circulation of digestive enzymes. *Science* **189**, 472–474, 1975.

7. Rubinstein E, *et al.*, Antibacterial activity of the pancreatic fluid. *Gastroenterol* **88**, 927–932, 1985.

8. Oelgoetz AW, *et al.*, The treatment of food allergy and indigestion of pancreatic origin with pancreatic enzymes. *Am J Dig Dis Nutr* **2**, 422–426, 1935.

9. Carroccio A, *et al.*, Pancreatic enzyme therapy in childhood celiac disease: A double-blind prospective randomized study. *Dig Dis Sci* **40**, 2555–2560, 1995.

10. Innerfield I, *Enzymes in Clinical Medicine*. McGraw Hill, New York, 1960.

11. Horger I, Enzyme therapy in multiple rheumatic diseases. *Therapiewoche* **33**, 3948–3957, 1983.

12. Ransberger K, Enzyme treatment of immune complex diseases. *Arth Rheum* **8**, 16–19, 1986.

13. Steffen C, *et al.*, Enzyme therapy in comparison with immune complex determinations in chronic polyarteritis. *Rheumatologie* **44**, 51–56, 1985.

14. Ransberger K and van Schaik W, Enzyme therapy in multiple sclerosis. *Der Kassenarzt* **41**, 42–45, 1986.

15. Hoefer-Janker H, The importance of vitamin A and proteolytic enzymes in cancer therapy. *Arz Praxis* **54**, 2805–2806, 1971.

16. Rokitansky O, Adjuvant enzyme treatment before and after breast cancer surgery. *Dr Med* **1**, 16, 1980.

17. Dean DH and Hiramoto RN, Weight loss during pancreatin feeding of rats. *Nutr Rep Intl* **29**, 167–172, 1984.

50 Spleen Extracts

1. Minter MM, Agranulocytic angina: Treatment of a case with fetal calf spleen. *Texas State J Med* **2**, 338–343, 1933.

2. Gray GA, The treatment of agranulocytic angina with fetal calf spleen. *Texas State J Med* **29**, 366–369, 1933.

3. Greer AE, Use of fetal spleen in agranulocytosis: Preliminary report. *Texas State J Med* **28**, 338–343, 1932.

4. Fridkin M and Najjar VA, Tuftsin: Its chemistry, biology, and clinical potential. *Crit Rev Biochem Mol Biol* **24**, 1–40, 1989.

5. Diezel W, *et al.*, The effect of splenopentin (DA SP-5) on *in vitro* myelopoiesis and on AZT-induced bone marrow toxicity. *Int J Immunopharmac* **15**, 269–273, 1993.

6. Rastogi A, *et al.*, Augmentation of human natural killer cells by splenopentin analogs. *FEBS Letters* **317**, 93–95, 1993.

7. Volk HD, *et al.*, Immunorestitution by a bovine spleen hydrosylate and ultrafiltrate. *Arzneim Forsch* **41**, 1281–1285, 1991.

8. He SW, Effect of splenectomy on phagocytic function of leukocytes. *Chung Hua Wai Ko Tsa Chih* **27**, 354–381, 1989.

9. Spirer Z, *et al.*, Decreased tuftsin concentrations in patients who have undergone splenectomy. *Br Med J* **2**, 1574–1576, 1977.

10. Corazza GR, *et al.*, Tuftsin deficiency in AIDS. *Lancet* **i**, 12, 13, 1991.

11. Spirer Z, The role of the spleen in immunity and infection. *Adv Pediatrics* **27**, 55–88, 1980.

51 Thymus Extracts

1. Cazzola P, Mazzanti P, and Bossi G, *In vivo* modulating effect of a calf thymus acid lysate on human T lymphocyte subsets and CD4+/CD8+ ratio in the course of different diseases. *Curr Ther Res* **42**, 1011–1017, 1987.

2. Kouttab NM, Prada M, and Cazzola P, Thymomodulin: Biological properties and clinical applications. *Medical Oncology and Tumor Pharmacotherapy* **6**, 5–9, 1989.

3. Fiocchi A, *et al.*, A double-blind clinical trial for the evaluation of the therapeutic effectiveness of a calf thymus derivative (Thymomodulin) in children with recurrent respiratory infections. *Thymus* **8**, 831–839, 1986.

4. Galli M, *et al.*, Attempt to treat acute type B hepatitis with an orally administered thymic extract (Thymomodulin): Preliminary results. *Drugs Exp Clin Res* **11**, 665–669, 1985.

5. Bortolotti F, *et al.*, Effect of an orally administered thymic derivative, Thymodulin, in chronic type B hepatitis in children. *Curr Ther Res* **43**, 67–72, 1988.

6. Valesini G, *et al.*, A calf thymus lysate improves clinical symptoms and T-cell defects in the early stages of HIV infection: Second report. *Eur J Cancer Clin Oncol* **23**, 1915–1919, 1987.

7. Kang SD, Lee BH, Yang JH, and Lee CY, The effects of calf-thymus extract on recovery of bone marrow function in anticancer chemotherapy. *New Med J (Korea)* **28**, 11–15, 1985.

8. Marzari R, *et al.*, Perennial allergic rhinitis: Prevention of the acute episodes with Thymomodulin. *Min Med* **78**, 1675–1681, 1987.

9. Genova R and Guerra A, Thymomodulin in management of food allergy in children. *Int J Tiss React* **8**, 239–242, 1986.

10. Cavagni G, *et al.*, Food allergy in children: An attempt to improve the effects of the elimination diet with an immunomodulating agent (thymomodulin): A double-blind clinical trial. *Immunopharmacol Immunotoxicol* **11**, 131–142, 1989.

52 Thyroid Extracts

1. Petersdorf, R., *et al.* (eds.), *Harrison's Principles of Internal Medicine.* McGraw-Hill, New York, NY, 1983, pp. 614–623.

2. Mazzaferri EL, Adult hypothyroidism. *Postgraduate Medicine* **79**, 64–72, 1986.

3. Barnes BO and Galton L, *Hypothyroidism: The Unsuspected Illness.* Thomas Crowell, New York, NY, 1976.

4. Langer SE and Scheer JF, *Solved: The Riddle of Illness.* Keats, New Canaan, CT, 1984.

5. Gold M, Pottash A, and Extein I, Hypothyroidism and depression, evidence from complete thyroid function evaluation. *JAMA* **245**, 1919–1922, 1981.

6. Drinka PJ and Nolten WE, Review: Subclinical hypothyroidism in the elderly: To treat or not to treat? *Am J Med Sci* **295**, 125–128, 1988.

7. Banovac K, Zakarija M, and McKenzie JM, Experience with routine thyroid function testing: Abnormal results in "normal" populations. *J Florida Med Assoc* **72**, 835–839, 1985.

8. Rosenthal MJ, Hunt WC, Garry PJ, and Goodwin JS, Thyroid failure in the elderly: Microsomal antibodies as discriminate for therapy. *JAMA* **258**, 209–213, 1987.

9. Althaus U, Staub JJ, Ryff-De Leche A, *et al.*, LDL/HDL-changes in subclinical hypothyroidism: Possible risk factors for coronary heart disease. *Clinical Endocrinology* **28**, 157–163, 1988.

10. Dean JW and Fowler PBS, Exaggerated responsiveness to thyrotrophin releasing hormone: A risk factor in women with artery disease. *Brit Med J* **290**, 1555–1561, 1985.

11. Turnbridge WMG, Evered DC, and Hall R, Lipid profiles and cardiovascular disease in the Wickham area with particular reference to thyroid failure. *Clin Endocrinol* **7**, 495–508, 1977.

12. Joffe R, Roy-Byrne P, and Udhe T, Thyroid function and affective illness: A reappraisal. *Biol Psychiatry* **19**, 1685–1691, 1984.

13. Krupsky M, *et al.*, Musculoskeletal symptoms as a presenting sign of long-standing hypothyroidism. *Isr J Med Sci* **23**, 1110–1113, 1987.

14. Hochberg MC, *et al.*, Hypothyroidism presenting as a polymyositis/like syndrome. *Arth Rheum* **19**, 1363–1366, 1976.

15. Krause MV and Mahan LK, *Food, Nutrition, and Diet Therapy, 7th Edition.* WB Saunders, Philadelphia, PA, 1984, pp. 170–174.

16. Jennings IW, *Vitamins in Endocrine Metabolism.* CC Thomas, Springfield, IL, 1970.

17. Prasad A, Clinical, biochemical and nutritional spectrum of zinc deficiency in human subjects: An update. *Ntr Rev* **41**, 197–208, 1983.

18. Lennon D, Nagle F, Stratman F, *et al.*, Diet and exercise training effects on resting metabolic rate. *Int J Obesity* **9**, 39–47, 1985.

Index

A

Accessory nutrients, 9.
  See also Carnitine;
  Coenzyme Q$_{10}$; Flavo-
  noids; Probiotics
Accutane, 20
Acetic acid, 361
Acetylcholine
  in Alzheimer's disease, 140
  carnitine and, 290–291
  vitamin B$_1$ mimicking, 83
Achilles tendon, 431
Acne, 32, 416–417
  chromium and, 197–198
  retinoic acid and, 20
  zinc and, 187
Acne conglobata, 416
Acne vulgaris, 416
ACTH, melatonin and, 354
Activated riboflavin, 85
Acyclovir, 398
Acyl carrier protein (ACP), 115
Acyl-CoA, 283
Adrenal cortex, 381
  atrophy of, 383–384
Adrenal extracts, 381–385
  dosage, 384
  forms of, 384
  stress and, 381–383
Adrenal function
  exhaustion and, 383
  healthy function, 383–384
  vitamin B$_5$ and, 117
Adrenal gland, 377
Adventitia, 387
Advil, 368
Age spots, 417–418
Agglutinated sperm, 76
Aging. *See* Elderly persons;
  Symptoms of aging

AIDS, 418–419
  beta-carotenes and, 35
  carnitine and, 294
  coenzyme Q$_{10}$ and, 304
  lipoic acid and, 345–346
  NAC (n-acetylcysteine)
    and, 63
  pancreatic enzymes
    and, 397
  thymic hormone levels and,
    404
  thymus extracts and, 406
  tuftsin levels in, 402
  vitamin A and, 24, 31
  vitamin B$_6$ and, 107
  vitamin B$_{12}$ and, 132–133
  vitamin E and, 45
Akathisia, iron and, 211–212
Akne Treatment Cleanser, 417
Alarm reaction, 382
Alcohol and alcohol abuse,
    419–420
  biotin absorption, 114
  carnitine and, 292–293
  folic acid and, 126
  molybdenum and detoxi-
    fication, 219
  phosphatidylcholine and
    liver disease from, 130
  rosacea, 483
  sulfites in alcohol, 220
  vitamin B$_1$ deficiency, 82
  vitamin B$_6$ deficiency,
    100, 110
Aldehyde oxidase, 219
Aldose reductase, 74, 324
Aldosterone, 167, 381
Algal carotenes, 30
Algal polysaccharides, 310
Alkaline phosphatase, 371

Allergies. *See also* Food aller-
    gies; Sulfites
  essential fatty acids and,
    261–263
  glucocorticoids and, 381
  pancreatic extracts and, 396
  thymus activity and, 404
  thymus extracts and, 406
  vitamin C and, 67–68
Allicin, 437, 444
Allopathic medicine, 6–7
Alopecia, 111
Alpha-carotene, 27
Alpha-linolenic acid,
    242–243, 247
  breast cancer and, 267
  heart disease and, 259
Alpha-tocopherol, 33, 44, 46
Aluminum, 230
Alzheimer's disease, 420–422
  carnitine and, 290–291
  Ginkgo biloba, 357
  phosphatidylcholine sup-
    plementation for, 140
  silicon and, 230
Alzheimer's disease, *cont.*
  vitamin B$_1$ and, 83
  vitamin B$_{12}$ and, 128, 133–134
  zinc deficiency and, 188
American Cancer Society, 277
American College of Ad-
    vancement in Medicine
    (ACAM), 436
American Heart Associa-
    tion, 277
  diet, 359
Amino acids
  carnitine and errors in
    metabolism of, 294
  neurotransmitters, 102

Encyclopedia of Natural Medicine

by Michael T. Murray, N.D.,
and Joseph Pizzorno, N.D.
$19.95

The companion reference to the
Encyclopedia of Nutritional Supplements,
this bestselling volume explains the
principles of natural medicine and out-
lines their application through the safe
and effective use of herbs, vitamins,
minerals, diet, and nutrition. You'll
find extensive discussion of treatments
for more than seventy health problems.
Offering the best of naturopathic medicine, this comprehensive encyclopedia
is grounded in firm scientific principles
and represents countless hours of
enlightening research. Complete the
pair by ordering today!

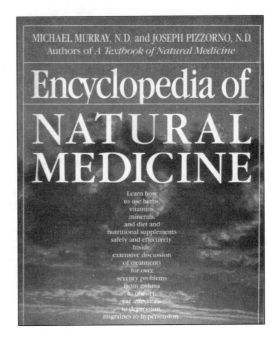

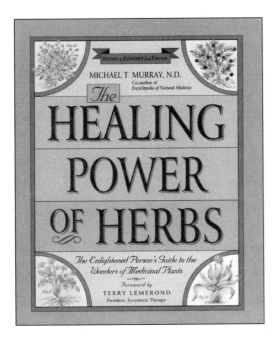

The Healing Power of Herbs—
The Enlightened Person's Guide to
the Wonders of Medicinal Plants

Revised & Expanded 2nd Edition

by Michael T. Murray, N.D.
$15.95

Enlightened consumers of health
products want more than just pills that
block out symptoms. Some of the most
powerful preventatives for ailments
are not located in prescription drugs
but in common herbs found in your
kitchen or your local health food
store. In this up-to-date and carefully
researched book on botanical medicine, Dr. Murray brings you the latest
scientific findings about the power and
efficacy of medicinal herbs.

To Order Books

Please send me the following items:

Quantity	Title	Unit Price	Total
_____	_____	$ _____	$ _____
_____	_____	$ _____	$ _____
_____	_____	$ _____	$ _____
_____	_____	$ _____	$ _____
_____	_____	$ _____	$ _____

Subtotal $ _____

Deduct 10% when ordering 3-5 books $ _____

7.25% Sales Tax (CA only) $ _____

8.25% Sales Tax (TN only) $ _____

5.0% Sales Tax (MD and IN only) $ _____

Shipping and Handling* $ _____

Total Order $ _____

Shipping and Handling depend on Subtotal.

Subtotal	Shipping/Handling
$0.00–$14.99	$3.00
$15.00–$29.99	$4.00
$30.00–$49.99	$6.00
$50.00–$99.99	$10.00
$100.00–$199.99	$13.50
$200.00+	Call for Quote

Foreign and all Priority Request orders:
Call Order Entry department
for price quote at 916/632-4400

This chart represents the total retail price of books only
(before applicable discounts are taken).

By Telephone: With MC or Visa, call 800-632-8676, 916-632-4400. Mon-Fri, 8:30-4:30.
WWW {http://www.primapublishing.com}

Orders Placed Via Internet E-mail {sales@primapub.com}
By Mail: Just fill out the information below and send with your remittance to:

Prima Publishing
P.O. Box 1260BK
Rocklin, CA 95677

My name is _____

I live at _____

City_____ State_____ Zip _____

MC/Visa#_____ Exp._____

Check/Money Order enclosed for $_____ Payable to Prima Publishing

Daytime Telephone _____

Signature _____